Magnetic Resonance Imaging in Orthopedic Sports Medicine

Magnetic Resonance Imaging in Orthopedic Sports Medicine

Edited by

Robert A. Pedowitz, MD, PhD
Department of Orthopaedics and Sports Medicine, University of South Florida College of Medicine, Tampa, FL, USA

Christine B. Chung, MD
Department of Radiology, University of California, San Diego, CA, USA

Donald Resnick, MD
Department of Radiology, University of California, San Diego, CA, USA

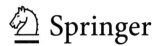 Springer

Editors
Robert A. Pedowitz, MD, PhD
Department of Orthopaedics and Sports Medicine, University of South Florida College of Medicine, Tampa, FL, USA

Christine B. Chung, MD
Department of Radiology, University of California, San Diego, CA, USA

Donald Resnick, MD
Department of Radiology, University of California, San Diego, CA, USA

ISBN 978-0-387-48897-4   e-ISBN 978-1-387-48898-1
DOI: 10.1007/978-1-387-48898-1

Library of Congress Control Number: 2008923736

Printed on acid-free paper

9 8 7 6 5 4 3 2 1

springer.com

Preface

.

This book grew from the commonsense notion that orthopedic surgeons and sports medicine clinicians need to understand the practical application and interpretation of magnetic resonance imaging (MRI) for the sake of their clinical practices, while radiologists need broad clinical perspective in order to provide the best and most accurate MRI information upon which patient care decisions must be made. As obvious as that notion might be, relatively little emphasis was placed upon genuine, interdisciplinary MRI education for practicing doctors, especially at the early advent of MRI technology. This need is now much better recognized, evidenced by the growth of excellent lecture-based educational opportunities. Examples include interdisciplinary instructional courses taught by both radiologists and orthopedic surgeons at the Radiological Society of North America and the American Academy of Orthopaedic Surgeons over the last half decade.

What has been missing from the educational landscape has been a focused, practical reference that would integrate the basic needs of radiologists and clinicians alike. This was the impetus for the current book, which has been an extraordinary cooperative venture by authors who were asked to bridge that gap in a single resource: orthopedic surgeons and sports medicine specialists writing for the sake of their radiology colleagues, and radiologists writing for the benefit of their clinician partners.

We sincerely hope that you will find the information in *Magnetic Resonance Imaging in Orthopedic Sports Medicine* stimulating, useful, and efficient. Our ultimate hope is that it will benefit the quality of service provided by clinicians and radiologists alike.

Robert A. Pedowitz, MD, PhD
Christine B. Chung, MD
Donald Resnick, MD

Acknowledgments

This book would not have been possible without the vision and support of Springer and our lead editor, Rob Albano, who has patiently allowed this project to evolve and mature. We sincerely appreciate the efforts of our lead editorial assistant, Sadie Forrester. Finally, and most importantly, we would like to thank our coauthors for the time and energy given to this venture. They are the foundation of this book, and we deeply respect their passion and commitment to excellence in education and patient care.

Robert A. Pedowitz, MD, PhD
Christine B. Chung, MD
Donald Resnick, MD

Contents

Contributors

Michael J. Angel, MD
Department of Orthopaedic Surgery, Long Island Jewish Medical Center, New Hyde Park, NY, USA

Romulo Baltazar, MD
Department of Radiology, Maimonides Medical Center, Brooklyn, NY, USA

Javier Beltran, MD, FACR
Department of Radiology, Maimonides Medical Center, Brooklyn, NY, USA

Jenny T. Bencardino, MD
Franklin and Seidelmann Subspecialty Radiology, Melville, NY, USA

Robert Downey Boutin, MD
Musculoskeletal Imaging, Medical Director, Med-Tel International, Davis, CA, USA

Mark D. Bracker, MD
Department of Family and Preventive Medicine, University of California, San Diego, CA, USA

Douglas Chang, MD, PhD
Department of Orthopaedic Surgery, University of California, San Diego, CA, USA

Weiling Chang, MD
Sharp-Grossmont Hospital, La Mesa, CA, USA

Christine B. Chung, MD
Department of Radiology, University of California, San Diego, CA, USA

Ali Dalal, BS
Department of Orthopaedic Surgery, University of California, San Diego, CA, USA

Steven R. Garfin, MD
Department of Orthopaedic Surgery, University of California, San Diego, CA, USA

Garry E. Gold, MD
Department of Radiology, Stanford University School of Medicine, Stanford, CA, USA

Carlos A. Guanche, MD
Southern California Orthopedic Institute, Van Nuys, CA, USA

Choll W. Kim, MD, PhD
Department of Orthopaedic Surgery, University of California, San Diego, CA, USA

Benjamin May, MD
Department of Radiology, Maimonides Medical Center, Brooklyn, NY, USA

Matthew Meunier, MD
Department of Orthopaedic Surgery, University of California, San Diego, CA, USA

Theodore T. Miller, MD
Department of Radiology and Imaging, Hospital for Special Surgery, New York, NY, USA

Patrick J. Murray, MD
Department of Orthopaedics, Baylor College of Medicine, Houston, TX, USA

Mini N. Pathria, MD, FRCP(C)
Department of Radiology, University of California San Diego Medical Center, San Diego, CA, USA

Robert A. Pedowitz, MD, PhD
Department of Orthopaedics and Sports Medicine, University of South Florida College of Medicine, Tampa, FL, USA

Cheryl A. Petersilge, MD
Departments of Radiology and Orthopedic Surgery, Case Western Reserve University School
of Medicine; Marymount Hospital, Cleveland Clinic Health System, Cleveland, OH, USA

Margie Pohl, FRACS
British Columbia's Foot and Ankle Clinic, Providence Health Care, Vancouver, BC, Canada.

Sean T. Powell, MD
San Jose-O'Connor Hospital Family Medicine Residency Program, San Jose, CA, USA

Donald Resnick, MD
Department of Radiology, University of California, San Diego, CA, USA

Catherine Robertson, MD
Department of Orthopaedic Surgery, University of California, San Diego, San Diego, CA, USA

Zehava S. Rosenberg, MD
Department of Radiology, Hospital for Joint Diseases–NYU Medical Center, New York, NY, USA

Marc R. Safran, MD
Departments of Orthopedic Surgery and Sports Medicine, Stanford University, Stanford, CA, USA

Ryan Serrano
Occidental College, Los Angeles, CA, USA

Nicholas A. Sgaglione, MD
Department of Orthopaedics, North Shore University Hospital, Great Neck, NY, USA

Benjamin Shaffer, MD
Department of Orthopedics, Georgetown University; Partner, Washington Orthopedics and Sports Medicine; Head
Team Physician/Medical Director, Washington Nationals and Washington Capitals NHL teams, Washington, DC, USA

Steven Sharon, MD
Musculosketetal MRI, Atlantic Radiologic Imaging, Staten Island, NY, USA

Lynne S. Steinbach, MD
Departments of Radiology and Orthopaedic Surgery, University of California San Francisco,
San Francisco, CA, USA

Joshua N. Steinvurzel, MD
Department of Orthopaedic Surgery, University of California, San Diego, CA, USA

Nicolas Theumann, MD
Service de Radiodiagnostic et Radiologie Interventionnelle, Lausanne, Switzerland.

Hamid Torshizy, MD
Division of Musculoskeletal Radiology, Department of Radiology, University of California
San Diego School of Medicine and VA San Diego Healthcare Systems, San Diego, CA, USA

Sailaja Yadavalli, MD, PhD
Department of Diagnostic Radiology, William Beaumont Hospital, Royal Oak, MI, USA

Alastair S.E. Younger, MB ChB, Msc, ChM, FRCSC
British Columbia's Foot and Ankle Clinic, Providence Health Care, Vancouver, British Columbia;
Division of Lower Extremity Reconstruction and Oncology, Department of Orthopaedics,
University of British Columbia, Vancouver, British Columbia, Canada

1
Muscle

A. Radiologic Perspective: Magnetic Resonance Imaging of Muscle

Robert Downey Boutin

Muscles give us both stability and power for all body movements. However, muscle contractions do more than enable our activities of daily living; they also allow us to exercise, which is associated with beneficial effects on longevity, general health, self-esteem, and mood.[1,2] With exercise, however, there is also the possibility of injury.

Traumatic insults to muscle in athletes are commonplace. In one study of 2873 adolescents, for example, the rate of injuries requiring medical attention was 40 injuries/100 adolescents/year, with an even higher rate of injuries resulting in time lost from sports (50 injuries/100 adolescents/year).[3] With regular recreational activities in adults, the annual injury rate is approximately 6%, and approximately 62% of all sports injuries reportedly result in time taken off work.[4] Elite athletes also may be injured. Indeed, the overall level of injury to professional soccer players is approximately 1000 times higher than in industrial occupations that are typically regarded as high risk (e.g., construction, mining).[5]

Athletic injuries to muscle have a wide variety of causes, treatments, and prognoses. Given that the cause and severity of injuries may be difficult to determine clinically in some cases, magnetic resonance imaging (MRI) is utilized increasingly in identifying the anatomic location and severity of various pain generators in athletes. In so doing, MRI is increasingly playing a key role in influencing treatment, predicting prognosis, assessing therapeutic response, and detecting potential treatment complications. After reviewing the principal indications for imaging of muscle and commonly used MRI techniques, this chapter reviews normal compartmental anatomy, normal anatomic variations, sports-related muscle injuries, and major differential diagnoses.

General Techniques and Indications for Imaging of Muscle

Common imaging techniques available to assess sports-related muscle injuries include radiography, computed tomography (CT), sonography, and MRI. Although these techniques can have complementary roles in achieving the correct diagnosis, each of these imaging methods has particular indications, strengths, and limitations.

Radiography remains the most common initial imaging test of choice to evaluate symptomatic patients. Not only does radiography allow relatively inexpensive screening for many osteoarticular derangements (e.g., fractures, arthritis), it also displays abnormal radiodensities in musculotendinous structures (e.g., heterotopic ossification, calcium hydroxyapatite crystal deposition).

Computed tomography facilitates the diagnosis of abnormalities such as those detected by radiography. Compared to radiography, the cross-sectional display allows for more precise evaluation of certain muscle derangements, including the characterization of mineralized matrix (e.g., calcification versus ossification, heterotopic ossification versus osteosarcoma). Although CT is commonly helpful in the workup of suspected heterotopic ossification, it is otherwise not commonly used for imaging muscle because (1) it has limited contrast resolution for examining muscle, and (2) it involves exposure of the patient to radiation (which is a known carcinogen and a particular drawback in younger patients). The actual radiation dose varies substantially with the scan technique, but the United States Food and Drug Administration estimates that an effective dose of 10 mSv (typical for a pelvic CT scan) may carry a 1 in 2000 lifetime risk of inducing fatal cancer, a risk that is important to consider for athletic injuries that are not life threatening.[6] Other experts conclude from the latest data that the risk of developing cancer from a single body CT scan with a 10 mSv dose is even higher: 1 in 1000 for an adult and 1 in 550 for a child.[7]

Sonography can be helpful in the diagnosis of disorders affecting muscles. Prime indications for sonography include (1) differentiation between cystic and solid lesions, (2) interrogation of soft tissue vascularity, and (3) dynamic examination of musculotendinous structures. However, potential practical disadvantages of sonography commonly include that it is regarded as an operator-dependent technique with limited contrast resolution and limited tissue penetration.

TABLE 1.1. Potential indications for MRI of muscle in athletes and other patients.

- To facilitate prompt diagnosis when necessary for initiating proper management for athletic injuries, particularly when the clinical diagnosis is uncertain
- To characterize the severity of injury or the presence of complications (when these considerations may affect management)
- To evaluate for uncommon sources of muscle pain in patients with an atypical clinical presentation or recalcitrant symptoms
- To provide objective documentation of the presence, progression, or resolution of a muscle disorder (e.g., patient is a poor historian, medicolegal situations)
- To display preoperative localization or planning information
- To help predict the prognosis (e.g., estimate recovery time) in athletes
- To investigate a soft tissue mass in a patient without a clear history of trauma
- To assess for an underlying structural cause of muscle weakness or neuropathy
- To evaluate the location, extent, and other manifestations of infection
- To assess the location and extent of myopathy, especially when it can help establish a diagnosis, guide choice of a biopsy site, or assess treatment response

Compared to MRI, for example, sonography is less sensitive at detecting nonacute hamstring strains,[8] less accurate in diagnosing atrophy in the supraspinatus and infraspinatus muscles,[9] and less suited to comprehensively assessing a region for potential pain generators (e.g., stress fracture, internal derangement).

Magnetic resonance imaging is commonly regarded as the advanced imaging test of choice for muscle. Although MRI of sports-related muscle injuries is a nascent field and has limitations (e.g., dynamic and functional capabilities are not routinely evaluated), the advantages of MRI include the lack of ionizing radiation, excellent soft tissue contrast resolution, and multiplanar tomographic display. Magnetic resonance imaging facilitates the diagnostic process by detecting alterations in muscle size, shape, and signal intensity. Potential indications for MRI of muscle in athletes and other patients are listed in Table 1.1.

Common Magnetic Resonance Imaging Techniques

Routine Magnetic Resonance Imaging Protocol

Although MRI protocols used to assess muscle disorders vary considerably, these exams commonly include a combination of pulse sequences in both long-axis (sagittal or coronal) and short-axis (axial) planes. Long-axis images (parallel to long bones) are prescribed with a field of view sufficient to provide an overview of the proximal-to-distal extent of a muscle disorder. Axial images enable cross-sectional evaluation of individual muscles, compartments, and neurovascular structures. Compared to the long-axis images, the axial images often utilize a smaller field of view that facilitates higher spatial resolution. One example of a routine screening exam for

muscle disorders or masses includes five pulse sequences: long axis T1-weighted and fast spin echo (FSE) inversion recovery (IR) images, as well as axial T1-weighted, FSE T2-weighted, and FSE fat-suppressed T2-weighted images.

Another, more abbreviated MRI protocol to evaluate muscle injuries using four pulse sequences also is commonly reported in clinical practice. For example, for a suspected hamstring strain,[8] FSE proton density (repetition time [TR]/echo time [TE]eff, 5000–6500/45) and FSE IR (TR range/TE range, 4000/35–55; inversion time, 120 ms) images may be acquired in both long-axis and axial planes (using a phased-array shoulder surface coil with a 20-cm field of view, 5-mm section thickness, no interslice gap, and two signals acquired). Regardless of the particular pulse sequences utilized, placement of a skin marker at the maximal site of symptoms facilitates direct correlation between the clinical and imaging findings.

Supplemental Magnetic Resonance Imaging Techniques

Other MRI techniques also may prove helpful in establishing a diagnosis, including contrast-enhanced imaging and gradient-echo imaging. Although intravenous gadolinium-based contrast material is generally not helpful for the routine MRI assessment of sports-related muscle injuries,[10] it may be helpful in some circumstances.[11–13] Contrast material is indicated most commonly for reasons other than typical muscle injuries in athletes, such as characterization of (1) synovitis,[14] (2) soft tissue necrosis (e.g., myonecrosis), and (3) certain mass lesions (e.g., differentiation of solid versus cystic lesions; identifying optimal biopsy sites that are free of necrosis or have active areas of inflammation; evaluating an operative bed for recurrence after sarcoma resection).

Gradient-echo imaging can be particularly useful for intentionally accentuating paramagnetic effects. Although these effects may result in "blooming" or susceptibility artifact that obscures adjacent anatomic structures and does not contribute to making a diagnosis in most athletic injuries, this phenomenon can help in honing a differential diagnosis by calling attention to hemosiderin, gas, ferromagnetic foreign bodies, or prior surgery (even on low-resolution localizer images). Fast gradient-echo images can be used to provide high temporal resolution for assessing anatomic and pathologic changes in muscle. For example, muscle contraction during the MRI examination may demonstrate retraction of a torn muscle, dynamic nerve entrapment,[15] or dynamic muscle herniation through a fascial defect.[16]

Experimental Magnetic Resonance Imaging Techniques

Promising pulse sequences used for studying muscle include several dynamic and functional techniques. Dynamic techniques with phase contrast imaging allow real-time imaging at several frames per second and may prove useful in both biomechanical and clinical analysis of muscle contraction in vivo (e.g., quantitative measurement of three-dimensional muscle velocities).[17,18] Magnetic resonance elastography can simultaneously measure muscle stiffness and temperature,[19] and is sensitive to both muscle morphology (e.g., unipennate, longitudinal) and fiber composition (e.g., type I or II).[20]

Functional muscle MRI has been used to study muscle activation patterns associated with various sports, optimal sports performance, overuse injuries, and treatment interventions (e.g., physical therapy, anterior cruciate ligament [ACL] reconstruction).[21–27] BOLD (blood oxygenation level dependent) MRI produces contrast from changes in the microvascular ratio of oxyhemoglobin (a diamagnetic substance) to deoxyhemoglobin (a paramagnetic substance) that occur with maneuvers such as exercise, oxygen administration, or certain medications (e.g., vasodilators).[28] Evaluation of the microcirculation of normal and diseased skeletal muscle may provide insights into such diverse topics as muscle fiber composition in athletes and vascular insufficiency.[29]

The functional MRI technique known as T2 mapping displays the spatial patterns of muscle recruitment and the intensity of muscle activation immediately after exercise. This transient activity-induced T2 hyperintensity occurs after as few as one or two contractions[30] and normally resolves within 30 minutes.[26] Increased T2 signal may be related partly to osmotically driven shifts of muscle water that increase the volume of the intracellular space and metabolic end products that cause postexercise intracellular acidosis.[26] (Whereas surface electromyography [EMG] is biased by activity in superficially located muscles and detects electrical activity, T2 mapping displays a global overview of metabolic activity in muscle.[31]) After completion of a training program, MRI demonstrates that individuals performing a given exercise use less muscle volume,[32] and that the exercise-induced T2 hyperintensity in muscle is reduced.[33] Magnetic resonance imaging also can be utilized to assess the whole body mass and distribution of both muscle and fat, both in athletes and in patients with muscle disorders.[34–36]

Normal Anatomy

The fundamental structural element of skeletal muscle is the muscle fiber. Within each fiber, the contractile proteins myosin and actin are incorporated into thick and thin filaments, respectively, which are arrayed in longitudinally repeated banding patterns termed sarcomeres.[37] On a standard MR image, a single pixel includes approximately 100 muscle fibers,[26] and a typical motor neuron in the lower extremity innervates approximately 400 muscle fibers.

The architecture of the fibers in any particular muscle is directly related to the muscle's function and mechanical behavior. For example, the maximal force that can be produced by a muscle is proportional to the physiologic cross-sectional area of that muscle. On the other hand, the speed and amount of shortening in any given muscle is proportional to the length of its fibers. Imaging can be used to measure muscle contraction, muscle thickness, pennation angle, and fascicle length.[38–40]

Compartmental Anatomy

Compartments are distinct domains bordered by tissues (e.g., fascia, cortical bone) that tend to constrain the spread of pathologic processes (e.g., compartment syndrome, infection, neoplasm). Knowledge of compartmental anatomy is of particular importance in interpreting MRI exams of muscle, and the work of others is summarized here.[41–44] In the upper extremity, the mid-arm has two muscular compartments divided by the humerus and intermuscular septum: anterior (biceps, brachialis, and coracobrachialis) and posterior (triceps). The forearm has been depicted as containing a variable number of compartments, although dividing the volar, dorsal, and mobile wad muscles into three compartments is used commonly.

In the pelvis, each muscle is considered to be a separate compartment. In the lower extremity, three compartments are present in the mid-thigh: anterior (quadriceps and sartorius), posterior (hamstrings), and medial (adductors and gracilis). In the leg, four compartments are present: anterior (tibialis anterior, extensor hallucis longus, extensor digitorum longus, and peroneus tertius); lateral (peroneus brevis and peroneus longus); superficial posterior (soleus, gastrocnemius, and plantaris); and deep posterior (tibialis posterior, flexor digitorum longus, flexor hallucis longus, and popliteus). The ankle and dorsum of the foot are considered extracompartmental, but the plantar portion of the foot is divided into three compartments: medial, central, and lateral.

Anatomic Variations in Muscles

Anatomic variations in muscle are very common.[45] The multitudinous anomalies that have been described may be divided conceptually into those muscles that are (1) absent; (2) doubled; (3) divided into two or more parts; (4) deviant in course; (5) joined to a neighboring muscle; (6) altered in size or shape (e.g., the distribution of the fleshy and tendinous portions); or (7) completely new, "extra" muscles.[46]

Anomalous muscles are usually of no clinical significance. However, these anatomic variations can become crucially important in many situations,[45,47] including when they are (1) misdiagnosed clinically as a palpable neoplasm or a torn, retracted muscle; (2) compressing a neurovascular structure (e.g., causing compressive neuropathy); (3) contributing to chronic compartment syndrome; (4) subjected to various insults (e.g., strain injury); or (5) encountered during surgery (e.g., surgical anatomy implications, potential for harvest of accessory tissue).

TABLE 1.2. Muscle variations and their prevalence*.

Muscle Variation	Prevalence (%)
Upper extremity	
Biceps	8–20
Pronator teres	8
Anconeus epitrochlearis	5–25
Palmaris longus	11–13
Flexor digitorum superficialis	14
Abductor digiti minimi	24
Lumbricals	20
Pelvis and lower extremity	
Piriformis	15
Gastrocnemius	3–5
Peroneus quartus	10–22
Accessory flexor digitorum longus	2–8
Accessory soleus	1–6
Peroneocalcaneus internus	1

* Although most variations are not clinically significant, they become important most commonly when they are misdiagnosed clinically as a soft tissue neoplasm or when they compress an adjacent nerve or blood vessel.

Anatomic variations are generally underdiagnosed in daily practice. Magnetic resonance imaging facilitates the diagnosis of an anomalous muscle by demonstrating its characteristic morphology, origin, insertion, and course relative to adjacent anatomic structures. However, anomalous muscles are often inconspicuous with imaging, since these muscles have the same signal intensity as neighboring skeletal muscles (assuming the anomalous muscle is undisturbed by trauma or other insults).

Although variations in musculotendinous anatomy can occur throughout the body, these muscles come to clinical attention most commonly in the wrist, hand, and ankle regions. For example, in one study examining the volar aspect of 42 normal wrists,[48] MRI demonstrated a total of 23 muscle variations. In the ankle region, three anomalous muscles are encountered with regularity[47,49]: (1) peroneus quartus (prevalence, 10% to 22%), (2) flexor digitorum accessorius longus (prevalence, 2% to 8%), and (3) accessory soleus (prevalence, 1% to 6%). A few of the most common, clinically significant musculotendinous variations are listed in Table 1.2.

Common Sports-Related Muscle Disorders

General categories of athletic muscle disorders include biomechanical overload during muscle contraction (e.g., strain), blunt trauma (e.g., contusion), hemorrhage, heterotopic ossification, delayed-onset muscle soreness, penetrating trauma (e.g., laceration), muscle herniation, compartment syndrome, and denervation. Strains and contusions reportedly comprise about 90% of all sports-related muscle injuries,[50] and are emphasized in the discussion below with the related topics of muscle hemorrhage and heterotopic ossification.

Overview of Muscle Strain Injuries

Risk Factors

Magnetic resonance imaging is used commonly to study how the characteristics of strain injuries vary depending on the athlete's sport, strength, endurance, technique, and expertise. In general, research has shown that the strongest risk factor for developing a muscle strain injury is a recent history of that same injury, and the next strongest risk factor is a past history of the same injury.[51] For example, studies have shown a two to seven times increase in hamstring strains occurring in athletes with a prior history of such thigh injuries, and recurrence rates generally ranging from 12% to more than 30%.[51–58] Other risk factors for muscle strain injuries may include low muscle strength (or muscle strength imbalances), limited flexibility, inadequate warm up, poor technique,[53] and muscle fatigue.[59–63] Concentric-only resistance training also increases the vulnerability of muscle to eccentric exercise-induced injury, and MRI has been used to objectively document the more widespread muscle injury in this situation.[64]

Mechanisms of Injury

Why do muscles tear? Strain injuries commonly occur when a powerful muscle contraction is combined simultaneously with forced lengthening of the musculotendinous unit. Many specific biomechanical variables have been proposed, including fiber strain magnitude, peak joint torque, and starting muscle length.[65] Empirically, we know that muscle strains most commonly occur in the lower extremity muscles when recruited to sprint, kick, jump, or pivot.[51,53,57,60,66]

Different types of athletes may have very different injury mechanisms and prognoses. For example, the two mechanisms commonly implicated for hamstring strains in Australian football players are sprinting/acceleration (81%) and kicking (19%).[66] However, in sprinters and dancers,[66] one study showed that all elite sprinters sustained their hamstring strains during high-speed sprinting, whereas all professional dancers were injured while performing slow stretching-type exercises (rather than powerful muscle contractions). While the initial loss of flexibility and strength was greater in sprinters than in dancers (p < .05), the sprinters recovered to preinjury performance levels more quickly (median 16 weeks [range 6–50] for the sprinters versus 50 weeks [range 30–76] for the dancers). Because the recovery interval is variable, MRI has been used to help predict recovery time (see below).

Magnetic Resonance Imaging Diagnosis and Grading of Strain Injuries

Muscle strains may be graded along a spectrum of injury, from mild (grade 1, microscopic injury) to moderate (grade 2, macroscopic partial tear) to severe (grade 3, complete tear). Mild and moderate strain injuries are far more common than complete tears.

Grade 1 Injury

Mild (grade 1) strains are characterized by microscopic injury to the muscle (also defined as less than 5% of fibers injured, without gross fiber discontinuity). While clinical examination reveals no significant loss in strength or range of motion in most cases, MRI displays hyperintense signal on fluid-sensitive images due to edema and hemorrhage in the acute setting. This edema and hemorrhage may be seen focally or diffusely in muscle, and reflects the severity of the injury. Edema-like signal characteristically tracks along muscle fascicles creating a feathery margin that reflects the muscle architecture (Fig. 1.1).

Grade 2 Injury

With moderate (grade 2) strains, some muscle fibers are torn, but there is continuity of some fibers near the site of injury. (Partial tears may be further subdivided, and considered high grade if more than 70% of the fibers are torn, moderate if 30% to 70% of the fibers are torn, and low grade if less than 30% of the fibers are torn.[67]) The presence of a hematoma at the musculotendinous junction (MTJ) is regarded as essentially pathognomonic of a grade 2 strain injuries.[68,69] In addition, a rim of perifascial high signal intensity may track around the muscle, particularly when there is disruption of the epimysium. Perifascial (intermuscular) edema and blood are common, occurring in approximately 68%[70] to 87%[71] of athletes studied with acute incomplete tears. This fluid signal intensity commonly tracks along soft tissue planes into more distal and dependent positions (due to gravity). When blood tracks into the subcutaneous fat layer beneath the skin, this commonly results in ecchymosis.

Grade 3 Injury

With a complete tear, MRI displays discontinuity of all fibers at the level of injury, with or without retraction of the torn fibers (Fig. 1.2). Even when there is not gross retraction, torn fibers may appear slightly lax upon careful inspection. Focal collection of fluid-like signal intensity or hematoma typically is identified in the gap created by a recent tear.

Magnetic Resonance Imaging Report Checklist

The checklist of MRI findings that should be reported for muscle injuries generally includes at least five features: (1) the name of the injured muscle(s); (2) the site(s) of injury within the muscle (e.g., musculotendinous junction); (3) the extent of injury (e.g., injury grade, length of injured muscle in centimeters on long-axis FSE-IR images, the amount of retraction in any torn fibers); (4) any focal fluid collection, hematoma, or heterotopic ossification; and (5) any other findings that may have treatment implications, prognostic implications, or indicate the acuity/chronicity of the injury (e.g., muscle atrophy, fibrosis). Pertinent negative findings (e.g., normal bone) and any practical imaging differential diagnosis also are appropriate.

Natural History of Muscle Injury on Magnetic Resonance Imaging

The MRI findings of strain injuries vary with time, and MRI can distinguish between acute and nonacute injuries.[72] Muscle healing generally occurs through three interrelated, time-dependent phases: (1) degeneration and inflammation, (2) muscle regeneration and repair, and (3) remodeling.[73–75] The phases of the healing response tend to be similar regardless

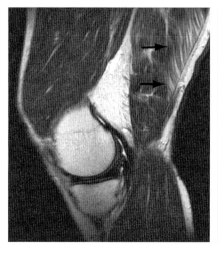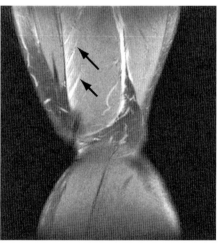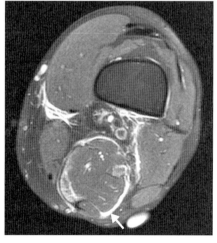

A   B   C

Fig. 1.1. Grade 1 strain in the distal semimembranosus in a 40-year-old man, 3 days after an injury that occurred while sprinting during a lacrosse game. Sagittal fast spin echo (FSE) T2-weighted (A) and coronal fat-suppressed FSE proton-density (PD) images (B) show a feathery pattern of high signal intensity adjacent to the musculotendinous junction (MTJ) (arrows). (C) Axial fat-suppressed FSE PD image shows prominent perifascial fluid signal (arrows) that is characteristic of a recent injury (adjacent to the skin marker).

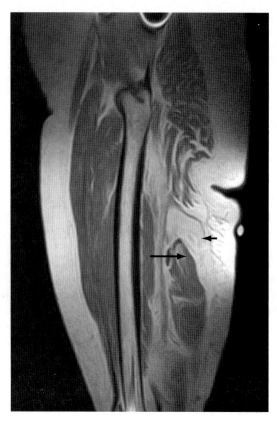

FIG.1.2. Complete proximal biceps femoris tear, 2 weeks after injury. Sagittal T1-weighted image shows retraction of torn hamstring fibers into the mid-thigh (long arrow), with the high signal intensity hematoma in the gap (short arrow) created by the tear (at the level of the skin marker).

of the type of insult to muscle (e.g., strain, contusion, and laceration), although the intensity and ultimate outcome may vary.

Acute Phase

Acutely, hemorrhage at the site of injury is followed by muscle degeneration/necrosis and inflammatory cell response with edema that begins in earnest by day 2.[76] With MRI, T2 hyperintensity peaks at 24 hours to 5 days after a muscle strain injury.[10] The edema-like signal on fluid-sensitive images tends to become less conspicuous over time, generally resolving by 6 to 10 weeks. Although a markedly abnormal scan at 6 weeks after injury may predict an increased risk of reinjury,[77] persistent abnormalities may be displayed by MRI at 6 weeks in 36% of athletes,[78] even though most athletes have returned to competition. Functional MRI techniques (e.g., MR elastography) ultimately may prove helpful in evaluating the viscoelastic properties of injured muscle for diagnostic and prognostic purposes.

Nonacute Phase

Microscopically, muscle regeneration and fibrosis (scarring) begins by day 7 to 10.[60,75,76] With MRI, scar tissue may become visible as early as day 14.[79] At this time point, the scar has matured enough so that it is no longer the weakest link;

rather, if loaded to failure, the rupture usually occurs within the muscle tissue adjacent to the newly formed "mini"–musculotendinous junctions between the regenerated myofibers and the scar tissue.[75] Over time, scar tends to become more organized and well defined. Fibrosis is characteristically seen on MRI as low signal intensity on all pulse sequences, but may be inconspicuous.

With fibrosis, there is tissue retraction (volume loss) and the ability of the muscle to lengthen is reduced, which presumably makes the muscle more susceptible to recurrent strain.[73,75] In part by inhibiting scar formation, the direct injection of specific growth factors into injured muscle may significantly improve the speed and degree of recovery.[74] Thus, MRI ultimately may be used to diagnose muscle injuries, as well as to guide percutaneous injections in the future.

In the chronic setting, residual hematoma also may cause low signal intensity owing to the presence of hemosiderin, most prominently on gradient echo images.

Anatomy at Risk

Where do muscles tear? When a musculotendinous unit is strained to the point of failure, the "weak link" in the chain formed by muscle, tendon, and bone tends to vary depending on the age of the athlete. Although the subject of this chapter is muscle (rather than bone or tendon), it is worth noting that there tend to be three entirely different target sites for these non–contact injuries, depending on whether the athlete is a child, a young adult, or an older adult:

- In children and adolescents, the weak link tends to be located at the physeal (growth) plate, and therefore injury caused by excessive tension on the muscle-tendon-bone chain tends to result in apophyseal avulsion fractures (Fig. 1.3).
- In young adult athletes, the biomechanically weak link tends to be near the MTJ, and therefore this is the classic site for muscle strains in this age group (Fig. 1.1).
- In older adults with tendinosis, biomechanical overload of the musculotendinous unit commonly results in fibers tearing at sites that are structurally weakened by tendon degeneration (Fig. 1.4).

Potential Clinical Relevance of Magnetic Resonance Imaging Results

Because there are exceptions to these age-group generalizations, MRI is commonly indicated to help guide management decisions by pinpointing the location of injury in the muscle–tendon–bone chain and defining the severity of injury. In particular, MRI objectively documents injuries that may be amenable to surgical repair, including tendon tears, tendon avulsions, and certain osseous avulsions. Magnetic resonance imaging also has been advocated in the preoperative workup for a minority of patients with persistent pain and functional limitations that may be related to heterotopic ossification, extensive recurrent strain, musculotendinous fibrosis, or adjacent soft tissue adhesions. For example, in the setting of a

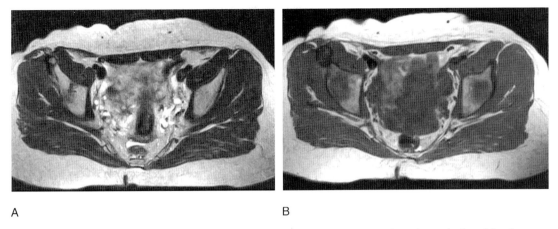

Fɪɢ. 1.3. (A) In an older patient, axial FSE T2-weighted image shows an old, small, well-corticated, ununited avulsion fragment at the right anterior inferior iliac spine. (B) More inferiorly, axial T1-weighted image demonstrates prominent low signal intensity owing to the presence of fibrosis and mineralization.

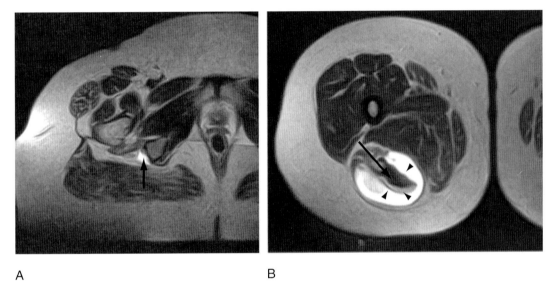

Fɪɢ. 1.4. Tear through area of tendinosis in proximal hamstring tendon in a 61-year-old woman during low-energy trauma while shopping. (A) Axial FSE T2-weighted image shows high signal intensity fluid abutting the ischial tuberosity (arrow) (the site of origin of the hamstring tendons). (B) More distally, axial FSE T2-weighted image demonstrates the torn, degenerated hamstring tendon fibers (arrow) surrounded by high signal intensity fluid (arrowheads).

chronic hamstring tear, surgical repair may be technically demanding and possibly have suboptimal results, because (1) the sciatic nerve is commonly encased in dense scar tissue that causes adherence of the nerve to the torn hamstrings and (2) fibrosis and retraction of chronic tears may make mobilization of the tendon back to the ischial tuberosity for repair difficult.[80,81]

Although most muscle strains can be managed conservatively,[82] confirming the diagnosis of a muscle strain with MRI is potentially important because other entities in the clinical differential diagnosis may be treated very differently (e.g., stress fracture, compartment syndrome). In addition, an accurate diagnosis is important because a specific graded supervised rehabilitation program is considered crucial to minimizing morbidity,[10,58,59] including osteoarthritis.[83] The "muscle dysfunction hypothesis"[83]

reasons that properly contracting muscles are the main force absorber for a joint, and that muscle injury can cause muscle dysfunction that leads to articular biomechanical overload and premature osteoarthritis. For example, this hypothesis suggests that muscle dysfunction (rather than primary cartilage "wear and tear") is the reason that soccer players are at increased risk for hip osteoarthritis compared to distance runners. (Soccer players, unlike distance runners, suffer relatively frequent groin muscle strains and quadriceps contusions.)

Commonly Strained Muscles

The three biomechanical characteristics that commonly put certain musculotendinous structures at risk for strain injury are that they (1) undergo eccentric contraction, (2) cross two joints, and

(3) have a high proportion of fast twitch fibers. The most commonly strained muscles are in the lower extremity, and include the hamstrings, quadriceps, adductors, and triceps surae. Less commonly, strain injuries occur elsewhere, including the anterior chest wall (e.g., pectoralis major[67]), the upper extremity (e.g., triceps[84]), the abdominal wall (e.g., internal oblique muscle in cricket and tennis players[85–87]), and the paravertebral musculature (e.g., in windsurfers and other athletes[88,89]).

Hamstrings Strain

Anatomy and Mechanism of Injury

The hamstring muscle complex (i.e., biceps femoris, semitendinosus, and semimembranosus) spans two joints, and functions primarily to flex the knee and extend the hip. Sprinting athletes sustain hamstring strains with an incidence rate of almost 25%.[90] A recent biomechanical study[90] suggests that the hamstrings are most vulnerable to injury during a 130-ms period during the late swing phase of sprinting (immediately before foot contact) when the muscle is active, loaded, and elongating while resisting knee extension. It is at this time when the biceps femoris long head is particularly susceptible to an eccentric (lengthening) contraction injury, reaching a peak length that is 12% beyond the length seen in an upright posture and significantly exceeding the maximum length of the medial hamstrings (p<.01).[91] The hamstrings musculature—and, in particular, the biceps femoris long head—also may be prone to strain injuries for at least four additional reasons: (1) it has a high proportion of powerful fast twitch (type II) fibers,[92] (2) it is often relatively weak (compared to the antagonist quadriceps and iliopsoas muscles),[93] (3) it crosses two joints (and therefore is subject to increased stretch and force production extrinsically as both a hip extensor and a knee flexor),[92] and (4) the biceps femoris has two heads with dual innervation and extensive attachments[94,95] that may result in asynchronous contraction.[58]

Magnetic Resonance Imaging Findings

In the hamstrings, as elsewhere, distraction injuries in young adults target the muscle (rather than the bone or tendon attachments)[71]. For example, in one study that included 30 athletes with hamstring injuries,[70] the MTJ of the muscle was involved in 93% (along the intramuscular MTJ in 24 cases and isolated at the muscle ends in four cases), with only 7% of injuries that extended to the eccentrically epimysium.

In another MRI study that imaged 179 acute hamstring injuries in athletes with a mean age of 28 years,[96] 154 injuries (86%) were located within muscle. In contrast, only 21 occurred at the proximal tendon–bone attachment (16 avulsions and five partial tears), and only four occurred at the distal tendon attachment (all avulsions). (The two osseous avulsions that occurred were located at the ischium in skeletally immature adolescent athletes.) Of the muscle injuries, the most commonly injured constituent was the biceps femoris (more than 80%), with far fewer injuries involving the semimembranosus (14%) or semitendinosus (6%). Within any given muscle, strain injuries were centered most commonly near the intramuscular MTJ. In the biceps femoris, for example, 61% involved the MTJ, 35% involved the myofascial junction (i.e., eccentrically, at the junction of muscle and its epimysial covering), and 4% had only intramuscular hematomas.

Other MRI studies of hamstring injuries in young adult athletes also have found a particular propensity for the following: (1) partial tears (far more common than complete tears), (2) injuries preferentially involving the biceps femoris long head (far more common than in the biceps femoris short head or the "medial" hamstrings), and (3) injuries involving the MTJ (far more common within the muscle belly than at the ends of the muscle).[71,97] Multiple hamstring muscles may be injured in up to 33%[71] to 40%[70] of cases.

Quadriceps Strain

Anatomy and Mechanism of Injury

The quadriceps muscles (i.e., rectus femoris and vastus muscles) function primarily to flex the hip and extend the knee. Quadriceps strain injuries commonly occur during sprinting and kicking (e.g., in track and field, football, soccer).[10,98] The rectus femoris crosses two joints, has a high proportion of type 2 fibers, and is by far the most commonly strained quadriceps muscle. The vastus muscles effectively cross only the knee joint, are composed of predominantly type 1 fibers, and are strained only occasionally.

Magnetic Resonance Imaging Findings

Rectus femoris strains in young adults typically are incomplete tears along the MTJ (more commonly along the deep MTJ within the muscle belly than at the ends of the muscle) (Fig. 1.5). These injuries classically target the muscle near the hypointense central tendon and are associated acutely with surrounding hyperintense signal on axial T2 images; this concentric appearance on MRI has been termed an acute "bull's eye" sign.[10] Interestingly, the mean recovery interval is much longer for these rectus femoris strains located centrally (along the central tendon) than those located peripherally (even when their size is larger) (27 days vs. 9 days).[10]

In older adults (at least 40 to 50 years of age), biomechanical failure of the quadriceps more often occurs at the distal tendon near the patellar attachment. Spontaneous or bilateral distal quadriceps tendon ruptures are almost always associated with underlying tendinopathy or enthesopathy,[99] often coupled with known risk factors for tendinopathy (e.g., corticosteroids, chronic renal disease, or diabetes),[100,101] although exceptions do occur rarely in athletes.[102,103] Microscopic analysis of spontaneously ruptured quadriceps tendons reveals that

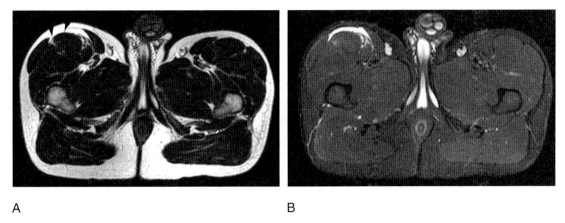

A   B

FIG. 1.5. Rectus femoris strain in a 24-year-old man, 1 day after sudden pain associated with kicking the ball during a soccer game. Axial FSE T2-weighted (A) and axial FSE inversion recovery (IR) (B) images of the proximal thighs show a mild rectus femoris strain, with high signal intensity surrounding the central tendon, as well as adjacent perifascial fluid signal (arrowheads).

collagen fiber diameter is significantly smaller than in normal tendons (−24%; p <.00001).[104] Failure of the rectus femoris at its tendinous origin (direct head) has been reported rarely in professional football kickers (without subjacent osseous avulsion).[105] In adolescent athletes, avulsion of the anterior inferior iliac spine is the second most common site for apophyseal avulsions in the pelvis (only ischial tuberosity avulsions at the hamstring origin are more common).

Adductor Strain

Anatomy and Mechanism of Injury

The thigh adductor muscles function primarily to adduct the hip. Adductor injuries are thought to result commonly from biomechanical overload when forced abduction of the lower extremity occurs during eccentric contraction of adductor muscles.[106] Groin strains are relatively common and potentially disabling athletic injuries that are associated with sports requiring rapid changes in direction (e.g., hockey,[54,107] soccer,[108] Australian football,[109] American football,[51,110] rugby[111,112]).[113] In the National Hockey League, for example, muscle strains in the groin or adjacent abdominal regions occur with an incidence of up to 20 injuries per 100 players per year, with 25 player games missed per year on each team and a large proportion of recurrent injuries (24%).[54]

Magnetic Resonance Imaging Findings

Adductor musculotendinous injuries are observed most commonly at the adductor longus, with injuries less commonly reported at the gracilis,[11,114] adductor magnus,[115] adductor brevis,[115,116] and iliacus[117] (Fig. 1.6). In part because the site and severity of injury are variable, experts have highlighted the importance of individualized diagnosis and treatment.[118] Magnetic resonance imaging helps differentiate patients with acute adductor injuries into those with partial tears in the muscle (who may be managed nonoperatively)[116] versus those with avulsions or complete

tears of the tendon (who potentially may be treated with operative repair).[106] Chronic overuse and other factors (e.g., fluoroquinolone antibiotics, such as ciprofloxacin) may predispose the tendon or enthesis to mucinous degenerative change, with rupture or avulsion seen even in young individuals by MRI.[11,106,119–121] Adductor strains that are treated improperly may become chronic and hamper athletes from playing at their full potential.[113]

Chronic groin pain in athletes, sometimes referred to as "athletic pubalgia," can be a vexing clinical problem with a particularly long clinical differential diagnosis (Table 1.3).[11,122–126] Although imaging definitely does not solve all diagnostic conundrums, MRI has been promoted as the imaging modality of choice to facilitate prompt and specific diagnosis in many cases.[127]

Triceps Surae Strain

Anatomy and Mechanism of Injury

Several muscles and tendons at the posterior aspect of the knee and calf contribute to knee flexion, ankle dorsiflexion, or both. The most common muscular strain in the calf affects the medial head of the gastrocnemius muscle,[128] which may be due to differential patterns of muscle activation, distinct anatomic variations in the gastrocnemius-soleus junction, and differential strain during contractions[129] (Fig. 1.7). Substantial injuries to other muscles in this region also may occur, including elsewhere in the triceps surae (composed of the gastrocnemius and soleus), the plantaris, and the popliteus (Figs. 1.8 and 1.9).

The classic clinical history is sudden onset of sharp pain in young and middle-aged adult athletes participating in a racquet sport, skiing, or running. However, calf muscle strains also may occur in deconditioned individuals during mundane daily activities, such as running to catch a bus or climbing stairs.[128] Consequently, calf injuries may be underdiagnosed clinically.[130]

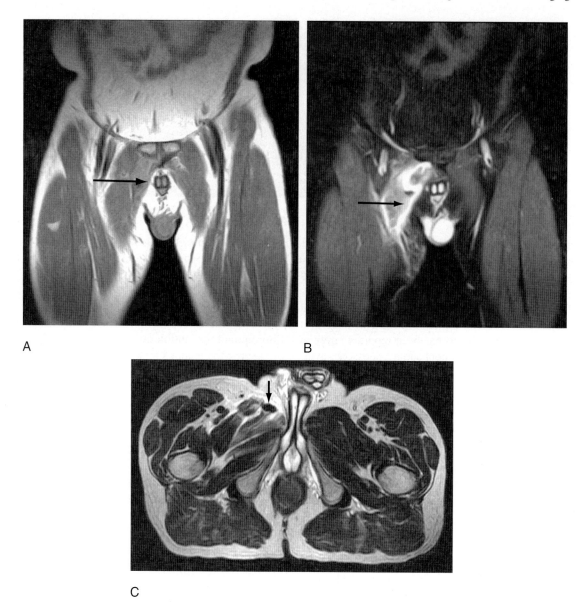

FIG. 1.6. Adductor avulsion in a 54-year-old man, 2 days after a bowling injury. Coronal T1-weighted (A) and coronal FSE IR (B) images show abnormal increased signal intensity outlining torn adductor fibers (arrow) and site of origin on the pubis. (C) Axial FSE T2-weighted image demonstrates subtle laxity in both the avulsed adductor brevis tendon and in the adductor longus that has torn near the musculotendinous junction (MTJ) (arrow).

TABLE 1.3. Chronic groin pain in athletes: imaging may aid in narrowing the potentially long list of clinical differential diagnostic possibilities.

- Muscle or tendon derangements (e.g., adductors, lower abdominals)
- Osseous derangements (e.g., stress fracture of the pelvis or femoral neck; avulsion fracture; adductor insertion avulsion syndrome (thigh splints); infection; femoral head osteonecrosis)
- Articular derangements (e.g., osteitis pubis, femoral head osteochondral lesion, hip arthritis, labral tear, femoroacetabular impingement)
- Bursal derangements (e.g., iliopsoas bursitis)
- Hernias (e.g., inguinal hernia, obturator hernia, femoral hernia, prehernia complex)
- Genitourinary derangements (e.g., ureteral calculi, cystitis, epididymitis, prostatitis, ovarian pathology, endometriosis)
- Nerve derangements (e.g., obturator nerve or ilioinguinal nerve entrapment)
- Vascular or ischemic derangements (e.g., compartment syndrome)
- Mass (e.g., cyst)

Magnetic Resonance Imaging Findings

Although the diagnosis of a strain injury may be suspected clinically, MRI may be indicated to confirm the presumed diagnosis (objectively documenting both the location and extent of injury), help predict prognosis, and rule out the many other entities in the long clinical differential diagnosis (Table 1.4).[130] As shown in one MRI study of 23 injuries to the distal gastrocnemius,[131] most gastrocnemius injuries involve the MTJ (96%) and target the medial head (86%). Both MRI and sonography generally show that partial gastrocnemius tears are much more common than complete tears, often with collection of fluid signal seen between the medial gastrocnemius and the soleus at the mid-calf level[128,132,133] (Fig. 1.10).

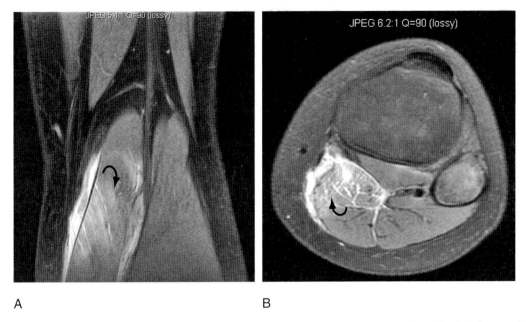

A   B

FIG. 1.7. Low-grade partial tear in the medial gastrocnemius. Coronal (A) and axial fat-suppressed FSE T2-weighted (B) images show high signal intensity collecting near the intramuscular tendon fibers and adjacent feathery signal that reflects muscle pennation (curved arrow).

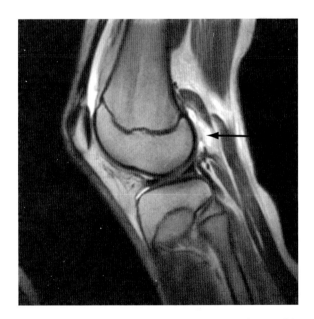

FIG. 1.8. Partial tear in the lateral gastrocnemius in an 18-year-old man, 1 week after acute-onset pain while running. Sagittal FSE T2-weighted image shows partial disruption of the proximal gastrocnemius fibers at the musculotendinous junction (MTJ) region (arrow).

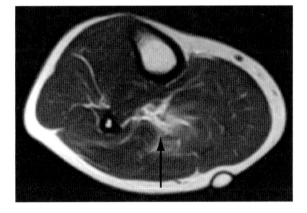

A

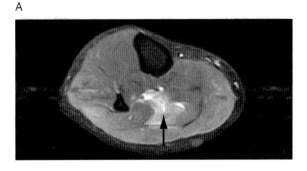

B

FIG. 1.9. Mild strain in the soleus muscle in a 40-year-old long-distance runner, 2 days after acute-onset pain while pushing off during a 9-mile run. Axial FSE T2-weighted (A) and axial FSE IR (B) images of the calf show feathery high signal intensity in the soleus muscle (arrow). Subsequently, he has strained the muscle twice more while running, and chronic pain has hampered his running.

'In a recent series of 75 strains in the calf,[134] most injuries were acute (80%) and had a hematoma (61%), with an average muscle injury size measured by MRI at 2.5 cm in width (range, 0.3 to 8 cm) and 5.5 cm in length (range, 1.5 to 12 cm). Most calf injuries (66%) were isolated to one muscle (54% were isolated to the gastrocnemius (usually the MTJ of the medial head), while 41% were

TABLE 1.4. Clinical differential diagnosis of calf pain may include many different etiologies.

- Muscle or tendon derangements (e.g., strain, contusion, hernia)
- Bursal derangements (e.g., ruptured Baker's cyst)
- Osseous derangements (e.g., stress fracture or stress reaction)
- Nerve derangements (e.g., nerve entrapment, radiculopathy, or referred pain)
- Vascular or ischemic derangements (e.g., compartment syndrome, venous thrombosis, thrombophlebitis, cystic adventitial disease, endartery stenosis of the popliteal artery)
- Mass (e.g., hematoma, heterotopic ossification, ganglion, nerve sheath tumor)

isolated to the soleus). The majority of patients who had strains at more than one site had a combination of gastrocnemius and soleus injuries. Risk factors in the form of Achilles tendinopathy or prior calf strain (often with scar tissue seen on MRI) were found in a substantial minority (27%) of patients.

Pectoralis Major Muscle

Anatomy and Mechanism of Injury

The pectoralis major is the largest, most superficial muscle in the anterior chest wall and forms the anterior fold of the axilla. This fan-shaped muscle originates primarily from the medial half of the clavicle, the sternum, and the first six costal cartilages.[135] The clavicular and sternal (sternocostal) heads decussate laterally, forming a tendon that inserts into the lateral lip of the humeral bicipital groove.

Pectoralis major injuries most commonly occur while the arm is abducted, extended, and externally rotated, often in combination with eccentric contraction, maximal contraction (e.g., a fall or high-demand athletic endeavor), or a direct blow (e.g., a motor vehicle accident). Although these injuries may occur in women[136,137] and the elderly,[138] a typical patient is a muscular male between the ages of 20 and 40 years who is injured while weight lifting (e.g., particularly bench pressing).[139] Anabolic steroid use is associated with tendon ruptures, likely because (1) steroids result in stiffer tendons that absorb less energy, and (2) the tendon is susceptible to injury owing to disproportionate hypertrophy of muscle tissue.

Magnetic Resonance Imaging Findings

Magnetic resonance imaging is highly valuable in helping to stratify patients into nonoperative versus operative treatment groups[136] (Figs. 1.11 and 1.12). (Although there is some debate,[140] nonsurgical management is recommended generally for proximal tears and elderly, sedentary patients, while surgery is favored for active patients with a high-grade or complete tear located distally, particularly at or near the enthesis.[141]) For most patients in whom the maximal area of interest is lateral to the nipple, a dedicated surface coil with a unilateral field of view (e.g., 18 to 22 cm) and 3- to 4-mm sections[67] are recommended.

Normally, the pectoralis major tendon should be identified inserting into the proximal humeral shaft within 1 to 1.5 cm inferior to the quadrilateral space.[142] Axial images are not expected to display the separate layers of the pectoralis major tendon,[143]

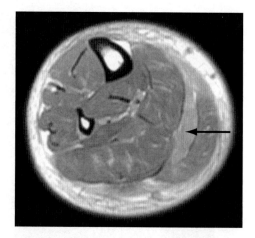

A

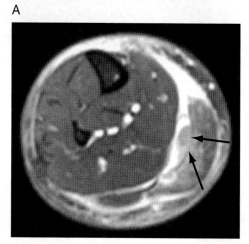

B

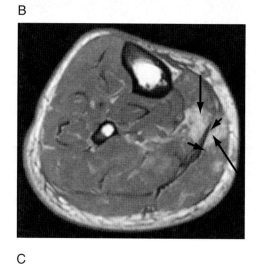

C

FIG. 1.10. Partial tear of the medial gastrocnemius in a 35-year-old man, 1 week after he recalls a sudden painful "snap" during push off. (A) Axial T1-weighted image shows a collection of increased signal intensity (arrow), consistent with hematoma, at the site of the tear. (B) Axial FSE IR image demonstrates the partial tear in the deep fibers of the medial gastrocnemius, near the junction with the soleus aponeurosis (arrows). (C) In a different patient, axial T1-weighted image shows findings of an old strain injury, with low signal intensity thickening of the aponeurosis owing to fibrosis (arrowhead) and high signal intensity adjacent to the aponeurosis owing to fat deposition (arrows).

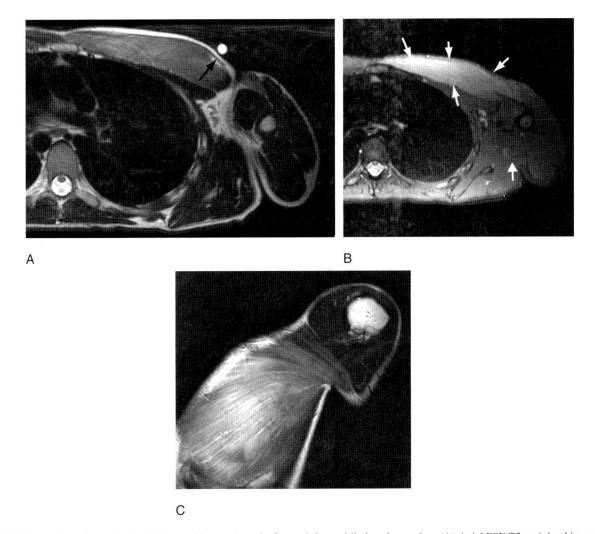

FIG. 1.11. Pectoralis major strain in a 19-year-old man, 1 week after an injury while bench pressing. (A) Axial FSE T2-weighted image demonstrates a low-grade partial tear near the musculotendinous junction (MTJ) (immediately adjacent to the skin marker) (arrow). Axial FSE IR (B) and coronal FSE T2-weighted (C) images show diffuse edema signal in the pectoralis major muscle (arrowheads).

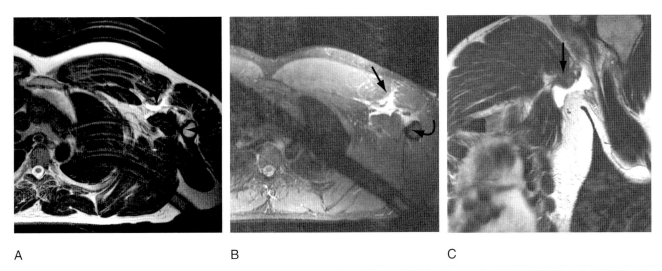

FIG. 1.12. Pectoralis major tendon tear in a 43-year-old man, 1 week after an injury while bench pressing. Axial FSE T2-weighted (A), axial FSE IR (B), and coronal FSE T2-weighted (C) images demonstrate a complete tear in the distal tendon. The torn tendon fibers (straight arrow) are retracted, lax, and surrounded by high signal intensity. Subtle ill-definition at the anterior humeral cortex (curved arrow) is secondary to periosteal stripping.

but thin oblique-coronal images prescribed parallel to the long axis of the tendon may be particularly helpful in grading of partial tears.[67] Low-grade partial tears most commonly are observed within the muscle belly or at the MTJ, in contradistinction to avulsions and complete tears. The sternal head (inferior and deep fibers) are torn most commonly.[136,139,143] Images should be inspected for a hyperintense T2 signal located immediately superficial to the humeral cortex; this finding is characteristically caused by periosteal stripping that occurs during tendon avulsion from its insertion site.[67]

The amount of retraction of torn fibers may vary substantially (e.g., 0 to 13 cm[67]). Retraction of torn fibers may be minimal in some cases because remnants of the clavicular head remain intact[144] or because fascia investing the muscle may remain continuous with the fascia of the brachium and the medial antebrachial septum.[141] Of note, MRI also can successfully diagnose recurrent pectoralis major tears after surgical repair.[144]

Accuracy of Clinical Evaluation vs. Magnetic Resonance Imaging Evaluation

How Accurate is Clinical Evaluation?

Although clinical evaluation is invaluable, clinical diagnoses of muscle strains are not entirely consistent or specific. Particularly when an athlete's clinical presentation is atypical or vague, accurate diagnosis can be very challenging, even for the most astute clinician. For example, in a study of professional athletes evaluated by highly experienced sports medicine physicians, MRI helped confirm the presence of hamstring strain in 9% of patients with an atypical history or clinical examination.[59,95]

Conversely, young athletes with posterior thigh pain who are diagnosed clinically with a hamstring strain may have etiologies other than simply a hamstring strain in 15% of cases,[56] and therefore a clinical differential diagnosis may be warranted.[58,95] For example, a partial list of clinical differential diagnostic considerations for posterior thigh pain[95] may include various musculotendinous derangements (e.g., hamstring strain, spasm/cramp, contusion, myositis ossificans, hernia, tendinopathy, enthesopathy); nerve entrapment (e.g., referred pain from the lumbosacral spine or sciatic nerve entrapment due to hematoma, anatomic muscle variation, piriformis conditions); vascular derangements (e.g., compartment syndrome, vascular claudication); osseous derangements (e.g., stress fracture of femur or pelvis, ischial tuberosity avulsion, thigh splints); neoplasms (e.g., bone tumor, soft tissue tumor such as a nerve sheath tumor); articular derangements (e.g., sacroiliitis); ligament injury (e.g., sacrospinous or sacrotuberous sprain); bursal derangements (e.g., ischiogluteal or semimembranosus bursitis); and infection.

How Accurate is Magnetic Resonance Imaging Evaluation?

There is no gold standard (e.g., surgical or pathologic evaluation) to verify the clinical or imaging diagnosis of strain injury in the vast majority of cases. However, there is empirical evidence that MRI is highly accurate in diagnosing clinically significant injuries—and not diagnosing injuries that are not clinically significant. Indeed, sudden onset of thigh pain is highly associated with a positive MRI exam (97%),[59] but insidious pain or stiffness does not correlate with positive MRI results in a substantial minority of athletes (e.g., 19%,[52] 31%,[72] and 45%[55] in recent studies).

Negative MRI exam results may be either true-negative or false-negative results. If the MRI is truly negative in a patient with pain, the patient may have had an injury other than a strain (e.g., a muscle cramp) in the exam field of view, or may have referred symptoms from a pain generator outside the field of view. Lumbosacral nerve root entrapment, for example, is a well-known cause of referred pain to the thigh. (Interestingly, such entrapment may actually predispose athletes to strain injuries.[51,145])

Magnetic resonance imaging may be falsely negative in an athlete with a strain injury because the exam has insufficient spatial or contrast resolution (and therefore does not detect small, slight, or nonacute injuries). In the athletes with thigh pain and a negative MRI exam, there is a substantial correlation with a history of back injury,[52] a hamstring injury in previous seasons (observed in 50% of athletes with negative MRI exams in one study[72]), and a prompt return to their sport.[55] In contrast, those athletes with thigh pain and a positive MRI have approximately a twofold[55] to threefold[52] increase in the number of days required for successful rehabilitation, and a substantially increased risk of reinjury to their hamstrings.[55] For example, in athletes studied with posterior thigh pain and suspected grade 1 hamstring strains,[55] the rehabilitation interval was significantly shorter for those with negative MRI exams than for those with muscles strains diagnosed by MRI (e.g., average of <7 days versus >20 days), and no MRI-negative athletes had recurrent injuries. Recent research indicates that MRI is a particularly useful predictor of the rehabilitation duration in cases of moderate or severe hamstring injuries (particularly those with an injured area measuring >6 cm in longitudinal length or >10% in cross section).[72]

Acute Strain and Predicting Prognosis

Clinical Prediction of Prognosis

The grade of the injury as assessed during clinical testing is generally a significant predictor of recovery time (p = .001) and one report indicates it is better than MRI for minor strains.[72] However, convalescence periods for strain injuries do vary considerably, reportedly from less than 1 week to more than 1 year.[59,96] For example, in a study of 68 hamstring strains in professional soccer players, the recovery period averaged 14 days, but the recovery period ranged from 1 day to 3 months.[146] Even for a strictly defined population of football players with only grade 1 hamstring strain injuries diagnosed clinically, the mean rehabilitation interval varied from less than 1 week to 3 weeks, depending on the presence and extent of hyperintense T2 signal in muscle.[55] In another study of clinical grading and prognosis,[72] the duration of recovery for hamstring strains was reported as follows:

• Grade 1: Predicted range, 0 to 21 days (mean, 7); actual range, 5 to 35 days (mean, 9)

• Grade 2: Predicted range, 14 to 35 days (mean, 24); actual range, 4 to 56 days (mean, 27)
• Grade 3: Surgery

Magnetic Resonance Imaging Prediction of Prognosis

A growing body of data that indicates clinical assessment may be supplemented by MRI evaluation and that MRI findings correlate significantly with a player's recovery time.[10,55,66,72,77] For example, in a 2-year study of 180 soccer players using MRI diagnostic criteria, the mean recovery time for acute hamstring strains was reportedly 9 days for a grade 1 injury, 18 days for a grade 2 injury, and 28 days for a grade 3 injury.[147] In this group, the longitudinal extent of the hyperintense short-tau inversion recovery (STIR) signal also was used to predict the recovery time (in days) with an accuracy of approximately 80%.

With MRI of acute strain injuries, rehabilitation time also may be predicted with three quantitative ways of measuring hyperintense signal on fat-suppressed, fluid-sensitive images: (1) the longitudinal length,[10,55,72,77] (2) the cross-sectional area,[10,55,70,72] and (3) the volume[70] of muscle involvement. Measurement of the longitudinal length of muscle involvement is the simplest parameter to obtain, and may be the best practical predictor of rehabilitation time.[55]

Cross-sectional area can be measured by selecting the transaxial fat-suppressed T2–weighted image with the greatest percentage of cross-sectional involvement.[10] In a study of quadriceps strains,[10] cross-sectional involvement of 1% to 14% correlated with a mean rehabilitation interval of less than 9 days, while 15% involvement generally predicted a mean rehabilitation interval of approximately 15 days (this increased to at least 30 days when the central tendon of the rectus femoris also was involved by MRI). (With respect to longitudinal involvement of the muscle, hyperintense signal measuring <13 cm had a mean overall rehabilitation interval of <10 days, versus injuries spanning >13 cm that had a rehabilitation interval of approximately 21 days [33 days when affecting the central tendon]).

The extent of injury displayed by MRI also helps predict which athletes are at increased risk of recurrent tear.[78] For example, hamstring muscle strains exceeding 50% to 55% of the cross-sectional area have an extremely high rate of recurrent tears within 2 years, as well as a significantly longer rehabilitation time.[95,148] When a recurrent injury occurs, rehabilitation time is significantly increased when compared to that for new injuries. For example, in a recent study on hamstring strains, the number of lost days for new injuries averaged 14 days, versus 25 days lost for recurrent injuries.[57]

Muscle Contusion

The mechanism of injury of muscle contusions is direct, blunt trauma. The consequent hemorrhage and edema commonly result in varying degrees of pain, swelling, limited range of motion, ecchymosis, and hematoma formation.[50] Heterotopic ossification occurs in approximately 9% of cases, and is associated with the initial injury grade.[149] Pseudolipomas also have been reported in soft tissue after contusion.[150]

Magnetic Resonance Imaging Findings

The most common area for athletic contusions is the quadriceps, and the vastus intermedius is the most characteristic muscle injured (Fig. 1.13). Fluid-sensitive images demonstrate hyperintense signal that may have a diffuse or geographic appearance, often with feathery margins

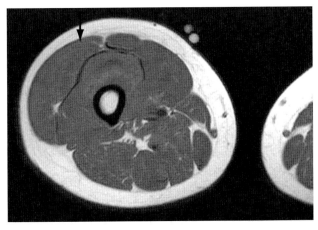
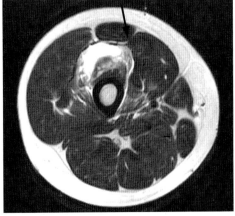

A   B

FIG. 1.13. Vastus intermedius muscle contusion in a 21-year-old man, 4 weeks after striking a tree with his thigh while snowboarding. (A) Axial T1-weighted image shows only minimal signal alteration (straight arrow) in the vastus intermedius muscle. (B) Axial FSE T2-weighted image demonstrates fluid signal collecting at the site of partial fiber disruption (straight arrow), with adjacent edema signal. T2* gradient echo imaging (not shown) did not show susceptibility artifact or otherwise contribute to the diagnosis in this case.

(due to capillary rupture and infiltrative bleeding). Unlike a muscle strain, the abnormal signal is usually not localized to the MTJ of muscles crossing two joints and the muscle volume may be more prominently increased from hemorrhage.

Given that contusions may have imaging features in common with strain (noncontact) injuries, the radiologist should make an effort to learn the mechanism of injury when interpreting images (e.g., with a patient interview or questionnaire, if the referring physician does not provide this information). The recovery time for lower extremity contusions reportedly tends to be significantly shorter than for strain injuries (mean time: 19 ± 9 days versus 26 ± 22 days).[151] The resolution of MRI findings tends to lag far behind functional recovery.[152]

Hemorrhage and Hematoma

Hemorrhage may occur interstitially in a nonfocal fashion within the substance of muscle (yielding edema-like signal in the acute setting) or may accumulate focally in the form of a hematoma. Bleeding into muscle occurs in association with a wide variety of disorders, including trauma, anticoagulation (e.g., heparin), bleeding diathesis (e.g., hemophilia), and focal vascular disorders (e.g., vascular malformation). Hemorrhage into muscle may result in pain, limited motion, anemia, a soft tissue mass, a compressive neuropathy, or compartment syndrome.

Magnetic Resonance Imaging Findings

The MRI appearance of blood is influenced by several variables, including the state of the hematoma itself (e.g., clot retraction, location, and size of the hematoma), the MRI technique (e.g., field strength, echo time, gradient echo technique), and the state of hemoglobin breakdown products. As hemoglobin breaks down, it sequentially forms specific iron compounds that influence the MRI appearance over time: oxyhemoglobin, deoxyhemoglobin, intracellular methemoglobin, extracellular methemoglobin, and hemosiderin.[153,154]

In general, hematomas have been reported as being acute (less than a week old, with intermediate T1 and decreased T2 signal intensity); subacute (1 week to 3 months old, with variable increased T1 and T2 signal intensity); and chronic (more than 3 months old, with variably increased signal that progressively becomes more hypointense from the periphery on all pulse sequences).[155] Most of the intramuscular hematomas that have been evaluated with MRI between 2 days[156] and 5 months[157] after injury display characteristics of methemoglobin, with increased signal intensity on both T1- and T2-weighted images.[158] Hemosiderin, the final iron-containing product of hemoglobin degradation, contributes to the progressive low signal intensity that is commonly most conspicuous at the periphery of chronic hematomas on all pulse sequences, with characteristic susceptibility ("blooming") artifact on gradient-echo images.

Intramuscular hematomas often resorb substantially over a period of 6 to 8 weeks,[159] but they may linger for many months.[160] Serous-appearing fluid from a hematoma occasionally may persist to form a pseudocyst (pseudotumor), characteristically at the MTJ.[161] These lesions are reported most commonly in the rectus femoris, but may be observed at other sites, including the hamstrings and triceps surae.

The clinical and imaging differential diagnosis of a benign hematoma sometimes includes a hemorrhagic neoplasm. When the lesion in question shows no contrast enhancement, this generally aids in excluding a neoplasm. Like neoplasms, however, posttraumatic hematomas may show variable contrast enhancement. Therefore, follow-up clinical and MRI evaluation may be indicated when the diagnosis of a probably benign hematoma is in doubt.

Heterotopic Ossification

Heterotopic ossification may be defined as the formation of nonneoplastic bone-like tissue in the soft tissues. A common location for heterotopic ossification is in muscle, where it is commonly referred to as myositis ossificans. The most common complaints involve pain, tenderness, swelling, a palpable mass, and nerve impingement.[50,162–165] Common predisposing factors for heterotopic ossification (found in 37% to 75% of patients) include trauma (e.g., contusion, surgery, burns); neurologic insults (e.g., spinal cord injury, traumatic brain injury, stroke); and conditions associated with a propensity for bone formation (e.g., diffuse idiopathic skeletal hyperostosis, ankylosing spondylitis).

Heterotopic ossification classically may evolve through three histologic, clinical, and radiologic phases: (1) an acute or pseudo-inflammatory phase; (2) a subacute or pseudotumoral phase; and (3) a mature, self-limited phase.[163] It is hypothesized that certain insults to soft tissue may trigger an early inflammatory cell reaction, as well as mesenchymal cell metaplasia that results in highly cellular areas of pleomorphic fibroblasts and osteoblasts. Osteoblasts then deposit osteoid in a centripetal fashion. This eventually gives rise to the recognizable zonal architecture that approximates native bone: a mature shell of compact bone surrounded peripherally cancellous bone centrally.

Magnetic Resonance Imaging Findings

Heterotopic ossification typically targets the large muscles in the hip, thigh, upper arm, and elbow regions. In the acute and subacute stages of heterotopic ossification, imaging examinations have a notoriously nonspecific appearance. During the first week, imaging exams commonly show only vague swelling. Within approximately 2 to 6 weeks after the onset of symptoms, radiography and CT demonstrate foci of nonspecific mineralization.[166,167] Both CT and MRI typically show an ill-defined mass that may be confused with a soft tissue sarcoma or infection. Periostitis may be present, although adjacent osseous destruction is absent.

Given that this early, immature mineralization is not diagnostic, short-term follow-up radiography or CT (repeated at an interval of approximately 4 weeks) is commonly used to confirm suspected heterotopic ossification. Although MRI is reportedly the most sensitive technique for identifying small, early lesions,[168] the diagnostic specificity of CT is far higher than that of MRI (because mineralization is not demonstrated as reliably by MRI). By 1 to 2 months after the onset of symptoms, CT typically shows a peripheral rind of mineralization.

With MRI, prior to lesion maturity, most heterotopic ossification is displayed as areas of nonspecific intermediate T1 signal intensity and hyperintense T2 signal intensity,[165,169] with ill-defined edema-like signal intensity and contrast enhancement commonly observed in the adjacent muscle and sometimes in the adjacent bone marrow.[164] (Prominent perilesional edema is not typical for soft tissue sarcomas, but is characteristic of traumatic and inflammatory processes.) Heterotopic ossification may show enhancement centrally or peripherally.[169] (Rim enhancement is not commonly seen with soft tissue neoplasms.[170]) Gradient-echo pulse sequences may be helpful in some cases for detecting areas of soft tissue mineralization, since they are more sensitive than spin-echo pulse sequences for this purpose.

In the mature form, the imaging findings that allow confident differentiation of heterotopic ossification from neoplasm include that the well-defined ossific mass is more mature peripherally than centrally, is not associated with underlying bone destruction, does not grow over time, and is associated with decreasing contrast enhancement over time. With maturity, heterotopic ossification on MRI generally appears well defined and inhomogeneous, with signal intensity that is isointense or hypointense to fat on all pulse sequences. In particular, T2 hyperintensity is uncommon, and approximately 85% of lesions have signal intensity that is equivalent to fat and cortical bone.[169] Heterotopic ossification matures over a period that is usually reported as 6 months to 1.5 years,[171–174] but ranging widely from 3.5 months to more than 5 years.[169] Resorption of the osseous mass may occur in some patients over a period of 1 year to more than 5 years.[167,169,175] Although bone scintigraphy was once the favored advanced imaging test to determine lesion maturity, CT and MRI are increasingly used to evaluate both lesion maturity and anatomic complications that may influence operative treatment (e.g., nerve impingement).[164]

Delayed-Onset Muscle Soreness

Delayed-onset muscle soreness (DOMS) refers to the pain and soreness in muscles that follows unaccustomed exertion.[176] Unlike strain injuries, patients with DOMS do not recall any one particular moment of trauma or experience an acute onset of pain. Rather, soreness typically begins the day after exertion and then subsides within 1 week. Activities requiring eccentric muscle contractions are common culprits (e.g., downhill hiking, certain types of manual labor).

Eccentric muscle contractions, in which the muscle lengthens as it exerts force, generate greater tension per cross-sectional area of active muscle than concentric contractions, which may result in injury to muscle tissue.[177]

Magnetic Resonance Imaging Findings

Magnetic resonance imaging displays hyperintense T2 signal indicative of interstitial edema. Muscle affected by DOMS shows good correlation between the signal intensity increases seen on fluid-sensitive MR images and the ultrastructural remodeling seen by electron microscopy[178] (e.g., loss of regular orientation of the Z bands in muscle).[179] This edema-like signal reportedly has a similar appearance to a mild strain, but may be more diffusely distributed in the muscle (i.e., less prone to target to the MTJ in a localized fashion). Although clinical history can allow for easy differentiation between these two entities in most instances, the abnormal signal intensity caused by DOMS may remain for up to 80 days,[180] and therefore the history of a provocative event may not be forthcoming.

Muscle Laceration

Lacerations are produced by a penetrating injury (e.g., a skate blade). Magnetic resonance imaging may prove useful in planning treatment with complex suture repair,[181] but also potentially for guiding the future application of treatments for enhancing muscle recovery (e.g., the antifibrosis agent relaxin[182] and stem cells[183,184]).

Magnetic Resonance Imaging Findings

Magnetic resonance imaging demonstrates the acute laceration as a sharply marginated zone of fiber discontinuity with associated T2 hyperintensity caused by hemorrhage and edema. In the chronic setting, volume loss in the muscle may be seen, sometimes with fibrotic tissue (displayed as low T2 signal intensity) and deposition of fat associated with atrophy (manifested as high T1 signal intensity).

Muscle Herniation

Muscle herniation refers to protrusion of muscle tissue through a focal fascial defect.[185–189] In athletes, these fascial defects may occur due to muscle hypertrophy (with or without chronic exertional compartment syndrome) or due to traumatic disruption of the fascial sheath. Herniations of muscle are seen typically as a small, superficial, soft tissue bulge that becomes more prominent and firm with muscle contraction. Most muscle herniations are asymptomatic, but they can cause substantial pain, cramping, and tenderness.[186,187] Although conservative management is usually adequate, imaging may be appropriate when the reported options for therapeutic interventions are under consideration (e.g., local injection of botulinum toxin, fasciotomy, fascial repair).

Magnetic Resonance Imaging Findings

Magnetic resonance imaging can display herniation of muscle (that typically appears normal in signal intensity) through discontinuous overlying fascia, thus allowing differentiation from a soft tissue neoplasm.[185,188] The outward bulging of muscle is often subtle, and may be elicited dynamically with muscle contraction during MRI or sonography.[16,186,189] Muscle herniations rarely may impinge upon an adjacent nerve or may become incarcerated. Although virtually any muscle can be affected, muscle hernias most commonly occur in the middle to lower portions of the leg, particularly involving the anterior and lateral compartment muscles.

Muscle Ischemia and Necrosis

Compartment Syndrome

Compartment syndrome is defined as elevated pressure in a relatively noncompliant anatomic space that can cause ischemia, pain, and potentially neuromuscular injury, including myonecrosis and rhabdomyolysis.[190–194] Muscle ischemia can result when elevated intracompartmental pressure exceeds the intravascular pressure of thin-walled small vessels and these vessels collapse, thereby decreasing the arteriovenous pressure gradient and impeding blood flow.

Compartment syndrome is classified generally as acute or chronic. Acute compartment syndrome occurs most commonly in association with fractures (particularly of the tibia) and soft tissue trauma (e.g., hemorrhage, severe contusion, iatrogenic insults, muscle rupture), and typically should be evaluated by direct percutaneous pressure measurement. For chronic compartment syndrome, direct pressure measurements and near-infrared spectroscopy measurements of oxygen saturation yield comparable results (sensitivities of 77% vs. 85%, respectively, and specificities of 83% vs. 67%, respectively).[194]

Chronic compartment syndrome results most commonly from exertional causes (e.g., exercise, occupational overuse); nonexertional causes (e.g., mass lesion, anomalous muscle, infection) are uncommon in athletes. Chronic exertional compartment syndrome (CECS) can occur secondary to exertion because chronic muscle activity causes muscle hypertrophy and transiently can swell muscle fibers up to 20 times their resting size, thus causing increased pressure in noncompliant compartments. Chronic exertional compartment syndrome in athletes most commonly occurs in the leg, thigh, and forearm, with characteristic locations that vary with the type of activity:

- Runners: anterior and deep posterior compartment of the leg; posterior compartment of the thigh
- Soccer players: deep posterior compartment of the leg
- Cyclists: deep posterior compartment of the leg; anterior compartment of the thigh
- Tennis players: flexor-pronator compartment of the forearm
- Motorcycle racers: flexor-pronator compartment of the forearm

Magnetic Resonance Imaging Findings

Magnetic resonance imaging can be used to study the location and extent of ischemic damage to muscle, with variable results.[194–200] Potential MRI indications that have been proposed include the diagnostic assessment of atypical cases (e.g., uncommon location or cause for compartment syndrome, borderline pressure measurements) and evaluation for an underlying lesion (e.g., hematoma, neoplasm) that may contribute to compartment hypertension and need to be addressed at surgery.

With acute compartment syndrome, diffuse edema-like signal and mildly increased muscle girth are common, occasionally with foci of hemorrhage. With impending compartment syndrome, gadolinium-enhanced T1–weighted images typically show avid contrast enhancement in the affected muscles.[197]

With CECS, diffuse edema-like signal and mildly increased muscle girth are common after exercise. The change in T2 signal intensity between pre-exercise and post-exercise images is significantly greater in compartments with post-exercise hypertension.[195–199] For example, in a study of 41 anterior compartments with CECS, T2 signal intensity increased by 28% (range 14–39%) following exercise, compared to an increase of 8% (range 0–9%) in the anterior compartments of controls and 4% (range 0–10%) in uninvolved superficial posterior compartments.[198]

The clinical differential diagnosis of stress-related anterior lower leg pain commonly includes CECS, bone stress injury, and traction periostitis. Interestingly, these three entities may occur separately or together. For example, in a recent study of 44 cases, there was no significant difference in bone findings between patients with and without CECS.[200]

Rhabdomyolysis

Rhabdomyolysis refers to acute muscle necrosis and leakage of muscle contents into the circulation.[201–205] The diagnosis of rhabdomyolysis can be defined clinically as muscle pain or weakness that is associated with myoglobinuria (classically with dark brown urine) and markedly elevated creatine kinase levels (e.g., higher than 10 times the upper limit of normal). Release of myoglobin and other metabolites from damaged muscle that potentially can result in acute renal failure (in 15–30% of all cases), electrolyte imbalance with cardiac arrest, and even death (3%).[201]

Multiple causative factors are present in 60% of all cases.[201] The most common insults causing rhabdomyolysis are excessive muscle activity, toxins (e.g., alcohol, illicit drugs, prescription medications such as statins), trauma (e.g., crush injury, bull riding, electrical injury), and muscle ischemia (e.g., compartment syndrome). Less commonly, an underlying myopathy or genetic metabolic derangement may be present (10% of all cases),[201] including occasionally in high-level athletes.[202] Exertional rhabdomyolysis may occur in individuals following strenuous activities (e.g., marathon running, weight lifting, military basic training, and even when excessive exercise is given as punishment for a child talking in class!).[204–206]

Magnetic Resonance Imaging Findings

Magnetic resonance imaging is the most sensitive imaging test to document the location and extent of muscle involvement in patients with rhabdomyolysis.[206] In one prospective study of patients with rhabdomyolysis,[207] abnormal muscles were demonstrated by sonography in 42% of patients, by CT in 62% of patients, and by MRI in 100% of patients. The principal MRI finding of rhabdomyolysis is diffuse edema-like signal in the involved muscle. The severity of the signal alterations correlates with the severity of the injury. Repeat MRI examinations show that the edema-like signal in mild cases resolves in parallel with the clinical course, likely representing the presence transient edema.[208]

Muscle Denervation

Muscle denervation can result in substantial pain, weakness, and disability. Denervation is caused most commonly by nerve fiber entrapment (e.g., by a disk herniation, mass, anomalous muscle, fibrous tissue) or trauma (e.g., mechanical stretch); other potential causes include inflammation (e.g., autoimmune), ischemia, nerve sheath tumor, systemic neuropathy, iatrogenic insults, and idiopathic causes.[209–213]

Magnetic Resonance Imaging Findings

Magnetic resonance imaging is used increasingly as an adjunct to clinical and EMG diagnosis of muscle denervation, as well as to determine its cause and distribution in many cases.[209–218] For example, MRI is useful in helping to diagnose denervation syndromes involving the brachial plexus[217] and the shoulder girdle,[209] including suprascapular neuropathy (e.g., due to a paralabral cyst), quadrilateral space syndrome, and Parsonage-Turner syndrome.

In the pelvis and lower extremity, MR neurography (utilizing high-resolution T1 and fat-suppressed fluid-sensitive images) has been used to study extraspinal neuropathic pain problems, including sciatica of non-disk origin[213] and foot drop.[211] For example, in a recent study of 239 consecutive patients with sciatica in whom standard diagnosis and treatment failed to effect improvement,[213] piriformis muscle asymmetry and sciatic nerve hyperintensity at the sciatic notch exhibited a 93% specificity and 64% sensitivity in distinguishing patients with piriformis syndrome from those without it who had similar symptoms (p < .01). With neurogenic foot drop, MRI of the leg can show distinct patterns of hyperintense signal in muscle that indicates whether denervation is caused by a derangement involving the peroneal nerve, L5 radiculopathy, or another lesion (e.g., a partial sciatic nerve lesion, or lesions involving the lumbosacral plexus or cauda equina).[211] In a prospective study of 40 consecutive patients with foot drop,[211] MRI and EMG were in agreement in 37 (93%) patients. (In three patients, MRI demonstrated more widespread involvement than did EMG, and there were no false-negative MRI results.) Other investigators[218] have shown that MRI has the potential to distinguish traumatic peripheral nerve injuries that recover through axonal regeneration versus those that do not (and therefore require surgical repair).

The signal intensity and morphology of muscle undergo well-described changes with subacute and chronic denervation.[209,214–216,218] After a nerve insult, changes generally are seen in muscle using MRI after approximately 2 weeks (although changes have been reported as early as 1 day in animals). In particular, these subacute changes in muscle are displayed as high signal intensity on fluid-sensitive images and normal signal intensity on T1–weighted images. T2 hyperintensity in muscle reportedly occurs because of an increase in the extracellular fluid volume or capillary enlargement.[215,216]

Although hyperintense T2 signal in muscle is not a specific finding by itself, a specific diagnosis is suggested in the appropriate clinical setting by involvement of a specific nerve territory and, classically, hyperintense T2 signal involving a peripheral nerve.[210,212,214,219] (Unlike a muscle strain injury, the hyperintense T2 signal in denervated muscles is not associated with perifascial edema.) The signal intensity changes of subacute muscle denervation can increase until at least 2 months (in an animal model) and are reversible. After reinnervation occurs, T2 hyperintensity peaks approximately 2 to 3 weeks later and normalizes by 6 to 10 weeks.

With chronic denervation, diminished bulk and fatty infiltration commonly occur in muscle. These atrophic changes are best displayed on T1-weighted MR images. Profound atrophic changes seen after chronic denervation may be irreversible.

Chronic denervation results most commonly in muscle volume loss, but pseudohypertrophy and true hypertrophy may occur in the affected extremity.[220–224] Both pseudohypertrophy and true hypertrophy may result in a palpable soft tissue mass that serves as an indication for MRI. Pseudohypertrophy may occur in denervated muscle when accumulation of fat and connective tissue causes paradoxical muscle enlargement and hyperintense T1 signal intensity due to adipose tissue. True hypertrophy may occur in synergistic muscles adjacent to the area of denervation; hypertrophied muscle is isointense with normal muscle.

Magnetic Resonance Imaging Differential Diagnosis

Skeletal muscle may be afflicted by a spectacular array of primary and systemic disorders. Magnetic resonance imaging helps establish a diagnosis or limited differential diagnosis by displaying abnormalities in muscle morphology and signal intensity that often target characteristic locations. Although these MRI abnormalities may be diagnostic in certain clinical settings, the human body responds to an infinite variety of insults to muscle with only a limited number of nonspecific biologic responses (e.g., edema, atrophy, fibrosis). In other words, since similar gross pathologic features may be caused by many different disorders (and MRI reflects these nonspecific gross pathologic changes), differential diagnosis may be necessary in some cases. As a first approximation, the physician may simplify the MRI differential diagnosis into three broad categories based on the presence of edema, fatty infiltration, or a mass.[225]

Muscle Edema Pattern

The muscle edema pattern refers to the presence of high T2 signal intensity in muscle. This pattern is most commonly due to a recent insult or a biologically active process. In athletes, edema-like signal is typically due to acute or subacute trauma (e.g., strain, contusion). Other, less common causes include muscular exertion (e.g., DOMS); various vascular insults (e.g., compartment syndrome, deep venous thrombosis, diabetic muscle infarction); rhabdomyolysis; subacute denervation; myositis (e.g., infectious, autoimmune); or recent iatrogenic insults (e.g., percutaneous injection of medication, surgery, radiation therapy).

In contradistinction to the "edema" pattern, the differential diagnosis for low T2 signal intensity in muscle commonly includes fibrosis, calcification, hemosiderin, gas, and foreign bodies.

Fatty Infiltration Pattern

The fatty infiltration pattern refers to the presence of fatty signal intensity (on all pulse sequences) in muscle, and is most commonly due to a nonacute muscle insult. In athletes, this pattern may be observed after a chronic high-grade musculotendinous injury (e.g., tendon tear), as well as with other insults causing chronic muscle disuse[226] or chronic denervation. For example, after a full-thickness rotator cuff tear, supraspinatus fatty infiltration and muscle atrophy are associated with chronicity and are proportional to the amount of musculotendinous retraction.[227] These supraspinatus muscle changes may be highly asymmetric, with the deep (scapular) fibers tending to undergo fatty infiltration, while the superficial (fascial) fibers primarily undergoing atrophy.[228] (Atrophy and fibrofatty infiltration result in a smaller, stiffer musculotendinous structure that alters its biomechanics and makes it prone to recurrent tear after repair.[229]) Fat also may be contained in other processes, such as mature heterotopic ossification and lipomatous lesions.

In addition to fatty tissue, hyperintense T1 signal in muscle may be caused by derangements containing methemoglobin (e.g., hematoma, hemorrhagic neoplasm), proteinaceous material (e.g., proteinaceous debris in a necrotic neoplasm), or certain paramagnetic materials (e.g., melanin in a metastatic melanoma, enhancement with gadolinium-based contrast material).

Mass Lesion Pattern

The MRI differential diagnostic category of the mass lesion pattern is considered when there is a space-occupying lesion. In athletes, this is most commonly due to trauma (e.g., hematoma, myositis ossificans). Although less common, other causes of masses may affect athletes, including neoplasms, infections (e.g., pyomyositis, parasitic infection), and muscular sarcoidosis.

Conclusion

Muscle disorders have a wide variety of causes, treatments, and prognoses. Given that clinical assessment may be difficult in some cases, MRI commonly aids in identifying the location, severity, and extent of pain generators in muscle. In so doing, MRI is increasingly playing a key role in helping limit the differential diagnosis, influencing the treatment, and predicting the prognosis for muscle disorders in athletes.

B. Orthopedic Perspective: Muscle and Tendon Disease

Sean T. Powell and Mark D. Bracker

Skeletal muscle pathology encountered in orthopedic and sports medicine may be acute, subacute/chronic, or a late complication as a result of previous injury. This section discusses common pathologic conditions of skeletal muscle with attention to pathophysiology, clinical features, evaluation, and management. Special attention is given to the use of MRI in the evaluation of these conditions.

Acute muscle pathology in orthopedic sports medicine can be a result of direct force to muscle tissue from an extrinsic source (contusion, laceration) or by indirect force due to excessive stretch (acute muscle strain). Further, it can be a result of damage to the muscle cells as a result of excessive exercise (exertional rhabdomyolysis) or ischemia (acute compartment syndrome) (Table 1.5).

Acute Muscle Strain

Definition and Pathophysiology

Acute muscle strains are the most common injuries to skeletal muscle encountered in sports medicine (Table 1.6).[230,231] An acute muscle strain is defined as a tear of muscle fibers at the MTJ caused by excessive stretch.[232,233] There is a continuum of severity of muscle strain injury ranging from disruption of few muscle fibers to complete tears of the MTJ with retraction of the resulting muscle segments. Grade I, mild strain, is characterized by disruption of fewer than 5% of the muscle fibers at the MTJ. Grade II, moderate strain, is characterized by rupture of greater than 5% but fewer than 100% of the

TABLE 1.5. Acute muscle pathology in orthopedic sports medicine.

Acute conditions	Local sequelae	Systemic sequelae
Acute muscle strain	Hematoma Fibrosis	None
Muscle contusion	Hematoma Myositis ossificans	None
Muscle laceration	Fibrosis	None
Exertional rhabdomyolysis	Acute compartment syndrome	Renal failure Disseminated intravascular coagulation (DIC) Electrolyte imbalance Hepatic failure
Acute compartment syndrome	Contracture Denervation	Rhabdomyolysis Renal failure

TABLE 1.6. Strain and contusion injuries in sports.

	Injury type			
	DOMS	Partial strain	Complete strain	Contusion
Mechanism	Repetitive stretch	Single stretch	Single stretch	Blunt trauma
Pain	After 24–72 hours	Immediate	Immediate	Immediate
Site	Muscle belly	MTJ	MTJ or muscle belly	Muscle belly
Bleeding	None	May escape	May escape	Confined to injury site
Surgery	No	No	Possible	Possible

DOMS, delayed-onset muscle soreness; MTJ, musculotendinous junction.
Source: Adapted from Best,[283] with permission of Cambridge University Press.

muscle fibers. Grade III, severe strain, is characterized by a complete rupture of the MTJ.[234–237] On the field and in the trainer's office, acute muscle strains are commonly known as muscle "pulls" or "tears."

Acute muscle strain injuries are caused by a single excessive force that stresses the muscle beyond its ability to withstand the force.[231,234] Extensive research has shown that in adults, the site of muscle strain occurs most commonly at or near the MTJ, where muscle fibers attach to the connective tissue that connects muscle cells to bone (Fig. 1.14). The susceptibility of the MTJ occurs because this structure is thought to constitute the weakest point in the musculotendinous unit in adults.[230,231] In skeletally immature patients, the weakest point in this mechanical chain is the apophysis, or growing part of bone. This explains why this age group is more likely to suffer apophyseal avulsion injuries than adults.[235]

Pathophysiologically, the tearing of muscle fibers and blood vessels in an acute muscle strain causes an accumulation of blood and debris from necrotic muscle cells at the site of the injury. This results in the formation of a hematoma in the defect caused by the strain injury. An inflammatory reaction then occurs over the next 24 to 48 hours in which inflammatory cells migrate to the area and phagocytose the muscle cell debris and blood clot. Pain and swelling result from inflammatory mediators released at the site of injury and increased capillary permeability. After the inflammatory phase, the healing phase begins. The healing phase of an acute muscle strain can be viewed as a balance between two competing processes: recovery and regeneration of muscle fibers versus the for-

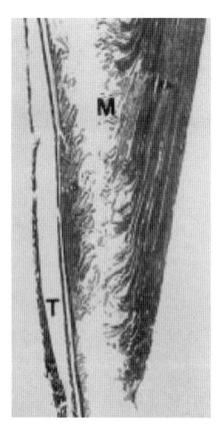

FIG. 1.14. Histologic appearance of an extensor digitorum longus muscle specimen obtained immediately after strain injury. Note limited rupture of the most distal fibers near the myotendinous junction. M, intact muscle fibers; T, tendon. (Masson stain, original magnification × 1.75.) (From Noonan and Garrett.[321] © 1997, with permission from Elsevier.).

mation of dense scar tissue.[237] Regeneration of muscle fibers is achieved through the mobilization of satellite cells from the basal lamina of the myofiber. Satellite cells are a pool of cells that proliferate and fuse to form new myotubules in the event of injury to the muscle.[238] The goal of treatment is to maximize muscle regeneration across the defect while minimizing fibrous scar formation and contracture, giving the patient the best possible functional outcome.

Eccentric muscle contractions are implicated as the cause of most muscle strain injuries. As opposed to concentric contraction, wherein the muscle shortens as it contracts, or isotonic contraction, wherein the muscle remains a constant length, during eccentric contraction the muscle stretches, or is being mechanically lengthened as it is contracting.[233,239] The result is that the muscle is subjected to greater forces, which lead to muscle failure and rupture of myofibers at the MTJ. Eccentric contractions are common in speed sports in which bursts of acceleration or jumping are necessary, such as track, basketball, football, soccer, and rugby.[230,231]

Muscles that cross two joints, contain a higher proportion of type II (fast-twitch) fibers, and those subjected to eccentric contraction in the course of activity are most vulnerable to acute muscle strain. Particular muscles include the gastrocnemius, the rectus femoris, the hamstrings (particularly the biceps femoris), the hip adductors, the biceps brachii, and the pectoralis major.[231,232,233,239] Strain injuries may also affect the paraspinous muscles in the lumbar and cervical regions.[232]

Based on extensive clinical and athletic experience, previous muscle injury and fatigue are thought to be risk factors for strain injury, whereas conditioning, stretching and warm-up are thought to be protective. Research on animal models and a limited number of clinical trials have served to validate these long-held beliefs about muscle strain injuries. Experiments on rabbit muscle have shown that muscle subjected to nondisruptive myotendinous injury was more susceptible to strain injury than control muscle.[240] Further studies have demonstrated that muscle subjected to repeated contraction is able to absorb less energy before reaching the degree of stretch that causes injury, suggesting that muscle fatigue is a risk factor for muscle strain injury.[241] In another study, isometrically conditioned muscles required more force to induce strain injury than contralateral controls, suggesting that isokinetic stretching prior to activity may be protective against strain.[242] Finally, experiments by Noonan and colleagues[230] showed that warming of muscle might be protective against strain injury. The conclusions drawn from these experiments are that warm, stretched muscle is less likely to suffer strain injury than previously injured, cold, unprepared muscle.

Clinical Presentation

The typical presentation of an acute muscle strain injury is acute muscle pain after an episode of severe loading of a muscle. The pain often occurs after a maneuver in a speed sport. The history may reveal onset of pain after a specific movement that the patient can either describe or simulate. The patient might have heard a pop or felt a tear at the time of the injury. The patient might report a history strain injury to the same muscle group in the past (Fig. 1.15).

The physical examination varies depending on the severity of the patient's muscle strain. In all cases, the physical exam reveals tenderness over the MTJ of the strained muscle. As the MTJ is often a vast structure, spanning up to half the length of the muscle belly itself, a large area might be tender on examination.

In grade I strains, the patient presents with tenderness and pain reproducible with use of the muscle or passive stretch. However, there are no clinically apparent deficits in strength or motion.[235] Clinicians must recognize that strength or motion testing may be limited in the clinical setting due to guarding secondary to pain. Grade II strains have the same clinical findings as grade I strains, with increased pain and the possible presence of ecchymosis at the site of the injury due to the extravasation of blood from the strain site outside of the perimysium into the subcutaneous space. The presence of an ecchymosis suggests an injury that has been present for at least 1 day.[231]

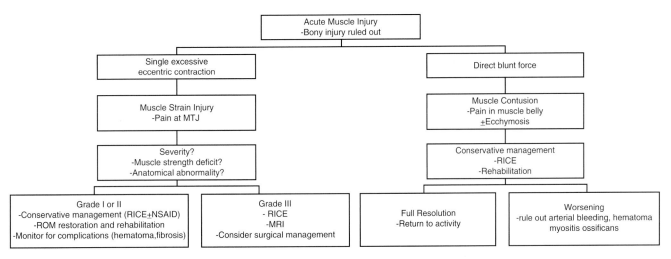

FIG. 1.15. Treatment algorithm for acute muscle injury. MTJ, musculotendinous junction; RICE, rest, ice, compression, and elevation.

In the presence of a grade II or III strain, a defect in the muscle at the site of the strain may be palpable, although this is an inconsistent finding. The palpation of a defect may be more difficult in the presence of a hematoma or collection of fluid in the defect.[235,243]

Grade III muscle strains are sometimes clinically evident due to the presence of the retracted segment of the muscle as a palpable pseudomass and grossly distorted anatomy with a significant deficit in muscle strength (Fig. 1.16).[230,235]

The differential diagnosis includes other soft tissue injuries, such as ligamentous sprains, bursitis, or tendon rupture; bony injuries, such as avulsion fractures, stress fractures, and apophysitis; joint conditions, such as sacroiliitis; and unrelated muscle conditions, such as myositis ossificans.

Evaluation

Clinical assessment of acute muscle strain injury can be challenging due to patient pain, guarding, and recruitment of syn-

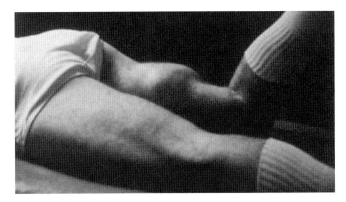

FIG. 1.16. Clinical photograph of an athlete with a severe hamstring strain. Note the pseudomass in the right posterior thigh. (From Clanton and Coupe.[237] © 1998 American Academy of Orthopaedic Surgeons, with permission.).

ergist muscles interfering with clinical examination of strength in the affected muscle.[232] As a result, imaging is often sought to determine the extent of injury and the prognosis, and to evaluate healing lesions. Of the existing imaging modalities, ultrasound, computed tomography, and MRI have all been used to evaluate acute muscle strain injuries.[232,234] Plain radiographs are of little value in the setting of muscle strain injury except to rule out bony injuries including avulsion injury.[244] Ultrasound, which is less costly and more universally available than MRI, is considered an appropriate imaging modality for muscle strain injury.[234] One study of Australian football players showed ultrasound to be as sensitive as MRI in detecting acute hamstring strain injury, but not as sensitive for evaluating healing injuries.[245] Ultrasound is thought to be an appropriate substitute for MRI in situations where MRI is prohibitively expensive or inconvenient, or when there are contraindications to MRI.

Due to its superior resolution, the ability to rule out injuries to adjacent structures, and the lack of dependence on a competent operator, MRI is the imaging modality of choice for muscle strain injuries.[233,235] Magnetic resonance imaging has been shown to be sensitive for detecting muscle edema, inflammation, and hemorrhage that occurs in muscle strain injury. Furthermore, MRI is useful in muscle strain injury because of its ability to rule out pathology to adjacent structures and thereby narrow the differential diagnosis.[232] Most cases of grade I or II muscle strain do not warrant MRI investigation. However, MRI does have a place in several clinical situations: (1) evaluation of injuries wherein the possibility of severe (grade III) strain exists, (2) surgical planning, (3) evaluation of high-level and professional athletes to achieve accurate prognosis, and (4) evaluation of healing lesions for complications.

When the possibility of severe strain exists, MRI is warranted. Patients with grade III strains may benefit from surgical correction of their injury. As a result, MRI must be obtained if the possibility of a severe strain cannot be ruled out so that the patient receives appropriate management.

Magnetic resonance imaging also is warranted in the setting of a known severe muscle strain. In this setting, the exquisite anatomic detail afforded by MRI is invaluable in planning the proper approach and repair. The goal of surgery is to preserve the length of the muscle, thereby preserving force generation. Magnetic resonance imaging is increasingly utilized in the evaluation of high-level and professional athletes as a prognostic tool. In this special population, accurate prognosis is important in team dynamics and in preventing future injury that may shorten a player's career.

Studies in this area have investigated whether MRI is superior to clinical examination in prognosticating the duration of disability due to strain injury. One study of clinically diagnosed hamstring strains in professional Australian football players showed that strains associated with MRI findings were correlated with longer recovery times than MRI-negative injuries, suggesting that MRI has value in prognosticating recovery time in this population.[246] However, a recent cohort study of 58 professional Australian football players comparing clinical evaluation and MRI as prognostic tools showed that clinical evaluation was more accurate than MRI in predicting length of time before return to play. However, the authors point out that MRI appears to be useful as a prognostic tool in moderate and severe strains.[247] Studies have also investigated MRI as a replacement for field testing to determine if patients are ready to return to competition. One systematic review, however, found that the evidence is insufficient to use MRI in this capacity.[248]

The last indication for MRI in the clinical setting is for patients with suspected complications of muscle strain injury. Patients with symptoms that recur or worsen when they were expected to improve might benefit from MRI evaluation. Possible complications include chronic strain, which is commonly encountered after premature return to competition; hematoma, which may benefit from surgical drainage; fibrous adhesion formation; and myositis ossificans, a rare complication of muscle strains (seen more commonly in muscle contusions), which will be discussed later.

Management

For mild or moderate muscle strains, conservative (i.e., nonsurgical) management is indicated. There are three components of conservative management: acute care, rehabilitation, and prevention of reinjury. In the acute setting of a mild or moderate strain, the goal of treatment is to limit hematoma formation and swelling while providing an environment conducive to muscle repair and regeneration. To that end, acute care of a muscle strain injury entails a short period of relative rest (followed by early mobilization), cryotherapy (ice), compression, and elevation (the "RICE" regimen).[237,249] Pain management using nonsteroidal antiinflammatory drugs (NSAIDs) is controversial. Other therapeutic modalities examined for acute muscle strain injury include therapeutic ultrasound and hyperbaric oxygen, which need further study despite some promise for treating muscle strain injuries.

Relative rest in the acute phase after muscle strain injury is an effective means of pain control and allows the regeneration of muscle fibers across the MTJ. A short period of relative rest after injury also prevents further injury to the MTJ. After a period of 3 to 7 days of rest, most sources recommend mobilization of injured muscles in order to prevent atrophy and help align regenerating muscle fibers. Järvinen and Lehto[250] examined the effects of early mobilization, immobilization, and mobilization following a short immobilization period in ruptured rat gastrocnemius muscle. In the study, the investigators found that mobilization after a short period (1 week) of immobilization resulted in better alignment of healing muscle fibers and good functional results. As a result, the current recommendation for treatment of muscle strain injuries is a short period of immobilization followed by early mobilization of the area involved to recover proprioception, approximate physiologic tissue planes, and prevent atrophy.

Cryotherapy (application of ice or cold pack) is a mainstay in the treatment of soft tissue injuries in sports medicine. Despite the ubiquitous use of cryotherapy, according to a recent systematic review, controlled trials are lacking in the case of muscle strain and contusion injury.[251] The beneficial effects of cryotherapy are likely from a combination of decreasing inflammation and desensitizing local pain receptors.[244] Elevation presumably causes a decrease in hydrostatic pressure at the site of the lesion, thereby lessening edema. The use of elevation is a cornerstone of treatment for acute muscle strain, but studies confirming its efficacy are lacking.

Treatment of muscle strain injury with compression is thought to be beneficial by limiting hematoma formation and swelling with mechanical pressure. Compression is commonly used and is unlikely to cause harm. In one of the only studies of compression in the treatment of muscle injury, a group of patients treated with maximal compression in acute muscle strain and contusion injuries failed to show any benefit from maximal compression compared to a control group, both in the size of hematoma and in time to recovery. However, almost every patient in the control group used some form of submaximal compression to treat the lesions, so submaximal compression cannot be discredited as a treatment modality based on the study.[252]

Nonsteroidal antiinflammatory drugs are prescribed commonly for patients with muscle strain injury for pain control. These medications produce analgesia by inhibiting cyclooxygenase enzymes, thereby decreasing prostaglandin production. Theoretical concern exists as to whether these medications inhibit the proper healing of muscle strain injuries because they inhibit the synthesis of inflammatory mediators involved in the healing process. Much of the concern regarding NSAIDs in muscle injury comes from a study by Mishra et al.,[253] in which rabbit muscles were subjected to muscle injury caused by repetitive eccentric contractions. In the study, a group of animals treated with flurbiprofen for 6 days showed enhanced recovery of muscle tension at 3 and 7 days, but had deficits compared to the untreated control group at 28 days. The finding that the NSAID-treated group showed deficits at 28 days suggests the possibility that NSAIDs interfere with muscle repair leading to long-term deficits.

In a study of rabbit muscle subjected to strain injury, the group treated with NSAID therapy (piroxicam) showed a significant increase in contractile force at 1 day compared to untreated control muscles. However, there was no difference in contractile force between the two groups at 2, 4, and 7 days, and no significant difference was ever observed in tensile strength between the groups.[254] Further animal studies have found no evidence that NSAIDs negatively affect satellite cell proliferation.[255] There are comparably fewer studies of NSAIDs for acute muscle strains in human subjects. In a double-blind, placebo-controlled randomized trial, human subjects with acute hamstring strains were divided into three groups: one receiving physiotherapeutic treatment alone, one receiving meclofemate (an NSAID) plus physiotherapeutic treatment, and one receiving diclofenac (an NSAID) plus physiotherapeutic treatment. In the trial, the investigators found no significant differences in pain, swelling, or muscle performance between the three groups over the course of 1 week.[256] The consensus regarding NSAID therapy in muscle strain injuries is that short-term therapy is likely to be safe, but there is little evidence of efficacy. In addition, long-term use of NSAIDs should be discouraged due to possible negative effects on muscle strength and side effects such as renal failure and gastrointestinal (GI) bleeding.

Therapeutic ultrasound has been suggested as a treatment for muscle strain injury. To date, studies have failed to show a benefit from therapeutic ultrasound in the healing of acute muscle strain injuries.[257] Alternatively, hyperbaric oxygen has been suggested as a treatment modality for acute muscle strain injuries based on the theory that satellite cell proliferation (and therefore muscle regeneration) is enhanced by high oxygen tension. Although one study showed promising results in a rat model, the authors pointed out that further study is necessary.[258]

For treating severe (grade III) muscle strains, operative treatment is recommended to preserve muscle length and prevent fibrous contracture.[249] However, there is now some suggestion that nonoperative treatment, with up to 2 weeks of immobilization to ensure approximation of wound edges, achieves results equivalent to surgery in cases of severe strain. In a study by Almekinders,[259] rat muscle treated with surgical repair was shown to recover passive strength to a greater degree at 1 week than muscle treated with splinting only. However, by 2 weeks no differences were noted between the surgical or splinted groups. It is unclear how applicable the study is to the treatment of human strain injuries, as this study employed a rat model with an artificial muscle transection injury. Currently, surgical management of muscle strain injury should be considered in cases of severe (grade III) muscle strain injury, full avulsion of the musculotendinous unit from bone, and bony avulsion with 2 cm or more of displacement.[235,237] Additionally, surgery should be considered in patients with a history of muscle strain injury with persistent pain with extension of the affected muscle. Such a finding suggests that a fibrous scar has formed, leading to limited movement and pain.[238]

Muscle Contusion and Laceration

Definition and Pathophysiology

Muscle contusions and lacerations differ from muscle strain injuries in that they represent acute muscle injuries caused by a direct blow to muscle rather than by excessive stretch (see Table 1.6). Contusions and lacerations differ from each other, as contusions are caused by direct force from a blunt object while lacerations are caused by penetrating trauma (see Fig. 1.15). Since muscle lacerations are not typically encountered in sports medicine, these injuries are not discussed in detail in this chapter.

A muscle contusion occurs when a blunt object strikes a muscle. The result is rupture of myofibers and blood vessels at the site of the injury. As in the case of muscle strain injuries, this causes a local collection of blood and cell debris, which is gradually resorbed by phagocytes in the subsequent inflammatory response. The final stage involves regeneration of muscle fibers from recruitment of satellite cells.[233]

Muscle contusion injuries are common in contact sports, particularly in sports in which participants wear little protective padding. As a result, contusions are common in Australian football, rugby, and soccer. Protective padding aims to prevent muscle contusion injuries, as it serves to distribute the kinetic energy of the inciting blow over a greater surface area. Illustrating this point, a prospective study of padding in Australian football players showed that the group that wore protective thigh padding suffered significantly fewer contusion injuries than the control group.[260]

In a landmark study of muscle contusion injuries, Jackson and Feagin[261] proposed a grading system for contusion severity. The grading system is based on the resultant limitation of range of motion of the knee joint 12 to 24 hours postinjury. In this system, mild contusions are those that leave the patient with near-normal range of motion and normal gait. Moderate contusions leave the patient with less than 90 degrees of knee flexion and antalgic gait. Severe contusions are marked by less than 45 degrees of knee flexion and a prominent limping gait.

Clinical Presentation

The presentation of a muscle contusion injury is pain and swelling in a muscle at the site of blunt trauma. The history is likely to reveal a blunt injury to the site of the contusion. Physical examination reveals tenderness, discoloration, and swelling at the site of the injury. Depending on the severity of the injury, there may be decreased range of motion at the adjacent joints and inability to bear weight on the extremity.[261] If blood escapes the muscle belly and tracks into more superficial fascial planes, ecchymosis will be present. The differential diagnosis of muscle contusion injury includes arterial rupture, muscle strain injury, bony injury, abscess, tumor, compartment syndrome, and myositis ossificans.

Evaluation

As in the case of muscle strain injury, in suspected uncomplicated muscle contusion evaluation is rarely necessary beyond the history and physical examination. However, there are situations in which clinical imaging is warranted in the evaluation of possible muscle contusion injury. For the same reasons as in muscle strain injury, MRI is the imaging modality of choice for muscle contusion injuries.[235]

Situations in which suspected muscle contusion injury warrant further investigation with imaging include (1) in the context of absent or remote history of trauma to the area, and (2) suspected complications such as persistent hematoma or myositis ossificans. A remote or absent history of trauma to an area that resembles a clinical muscle contusion injury suggests the possibility of soft tissue malignancy. Given this possibility, it is absolutely essential to obtain an MRI to rule out these potentially life-threatening conditions.

In a patient with a suspected muscle contusion injury who has not responded to conservative treatment in the expected timeframe, there is concern for the complications of muscle contusion injury such as persistent hematoma or myositis ossificans. Imaging may be a useful adjunct to rule out such complications. Myositis ossificans, which is discussed later, may be imaged with plain radiographs, CT, nuclear scans, or MRI.[235] A patient with suspected muscle contusion injury whose affected limb continues to swell after 48 hours suggests the possibility of arterial injury.[261] In that situation, arteriography or CT may be used to rule out arterial bleeding.

Management

Most muscle contusion injuries are self-limited and, with treatment, the duration of disability is proportional to the severity of the injury, ranging from 13 days on average for mild contusions to 21 days on average for severe contusions.[262] In one study, muscle contusion injuries were noted to have a time to recovery (based on time to pain-free field testing) of 19 ± 9 days, which was significantly shorter than time to recovery for strain injuries (26 ± 22 days).[252]

In the acute phase of conservative treatment, the goal is to limit hematoma formation in the affected muscle. To that end, the RICE regimen is the mainstay of acute treatment for muscle contusion injuries. Clinical trials have shown benefits of short-term immobilization of contusion injuries in flexion followed by early mobilization at 24 to 48 hours depending on the severity of the contusion injury.[262] Studies have shown that prolonged immobilization leads to decreased muscle mass over time and should be avoided. Cryotherapy is a ubiquitous and well-accepted treatment modality in sports medicine, as discussed previously. Compression is thought to limit the size of hematoma formation, and is considered a cornerstone of treatment for muscle contusion injury.

As in the case of muscle strain injuries, the use of NSAIDs in the treatment of muscle contusion injuries is controversial. Although these agents are generally well tolerated and produce analgesia, they inhibit the inflammatory pathway and therefore theoretically interfere with healing of muscle contusion injuries. A study using a rat model of muscle contusion injury found that animals treated with NSAIDs showed a delay in the inflammatory response and decreased tensile strength compared to controls.[263] One of the major studies on the treatment of muscle contusion injuries in humans did not employ NSAID therapy as part of its protocol.[262] The consensus is that NSAID therapy is unlikely to be of benefit in uncomplicated muscle contusion injury, particularly in long-term muscle strength.

Corticosteroids and anabolic steroids have been investigated as treatment modalities for muscle contusion injury. Corticosteroids, like NSAIDs, inhibit the inflammatory process and thus carry the same risk of affecting the healing process. One study in a rat model showed increased muscle strength in animals treated with corticosteroids at day 2 compared to controls. However, decreased muscle strength was observed in this group compared to controls at day 7. From these data, corticosteroids seem to cause damage to healing muscles and should not be used in muscle contusion injury. The study also investigated the use of anabolic steroids in muscle contusion injury. They found that muscles treated with anabolic steroids were significantly stronger than control muscles. The authors recommend further study into the use of anabolic steroids for contusion injuries.[264]

After the acute phase of treatment, the next phase is aimed at recovering a full range of motion followed by strength in the affected muscle. To this end, pain-free range of motion and strengthening exercises are recommended. Return-to-play criteria are different depending on which muscle is affected by a contusion injury, but for quadriceps contusion one study recommended that patients need to demonstrate 120 degrees of knee flexion and be free of atrophy or weakness before returning to athletic activity.[262]

Complications arising from contusion injury should be suspected if the patient fails to improve in the expected timeframe or experiences worsening symptoms. Complications of muscle contusion injury include heterotopic ossification (myositis ossificans; see later discussion), persistent hematomas, and compartment syndrome. Persistent hematomas may be surgically drained for symptomatic relief and to prevent further complications such as abscess formation (see Table 1.6).[252,265]

Exertional Rhabdomyolysis

Definition and Pathophysiology

Rhabdomyolysis refers to a condition of destruction of skeletal muscle cells with resultant spilling of intracellular contents into the systemic circulation.[266] Although serum elevation of muscle cell markers such as creatine kinase (CK), lactate dehydrogenase (LDH), and aspartate aminotransferase (AST) have been shown to occur in athletes undergoing heavy exercise, suggesting some degree of muscle injury, rhabdomyolysis refers to a condition wherein severe, large-scale destruction of skeletal muscle causes a fulminate illness requiring hospitalization to prevent cardiac arrest, acute renal failure, and death.[266]

Broadly, there are two categories of causes of rhabdomyolysis: nonexertional and exertional. Nonexertional causes of rhabdomyolysis are numerous, and include crush injury, thermal injury, hereditary metabolic derangements (e.g., McArdle's disease), skeletal muscle abnormalities (e.g., Duchenne's muscular dystrophy), infections (such as HIV), alcohol ingestions, and medications (e.g., hepatic hydroxymethylglutaryl coenzyme A [HMG CoA] reductase inhibitors). The exertional form of rhabdomyolysis is addressed here, as it is more common in sports medicine.

Exertional rhabdomyolysis is caused by overexertion of large muscle groups leading to disruption of cellular membranes and subsequent release of intracellular contents into the circulation. Although exertional rhabdomyolysis has been observed in well-trained athletes, untrained athletes taking part in strenuous exercise are at higher risk for this condition. Additional risk factors include dehydration, high altitude, eccentric exercise, illness, hyperthermia, underlying myopathy, and use of medications that impair the body's normal cooling mechanisms or produce dehydration (e.g., anticholinergic medications, diuretics).[267]

The release of muscle cell contents in rhabdomyolysis leads to hyperkalemia, hyperphosphatemia, hypo- or hypercalcemia, and myoglobinuria. Complications associated with rhabdomyolysis include cardiac arrest due to hyperkalemia, acute renal failure, hepatic failure, disseminated intravascular coagulation due to the presence of necrotic tissue and phospholipid release, and compartment syndrome. Acute renal failure in rhabdomyolysis is caused by precipitation of myoglobin in the renal tubules, dehydration, and disordered renal hemodynamics. Hepatic failure results from the release of hepatotoxic compounds from skeletal muscle. Compartment syndrome may occur as a result of increased pressure in an osseofascial compartment leading to muscle ischemia.

Clinical Presentation

Patients with exertional rhabdomyolysis present with profound weakness, pain, and swelling in affected muscles (Fig. 1.17). The symptoms may present up to several days after the inciting exercise and are related to breakdown of affected muscles. Additionally, patients may have systemic symptoms such as malaise and fever caused by the inflammatory reaction to the necrotic muscle tissue. Finally, patients will likely report dark, tea- or cola-colored urine, indicative of myoglobinuria. The history in the case of exertional rhabdomyolysis likely reveals intense or unaccustomed exercise activity in the days before symptoms began. Physical examination reveals stiffness, weakness, or decreased range of motion in affected muscle groups.[268]

The differential diagnosis for muscle pain with dark urine includes "march hemolysis," muscle conditions such as delayed-onset muscle soreness, muscle strain, and compartment syndrome with a superimposed cause of dark urine (hepatitis, hemolysis, phenazopyridine ingestion, malaria, or genitourinary pathology).[268]

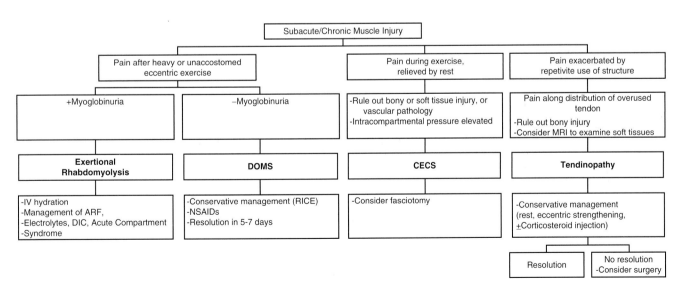

FIG. 1.17. Treatment algorithm for subacute and chronic muscle injury. ARF, acute renal failure; CECS, chronic exertional compartment syndrome; DIC, disseminated intravascular coagulation; DOMS, delayed-onset muscle soreness; NSAID, nonsteroidal antiinflammatory drug; RICE, rest, ice, compression, and elevation.

Evaluation

Confirmation of the diagnosis of rhabdomyolysis is based on laboratory measurements, which indirectly confirm the presence of muscle cell necrosis. Serum tests reveal elevated creatine kinase (CK), indicative of muscle cell contents in the systemic circulation. Sequential serum CK measurements can be used to follow the ongoing destruction of muscle cells as well as resolution of muscle necrosis. Interestingly, serum CK measurements seem to peak at different time points depending on the nature of the inciting exercise. Predominantly concentric exercise causes an immediate but mild rise in CK with a peak at about 24 hours. Predominantly eccentric exercise causes a robust rise in CK beginning at 2 days and peaking in 5 to 6 days.[268]

Urine tests indicated in rhabdomyolysis include dipstick and microscopic urinalysis. Urine dipstick shows a positive orthotoluidine test, indicative of heme-containing compounds in the urine. In rhabdomyolysis, this finding occurs in the context of urine negative for red blood cells on microscopy, suggesting myoglobinuria.

Although not typically indicated, imaging has been used to further evaluate patients with acute exertional rhabdomyolysis. Ultrasound, CT, and MRI have been investigated for this purpose. According to one study, MRI has the greatest sensitivity of the three for detecting nonspecific changes consistent with rhabdomyolysis (100% for MRI versus 62% for CT and 42% for ultrasound).[269] The MRI findings in rhabdomyolysis that were seen in the study were areas of increased signal intensity, a nonspecific finding suggesting muscle edema. Because the findings in rhabdomyolysis are nonspecific, MRI can support the diagnosis of rhabdomyolysis only in the context of the full clinical picture. However, it was also suggested that MRI aids in the treatment of rhabdomyolysis when compartment syndrome exists and fasciotomy is indicated.[269,270] As a side note, MRI is also recommended by some authors for evaluating a patient with acute renal failure of unknown etiology in order to rule out rhabdomyolysis, due to its sensitivity for detecting rhabdomyolysis.[271]

Management

Management of rhabdomyolysis is aimed at support of urine output to prevent acute renal failure. As a result, aggressive intravenous hydration is the mainstay of treatment. Alkalinization of the urine by addition of sodium bicarbonate to intravenous fluids and use of mannitol are suggested by some sources to further facilitate excretion of myoglobin, but their use is controversial and not generally considered necessary.[272,273]

Treatment of electrolyte imbalances is also important in rhabdomyolysis. Hyperkalemia should be managed using insulin and dextrose infusion or sodium polystyrene sulfonate (Kayexalate) as the clinical picture dictates. Hyperphosphatemia can be treated with oral phosphate binders. Hypocalcemia is generally not necessary to correct with exogenous calcium supplementation, as it tends to resolve spontaneously as calcium is mobilized from necrotic muscle tissue.[274]

Exertional rhabdomyolysis may be complicated by acute renal failure, disseminated intravascular coagulation (DIC), or compartment syndrome. Complications should be treated as they arise. Acute renal failure is treated with dialysis as indicated. Disseminated intravascular coagulation is treated with fresh frozen plasma or platelet infusion if bleeding occurs. Compartment syndrome, as will be discussed in the next section, is treated with fasciotomy to relieve increased intracompartmental pressure and prevent contracture.

Acute Compartment Syndrome

Definition and Pathophysiology

Compartment syndromes are caused by excessive pressure buildup in an osseofascial compartment, leading to muscle and nerve ischemia. If untreated, compartment syndromes lead to muscle fibrosis and contracture. Excess pressure in an osseofascial compartment might be a result of hemorrhage or edema and leads to collapse of capillaries supplying the muscle and nerve cells. The result is ischemic myoneural necrosis, with increasing edema causing a vicious cycle of increasing compartment pressure ultimately leading to a contracted, useless limb (Volkmann's contracture).

Compartment syndromes may be acute or chronic. In the acute setting, compartment syndromes usually present as complications of fracture or crush injury as the result of blood and edema in a relatively noncompliant osseofascial compartment. Fractures of the distal humerus, proximal radius, and tibia are associated with a high risk of compartment syndrome. Acute compartment syndromes may also be a complication of athletic muscle injury, as cases caused by muscle strain, rupture, contusion, and rhabdomyolysis have been reported.[270,275] Further, cases related to muscle edema from exercise in the absence of injury have been reported.[235]

Clinical Presentation

Patients with acute compartment syndrome present with deep pain or pressure localized to the affected compartment. The history most likely is notable for trauma, fracture, recent surgery, or athletic injury. Classically, physical examination findings associated with acute compartment syndrome have been termed the "6 P's": pain exacerbated by passive stretch of involved muscle groups, pink skin due to vasodilation, paresis due to nerve ischemia, paresthesias (as a result of nerve ischemia), and "pulses." Contrary to established dogma regarding pulses in compartment syndrome, distal pulses are usually present in the early stages of the disease because pressures must be very high to occlude flow in the large arteries.[276]

The differential diagnosis of acute compartment syndrome includes arterial occlusion, deep vein thrombosis (DVT), and neuropathy of the affected limb.

Evaluation

The gold standard diagnostic modality for acute and chronic compartment syndromes is intracompartmental pressure measurement. In the acute setting, such measurements may be made with a variety of devices. Elevated intracompartmental pressure confirms the diagnosis of acute compartment syndrome. Controversy exists as to what is considered a "threshold pressure" above which a clinically significant compartment syndrome exists and how long such a pressure must be sustained within a compartment for damage to occur. However, studies have shown that the threshold pressure is around 30 to 40 mm Hg.[276]

Acute compartment syndromes represent a situation in which limbs are acutely threatened. It is for this reason that imaging evaluations are rarely undertaken in this setting. However, MRI has been shown to be sensitive for detecting nonspecific changes in muscle attributable to compartment syndrome and could therefore theoretically be used to evaluate patients for compartment syndrome when clinical doubt exists.[234,235]

Management

The goal of treatment of acute compartment syndrome is to relieve the pressure and preserve the neuromuscular function of the affected limb. Although the definitive treatment for compartment syndromes is fasciotomy of the affected compartment, some compartment syndromes have been shown to resolve with conservative treatment.[277] If conservative treatment fails, immediate fasciotomy of the affected compartment is indicated to salvage the use of the limb (Figs. 1.18 and 1.19).[276]

Subacute and chronic conditions of muscle and tendon in orthopedic sports medicine are typically related to overuse of the musculotendinous unit. Pathology may be due to eccentric contractions (e.g., delayed-onset muscle soreness), muscle ischemia (e.g., chronic exertional compartment syndrome), or degeneration of tendons due to overuse (e.g., tendinopathy). Additionally, chronic conditions of muscle may be due to late complications of acute and subacute or chronic muscle pathology (e.g., myositis ossificans) (Table 1.7).

Delayed-Onset Muscle Soreness

Definition and Pathophysiology

Delayed-onset muscle soreness (DOMS) is a condition of temporary muscle pain and weakness that results from reversible damage to muscle cells. It is most often caused by unaccustomed or heavy exercise, specifically exercise involving eccentric muscle contractions, and is familiar to athletes at all skill levels (Table 1.7). Although similar to muscle strain injuries in mechanism of injury (eccentric exercise), DOMS has a more gradual time course and a different pathophysiology than muscle strain injury.

Pathophysiologically, several models have been forwarded to account for DOMS. However, none of the models alone can perfectly account for the pathophysiologic changes associated with DOMS. Therefore, an integrated model has been put forward in the literature.[278] The integrated model holds that the changes leading to DOMS result from microstructural damage to muscle as a result of eccentric contractions. Rather than causing tearing of muscle fibers at the MTJ as in acute strain injury, in DOMS these forces cause damage in the microstructure of type II muscle fibers. Studies of muscle biopsy specimens after eccentric contraction have revealed a characteristic damage pattern to muscle structure in DOMS referred to as "Z-line streaming."[278,279] Further, damage to the muscle architecture results in calcium accumulation within the damaged tissue. This activates proteolytic enzymes, further damaging the muscle. These events account for the rise in serum CK (a marker of skeletal muscle damage) observed in DOMS.

Several hours after the initial damage to the muscle, there is an inflammatory reaction in which neutrophils are recruited to the site of injury. Neutrophils in turn phagocytose cellular debris and release oxidative substances causing further muscle damage. Monocytes, precursors to macrophages, are attracted to the site and produce inflammatory mediators that give rise to pain. In addition, increased pressure in the muscle caused by increased capillary permeability in the inflammatory reaction results in pain. The symptoms resolve over the course of 5 to 7 days, although studies have shown that evidence of DOMS in MRI scans (increased T2 signal indicating muscle edema) may persist even months past the resolution of symptoms.[280] The significance of this finding is not clear.

Clinical Presentation

The patient with DOMS presents with muscle pain and decreased strength in the affected muscles. Patients describe the pain as an "ache" and may report muscle stiffness or weakness. The history includes a bout of unaccustomed or heavy exercise, heavy manual labor, or other activity that incorporates eccentric muscle contraction prior to the onset of symptoms. Unlike patients with acute muscle strain injuries, patients with DOMS do not recall a dramatic "pop" or "tear" with immediate pain. Physical exam reveals tenderness over the affected muscle (sometimes localizing to the MTJ but possibly generalizing to the whole muscle), possible edema, and decreased strength or range of motion.[281]

The differential diagnosis for DOMS includes muscle strain, muscle contusion, exertional rhabdomyolysis, compartment syndrome, tendinopathy, referred pain, neuropathic pain, DVT, and bony or ligamentous injury.

Evaluation

Since DOMS is a self-limited condition, a patient with history and physical exam strongly suggestive of DOMS requires no further workup. Depending on the clinical picture, the workup

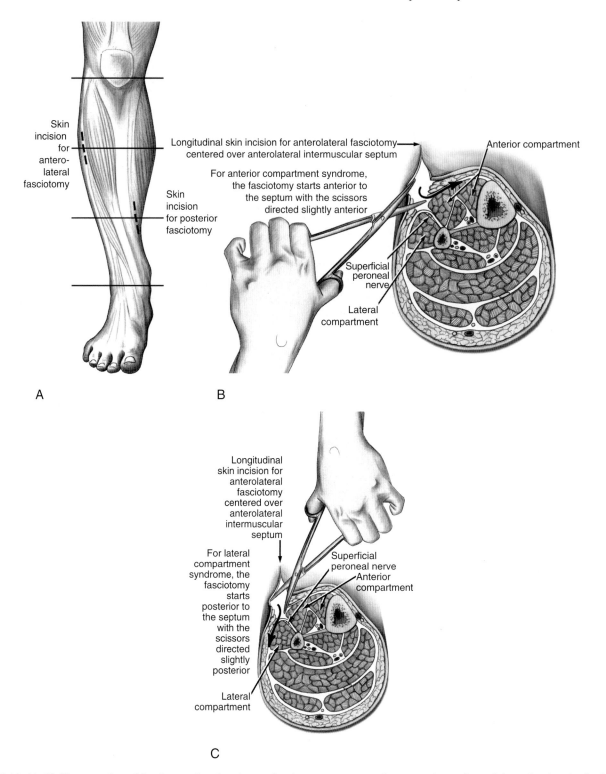

Fig. 1.18. (A–C) The anterolateral fasciotomy for chronic exertional compartment syndrome can be performed through a longitudinal skin incision centered over the anterolateral intermuscular septum. The skin incision should be at the junction of the proximal and middle thirds of the leg. In the anterior compartment, the fasciotomy should begin anterior to the septum, with scissors directed anteriorly, in order to avoid injury to the superficial peroneal nerve. In the lateral compartment, the fasciotomy should start posterior to the septum, with scissors directed slightly posterior. (From Johnson DH, Pedowitz RA. Practical Orthopaedic Sports Medicine and Arthroscopy. Philadelphia: Lippincott Williams & Wilkins, 2006, with permission.).

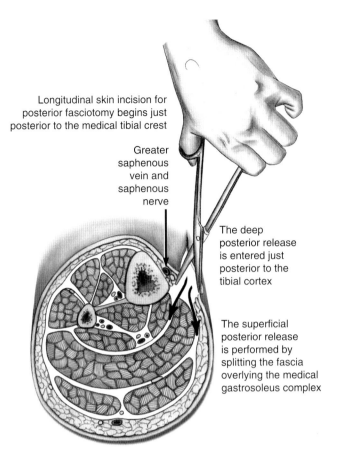

Longitudinal skin incision for posterior fasciotomy begins just posterior to the medical tibial crest

Greater saphenous vein and saphenous nerve

The deep posterior release is entered just posterior to the tibial cortex

The superficial posterior release is performed by splitting the fascia overlying the medical gastrosoleus complex

FIG. 1.19. The posterior fasciotomy for chronic exertional compartment syndrome begins with a skin incision just posterior to the medial tibial crest, at the junction of the middle and distal thirds of the leg. Care should be taken to protect the saphenous nerve and vein. The superficial posterior release is performed by splitting the fascia overlying the medial gastrosoleus complex. The deep posterior compartment is entered just posterior to the tibial cortex. Scissors should be slightly open during the fasciotomy in order to avoid injury to perforating vessels and / or the posterior tibial neurovascular structures. (From Johnson DH, Pedowitz RA. Practical Orthopaedic Sports Medicine and Arthroscopy. Philadelphia: Lippincott Williams & Wilkins, 2006, with permission.).

may include plain radiographs (to exclude bony injury), urinalysis (to exclude exertional rhabdomyolysis), compartmental pressure measurement (to exclude compartment syndrome), or ultrasound (to exclude DVT).

TABLE 1.7. Subacute or chronic muscle pathology.

Subacute/chronic conditions	Local sequelae	Systemic Sequelae
Delayed-onset muscle soreness (DOMS)	Protection against future DOMS	None
Chronic exertional compartment syndrome (CECS)	Denervation Contracture	None
Overuse injury/tendinopathy	Tendon rupture	None
Myositis ossificans	Decreased ROM	None

Magnetic resonance imaging has been shown to be sensitive for DOMS-related changes and has been used to study DOMS pathogenesis.[282] However, MRI is not generally warranted in the clinical workup of DOMS except to exclude DVT, ligamentous injury, and other soft tissue injury. Magnetic resonance imaging in DOMS shows increased signal on T2 sequences suggestive of muscle edema. These are nonspecific findings that are also consistent with grade 1 muscle strain injuries. It is therefore believed that DOMS may be most reliably differentiated from acute muscle strain injury on the basis of the patient's history. It must also be noted that changes attributable to DOMS in MR images may persist long past resolution of symptoms.

Management

Delayed-onset muscle soreness is a self-limited condition. Classically, symptoms begin shortly after the inciting exercise, peak in 24 to 72 hours, and in most patients resolve fully in 7 days with no residual loss of function.[230,232,283] In the meantime, management has classically consisted of rest, cryotherapy, compression, and NSAIDs. Electric nerve stimulation and massage have been studied for the treatment of DOMS with mixed results, while pre- or postexercise stretching and hyperbaric oxygen have demonstrated no benefit. Fortunately, due to the "repeated bout" effect, an episode of DOMS might be protective against future recurrences after eccentric exercise.

Relative rest is indicated in the management of DOMS to prevent further injury. However, as in the case of acute muscle strain, total immobilization is not thought to be beneficial. Gentle isometric stretching aimed at increasing range of motion (ROM) are thought to help align muscle fibers for proper healing. Cryotherapy is used in the management of DOMS primarily for its analgesic effects and is unlikely to cause harm if used in moderation. However, in one study of cryotherapy for DOMS, immersion of an affected arm in a cold water bath showed no effect on muscle soreness, torque generation, or muscle girth compared to contralateral control arms.[284] Compression is a commonly employed modality for DOMS. One study showed that continuous compression is beneficial in DOMS in decreasing subjective pain, CK elevation, swelling, and force generation compared to control.[285] Another study found that intermittent compression is beneficial in decreasing stiffness and pain associated with DOMS.[286]

The use of NSAIDs for muscle injuries, as previously discussed, is controversial due to the potential for these drugs to interfere with the healing process or cause adverse side effects. Mishra et al.[253] observed decreased muscle strength in a rat model treated with NSAIDs after muscle injury, which suggests that NSAIDs may have a deleterious effect on muscle healing from DOMS. Clearly, further study in this area is indicated. However NSAID therapy for DOMS has been studied with reference to several investigational indices, including subjective pain, functional testing, measurements of muscle girth and edema (radiologically and clinically), serum markers (generally using serum CK, which is thought to be a marker of muscle damage), and microscopic evidence of inflammation. Additionally, studies have examined the use of NSAIDs administered after the onset of DOMS[281,287–289] or both before and after the onset of symptoms.[290,291] Most studies show a subjective decrease in pain in patients using oral or topical NSAIDs compared to placebo.[281,287–289,291] Some studies also show a benefit in increased muscle strength or decreased swelling as measured by MRI.[287,288] Most studies also showed a significant decrease in serum CK rise in the treatment group, suggesting that NSAIDs protect against muscle damage in DOMS,[289,291] but some studies show no difference between groups.[288,290] One study of eight men treated with naproxen sodium after eccentric exercise failed to show a benefit of treatment in serum CK, muscle strength at 24 hours, and pain.[290] Most of these trials did not report any adverse drug reactions related to NSAID use.

In one trial, patients in the treatment group received diclofenac for a total of 27 days, which was much longer than in any other trial. In this trial, there were no significant differences in adverse drug reactions observed between the treatment and control groups.[291] Studies have yielded mixed results on the efficacy of NSAIDs, although the preponderance of evidence seems to suggest that short courses of these drugs starting before or after onset of symptoms of DOMS tend to be beneficial in attenuating soreness, muscle weakness, and muscle damage. Although there is still a questionable risk of long-term damage to muscle as a result of NSAID treatment, short courses seem to be well tolerated.

Electrical stimulation for treating DOMS has been studied by several investigators. So far, the results have been mixed. In one study, transcutaneous electrical nerve stimulation (TENS) seemed to have an analgesic effect on DOMS at 24 and 48 hours.[292] However, a more recent placebo-controlled trial of TENS showed no significant effect on DOMS-related pain.[293] Massage has been shown to be effective for DOMS in some studies, including a study in which massage 2 hours after exercise improved pain scores at 48 hours.[294] Some studies show no benefit, possibly because of variation in massage techniques. One systematic review showed insufficient evidence to recommend hyperbaric oxygen treatment, and even found evidence that hyperbaric oxygen may increase interim pain in DOMS.[295] Pre- and postexercise static stretching has been shown not to be effective in preventing or limiting pain associated with DOMS, as has topical heat application.[278,296]

Fortunately for patients suffering from DOMS, bouts of exercise that induce muscle damage appear to induce adaptations that are protective against future muscle damage and DOMS. This process is called the "repeat bout" effect. One study showed that one bout of downhill running (commonly used in DOMS studies because it causes eccentric gastrocnemius and soleus contractions) significantly decreased pain and CK elevations when the exercise was repeated at 3 and 6 weeks.[297]

Chronic Exertional Compartment Syndrome

Definition and Pathophysiology

Chronic exertional compartment syndrome (CECS) is a condition of exercise-induced pain in an osseofascial compartment as a result of pathologically elevated intracompartmental pressure (see Table 1.7). Typically, the condition presents in the compartments of the leg (anterior, posterior, deep posterior, and lateral), although presentation in other compartments is possible. For the most common form of CECS discussed in the literature (anterior leg CECS), the cardinal symptom is chronic, exercise-induced leg pain.

The pathophysiology of CECS is not as clear as that of acute compartment syndrome. Although some studies have provided evidence for muscle ischemia giving rise to the pain associated with CECS (a similar mechanism to the mechanism of acute compartment syndrome), some studies have refuted such a model.[298–300] Other studies have suggested that patients with CECS have pathologically thickened fascia, which predisposes them to CECS.[299]

Clinical Presentation

The patient with CECS presents with chronic, exercise-related pain. Typically patients are young and athletic; the mean age in one study was 26.[301] The pain may be described as "pressure," "aching," or "sharp," and localizes to the involved compartment(s). Historically, the pain occurs after exercise of the involved muscles and resolves with rest. The pain may progress over time, causing the patient to be able to tolerate progressively less exercise before onset of pain. Other symptoms of CECS include muscle weakness and paresthesias that are likely related to compromised nerve function.

Physical examination is typically unrevealing in patients with CECS, particularly when they are asymptomatic. Pain to palpation of involved muscles, muscle hypertrophy, and palpation of muscle hernias (which occur in 20% to 60% of patients) are possible physical exam findings.[299,301]

There is a broad differential diagnosis for CECS (particularly in a patient presenting with leg pain). The differential includes muscle strain injury, DOMS, medial tibial stress syndrome (tibial periostitis), stress fracture, tendon pathology, peripheral vascular disease, peroneal nerve apraxia, peripheral neuropathy, DVT, spinal stenosis, and lumbar herniated nucleus pulposus.

Evaluation

The lack of physical examination findings in CECS has prompted many investigators to validate objective means to make the diagnosis. In contrast to acute compartment syndrome, where plain radiographs are of little value, plain radiographs are indicated to rule out bony pathology such as stress fractures in CECS. As in acute compartment syndrome, the gold standard diagnostic modality for CECS is intracompartmental pressure measurement. In CECS, investigators have emphasized pressure measurements after exercise, preferably that which reproduces symptoms. The most widely accepted pressure measurement criteria for CECS are those set forward by Pedowitz et al.[301] Their study identified three criteria: a preexercise resting intracompartmental pressure ≥15 mm Hg, a 1 minute postexercise pressure 30 mm Hg, or a 5-minute postexercise pressure 20 mm Hg. The study suggested that application of these criteria combined with a history suggestive of CECS should result in less than a 5% false-positive rate in the diagnosis of CECS. The authors recommend repeat pressure measurement and clinical judgment in equivocal cases.

Since intracompartmental pressure (ICP) measurements are invasive and to some degree depend on operator technique, other modalities to make the diagnosis of CECS have been studied. For this purpose, MRI and near-infrared spectroscopy (NIRS) have been examined in several studies. In an early study of MRI for CECS, the investigators found that MRI had promise as a diagnostic modality but concluded at the time that MRI was not indicated in the workup of CECS.[298] The most recent such study was a prospective study comparing intracompartmental pressure measurement, MRI, and NIRS for diagnosis of CECS.[302] The presence of CECS in the study was confirmed by resolution of symptoms after fasciotomy. The investigators found ICP and NIRS to have similar sensitivity and specificity for diagnosing CECS (77% for pressure measurement, 85% for NIRS), while MRI had unacceptably low specificity at similar levels of sensitivity (17% specificity at 86% sensitivity using a change in T2 ratio). The authors conclude that the study validated the diagnostic value of pressure measurement and NIRS but that MRI was less suitable for this purpose.

Another noninvasive method for diagnosing CECS that has been studied is thallium-201 single photon emission tomography (SPET) scanning, which could theoretically detect ischemia in a compartment affected by CECS. Unfortunately, a prospective study of 34 patients showed no qualitative or quantitative difference between patients with CECS. This finding suggests that thallium-201 SPET has no role in the diagnosis of CECS.[300]

Management

As in acute compartment syndrome, the definitive treatment of CECS is fasciotomy of involved compartments. Although conservative management may be attempted in CECS patients willing to decrease their exercise routine, the benefits of pain-free exercise generally outweigh the risks of surgery.

Many studies have been performed to examine outcomes of surgical management of CECS. Although the studies are difficult to compare because of different examined outcomes, most report postoperative success over the follow-up period.

In one series of 100 patients, of which 70 were treated with fasciotomy, surgical treatment resulted in a 90% rate of cure or significant functional improvement at 4.5 months after surgery.[303] In another study, fasciotomy was performed in 53 patients with convincing history and raised tissue pressure measurements (not using the Pedowitz et al.[301] criteria) and 18 patients with convincing history only. The study reports a marked reduction in symptoms in 87% of patients at 2 years postoperatively.[304] These studies concur with the usual success rates in studies of operative treatment of CECS that ranged from 42% to 92% in a recent review.[299]

Overuse Injuries/Tendinopathy

Definition and Pathophysiology

Overuse injuries in the medical literature are a heterogeneous group of disorders. This designation encompasses injuries to bones, nerves, ligaments, and the musculotendinous unit (see Table 1.7). The common thread is that in such chronic injuries the pathology results from overuse of an anatomic structure. Overuse injuries are commonly encountered in sports and occupational medicine, and are often named after the inciting sport (e.g., Little Leaguer's elbow, tennis elbow). Such nomenclature does not refer to the underlying pathologic process, and therefore is not employed in this discussion. This discussion is limited to injuries most commonly encountered in sports medicine that affect the tendon portion of the musculotendinous unit. Specifically, examples of such pathology that are discussed here include medial epicondylitis (golfer's elbow), lateral epicondylitis (tennis elbow), patellar tendinopathy (jumper's knee), and Achilles tendinopathy.

Pathophysiologically, tendinopathies are overuse injuries that result in degeneration of the overused tendon. Studies of affected tendons demonstrate separation of collagen fibers and loss of parallel orientation (Fig. 1.20). There is also an increase in type III collagen (indicative of an ongoing repair process) and an increase in mucoid ground substance.[305,306] These pathologic findings highlight the problems encountered in the nomenclature associated with overuse tendon injuries. Although commonly referred to as "tendonitis," implying an underlying inflammatory etiology, such injuries usually lack an inflammatory component in the chronic state. As a result, some authors have suggested that using the term tendinopathy or tendinosus is more accurate.[306] Such nomenclature is used in this discussion. Theoretically, any tendon is susceptible to tendinopathy, but tendons that are subjected to overuse, such as those mentioned above, are those classically affected.

Clinical Presentation

A patient with tendinopathy presents with chronic pain localized to the involved tendon. The pain is aggravated by use. The history

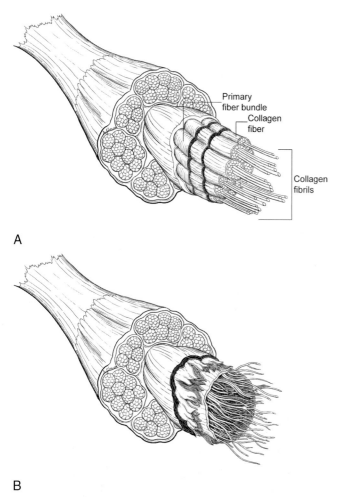

A

B

Fig. 1.20. (A) Artist's depiction of the structure of a healthy tendon. Note the tightly organized collagen fibrils. (B) A tendinopathic tendon, showing degenerative connective tissue changes and disordered collagen fibrils.

may reveal overuse of the tendon due to athletic activity (e.g., pain localizing to the lateral aspect of the elbow exacerbated by tennis). There will be a history of chronic symptoms. Physical exam reveals tenderness along the length of the involved tendon, possible erythema overlying the tendon, and possible muscle weakness. In many cases of tendinopathy, provocative tests that involve loading of the suspected tendon may be used to reproduce the patient's symptoms, making the diagnosis clear.

The differential diagnosis for tendinopathy includes bony or ligamentous injury, arthritis or other intraarticular pathology, DOMS, old muscle strain injury, apophyseal avulsion injury, nerve entrapment, or abscess.

Evaluation

Often tendinopathy is evident based on the history and physical exam findings, including provocative maneuvers. However, if history and physical examination are equivocal, or the patient has failed medical intervention and surgery is deemed appropriate, clinical imaging is warranted. Plain radiographs are used in

such injuries to rule out bony avulsion injuries and intraarticular bodies. To visualize the tendon itself, ultrasound, CT, and MRI have been studied in the literature. Of these imaging modalities, MRI is considered the modality of choice.

Ultrasound examination of the patellar tendon was shown to demonstrate degenerative change in all 28 knees that underwent surgical repair in one study. In the same study, MRI was equally effective in demonstrating degenerative changes in the same patients.[307] In another study of patellar tendinopathy, ultrasound demonstrated degenerative changes in all 16 patients, CT demonstrated similar findings, and MRI showed focal enlargement of the tendon in all cases with high-intensity lesions in 88% of cases.[308] In another study comparing MRI findings with pathologic specimens in patients with confirmed patellar tendinopathy, MRI showed findings in all diseased tendons, including focal thickening (11 out of 11 tendons), and abnormal signal intensity on T2–weighted images (10 out of 11 tendons).[309] These findings suggest that in patellar tendinopathy, all modalities may be useful to demonstrate degenerative changes. The choice of specific modality depends on individual factors; MRI has the benefit of being able to rule out pathology in adjacent structures and with its exquisite resolution is appropriate for surgical planning. Ultrasound, on the other hand, is inexpensive and quick and may be warranted when MRI is unavailable.

Studies of lateral elbow tendinopathy ("lateral epicondylitis") have demonstrated that ultrasound and MRI are useful imaging modalities. One study of 20 cases of elbow tendinopathy showed MRI findings to correlate well with the histopathologic findings. The study authors suggest that MRI is the appropriate imaging modality for surgical planning.[310]

Management

Management of tendinopathy is aimed at restoring healthy tendon architecture through the synthesis of new collagen. To that end, tendinopathies are treated with relative rest, cryotherapy, and eccentric strengthening exercise. Analgesia with local steroid injection or NSAID therapy remains controversial, as tendinopathies are considered to represent a degenerative rather than inflammatory process. Massage, orthotic devices, and therapeutic ultrasound are of uncertain benefit in the management of tendinopathy. Extracorporeal shock wave therapy (ESWT) has been shown to be of no benefit. Surgery is used in cases of tendinopathy that fail medical management, although controlled trials showing the efficacy of surgery are lacking.

Relative rest is used in the management of tendinopathy to protect degenerative tendons from further injury or rupture. However, no studies exist to guide clinicians on the duration or intensity of rest. Patients should be instructed to avoid activities that exacerbate their symptoms. Cryotherapy is used in tendinopathy to ease pain and allow for early mobilization. Eccentric strengthening exercises are thought to help align tendons properly and aid in the synthesis of new collagen. Given that there is little evidence of acute inflammation in the pathogenesis of tendinopathy, the use of NSAIDs and corticosteroids remains suspect. A recent Cochrane review of NSAID therapy for lateral elbow tendinopathy found that while topical NSAID therapy seems to be effective for short-term pain relief, there is insufficient evidence to recommend for or against oral NSAID therapy. The review further stated that injected corticosteroid therapy appears to be more effective than oral NSAIDs at controlling pain in lateral elbow tendinopathy in the short term.[311]

A Cochrane systematic review of rotator cuff tendinopathy concluded that subacromial steroid injection appears better than placebo but failed to demonstrate benefit over NSAIDs in a small number of trials.[312] A systematic review of injected corticosteroids for lateral elbow tendinopathy found statistically significant improvement in pain, global improvement, and grip strength compared to placebo and injected local anesthetics in the short term (<6 weeks). However, for intermediate and long-term outcomes (≥6 weeks), no benefits were found.[313]

Deep tissue friction massage failed to show a pain control benefit in lateral epicondylitis in a systematic review.[314] Orthotic devices are often used in the treatment of tendinopathy to absorb or dampen forces that put stress on degenerative tendons. A systematic review found that the use of orthotic devices in lateral elbow tendinopathy was inconclusive due to the limited number of randomized controlled trials.[315] Finally, another systematic review found insufficient evidence to recommend or discourage acupuncture for lateral elbow tendinopathy, although two small trials have demonstrated a short-term pain control benefit.[316] Extracorporeal shock wave therapy was shown in a systematic review of nine placebo-controlled trials to provide "little or no benefit in terms of pain and function in lateral elbow pain."[317]

Surgery is often pursued in patients with tendinopathy who have failed medical management. The aim of surgery in tendinopathy is to excise degenerative tissue from tendons. Although surgery is reported to be effective in some forms of tendinopathy, few controlled trials exist. A Cochrane review of surgery for lateral elbow tendinopathy found that no conclusion could be drawn regarding surgical treatment for this condition as no controlled trials were available.[318]

Myositis Ossificans

Definition and Pathophysiology

Myositis ossificans is a condition of heterotopic bone formation at a site of previous muscle trauma.[319] In sports medicine, myositis ossificans is most often encountered as a late complication of muscle contusion injury, and it is this presentation of myositis ossificans ("myositis ossificans traumatica") that is the subject of this discussion.

The development of myositis ossificans at the site of previous muscle trauma is thought to be a result of progressive organization and ossification of an intramuscular hematoma. The process has been divided into three stages: acute, subacute, and chronic.[6] The stages represent differing stages of organization of the hematoma and display different findings on imaging studies.

Myositis ossificans may present in any muscle, but large muscles such as the quadriceps are most often affected.[235] A study of quadriceps contusion injuries in West Point cadets found several risk factors for the development of myositis ossificans. Risk factors included range of knee flexion <120 degrees, injury secondary to playing football, a history of previous quadriceps injury, delay in treatment greater than 72 hours, and ipsilateral knee effusion. Patients with more risk factors were found to be at greater risk.[262] The incidence of myositis ossificans in the study was 9% overall, with a 17% incidence in patients with moderate and severe contusions.[262]

Clinical Presentation

A patient with myositis ossificans typically presents after acute blunt muscle trauma, although sometimes there is only a distant or forgettable trauma history (see Table 1.7). Patients report a failure of conservative management of their contusion injury or an acute worsening of pain after initial improvement.[319] They might also note swelling, heat, limited ROM of the adjacent joint, or a mass. Physical examination reveals swelling, heat, induration, and possibly a palpable mass over the involved muscle belly. Range of motion might be affected, and the patient might have a strength deficit secondary to pain. The differential diagnosis of myositis ossificans includes hematoma, abscess, osteomyelitis, or sarcoma.

Evaluation

Evaluation of suspected myositis ossificans may begin with laboratory tests. Serum alkaline phosphatase is typically elevated, as is erythrocyte sedimentation rate (ESR). These tests are not specific for myositis ossificans.

Clinical imaging may help make the diagnosis of myositis ossificans. Using imaging, myositis ossificans may be differentiated from sarcoma or abscess. Plain radiographs, CT scans, MRI, and nuclear bone scanning have been examined for this purpose. In all modalities, images of the affected area change over time as the lesion matures. In the acute stage, radiographs, CT images, and MRI show nonspecific changes. At this time, nuclear medicine bone scans have been shown to be more sensitive to detect myositis ossificans. In such scans, the lesion demonstrates increased tracer uptake. In the subacute stage, plain radiographs, CT scans, and MRI show a mass with irregular calcification that may be confused with a sarcoma. Finally, in the chronic stage, plain radiographs, CT images, and MRI show a mass resembling native bone. Nuclear bone scans show decreased uptake of radioactive tracer, suggestive of decreased metabolic activity. This finding, combined with a lack of invasion of adjacent structures and discontinuity with the adjacent bone, suggests a benign process such as myositis ossificans versus sarcoma.

Imaging findings in myositis ossificans can help inform the decision whether to biopsy a suspicious lesion. In myositis ossificans, biopsy is generally avoided in the acute and subacute stages due to possible exacerbation of the ossification process.[235] For this reason, surgical evaluation of myositis ossificans is contraindicated until the lesion reaches a stage of decreased metabolic activity. Lesions suspicious for sarcoma in imaging studies and those without a suspected precipitating cause suggesting myositis ossificans should be biopsied to exclude malignancy.

Management

Myositis ossificans in its acute and subacute stages is treated just like muscle contusion injury, using the RICE regimen. Treatments shown to prevent heterotopic ossification related to total hip arthroplasty such as NSAIDs (indomethacin and naproxen) and bisphosphonates are recommended by some authors.[319–321] However, no study has examined the use of these medications for myositis ossificans specifically. Additionally, radiation therapy is considered effective in the prevention of heterotopic ossification, but is generally not used in myositis ossificans.

Surgical resection of myositis ossificans is generally not indicated. Studies show that the presence of ossification does not affect ROM or limit activity.[262] Further, myositis ossificans may spontaneously resorb over the course of several years, obviating the need for surgery.[319] Complications of myositis ossificans include joint ankylosis, nerve entrapment, and limited ROM caused by masses of heterotopic bone. When such complications arise, surgery may be warranted. As mentioned previously, before surgery on myositis ossificans is undertaken, studies must be conducted to show that the lesion has reached its mature stage so that exacerbation of symptoms does not result.

References

1. Kujala UM. Benefits of exercise therapy for chronic diseases. Br J Sports Med 2006;40:3–4.
2. Ekeland E, Heian F, Hagen KB. Can exercise improve self esteem in children and young people? A systematic review of randomised controlled trials. Br J Sports Med 2005;39:792–8.
3. Emery CA, Meeuwisse WH, McAllister JR. Survey of sport participation and sport injury in Calgary and area high schools. Clin J Sport Med 2006;16:20–6.
4. Schneider S, Seither B, Tonges S, et al. Sports injuries: population based representative data on incidence, diagnosis, sequelae, and high risk groups. Br J Sports Med 2006;40:334–9.
5. Hawkins RD, Fuller CW. A prospective epidemiological study of injuries in four English professional football clubs. Br J Sports Med 1999;33:196–203.
6. United States Food and Drug Administration. Center for Devices and Radiological Health. Whole body scanning using computed tomography (CT). What are the radiation risks from CT? http://www.fda.gov/cdrh/ct/risks.html.
7. Semelka RC. Imaging x-rays cause cancer: a call to action for caregivers and patients, 2006. http://www.medscape.com/viewprogram/5063.
8. Connell DA, Schneider-Kolsky ME, Hoving JL, et al. Longitudinal study comparing sonographic and MRI assessments of acute and healing hamstring injuries. AJR Am J Roentgenol 2004;183:975–84.
9. Strobel K, Hodler J, Meyer DC, et al. Fatty atrophy of supraspinatus and infraspinatus muscles: accuracy of US. Radiology 2005;237:584–9.
10. Cross TM, Gibbs N, Houang MT, et al. Acute quadriceps muscle strains: magnetic resonance imaging features and prognosis. Am J Sports Med 2004;32:710–9.
11. Robinson P, Barron DA, Parsons W, et al. Adductor-related groin pain in athletes: correlation of MR imaging with clinical findings. Skeletal Radiol 2004;33:451–7.
12. el-Noueam KI, Schweitzer ME, Bhatia M, et al. The utility of contrast-enhanced MRI in diagnosis of muscle injuries occult to conventional MRI. J Comput Assist Tomogr 1997;21:965–8.
13. Mellerowicz H, Lubasch A, Dulce MC, et al. Diagnosis and follow-up of muscle injuries by means of plain and contrast-enhanced MRT: experimental and clinical studies. Rofo 1997;166:437–45.
14. Grainger AJ, Rhodes LA, Keenan AM, et al. Quantifying perimeniscal synovitis and its relationship to meniscal pathology in osteoarthritis of the knee. Eur Radiol 2007;17(1):119–24.
15. Pla ME, Dillingham TR, Spellman NT, et al. Painful legs and moving toes associates with tarsal tunnel syndrome and accessory soleus muscle. Mov Disord 1996;11:82–86.
16. Kendi TK, Altinok D, Erdal HH, et al. Imaging in the diagnosis of symptomatic forearm muscle herniation. Skeletal Radiol 2003;32:364–6.
17. Quick HH, Ladd ME, Hoevel M, et al. Real-time MRI of joint movement with true FISP. J Magn Reson Imaging 2002;15:710–15.
18. Sinha S, Hodgson JA, Finni T, et al. Muscle kinematics during isometric contraction: development of phase contrast and spin tag techniques to study healthy and atrophied muscles. J Magn Reson Imaging 2004;20:1008–19.
19. Le Y, Glaser K, Rouviere O, et al. Feasibility of simultaneous temperature and tissue stiffness detection by MRE. Magn Reson Med 2006;55:700–5.
20. Bensamoun SF, Ringleb SI, Littrell L, et al. Determination of thigh muscle stiffness using magnetic resonance elastography. J Magn Reson Imaging 2006;23:242–7.
21. Akima H, Kinugasa R, Kuno S. Recruitment of the thigh muscles during sprint cycling by muscle functional magnetic resonance imaging. Int J Sports Med 2005;26:245–52.
22. Hug F, Bendahan D, Le Fur Y, et al. Heterogeneity of muscle recruitment pattern during pedaling in professional road cyclists: a magnetic resonance imaging and electromyography study. Eur J Appl Physiol 2004;92:334–42.
23. Takeda Y, Kashiwaguchi S, Matsuura T, et al. Hamstring muscle function after tendon harvest for anterior cruciate ligament reconstruction: evaluation with T2 relaxation time of magnetic resonance imaging. Am J Sports Med 2006;34:281–8.
24. Takeda Y, Kashiwaguchi S, Endo K, et al. The most effective exercise for strengthening the supraspinatus muscle: evaluation by magnetic resonance imaging. Am J Sports Med 2002;30:374–81.

25. Yanagisawa O, Niitsu M, Yoshioka H, et al. MRI determination of muscle recruitment variations in dynamic ankle plantarflexion exercise. Am J Phys Med Rehabil 2003;82:760–5.

26. Patten C, Meyer RA, Fleckenstein JL. T2 Mapping of Muscle. Semin Musculoskelet Radiol 2003;7:297–307.

27. Green RAR, Wilson DJ. A pilot study using magnetic resonance imaging to determine the patterns of muscle group recruitment by rowers with different levels of experience. Skeletal Radiol 2000;29:196–203.

28. Noseworthy MD, Bulte DP, Alfonsi J. BOLD magnetic resonance imaging of skeletal muscle. Semin Musculoskelet Radiol 2003;7:307–15.

29. Ledermann HP, Schulte AC, Heidecker HG, et al. Blood oxygenation level-dependent magnetic resonance imaging of the skeletal muscle in patients with peripheral arterial occlusive disease. Circulation 2006;113:2929–35.

30. Meyer RA, Towse TF, Reid RW, et al. BOLD MRI mapping of transient hyperemia in skeletal muscle after single contractions. NMR Biomed 2004;17:392–8.

31. Price TB, Kamen G, Damon BM, et al. Comparison of MRI with EMG to study muscle activity associated with dynamic plantar flexion. Magn Reson Imaging 2003;21:853–61.

32. Ploutz LL, Tesch PA, Biro RL, et al. Effect of resistance training on muscle use during exercise. J Appl Physiol 1994;76:1675–81.

33. Conley MS, Stone MH, Nimmons M, et al. Resistance training and human cervical muscle recruitment plasticity. J Appl Physiol 1997;83:2105–211.

34. Abe T, Kojima K, Kearns CF, et al. Whole body muscle hypertrophy from resistance training: distribution and total mass. Br J Sports Med 2003;37:543–5.

35. Ozsarlak O, Parizel PM, De Schepper AM, et al. Whole-body MR screening of muscles in the evaluation of neuromuscular diseases. Eur Radiol 2004;14:1489–93.

36. O'Connell MJ, Powell T, Brennan D, et al. Whole-body MR imaging in the diagnosis of polymyositis. AJR Am J Roentgenol 2002;179:967–71.

37. Brooks SV. Current topics for teaching skeletal muscle physiology. Adv Physiol Educ 2003;27:171–82.

38. Hodges PW, Pengel LH, Herbert RD, et al. Measurement of muscle contraction with ultrasound imaging. Muscle Nerve 2003;27:682–92.

39. Kubo K, Kanehisa H, Azuma K, et al. Muscle architectural characteristics in young and elderly men and women. Int J Sports Med 2003;24:125–30.

40. Heemskerk AM, Strijkers GJ, Vilanova A, et al. Determination of mouse skeletal muscle architecture using three-dimensional diffusion tensor imaging. Magn Reson Med 2005;53:1333–40.

41. Toomayan GA, Robertson F, Major NM, et al. Upper extremity compartmental anatomy: clinical relevance to radiologists. Skeletal Radiol 2006;35:195–201.

42. Toomayan GA, Robertson F, Major NM. Lower extremity compartmental anatomy: clinical relevance to radiologists. Skeletal Radiol 2005;34:307–13.

43. Anderson MW, Temple HT, Dussault RG, et al. Compartmental anatomy: relevance to staging and biopsy of musculoskeletal tumors. AJR Am J Roentgenol 1999;173:1663–71.

44. Boles CA, Kannam S, Cardwell AB. The forearm: anatomy of muscle compartments and nerves. AJR Am J Roentgenol 2000;174:151–9.

45. Bergman RA, Afifi AK, Miyauchi R. Illustrated encyclopedia of human anatomic variation. Anatomic Atlases. Revised 2004. http://www.anatomyatlases.org/AnatomicVariants/AnatomyHP.shtml.

46. Kopsch F. Rauber's Lehrbuch der Anatomie des Menschen. Leipzig: Thieme, 1908.

47. Boutin RD. Anatomy and MR imaging of sports-related muscle injuries. In: Buckwalter KA, Kransdorf MJ, eds. RSNA Categorical Course in Diagnostic Radiology: Musculoskeletal Imaging—Exploring New Limits. Oak Brook, IL: Radiological Society of North America, 2003:7–24.

48. Zeiss J, Guilliam-Haidet L. MR demonstration of anomalous muscles about the volar aspect of the wrist and forearm. Clin Imaging 1996;20:219–21.

49. Cheung Y, Rosenberg ZS. MR imaging of the accessory muscles around the ankle. Magn Reson Imaging Clin North Am 2001;9:465–73.

50. Beiner JM, Jokl P. Muscle contusion injury and myositis ossificans traumatica. Clin Orthop Relat Res 2002;403(suppl):S110–9.

51. Orchard JW. Intrinsic and extrinsic risk factors for muscle strains in Australian football. Am J Sports Med 2001;29:300–3.

52. Verrall GM, Slavotinek JP, Barnes PG, et al. Clinical risk factors for hamstring muscle strain injury: a prospective study with correlation of injury by magnetic resonance imaging. Br J Sports Med 2001;35:435–9.

53. Bahr R, Holme I. Risk factors for sports injuries–a methodological approach. Br J Sports Med 2003;37:384–92.

54. Emery CA, Meeuwisse WH, Powell JW. Groin and abdominal strain injuries in the National Hockey League. Clin J Sport Med 1999;9:151–6.

55. Gibbs NJ, Cross TM, Cameron M, et al. The accuracy of MRI in predicting recovery and recurrence of acute grade one hamstring muscle strains within the same season in Australian Rules football players. J Sci Med Sport 2004;7:248–58.

56. Upton PA, Noakes TD, Juritz JM. Thermal pants may reduce the risk of recurrent hamstring injuries in rugby players. Br J Sports Med 1996;30:57–60.

57. Brooks JH, Fuller CW, Kemp SP, et al. Incidence, risk, and prevention of hamstring muscle injuries in professional rugby union. Am J Sports Med 2006;34(8):1297–306.

58. Woods C, Hawkins RD, Maltby S, et al. The Football Association Medical Research Programme: an audit of injuries in professional football—analysis of hamstring injuries. Br J Sports Med 2004;38:36–41.

59. Verrall GM, Slavotinek JP, Barnes PG, et al. Diagnostic and prognostic value of clinical findings in 83 athletes with posterior thigh injury: comparison of clinical findings with magnetic resonance imaging documentation of hamstring muscle strain. Am J Sports Med 2003;31:969–73.

60. Kirkendall DT, Garrett WE Jr. Clinical perspectives regarding eccentric muscle injury. Clin Orthop Relat Res 2002;403 Suppl:S81–9.

61. Mair SD, Seaber AV, Glisson RR, et al. The role of fatigue in susceptibility to acute muscle strain injury. Am J Sports Med 1996;24:137–43.

62. Gabbe BJ, Finch CF, Bennell KL, et al. Risk factors for hamstring injuries in community level Australian football. Br J Sports Med 2005;39:106–10.

63. Gabbe BJ, Bennell KL, Finch CF, et al. Predictors of hamstring injury at the elite level of Australian football. Scand J Med Sci Sports 2006;16:7–13.

64. Ploutz-Snyder LL, Tesch PA, Dudley GA. Increased vulnerability to eccentric exercise-induced dysfunction and muscle injury after concentric training. Arch Phys Med Rehabil 1998;79:58–61.

65. Butterfield TA, Herzog W. Effect of altering starting length and activation timing of muscle on fiber strain and muscle damage. J Appl Physiol 2006;100:1489–98.

66. Askling C, Saartok T, Thorstensson A. Type of acute hamstring strain affects flexibility, strength, and time to return to pre-injury level. Br J Sports Med 2006;40:40–4.

67. Connell DA, Potter HG, Sherman MF, el al. Injuries of the pectoralis major muscle: evaluation with MR imaging. Radiology 1999;210:785–91.

68. Palmer WE, Kuong SJ, Elmadbouh HM. MR imaging of myotendinous strain. AJR Am J Roentgenol 1999;173:703–79.

69. Palmer WE. Myotendinous unit: MR imaging diagnosis and pitfalls. In: Buckwalter KA, Kransdorf MJ, eds. RSNA Categorical Course in Diagnostic Radiology: Musculoskeletal Imaging—Exploring New Limits. Oak Brook, IL: Radiological Society of North America, 2003:25–35.

70. Slavotinek JP, Verrall GM, Fon GT. Hamstring injury in athletes: using MR imaging measurements to compare extent of muscle injury with amount of time lost from competition. AJR Am J Roentgenol 2002;179:1621–8.

71. De Smet AA, Best TM. MR imaging of the distribution and location of acute hamstring injuries in athletes. AJR Am J Roentgenol 2000;174:393–9.

72. Schneider-Kolsky ME, Hoving JL, Warren P, et al. A comparison between clinical assessment and magnetic resonance imaging of acute hamstring injuries. Am J Sports Med 2006;34:1008–15.

73. Huard J, Li Y, Fu FH. Muscle injuries and repair: current trends in research. J Bone Joint Surg Am 2002;84–A:822–32.

74. Menetrey J, Kasemkijwattana C, Day CS, et al. Growth factors improve muscle healing in vivo. J Bone Joint Surg Br 2000;82:131–7.

75. Jarvinen TA, Jarvinen TL, Kaariainen M, et al. Muscle injuries: biology and treatment. Am J Sports Med 2005;33:745–64.

76. Noonan TJ, Garrett WE Jr. Muscle strain injury: diagnosis and treatment. J Am Acad Orthop Surg 1999;7:262–9.

77. Connell DA, Burke F, Malara F, et al. Comparison of ultrasound and MR imaging in the assessment of acute and healing hamstring injuries (Abstract). Society of Skeletal Radiology Annual Meeting, 2003.

78. Koulouris G, Connell D. Imaging of hamstring injuries: therapeutic implications. Eur Radiol 2006;16:1478–87.

79. Greco A, McNamara MT, Escher RM, et al. Spin-echo and STIR MR imaging of sports-related muscle injuries at 1.5 T. J Comput Assist Tomogr 1991;15:994–9.

80. Klingele KE, Sallay PI. Surgical repair of complete proximal hamstring tendon rupture. Am J Sports Med 2002;30:742–7.

81. Orava S, Kujala UM. Rupture of the ischial origin of the hamstring muscles. Am J Sports Med 1995;23:702–5.

82. Sherry MA, Best TM. A comparison of 2 rehabilitation programs in the treatment of acute hamstring strains. J Orthop Sports Phys Ther 2004;34:116–25.

83. Shrier I. Muscle dysfunction versus wear and tear as a cause of exercise related osteoarthritis: an epidemiological update. Br J Sports Med 2004;38:526–35.

84. Singh RK, Pooley J. Complete rupture of the triceps brachii muscle. Br J Sports Med 2002;36:467–9.

85. Connell DA, Jhamb A, James T. Side strain: a tear of internal oblique musculature. AJR Am J Roentgenol 2003;181:1511–7.

86. Humphries D, Jamison M. Clinical and magnetic resonance imaging features of cricket bowler's side strain. Br J Sports Med 2004;38:E21.

87. Maquirriain J, Ghisi JP. Uncommon abdominal muscle injury in a tennis player: internal oblique strain. Br J Sports Med 2006;40:462–3.

88. Dyson R, Buchanan M, Hale T. Incidence of sports injuries in elite competitive and recreational windsurfers. Br J Sports Med 2006;40:346–50.

89. Bono CM. Low-back pain in athletes. J Bone Joint Surg Am 2004;86–A:382–96.

90. Heiderscheit BC, Hoerth DM, Chumanov ES, et al. Identifying the time of occurrence of a hamstring strain injury during treadmill running: a case study. Clin Biomech (Bristol, Avon) 2005;20:1072–8.

91. Thelen DG, Chumanov ES, Best TM, et al. Simulation of biceps femoris musculotendon mechanics during the swing phase of sprinting. Med Sci Sports Exerc 2005;37:1931–8.

92. Garrett WE Jr, Califf JC, Bassett FH 3rd. Histochemical correlates of hamstring injuries. Am J Sports Med 1984;12:98–103.

93. Yamamoto T. Relationship between hamstring strains and leg muscle strength. A follow-up study of collegiate track and field athletes. J Sports Med Phys Fitness 1993;33:194–9.

94. Burkett LN. Investigation into hamstring strains: the case of the hybrid muscle. J Sports Med 1975;3:228–31.

95. Koulouris G, Connell D. Hamstring muscle complex: an imaging review. Radiographics 2005;25:571–86.

96. Koulouris G, Connell D. Evaluation of the hamstring muscle complex following acute injury. Skeletal Radiol 2003;32:582–9.

97. Brandser EA, el-Khoury GY, Kathol MH, et al. Hamstring injuries: radiographic, conventional tomographic, CT, and MR imaging characteristics. Radiology 1995;197:257–62.

98. Straw R, Colclough K, Geutjens G. Surgical repair of a chronic rupture of the rectus femoris muscle at the proximal musculotendinous junction in a soccer player. Br J Sports Med 2003;37:182–4.

99. Hardy JR, Chimutengwende-Gordon M, Bakar I. Rupture of the quadriceps tendon: an association with a patellar spur. J Bone Joint Surg Br 2005;87:1361–3.

100. Ilan DI, Tejwani N, Keschner M, et al. Quadriceps tendon rupture. J Am Acad Orthop Surg 2003;11:192–200.

101. Shah MK. Simultaneous bilateral rupture of quadriceps tendons: analysis of risk factors and associations. South Med J 2002;95:860–6.

102. Shah M, Jooma N. Simultaneous bilateral quadriceps tendon rupture while playing basketball. Br J Sports Med 2002;36:152–3.

103. Katz T, Alkalay D, Rath E, et al. Bilateral simultaneous rupture of the quadriceps tendon in an adult amateur tennis player. J Clin Rheumatol 2006;12:32–3.

104. Jarvinen TA, Jarvinen TL, Kannus P, et al. Collagen fibres of the spontaneously ruptured human tendons display decreased thickness and crimp angle. J Orthop Res 2004;22:1303–9.

105. Hsu JC, Fischer DA, Wright RW. Proximal rectus femoris avulsions in national football league kickers: a report of 2 cases. Am J Sports Med 2005;33:1085–7.

106. Rizio L 3rd, Salvo JP, Schurhoff MR, et al. Adductor longus rupture in professional football players: acute repair

with suture anchors: a report of two cases. Am J Sports Med 2004;32:243–5.

107. Tyler TF, Nicholas SJ, Campbell RJ, et al. The association of hip strength and flexibility with the incidence of adductor muscle strains in professional ice hockey players. Am J Sports Med 2001;29:124–8.

108. Robinson P, White LM. The biomechanics and imaging of soccer injuries. Semin Musculoskelet Radiol 2005;9:397–420.

109. Orchard J, Seward H. Epidemiology of injuries in the Australian Football League, seasons 1997–2000. Br J Sports Med 2002;36:39–44.

110. Schlegel TF, Boublik M, Ho CP, et al. Role of MR imaging in the management of injuries in professional football players. Magn Reson Imaging Clin N Am 1999;7:175–90.

111. Gibbs N. Injuries in professional rugby league. A three-year prospective study of the South Sydney Professional Rugby League Football Club. Am J Sports Med 1993;21:696–700.

112. O'Connor D. Groin injuries in professional rugby league players: a prospective study. J Sports Sci 2004;22:629–36.

113. Nicholas SJ, Tyler TF. Adductor muscle strains in sport. Sports Med 2002;32:339–44.

114. Kalebo P, Karlsson J, Sward L, et al. Ultrasonography of chronic tendon injuries in the groin. Am J Sports Med 1992;20:634–9.

115. Orchard J, Best TM, Verrall GM. Return to play following muscle strains. Clin J Sport Med 2005;15:436–41.

116. Attarian DE. Isolated acute hip adductor brevis strain. J South Orthop Assoc 2000;9:213–5.

117. Sanders SM, Schachter AK, Schweitzer M, et al. Iliacus muscle rupture with associated femoral nerve palsy after abdominal extension exercises: a case report. Am J Sports Med 2006;34:837–9.

118. Tuite DJ, Finegan PJ, Saliaris AP, et al. Anatomy of the proximal musculotendinous junction of the adductor longus muscle. Knee Surg Sports Traumatol Arthrosc 1998;6:134–7.

119. Ippolito E, Postacchini F. Rupture and disinsertion of the proximal attachment of the adductor longus tendon. Case report with histochemical and ultrastructural study. Ital J Orthop Traumatol 1981;7:79–85.

120. Mouzopoulos G, Stamatakos M, Vasiliadis G, et al. Rupture of adductor longus tendon due to ciprofloxacin. Acta Orthop Belg 2005;71:743–5.

121. Sangwan SS, Aditya A, Siwach RC. Isolated traumatic rupture of the adductor longus muscle. Indian J Med Sci 1994;48:186–7.

122. Albers SL, Spritzer CE, Garrett WE Jr, et al. MR findings in athletes with pubalgia. Skeletal Radiol 2001;30:270–7.

123. Kluin J, den Hoed PT, van Linschoten R, et al. Endoscopic evaluation and treatment of groin pain in the athlete. Am J Sports Med 2004;32:944–9.

124. Brennan D, O'Connell MJ, Ryan M, et al. Secondary cleft sign as a marker of injury in athletes with groin pain: MR image appearance and interpretation. Radiology 2005;235:162–7.

125. Slavotinek JP, Verrall GM, Fon GT, et al. Groin pain in footballers: the association between preseason clinical and pubic bone magnetic resonance imaging findings and athlete outcome. Am J Sports Med 2005;33:894–9.

126. Boutin RD, Newman JS. MR imaging of sports-related hip disorders. Magn Reson Imaging Clin North Am 2003;11:255–81.

127. Nelson EN, Kassarjian A, Palmer WE. MR imaging of sports-related groin pain. Magn Reson Imaging Clin North Am 2005;13:727–42.

128. Delgado GJ, Chung CB, Lektrakul N, et al. Tennis leg: clinical US study of 141 patients and anatomic investigation of four cadavers with MR imaging and US. Radiology 2002;224:112–9.

129. Bojsen-Moller J, Hansen P, Aagaard P, et al. Differential displacement of the human soleus and medial gastrocnemius aponeuroses during isometric plantar flexor contractions in vivo. J Appl Physiol 2004;97:1908–14.

130. Johnston C, Ford S, Eustace S. MRI of calf pain in elite athletes. AJR 2006;186(suppl):A125(abst).

131. Weishaupt D, Schweitzer ME, Morrison WB. Injuries to the distal gastrocnemius muscle: MR findings. J Comput Assist Tomogr 2001;25:677–82.

132. Bianchi S, Martinoli C, Abdelwahab IF, et al. Sonographic evaluation of tears of the gastrocnemius medial head. J Ultrasound Med 1998;17:157–62.

133. Guillodo Y, Botton E, Saraux A, Le Goff P. Effusion between the aponeuroses (letter). J Ultrasound Med 1999;18:860–81.

134. Koulouris G, Jhamb A, Connell DA, et al. MR imaging findings of calf muscle injuries. AJR 2006;186(suppl):A41(abst).

135. Anderson JE. Grant's Atlas of Anatomy, 8th ed. Baltimore: Williams & Wilkins, 1983.

136. Zvijac JE, Schurhoff MR, Hechtman KS, et al. Pectoralis major tears: correlation of magnetic resonance imaging and treatment strategies. Am J Sports Med 2006;34:289–94.

137. Raske A, Norlin R. Injury incidence and prevalence among elite weight and power lifters. Am J Sports Med 2002;30:248–56.

138. Beloosesky Y, Grinblat J, Weiss A, et al. Pectoralis major rupture in elderly patients: a clinical study of 13 patients. Clin Orthop Relat Res 2003;413:164–9.

139. Aarimaa V, Rantanen J, Heikkila J, et al. Rupture of the pectoralis major muscle. Am J Sports Med 2004;32:1256–62.

140. Butler D. Pectoralis major muscle injuries: evaluation and management (letter). J Am Acad Orthop Surg 2006;14:259.

141. Petilon J, Carr DR, Sekiya JK, et al. Pectoralis major muscle injuries: evaluation and management. J Am Acad Orthop Surg 2005;13:59–68.

142. Lee J, Brookenthal KR, Ramsey ML, et al. MR imaging assessment of the pectoralis major myotendinous unit: An MR imaging-anatomic correlative study with surgical correlation. AJR Am J Roentgenol 2000;174:1371–5.

143. Carrino JA, Chandnanni VP, Mitchell DB, et al. Pectoralis major muscle and tendon tears: Diagnosis and grading using magnetic resonance imaging. Skeletal Radiol 2000;29:305–13.

144. Schachter AK, White BJ, Namkoong S, et al. Revision reconstruction of a pectoralis major tendon rupture using hamstring autograft: a case report. Am J Sports Med 2006;34:295–8.

145. Orchard JW, Farhart P, Leopold C. Lumbar spine region pathology and hamstring and calf injuries in athletes: is there a connection? Br J Sports Med 2004;38:502–4.

146. Chougle A, Batty PD, Hodgkinson JP. Audit of injuries in a premiership football squad over a 5-year period [letter]. J Sports Sci Med 2005;4:211–3 (http://www.jssm.org/b-v4n2.php).

147. Ward P. Brazilian radiologists take on soccer injuries. Diagn Imaging Eur 2005;21:18–21 (http://www.diagnosticimaging.com).

148. Verrall GM, Slavotinek JP, Barnes PG, et al. Assessment of physical examination and magnetic resonance imaging findings of hamstring injury as predictors for recurrent injury. J Orthop Sports Phys Ther 2006;36:215–24.

149. Ryan JB, Wheeler JH, Hopkinson WJ, et al. Quadriceps contusions. West Point update. Am J Sports Med 1991;19:299–304.

150. Theumann N, Abdelmoumene A, Wintermark M, et al. Post-traumatic pseudolipoma: MRI appearances. Eur Radiol 2005;15:1876–80.

151. Thorsson O, Lilja B, Nilsson P, et al. Immediate external compression in the management of an acute muscle injury. Scand J Med Sci Sports 1997;7:182–90.

152. Diaz JA, Fischer DA, Rettig AC, et al. Severe quadriceps muscle contusions in athletes. A report of three cases. Am J Sports Med 2003;31:289–93.

153. Bush CH. The magnetic resonance imaging of musculoskeletal hemorrhage. Skeletal Radiol 2000;29:1–9.

154. Rubin JI, Gomori JM, Grossman RI, et al. High-field MR imaging of extracranial hematomas. AJR Am J Roentgenol 1987;148:813–7.

155. Kransdorf MJ, Murphey MD. Imaging of Soft Tissue Tumors, 2nd ed. Philadelphia: Lippincott Williams & Wilkins, 2006.

156. Dooms GC, Fisher MR, Hricak H, et al. MR imaging of intramuscular hemorrhage. J Comput Assist Tomogr 1985;9:908–13.

157. De Smet AA, Fisher DR, Heiner JP, et al. Magnetic resonance imaging of muscle tears. Skeletal Radiol 1990;19:283–6.

158. De Smet AA. Magnetic resonance findings in skeletal muscle tears. Skeletal Radiol 1993;22:479–84.

159. El-Khoury GY, Brandser EA, Kathol MH, et al. Imaging of muscle injuries. Skeletal Radiol 1996;25:3–11.

160. Saotome K, Koguchi Y, Tamai K, et al. Enlarging intramuscular hematoma and fibrinolytic parameters. J Orthop Sci 2003;8:132–6.

161. Temple HT, Kuklo TR, Sweet DE, et al. Rectus femoris muscle tear appearing as a pseudotumor. Am J Sports Med 1998;26:544–8.

162. Kaplan FS, Glaser DL, Hebela N, et al. Heterotopic ossification. J Am Acad Orthop Surg 2004;12:116–25.

163. Bouchardy L, Garcia J. Magnetic resonance imaging in the diagnosis of myositis ossificans circumscripta. J Radiol 1994;75:101–10.

164. Hanquinet S, Ngo L, Anooshiravani M, et al. Magnetic resonance imaging helps in the early diagnosis of myositis ossificans in children. Pediatr Surg Int 1999;15:287–9.

165. Shirkhoda A, Armin AR, Bis KG, et al. MR imaging of myositis ossificans: variable patterns at different stages. J Magn Reson Imaging 1995;5:287–92.

166. Ackerman LV. Extra-osseous localized non-neoplastic bone and cartilage formation (so-called myositis ossificans). Clinical and pathological confusion with malignant neoplasms. J Bone Joint Surg 1958;40–A:279–98.

167. Renault E, Favier T, Laumonier F. Non-traumatic myositis ossificans circumscripta. Arch Pediatr 1995;2:150–55.

168. Parikh J, Hyare H, Saifuddin A. A review of the imaging features of post traumatic myositis ossificans using a multimodality approach with a particular emphasis on MRI. Radiological Society of North America Annual Meeting, Chicago, 2003.

169. Ledermann HP, Schweitzer ME, Morrison WB. Pelvic heterotopic ossification: MR imaging characteristics. Radiology 2002;222:189–95.

170. McCarthy EF, Sundaram M. Heterotopic ossification: a review. Skeletal Radiol 2005;34:609–19.

171. Kluger G, Kochs A, Holthausen H. Heterotopic ossification in childhood and adolescence. J Child Neurol 2000;15:406–13.

172. Lewallen DG. Heterotopic ossification following total hip Arthroplasty. Instr Course Lect 1995;44:287–92.

173. Tibone J, Sakimura I, Nickel VL, et al. Heterotopic ossification around the hip in spinal cord-injured patients. A long-term follow-up study. J Bone Joint Surg Am 1978;60:769–75.

174. Shehab D, Elgazzar AH, Collier BD. Heterotopic ossification. J Nucl Med 2002;43:346–53.

175. Coblentz CL, Cockshott WP, Martin RF. Resolution of myositis ossificans in a hemophiliac. J Can Assoc Radiol 1985;36:161–2.

176. Lieber RL, Friden J. Morphologic and mechanical basis of delayed-onset muscle soreness. J Am Acad Orthop Surg 2002;10:67–73.

177. Takarada Y. Evaluation of muscle damage after a rugby match with special reference to tackle plays. Br J Sports Med 2003;37:416–9.

178. Yu JG, Carlsson L, Thornell LE. Evidence for myofibril remodeling as opposed to myofibril damage in human muscles with DOMS: an ultrastructural and immunoelectron microscopic study. Histochem Cell Biol 2004;121:219–27.

179. Nurenberg P, Giddings CJ, Stray-Gundersen J, et al. MR imaging-guided muscle biopsy for correlation of increased signal intensity with ultrastructural change and delayed-onset muscle soreness after exercise. Radiology 1992;184:865–9.

180. Shellock FG, Fukunaga T, Mink JH, et al. Exertional muscle injury: evaluation of concentric versus eccentric actions with serial MR imaging. Radiology 1991;179:659–64.

181. Chance JR, Kragh JF Jr, Agrawal CM, et al. Pullout forces of sutures in muscle lacerations. Orthopedics 2005;28:1187–90.

182. Negishi S, Li Y, Usas A, et al. The effect of relaxin treatment on skeletal muscle injuries. Am J Sports Med 2005; 33:1816–24.

183. Li Y, Huard J. Differentiation of muscle-derived cells into myofibroblasts in injured skeletal muscle. Am J Pathol 2002;161:895–907.

184. Walter GA, Cahill KS, Huard J, et al. Noninvasive monitoring of stem cell transfer for muscle disorders. Magn Reson Med 2004;51:273–7.

185. Mellado JM, Perez del Palomar L. Muscle hernias of the lower leg: MRI findings. Skeletal Radiol 1999;28:465–9.

186. Bianchi S, Abdelwahab IF, Mazzola CG, et al. Sonographic examination of muscle herniation. J Ultrasound Med 1995;14:357–60.

187. Alhadeff J, Lee CK. Gastrocnemius muscle herniation at the knee causing peroneal nerve compression resembling sciatica. Spine 1995;20:612–4.

188. Zeiss J, Ebraheim NA, Woldenberg LS. Magnetic resonance imaging in the diagnosis of anterior tibialis muscle herniation. Clin Orthop 1989;244:249–53.

189. Beggs I. Sonography of muscle hernias. AJR Am J Roentgenol 2003;180:395–9.

190. Elliott KG, Johnstone AJ. Diagnosing acute compartment syndrome. J Bone Joint Surg Br 2003;85:625–32.

191. Olson SA, Glasgow RR. Acute compartment syndrome in lower extremity musculoskeletal trauma. J Am Acad Orthop Surg 2005;13:436–44.

192. Mohler LR, Styf JR, Pedowitz RA, et al. Intramuscular deoxygenation during exercise in patients who have chronic anterior compartment syndrome of the leg. J Bone Joint Surg Am 1997;79:844–9.

193. Fraipont MJ, Adamson GJ. Chronic exertional compartment syndrome. J Am Acad Orthop Surg 2003;11:268–76.

194. van den Brand JG, Nelson T, Verleisdonk EJ, et al. The diagnostic value of intracompartmental pressure measurement, magnetic resonance imaging, and near-infrared spectroscopy in chronic exertional compartment syndrome: a prospective study in 50 patients. Am J Sports Med 2005;33:699–704.

195. Eskelin MK, Lotjonen JM, Mantysaari MJ. Chronic exertional compartment syndrome: MR imaging at 0.1 T compared with tissue pressure measurement. Radiology 1998;206:333–7.

196. Kumar PR, Jenkins JP, Hodgson SP. Bilateral chronic exertional compartment syndrome of the dorsal part of the forearm: the role of magnetic resonance imaging in diagnosis: a case report. J Bone Joint Surg Am 2003;85–A:1557–9.

197. Rominger MB, Lukosch CJ, Bachmann GF. MR imaging of compartment syndrome of the lower leg: a case control study. Eur Radiol 2004;14:1432–9.

198. Verleisdonk EJ, van Gils A, van der Werken C. The diagnostic value of MRI scans for the diagnosis of chronic exertional compartment syndrome of the lower leg. Skeletal Radiol 2001;30:321–5.

199. Omar HA, Helms, CA, Bytomski J, et al. The role of MRI in the diagnosis of chronic exertional compartment syndrome. AJR 2006;186(suppl):A125(abst).

200. Kiuru MJ, Mantysaari MJ, Pihlajamaki HK, et al. Evaluation of stress-related anterior lower leg pain with magnetic resonance imaging and intracompartmental pressure measurement. Mil Med 2003;168:48–52.

201. Melli G, Chaudhry V, Cornblath DR. Rhabdomyolysis: an evaluation of 475 hospitalized patients. Medicine (Baltimore) 2005;84:377–85.

202. Krivickas LS. Recurrent rhabdomyolysis in a collegiate athlete: a case report. Med Sci Sports Exerc 2006;38:407–10.

203. Sheth NP, Sennett B, Berns JS. Rhabdomyolysis and acute renal failure following arthroscopic knee surgery in a college football player taking creatine supplements. Clin Nephrol 2006;65:134–7.

204. Clarkson PM. Case report of exertional rhabdomyolysis in a 12-year-old boy. Med Sci Sports Exerc 2006;38:197–200.

205. Moghtader J, Brady WJ Jr, Bonadio W. Exertional rhabdomyolysis in an adolescent athlete. Pediatr Emerg Care 1997;13:382–5.

206. Goubier JN, Hoffman OS, Oberlin C. Exertion induced rhabdomyolysis of the long head of the triceps. Br J Sports Med 2002;36:150–1.

207. Lamminen AE, Hekali PE, Tiula E, et al. Acute rhabdomyolysis: evaluation with magnetic resonance imaging compared with computed tomography and ultrasonography. Br J Radiol 1989;62:326–30.

208. Shintani S, Shiigai T. Repeat MRI in acute rhabdomyolysis: correlation with clinicopathological findings. J Comput Assist Tomogr 1993;17:786–91.

209. Elsayes KM, Shariff A, Staveteig PT, et al. Value of magnetic resonance imaging for muscle denervation syndromes of the shoulder girdle. J Comput Assist Tomogr 2005;29:326–9.

210. Moore KR, Tsuruda JS, Dailey AT. The value of MR neurography for evaluating extraspinal neuropathic leg pain: a pictorial essay. AJNR Am J Neuroradiol 2001;22:786–94.

211. Bendszus M, Wessig C, Reiners K, et al. MR imaging in the differential diagnosis of neurogenic foot drop. AJNR Am J Neuroradiol 2003;24:1283–9.

212. Filler AG, Maravilla KR, Tsuruda JS. MR neurography and muscle MR imaging for image diagnosis of disorders affecting the peripheral nerves and musculature. Neurol Clin 2004;22:643–82.

213. Filler AG, Haynes J, Jordan SE, et al. Sciatica of nondisc origin and piriformis syndrome: diagnosis by magnetic resonance neurography and interventional magnetic resonance imaging with outcome study of resulting treatment. J Neurosurg Spine 2005;2:99–115.

214. Fritz RC, Boutin RD. Magnetic resonance imaging of the peripheral nervous system. Phys Med Rehabil Clin North Am 2001;12:399–432.

215. Kikuchi Y, Nakamura T, Takayama S, et al. MR imaging in the diagnosis of denervated and reinnervated skeletal muscles: experimental study in rats. Radiology 2003;229:861–7.

216. Wessig C, Koltzenburg M, Reiners K, et al. Muscle magnetic resonance imaging of denervation and reinnervation: correlation with electrophysiology and histology. Exp Neurol 2004;185:254–61.

217. Raphael DT, McIntee D, Tsuruda JS, et al. Frontal slab composite magnetic resonance neurography of the brachial plexus: implications for infraclavicular block approaches. Anesthesiology 2005;103:1218–24.

218. Aagaard BD, Lazar DA, Lankerovich L, et al. High-resolution magnetic resonance imaging is a noninvasive method of observing injury and recovery in the peripheral nervous system. Neurosurgery 2003;53:199–203.

219. Bendszus M, Wessig C, Solymosi L, et al. MRI of peripheral nerve degeneration and regeneration: correlation with electrophysiology and histology. Exp Neurol 2004;188:171–7.

220. De Beuckeleer L, Vanhoenacker F, De Schepper A Jr, et al. Hypertrophy and pseudohypertrophy of the lower leg following chronic radiculopathy and neuropathy: imaging findings in two patients. Skeletal Radiol 1999;28:229–32.

221. Ilaslan H, Wenger DE, Shives TC, et al. Unilateral hypertrophy of tensor fascia lata: a soft tissue tumor simulator. Skeletal Radiol 2003;32:628–32.

222. de Visser M, Verbeeten B Jr, Lyppens KC. Pseudohypertrophy of the calf following S1 radiculopathy. Neuroradiology 1986;28:279–80.

223. Drozdowski W, Dzieciol J. Neurogenic muscle hypertrophy in radiculopathy. Acta Neurol Scand 1994;89:464–8.

224. Petersilge CA, Pathria MN, Gentili A, et al. Denervation hypertrophy of muscle: MR features. J Comput Assist Tomogr 1995;19:596–600.

225. May DA, Disler DG, Jones EA, et al. Abnormal signal intensity in skeletal muscle at MR imaging: patterns, pearls, and pitfalls. Radiographics 2000;20:S295–315.

226. Khalid M, Brannigan A, Burke T. Calf muscle wasting after tibial shaft fracture. Br J Sports Med 2006;40:552–3.

227. Gerber C, Meyer DC, Schneeberger AG, et al. Effect of tendon release and delayed repair on the structure of the muscles of the rotator cuff: an experimental study in sheep. J Bone Joint Surg Am 2004;86–A:1973–82.

228. Meyer DC, Pirkl C, Pfirrmann CW, et al. Asymmetric atrophy of the supraspinatus muscle following tendon tear. J Orthop Res 2005;23:254–8.

229. Safran O, Derwin KA, Powell K, et al. Changes in rotator cuff muscle volume, fat content, and passive mechanics after chronic detachment in a canine model. J Bone Joint Surg Am 2005;87:2662–70.

230. Noonan TJ, Best TM, Seaber AV, Garrett WE Jr. Thermal effects on skeletal muscle tensile behavior. Am J Sports Med 1993;21:517–22.

231. Garrett WE Jr. Muscle strain injuries: clinical and basic aspects. Med Sci Sports Exerc 1990;22:436–43.

232. Steinbach LS, Fleckenstein JL, Mink JH. Magnetic resonance imaging of muscle injuries. Orthopedics 1994;17:991–9.

233. Arrington ED, Miller MD. Skeletal muscle injuries. Orthop Clin North Am 1995;26:411–22.

234. De Marchi A, Robba T, Ferrarese E, Faletti C. Imaging in musculoskeletal injuries: state of the art. Radiol Med (Torino) 2005;110:115–31.

235. Boutin RD, Fritz RC, Steinbach LS. Imaging of sports-related muscle injuries. Radiol Clin North Am 2002;40:333–62,vii.

236. Bencardino JT, et al. Traumatic musculotendinous injuries of the knee: diagnosis with MR imaging. Radiographics 2000;20(Spec No):S103–20.

237. Clanton TO, Coupe KJ. Hamstring strains in athletes: diagnosis and treatment. J Am Acad Orthop Surg 1998;6:237–48.

238. Jarvinen TA, Jarvinen TL, Kaariainen M, Kalimo H, Jarvinen M. Muscle injuries: biology and treatment. Am J Sports Med 2005;33:745–64.

239. Nguyen B, Brandser E, Rubin DA. Pains, strains, and fasciculations: lower extremity muscle disorders. Magn Reson Imaging Clin North Am 2000;8:391–408.

240. Taylor DC, Dalton JD Jr, Seaber AV, Garrett WE Jr. Experimental muscle strain injury. Early functional and structural deficits and the increased risk for reinjury. Am J Sports Med 1993;21:190–4.

241. Mair SD, Seaber AV, Glisson RR, Garrett WE Jr. The role of fatigue in susceptibility to acute muscle strain injury. Am J Sports Med 1996;24:137–43.

242. Safran MR, Garrett WE Jr, Seaber AV, Glisson RR, Ribbeck BM. The role of warmup in muscular injury prevention. Am J Sports Med 1988;16:123–9.

243. Forster BB, Khan KM. A practical approach to magnetic resonance imaging of normal and injured tendons: pictorial essay. Can Assoc Radiol J 2003;54:211–20.

244. Noonan TJ, Garrett WE Jr. Muscle strain injury: diagnosis and treatment. J Am Acad Orthop Surg 1999;7:262–9.

245. Connell DA, et al. Longitudinal study comparing sonographic and MRI assessments of acute and healing hamstring injuries. AJR Am J Roentgenol 2004;183:975–84.

246. Gibbs NJ, Cross TM, Cameron M, Houang MT. The accuracy of MRI in predicting recovery and recurrence of acute grade one hamstring muscle strains within the same season in Australian Rules football players. J Sci Med Sport 2004;7:248–58.

247. Schneider-Kolsky ME, Hoving JL, Warren P, Connell D. A. A Comparison Between Clinical Assessment and Magnetic Resonance Imaging of Acute Hamstring Injuries. Am J Sports Med 2006;34:1008–15.

248. Orchard J, Best TM, Verrall GM. Return to play following muscle strains. Clin J Sport Med 2005;15:436–41.

249. O'Donoghue D. Injuries of the leg. In: Treatment of Injuries to Athletes. Philadelphia: WB Saunders, 1984 pp. 586–600.

250. Järvinen MJ, Lehto MU. The effects of early mobilisation and immobilisation on the healing process following muscle injuries. Sports Med 1993;15:78–89.

251. Bleakley C, McDonough S, MacAuley D. The use of ice in the treatment of acute soft-tissue injury: a systematic review of randomized controlled trials. Am J Sports Med 2004;32:251–61.

252. Thorsson O, Lilja B, Nilsson P, Westlin N. Immediate external compression in the management of an acute muscle injury. Scand J Med Sci Sports 1997;7:182–90.

253. Mishra DK, Friden J, Schmitz MC, Lieber RL. Anti-inflammatory medication after muscle injury. A treatment resulting in short-term improvement but subsequent loss of muscle function. J Bone Joint Surg Am 1995;77:1510–9.

254. Obremsky WT, Seaber AV, Ribbeck BM, Garrett WE Jr. Biomechanical and histologic assessment of a controlled muscle strain injury treated with piroxicam. Am J Sports Med 1994;22:558–61.

255. Thorsson O, Rantanen J, Hurme T, Kalimo H. Effects of nonsteroidal antiinflammatory medication on satellite cell proliferation during muscle regeneration. Am J Sports Med 1998;26:172–6.

256. Reynolds JF, Noakes TD, Schwellnus MP, Windt A, Bowerbank P. Non-steroidal anti-inflammatory drugs fail to enhance healing of acute hamstring injuries treated with physiotherapy. S Afr Med J 1995;85:517–22.

257. Rantanen J, Thorsson O, Wollmer P, Hurme T, Kalimo H. Effects of therapeutic ultrasound on the regeneration of skeletal myofibers after experimental muscle injury. Am J Sports Med 1999;27:54–9.

258. Best TM, Loitz-Ramage B, Corr DT, Vanderby R. Hyperbaric oxygen in the treatment of acute muscle stretch injuries. Results in an animal model. Am J Sports Med 1998;26:367–72.

259. Almekinders LC. Results of surgical repair versus splinting of experimentally transected muscle. J Orthop Trauma 1991;5:173–6.

260. Mitchell B. Efficacy of thigh protectors in preventing thigh haematomas. J Sci Med Sport 2000;3:30–4.

261. Jackson DW, Feagin JA. Quadriceps contusions in young athletes. Relation of severity of injury to treatment and prognosis. J Bone Joint Surg Am 1973;55:95–105.

262. Ryan JB, Wheeler JH, Hopkinson WJ, Arciero RA, Kolakowski KR. Quadriceps contusions. West Point update. Am J Sports Med 1991;19:299–304.

263. Jarvinen M, Lehto M, Sorvari T, et al. Effect of some anti-inflammatory agents on the healing of ruptured muscle: an experimental study in rats. J Sports Traumatol Rel Res 1992;14:19–28.

264. Beiner JM, Jokl P, Cholewicki J, Panjabi MM. The effect of anabolic steroids and corticosteroids on healing of muscle contusion injury. Am J Sports Med 1999;27:2–9.

265. Bonsell S, Freudigman PT, Moore HA. Quadriceps muscle contusion resulting in osteomyelitis of the femur in a high school football player. A case report. Am J Sports Med 2001;29:818–20.

266. Knochel JP. Exertional rhabdomyolysis. N Engl J Med 1972;287:927–9.

267. Walsworth M, Kessler T. Diagnosing exertional rhabdomyolysis: a brief review and report of two cases. Mil Med 2001;166:275–7.

268. Hamer R. When exercise goes awry: exertional rhabdomyolysis. South Med J 1997;90:548–51.

269. Lamminen AE, Hekali PE, Tiula E, Suramo I, Korhola O. A. Acute rhabdomyolysis: evaluation with magnetic resonance imaging compared with computed tomography and ultrasonography. Br J Radiol 1989;62:326–30.

270. Stock KW, Helwig A. MRI of acute exertional rhabdomyolysis—in the paraspinal compartment. J Comput Assist Tomogr 1996;20:834–6.

271. Nakahara K, et al. The value of computed tomography and magnetic resonance imaging to diagnose rhabdomyolysis in acute renal failure. Nephrol Dial Transplant 1999;14:1564–7.

272. Better OS, Rubinstein I, Winaver JM, Knochel JP. Mannitol therapy revisited (1940–1997). Kidney Int 1997;52: 886–94.

273. Homsi E, Barreiro MF, Orlando JM, Higa EM. Prophylaxis of acute renal failure in patients with rhabdomyolysis. Ren Fail 1997;19:283–8.

274. Sauret JM, Marinides G, Wang GK. Rhabdomyolysis. Am Fam Physician 2002;65:907–12.

275. McHale KA, Geissele A, Perlik PD. Compartment syndrome of the biceps brachii compartment following rupture of the long head of the biceps. Orthopedics 1991;14:787–8.

276. Mubarak SJ, Pedowitz RA, Hargens AR. Compartment syndromes. Curr Orthop 1989;3:36–40.

277. Robinson D, On E, Halperin N. Anterior compartment syndrome of the thigh in athletes—indications for conservative treatment. J Trauma 1992;32:183–6.

278. Cheung K, Hume P, Maxwell L. Delayed onset muscle soreness: treatment strategies and performance factors. Sports Med 2003;33:145–64.

279. Clarkson PM, Hubal MJ. Exercise-induced muscle damage in humans. Am J Phys Med Rehabil 2002;81:S52–69.

280. Shellock F, Fleckenstein J. Magnetic Resonance of muscle injuries. 2nd Ed. Philadelphia: Lippincott-Raven, 1997:1341–62.

281. Cannavino CR, Abrams J, Palinkas LA, Saglimbeni A, Bracker MD. Efficacy of transdermal ketoprofen for delayed onset muscle soreness. Clin J Sport Med 2003;13:200–8.

282. Nurenberg P, et al. MR imaging-guided muscle biopsy for correlation of increased signal intensity with ultrastructural change and delayed-onset muscle soreness after exercise. Radiology 1992;184:865–9.

283. Best TM. Muscle injury in athletes. In: Preedy V, Peters T, eds. Skeletal Muscle: Pathology, Diagnosis and Management of Disease. London: Greenwich Medical Media, 2002:49–60.

284. Paddon-Jones DJ, Quigley BM. Effect of cryotherapy on muscle soreness and strength following eccentric exercise. Int J Sports Med 1997;18:588–93.

285. Kraemer WJ, et al. Influence of compression therapy on symptoms following soft tissue injury from maximal eccentric exercise. J Orthop Sports Phys Ther 2001;31:282–90.

286. Chleboun GS, et al. Intermittent pneumatic compression effect on eccentric exercise-induced swelling, stiffness, and strength loss. Arch Phys Med Rehabil 1995;76:744–9.

287. Dudley GA, et al. Efficacy of naproxen sodium for exercise-induced dysfunction muscle injury and soreness. Clin J Sport Med 1997;7:3–10.

288. Lecomte JM, Lacroix VJ, Montgomery DL. A randomized controlled trial of the effect of naproxen on delayed onset muscle soreness and muscle strength. Clin J Sport Med 1998;8:82–87.

289. Tokmakidis SP, Kokkinidis EA, Smilios I, Douda H. The effects of ibuprofen on delayed muscle soreness and muscular performance after eccentric exercise. J Strength Cond Res 2003;17:53–59.

290. Bourgeois J, MacDougall D, MacDonald J, Tarnopolsky M. Naproxen does not alter indices of muscle damage in resistance-exercise trained men. Med Sci Sports Exerc 1999;31:4–9.

291. O'Grady M, et al. Diclofenac sodium (Voltaren) reduced exercise-induced injury in human skeletal muscle. Med Sci Sports Exerc 2000;32:1191–1196.

292. Denegar R, Huff C. High and low frequency TENS in the treatment of induced musculoskeletal pain: a comparison study. J Athl Train 1988;23:235–237.

293. Craig JA, Cunningham MB, Walsh DM, Baxter GD, Allen JM. Lack of effect of transcutaneous electrical nerve stimulation upon experimentally induced delayed onset muscle soreness in humans. Pain 1996;67:285–289.

294. Hilbert JE, Sforzo GA, Swensen T. The effects of massage on delayed onset muscle soreness. Br J Sports Med 2003;37:72–75.

295. Bennett M, Best TM, Babul S, Taunton J, Lepawsky M. Hyperbaric oxygen therapy for delayed onset muscle soreness and closed soft tissue injury. Cochrane Database Syst Rev 2005, Article number CD004713.

296. Jayaraman RC, et al. MRI evaluation of topical heat and static stretching as therapeutic modalities for the treatment of eccentric exercise-induced muscle damage. Eur J Appl Physiol 2004;93:30–38.

297. Byrnes WC, et al. Delayed onset muscle soreness following repeated bouts of downhill running. J Appl Physiol 1985;59:710–715.

298. Amendola A, et al. The use of magnetic resonance imaging in exertional compartment syndromes. Am J Sports Med 1990;18:29–34.

299. Shah SN, Miller BS, Kuhn JE. Chronic exertional compartment syndrome. Am J Orthop 2004;33:335–341.

300. Trease L, et al. A prospective blinded evaluation of exercise thallium-201 SPET in patients with suspected chronic exertional compartment syndrome of the leg. Eur J Nucl Med 2001;28:688–695.

301. Pedowitz RA, Hargens AR, Mubarak SJ, Gershuni DH. Modified criteria for the objective diagnosis of chronic compartment syndrome of the leg. Am J Sports Med 1990;18:35–40.

302. van den Brand JG, Nelson T, Verleisdonk EJ, van der Werken C. The diagnostic value of intracompartmental pressure measurement, magnetic resonance imaging, and near-infrared spectroscopy in chronic exertional compartment syndrome: a prospective study in 50 patients. Am J Sports Med 2005;33:699–704.

303. Detmer DE, Sharpe K, Sufit RL, Girdley FM. Chronic compartment syndrome: diagnosis, management, and outcomes. Am J Sports Med 1985;13:162–170.

304. Verleisdonk EJ, Schmitz RF, van der Werken C. Long-term results of fasciotomy of the anterior compartment in patients with exercise-induced pain in the lower leg. Int J Sports Med 2004;25:224–229.

305. Kneeland JP. MR imaging of muscle and tendon injury. Eur J Radiol 1997;25:198–208.

306. Maffulli N, Wong J, Almekinders LC. Types and epidemiology of tendinopathy. Clin Sports Med 2003;22:675–692.

307. Khan KM, et al. Patellar tendinosis (jumper's knee): findings at histopathologic examination, US, and MR imaging. Victorian Institute of Sport Tendon Study Group. Radiology 1996;200:821–827.

308. Davies SG, Baudouin CJ, King JB, Perry JD. Ultrasound, computed tomography and magnetic resonance imaging in patellar tendinitis. Clin Radiol 1991;43:52–56.

309. Yu JS, Popp JE, Kaeding CC, Lucas J. Correlation of MR imaging and pathologic findings in athletes undergoing surgery for chronic patellar tendinitis. AJR Am J Roentgenol 1995;165:115–118.

310. Potter HG, et al. Lateral epicondylitis: correlation of MR imaging, surgical, and histopathologic findings. Radiology 1995;196:43–46.

311. Green S, et al. Non-steroidal anti-inflammatory drugs (NSAIDs) for treating lateral elbow pain in adults. Cochrane Database Syst Rev 2002;2:CD003686.

312. Buchbinder R, Green S, Youd JM. Corticosteroid injections for shoulder pain. Cochrane Database Syst Rev 2003;1:CD004016.

313. Smidt N, et al. Corticosteroid injections for lateral epicondylitis: a systematic review. Pain 2002;96:23–40.

314. Brosseau L, et al. Deep transverse friction massage for treating tendinitis. Cochrane Database Syst Rev 2002;4:CD003528.

315. Struijs PA, et al. Orthotic devices for tennis elbow. Cochrane Database Syst Rev 2001;2:CD001821.

316. Green S, et al. Acupuncture for lateral elbow pain. Cochrane Database Syst Rev 2001;1:CD003527.

317. Buchbinder R, et al. Shock wave therapy for lateral elbow pain. Cochrane Database Syst Rev 2005;4:CD003524.

318. Buchbinder R, et al. Surgery for lateral elbow pain. Cochrane Database Syst Rev 2002;1:CD003525.

319. Beiner JM, Jokl P. Muscle contusion injury and myositis ossificans traumatica. Clin Orthop Relat Res 2002;403(suppl):S110–119.

320. Shehab D, Elgazzar AH, Collier BD. Heterotopic ossification. J Nucl Med 2002;43:346–353.

321. Noonan TJ, Garrett WE Jr. Muscle injury of the posterior leg. Foot Ankle Clin 1997;2:457–471.

2
Cartilage

A. Radiologic Perspective: Magnetic Resonance Imaging of Articular Cartilage—Conventional and Novel Imaging Techniques

Hamid Torshizy, Garry E. Gold, and Christine B. Chung

Traditionally, articular or hyaline cartilage has been described as a glistening layer of connective tissue that covers the articular surface of bones, acting mainly as a "shock absorber" for the lower extremity. This perception underscores the structural intricacy and functional importance of this tissue. Articular cartilage is a complex and dynamic tissue with unique properties and matrix constituents that are essential for normal joint function. Injuries and degenerative changes of articular cartilage result in significant morbidity and a diminished quality of life.[1] Advances in basic science research, novel therapeutic interventions, and imaging techniques have reaffirmed the pivotal importance of articular cartilage, and has changed the way we think about it and the various entities affecting it.

A vast spectrum of different pathophysiologic processes, including trauma, inflammatory arthritis, and primary osteoarthritis, are responsible for the irreversible loss of hyaline cartilage. However, the most common cause is osteoarthritis (OA), either of a degenerative primary etiology or secondary to trauma.[2]

Osteoarthritis

Osteoarthritis is an irreversible and chronic degenerative disorder of the joints characterized by gradual loss of hyaline cartilage and accompanying joint pain and dysfunction. It afflicts more than 20 million people in the United States, 10% of whom are adults over the age of 50.[3] It has been reported that nearly 2.0% of women and 1.4% of men per year develop radiographic signs of OA, though generally half of these cases lead to symptomatic disease.[4] In addition to being a leading cause of disability and dysfunction among the elderly, it is second only to heart disease as the leading cause of work disability.[5,6] This major public health issue is sure to increase further in our aging society.

The direct traditional medical costs and indirect economic and wage loss from arthritis in the United States are astounding, reaching in excess of $65 billion annually.[5] In fact, the total cost for arthritis, including OA, has been estimated to be over 2% of the United States gross domestic product.[7,8] While staggering amounts of money and resources are directed toward OA health care and research annually, the exact etiology of this important disease entity remains elusive. Osteoarthritis has long been considered the result of age or trauma. It is now thought that the etiology of OA is multifaceted, with mechanical, biomechanical, genetic, and various enzymatic factors implicated.

Assessment of cartilage injuries and osteoarthritis generally includes clinical, radiographic, and arthroscopic evaluation. Given that symptoms often do not parallel articular cartilage damage, clinical assessment can offer limited information about the integrity of articular cartilage.[8] In addition, radiographs mostly provide indirect and often inaccurate information regarding the integrity of articular cartilage, as evaluation of cartilaginous abnormalities is based on the severity of joint space narrowing.[9,10]

Arthroscopy is, and continues to be, the gold standard for diagnosing and monitoring the evaluation of cartilage damage and repair, as it allows direct visualization of the surface of cartilage. While arthroscopy is valued for the detection of gross morphologic defects such as surface irregularities and partial- and full-thickness defects, it does have deficiencies in the global evaluation of cartilage, specifically with regard to identification and characterization of less severe lesions. In this context, a complementary means of assessment is required which would (1) permit visualization of internal or mid-substance cartilage abnormalities,[11,12] (2) allow assessment of cartilage thickness, (3) provide an easily quantifiable or reproducible measure of overall severity of cartilage loss often needed for therapeutic interventions,[13] and (4) prove noninvasive and cost-effective. These qualities are afforded by imaging.[1,14,15]

Several imaging modalities exist for the evaluation of cartilage. Until recently, the limited capabilities of these various techniques in directly assessing the integrity of articular cartilage have limited the use of imaging in the assessment, diagnosis, and workup of articular cartilage pathology. However, magnetic resonance imaging (MRI) has emerged as the method of choice for the detection of cartilage abnormalities, such as OA, and for cartilage repair procedures.[16–25] To better understand the magnetic resonance (MR) appearance of articular cartilage, a discussion of its structure is necessary.

This chapter discusses the structure of articular cartilage, conventional MRI sequences and advances in MRI techniques used for the evaluation of both normal and abnormal articular cartilage, and imaging of surgical repair mechanisms of articular cartilage.

Structure and Function

Hyaline cartilage is an avascular, alymphatic, and aneural tissue with an extremely poor regenerative capacity. In general, it varies in thickness across different articulating surfaces, ranging from 1 to 7 mm in thickness with an average thickness of 2 to 3 mm.[26] The main function of cartilage is biomechanical in nature, and includes transmission and distribution of high loads with the ability to undergo reverse deformation, maintenance of contact stresses at acceptably low levels, promotion of a low-friction environment for movement at joints, and shock absorption.[27] Such versatility is a reflection of the complex and intricate organization of hyaline cartilage on a molecular level.

Articular cartilage is predominately composed of an extracellular matrix, which is composed primarily of type II collagen, water, large aggregating proteoglycans, and a relatively small number of chondrocytes.[28–31] In addition, other proteins, lipids, phospholipids, and various other collagens account for a minor component of its composition[28] (Table 2.1). Of note, the distribution of these components has been shown to vary not only across different joints, but also geographically within articular cartilage itself. They have also been shown to vary as a function of age.[32]

Chondrocytes are the major cellular component of hyaline cartilage, accounting for about 5% of the wet weight of hyaline cartilage.[28] Lacking direct cell-to-cell contact, each chondrocyte is separated from one another and from vascular and nervous systems, and thus must rely on diffusion of synovial fluids for nutrients.[31] During activities of loading and unloading, fluid is pumped into and out of cartilage, facilitating such diffusion.[26] Importantly, chondrocytes function to remodel the extracellular matrix through various catabolic and anabolic events. As a result, they are responsible for maintaining the structural and functional integrity of articular cartilage, as well as preserving its resilience.[33] Chondrocytes have limited

ability to replicate and regenerate, an important consideration for patients afflicted with cartilage loss.[15]

The extracellular matrix (ECM) of hyaline cartilage is a highly ordered structure composed predominately of water, collagen, and proteoglycans. Water is the most abundant component of the ECM, making up approximately 60% to 80% of the total weight.[34,35] The majority of water is held in place within the interstitial intrafibrillar space, located between the collagen-proteoglycan solid matrix, and is reversibly bound by negative charges on proteoglycans.[28] Water content is associated with various forces (discussed later) that are generated by negative charges and hydroxyl groups on the proteoglycans.[36] Water plays a pivotal role in the biomechanical properties of articular cartilage, providing hydraulic pressure that protects the structural integrity of cartilage under high loads and forces. In addition, it provides the ECM with its viscoelastic properties, ability to dissipate loads, and its reversible deformability properties.[28]

Proteoglycans are the third largest component of the ECM, constituting approximately 30% of the dry weight of the ECM.[35,37] They consist of a central core protein substituted with many hydroxyl groups and fixed, negatively charged carboxyl and sulfate groups attached to glycosaminoglycan (GAG) side chains. Further, proteoglycans are noncovalently bound to hyaluronic acid via link proteins, forming larger proteoglycan aggregates. Such tight packing and folding renders them relatively immobile within the collagen fibril meshwork, while at the same time producing electrostatic repulsion.[15,32] Collectively, these factors act to attract cations (mostly sodium) and result in net osmotic, ionic, and Donnan forces that attract water, generating a "swelling pressure" that allows cartilage to resist compression.[26,29]

Collagen is the second largest component of the ECM, constituting approximately 60% of the dry weight.[31,34] The majority of collagen in articular cartilage is type II, lining the surface of cartilage and creating a relatively impermeable membrane.[38] Different types of collagen serve to cross-link collagen fibrils, connect the collagen meshwork with proteoglycan aggregates, and facilitate communication between the ECM and chondrocytes.[38,39] This key interaction between collagen fibrils and proteoglycan aggregates creates a fiber-reinforced composite solid matrix that strengthens the structural framework of articular cartilage, while also providing tensional stability.[28,38] Collectively, the collagen meshwork acts to resist the "swelling pressure" mentioned earlier. Importantly, cartilage is not a uniform tissue. Across its thickness, from surface to subchondral bone, variations exist in its composition, organization, and mechanical properties.[29]

Classically, articular cartilage is structurally and functionally subdivided into four different histologic zones: (1) superficial or tangential zone; (2) middle or transitional zone; (3) deep or radial zone; and (4) the deepest zone, a zone of calcified cartilage (Fig. 2.1).

Apart from the depth at which they occur, variations in the orientation of the type II collagen fibrils have also been

TABLE 2.1. Components of cartilage.

Water
Chondrocytes
Collagen (primarily type II)
Hyaluronic acid
Glycosaminoglycans and aggrecans
Small proteoglycans

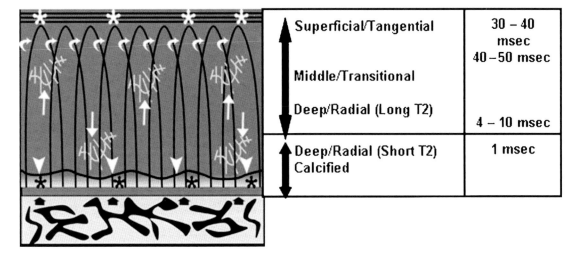

	Superficial/Tangential	30 – 40 msec
		40 – 50 msec
	Middle/Transitional	
	Deep/Radial (Long T2)	
		4 – 10 msec
	Deep/Radial (Short T2) Calcified	1 msec

FIG. 2.1. Diagram of the structure of articular cartilage. Arcades of collagen fibers (curved arrows) cross each other and are anchored in the subchondral bone (short black arrows) forming the extracellular matrix of cartilage. Large negatively charged macromolecules (glycosaminoglycans) (long white arrows) reside within the matrix. The four basic zones of cartilage include the superficial or tangential zone (white asterisks), the middle or transitional zone, the deep or radial zone, and the calcified layer of cartilage (black asterisks). The junction between the deep zone and that of calcified cartilage is denoted by the tidemark (white arrowheads). As noted, there is a zonal variation in T2 values with an order of magnitude of difference between the more superficial layers and the deeper radial and calcified layers.

used to categorize these zones. Of note, the various patterns of collagen fibrils in each zone are well suited to parallel the functional requirements of cartilage. For the purpose of this discussion these zones are discussed as separate entities; realistically, however, it is useful to think about these zones as gradual, continuous changes rather than discrete demarcated regions. In the following discussion, each zone is discussed separately in detail.

The superficial or tangential zone is the articulating surface (Fig. 2.1). It comprises approximately 10% to 20% of the articular cartilage thickness.[28] And while it has the highest collagen content, the collagen fibrils and chondrocytes are aligned parallel to the articular surface in a more highly ordered and dense fashion compared to deeper levels.[40] Chondrocytes in this layer are elongated or ellipsoid in appearance and express proteins, such as superficial zone protein (SZP), which lubricate the surface and provide a smooth gliding surface at the joint articulation as well as resist shear stresses.[28,32,41] While the proteoglycan concentration is relatively low, the water concentration is high, resulting in a thin layer of great tensile stiffness and strength, which further limits tissue permeability.[42,43] In fact, this zone has the lowest compressive modulus and deforms nearly 25 times more than the middle zone.[28]

Immediately beneath the superficial zone lies the middle or transitional zone (Fig. 2.1). This zone is so named because it represents a transition in morphology between the surface and deep zones. It comprises approximately 40% to 60% of the cartilage thickness.[28,44] The collagen fibrils are thicker, more loosely packed, and are aligned in an oblique fashion to the surface. It is this oblique orientation that is felt to be responsible for resistance to shearing forces.[29] At this level, the chon-

drocytes are rounder. This zone also has a higher compressive modulus than the superficial zone.[28]

Immediately under the middle zone lies the deep or radial zone, beneath which is the deepest zone or zone of calcified cartilage (Fig. 2.1). Together, these two zones comprise nearly 50% of the cartilage thickness.[44] The deep or radial zone is an uncalcified layer with collagen fibrils that are the thickest of any level and that are oriented perpendicular to the surface.[1] Its chondrocytes are arranged in a columnar-like fashion paralleling collagen fibers. Furthermore, this zone contains the lowest water and highest proteoglycan concentration, translating into the highest compressive modulus of any zone. Immediately beneath this zone is the deepest zone, a thin zone of calcified cartilage that contains a relatively small number of chondrocytes and collagen fibrils that function to attach cartilage to the underlying bone (Fig. 2.1).[45] The uncalcified radial zone is separated from the deeper zone of calcified cartilage by a tidemark, a basophilic line that represents where calcification ceases and where nonspecific tidemark molecule accumulate.[40,45–48]

It is not surprising that processes that lead to structural damage of cartilage have altered biomechanical properties. Recent advances in medical, pharmacologic, and surgical management of chondral abnormalities has necessitated, and resulted in, accompanying advances in noninvasive imaging methods for evaluating and monitoring such changes.

Magnetic Resonance Imaging

Magnetic resonance imaging has emerged as the modality of choice in evaluating chondral abnormalities. Given its superior soft tissue contrast and multiplanar capabilities, it has revolutionized the evaluation of articular cartilage abnormalities, while at the same time addressing several of the limitations of arthroscopy. Magnetic resonance imaging (1) provides in vivo morphologic information regarding thickness, volume, and three-dimensional configuration of cartilage; (2) provides in vivo biochemical information regarding collagen and extracellular matrix composition of hyaline cartilage, including the free water, proteoglycan, and sodium content; (3) is highly accurate in measuring cartilage volume, providing a quantitative and global marker for the progression of cartilage loss; (4) is non-invasive in nature, allowing for serial assessment of articular cartilage abnormalities without risk of injury and for follow-up of abnormalities in order to determine the natural history of the response to therapy; and (5) is cost-effective.[11,38,49,50]

The sheer complexity of the structure of articular cartilage necessitates the use of different techniques for its global evaluation. Optimal imaging characterization of articular cartilage necessitates the acquisition of images with high spatial resolution and signal-to-noise ratio (SNR). Furthermore, careful attention to MR acquisition parameters is necessary to ensure optimal contrast differentiating articular cartilage, joint fluid, and surrounding tissue structures. Limitations of MRI lie in the detection of early degenerative changes in the cartilage, changes that herald the presence of structural alteration at the macromolecular level.[51] While the emphasis to date has been on morphologic evaluation of articular cartilagen novel MR sequences will offer biochemical evaluation of cartilage components including techniques that reflect collagen and proteoglycan content. It is detection of abnormality at this level that will ultimately further the understanding of the etiology and progression of cartilage lesions, and begin an era of prevention of osteoarthritis, rather than palliation. The ensuing discussion focuses on the commonly used, existing MRI techniques, as well as advances in MRI in the evaluation of both normal articular detection and of lesion detection.

Conventional Magnetic Resonance Imaging Techniques

Conventional MRI has proven both sensitive and specific in the detection of chondral abnormalities, especially of high-grade lesions.[1,32,52–57] The MR classification system for grading chondral abnormalities is based on commonly used arthroscopic grading systems for cartilage lesions originally proposed by Outerbridge and Noyes (Table 2.2).[58,59] The Noyes system (not shown here) categorizes chondral lesions according to their diameter, depth, and location. Lesions are classified from 0% to 100% in severity, with healthy cartilage representing 100%. On the other hand, the Outerbridge classification schema (Table 2.2) takes into account the depth and size of the most severe chondral lesions.

Current MRI characterization of cartilage injury has focused on recognition of defects with regions of cartilage loss and gross morphologic alteration. In these regions of

TABLE 2.2. Magnetic resonance (MR) and modified outerbridge classification system of chondral abnormalities.

MR classification	Modified outerbridge classification
Grade 0: Normal intact cartilage	Grade 0: Normal intact cartilage
Grade 1: Normal contour ± abnormal signal	Grade 1: Chondral softening; intact surface; no other morphologic defects
Grade 2: Superficial fraying, erosion, or ulceration of <50% of thickness	Grade 2: Superficial fibrillation, fissuring, or ulceration involving <50% of thickness
Grade 3: Partial-thickness defect of ≥50% and <100% of thickness	Grade 3: Partial-thickness defect: fibrillation, fissuring, ulceration of chondral flap involving ≥50% but <100% of thickness
Grade 4: Full-thickness cartilage loss	Grade 4: Full-thickness defect: ulceration and bone exposure

tissue loss, characterizations of morphologic alterations are helpful in identifying the chronicity of lesions. Moreover, locations of lesions can be precisely described, and can help to determine stability, as well as etiology. Much less attention has been paid to the quality of the intact underlying cartilage itself. This is undoubtedly due in part to the structural complexity of cartilage, as well as to limitations in conventional imaging techniques in depicting intrasubstance changes within these deeper zones of articular cartilage. Several novel imaging techniques, discussed later, have allowed for detection of intrasubstance changes.

A multitude of different conventional pulse sequences are used for optimal evaluation of articular cartilage and chondral abnormalities (Table 2.3). These include T1-weighted spin echo (T1W SE), T2-weighted spin echo (T2W SE), fast spin echo (FSE), proton density, and fat-suppression techniques. In addition, magnetic resonance arthrography (MRA), computed tomography arthrography (CTA), and high field strength techniques further enhance morphologic evaluation. Currently there is no consensus on the single best articular cartilage sequence. Thus far, T2W FSE, fat-suppressed T1-weighted SE, three-dimensional (3D) spoiled gradient echo (GRE), proton density, and 3D double echo steady state (3D-DESS) sequences have demonstrated excellent sensitivity for the detection of higher grade chondral lesions.

These sequences, however, provide limited information regarding the biochemical and structural changes associated with early chondral lesions (grade 1), changes that precede gross morphologic changes.[60]

Numerous variations of these MR techniques exist, from changes in imaging parameters to changes in acquisition sequences. In addition, imaging protocols vary across institutions. Often, the selection of particular sequences depends on multiple factors, including clinicians' preferences, potential strengths and weaknesses of available vendor hardware platforms, and a host of different patient factors. And while we acknowledge that various other imaging sequences exist, the ensuing discussion focuses on the above-mentioned common techniques.

TABLE 2.3. Summary of selected conventional MR imaging techniques for cartilage evaluation.

MR technique	Grade detected (Outerbridge modified)	Morphology	Advantages	Disadvantages
T1W SE	2,3,4	+	Bone–cartilage interface delineation	Cartilage-joint fluid delineation; limited out-of-plane resolution
T2W SE	2,3,4	+	"Arthrogram-like" effect; internal cartilage detail	Decreased spatial resolution; poor SNR; lack of cartilage - subchondral bone delineation; limited out-of-plane resolution
FSE	2,3,4	+	Increased SNR and spatial resolution; short imaging times; insensitivity to magnetic susceptibility artifacts; simultaneous evaluation of other soft tissue structures	Limited out-of- plane resolution; blurring
Fat suppressed T1-weighted 3D SPGR	2,3,4	+	Thin sections; contrast at cartilage surface; increased resolution; superior in plane resolution; multiplanar reformatting capability	Long acquisition time; susceptibility to metal artifact and truncation artifact
MRA	2,3,4	+	Enhanced contrast between cartilage and joint fluid; optimal visualization of the articular surface contour	Invasive; time consuming
CTA	2,3,4	+		Invasive; time-consuming; poor soft tissue contrast
T2 parameter mapping	1,2,3,4	−	Quantitative assessment; assessment of early degenerative changes	Decreased SNR; time-consuming

CTA, computed tomography arthrography; FSE, fast spin echo; MRA, magnetic resonance arthrography; SE, spin echo; SNR, signal-to-noise ratio; SPGR, spoiled gradient echo; T1W, T1-weighted.

T1- and T2-Weighted Spin Echo Images

Intrinsic T1 and T2 relaxation times, reflections of local tissue properties, can be used to evaluate cartilage. On T1-weighted images, articular cartilage is homogeneous in appearance with intermediate signal intensity near that of muscle. While the dynamic range of contrast within cartilage is limited, the strength of this sequence lies in its delineation and characterization of the interfaces of cartilage and bone (Table 2.3).[60–65] Focal defects or chondral lesions within cartilage are identified by areas of hypointensity, a loss of the sharp interface of the chondral surface, frank defects within cartilage, or any combination of these findings.[62] Limitations exist in the depiction of cartilage–joint fluid interfaces, making identification of surface chondral abnormalities difficult.[66] This is especially the case in patients presenting with joint effusions. On T1W SE images, cartilage is characterized by a homogeneous, intermediate signal intensity that is isointense with muscle. Though T1W SE images offer limited interpretation with regard to articular cartilage, they may prove useful in the evaluation of the cartilage–subchondral interface.

T2-weighted spin echo (T2W SE) sequences have long been advocated in the assessment of cartilage, with a sensitivity of 48% to 100%, a specificity of 50% to 96%, and accuracy of 52% to 81% reported in studies of the patella.[38,67–70] On T2W SE images, articular cartilage has intermediate signal intensity, which contrasts with the high signal intensity of joint fluid and the low signal intensity of osseous cortex and fatty tissue. T2-weighted SE sequences take advantage of the arthrogram-like effect produced by the high signal intensity of joint fluid and the intermediate signal intensity of articular cartilage (Table 2.3). Together, this results in disparity in contrast that facilitates the accentuation of surface irregularities, such as fibrillation and fissuring, as well as internal defects within cartilage itself, which present as focal globular or linear regions of increased signal intensity with a background of articular cartilage of intermediate to low signal intensity.[64,71–73]

The disadvantages of this sequence include decreased spatial resolution as compared to T1-weighted images, a lack of contrast between cartilage and subchondral cortical bone, insensitivity to the intrinsically short T2 relaxation time of the zones of cartilage, and poor SNR.[51] In addition, T2W SE sequences are particularly susceptible to magic angle artifacts, leading to pitfalls of cartilage imaging and distortion of the zonal appearance of cartilage.[38] The addition of fat suppression to T1- and T2-weighted imaging increases the accuracy of cartilage evaluation and eliminates chemical shift artifacts.[62,68]

Fast Spin Echo Imaging and Fat Suppressed
T1-Weighted Three-Dimensional Spoiled
Gradient-Echo Imaging

Two clinically useful sequences imaging tools for evaluating chondral abnormalities include FSE and the fat-suppressed T1-weighted 3D spoiled gradient echo (SPGR) sequence (Figs. 2.2 and 2.3; Table 2.3).[26] The sensitivities and specificities of these acquisition techniques in detecting cartilage abnormalities has been reported to be between 81% and 94% and 94% and 99%, respectively.[52,54,74–78]

Fast Spin-Echo Imaging

Fast spin-echo imaging is a technique that is essentially a variant of spin-echo sequencing that incorporates the use of multiple echoes per repetition time to acquire data faster than conventional spin echo imaging (Fig. 2.2).

Fast spin-echo sequences have been advocated in the evaluation of articular cartilage pathology because they provide efficiency in image acquisition, along with an increase in the SNR and hence an increase in spatial resolution. They also allow for shorter image acquisition times (4 to 5 minutes), which

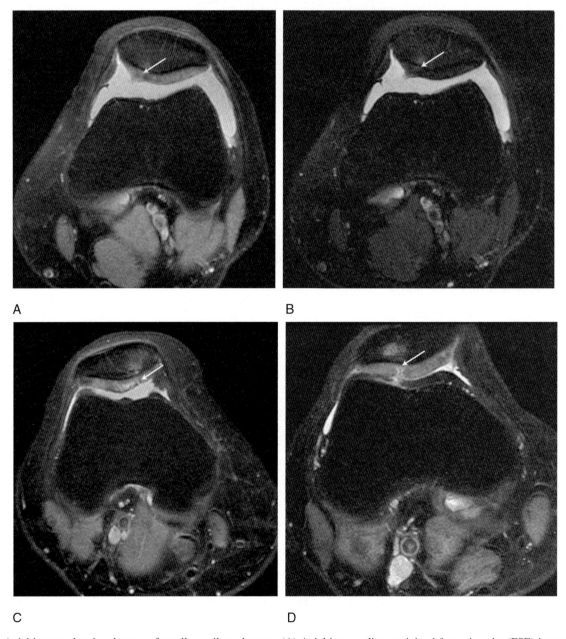

A   B

C   D

FIG. 2.2. Axial images showing degrees of patella cartilage damage. (A) Axial intermediate-weighted fast spin-echo (FSE) image showing superficial fibrillation and signal changes in the patellar cartilage (arrow). (B) Axial T2-weighted FSE image showing marrow edema at the same location (arrow). (C) Axial intermediate-weighted FSE image showing fissuring involving approximately 50% of the thickness of the cartilage. (D) Axial intermediate-weighted FSE image showing a full thickness cartilage fissure with bone marrow edema (arrow).

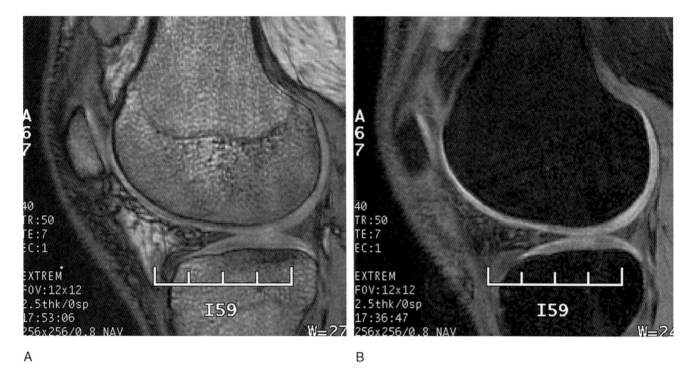

Fig. 2.3. Sagittal three-dimensional (3D) spoiled gradient echo (GRE) images of the knee obtained without (A) and with (B) fat suppression. Use of fat suppression or water-only excitation improves the dynamic range settings and allows demonstration of more detail in the cartilage.

can result in decreased patient discomfort and motion artifact (increasing patient compliance), and also enable the simultaneous evaluation of other soft tissue structures (menisci, ligaments, and tendons).

In addition, FSE sequences are relatively insensitive to magnetic susceptibility artifacts often encountered in patients who have undergone previous arthroscopic surgery and ligamentous reconstruction.[65] These artifacts, which are metallic remnants arising from surgical instrumentation, result in loss of cartilage signal and can obscure surrounding tissue signal intensity and anatomy.[26] The afforded insensitivity to magnetic susceptibility is an added benefit of FSE imaging that can provide the radiologist and surgeon with additional valuable information regarding prognosis and treatment options. Importantly, FSE sequences introduce magnetization transfer effect, which results in improved contrast between articular cartilage and adjacent tissues, as well as between normal and abnormal cartilage. The main limitation of FSE sequences is that they are two-dimensional in nature and, as a result, have limited out-of-plane resolution and limited capacity to perform multiplanar reconstructions, which are often vital in the evaluation of the curved structure of articular cartilage.[65]

Fat-Suppressed T1-Weighted Three-Dimensional Spoiled Gradient Echo Sequences

Of the routinely available imaging techniques, the highest accuracy for detection of chondral abnormalities have been reported with fat-suppressed T1-weighted 3D SPGR sequences.[52,65,68,74,76,78]

The sensitivity of this imaging technique in detecting chondral lesions has been reported to be as high as 93%.[77]

On fat-suppressed T1-weighted 3D SPGR sequences, normal articular cartilage demonstrates uniform high signal intensity throughout its thickness. Regions of altered morphology represent chondral abnormalities.[54,77,79] (Fig. 2.3).

Several studies have described the improved detection of articular cartilage lesions with fat-suppressed sequences in comparison to comparable sequences without fat suppression.[26] While T2 relaxation time is the major determinant of contrast between cartilage and fluid, fat suppression functions to increase contrast between cartilage (a non–lipid-containing tissue) and fatty bone marrow or subcutaneous fat (lipid-containing tissue). This is accomplished through the excitation of fat spins with subsequent dephasing prior to imaging.[80] On fat-suppressed images, cartilage demonstrates increased signal intensity (appears bright). The addition of fat suppression to T1-weighted imaging is useful in the evaluation of cartilage abnormalities. By suppressing fat, the gray scale of T1-weighted images is essentially "reset" to include a much narrower range of values allowing more contrast across the image, hence better delineation between cartilage and synovial fluid.[51] In addition, fat suppression also eliminates chemical-shift artifacts, which often distort the cartilage bone interface.[52,77]

Fat suppressed T1-weighted 3D SPGR sequences combine the aforementioned advantages of fat suppression with those of 3D imaging, which include increased resolution, superior in plane resolution, multiplanar reformatting capability, and small slice thickness.[26] In addition they increase the dynamic range of signal intensity of cartilage, allowing detection of more subtle changes in signal intensity. However, T1-weighted 3D SPGR sequences are more sensitive to magnetic susceptibility artifact and have longer acquisition times than FSE sequences. In addition, truncation artifact is most evident with this sequence.[81] Although FSE and T1-weighted 3D SPGR sequences have certain limitations, the advantages of one modality complement the disadvantages of the other, and vice versa. Thus, these modalities should be used together in such a complementary fashion when evaluating cartilage abnormalities.

Postarthrography Imaging

Magnetic Resonance Arthrography

Magnetic resonance arthrography has been advocated for the diagnosis of grade 2 to 4 chondral lesions (Table 2.3). An accuracy as high as 88% has been reported in the detection of chondral abnormalities using MRA.[38] Such accuracy is possible due to the enhanced contrast MRA affords between cartilage and intraarticular MR contrast agents.[66,72,82]

Most commonly, a prepared mixture of gadolinium-diethylenetriamine pentaacetic acid (Gd-DTPA) agent diluted to a 1 millimolar concentration with normal saline is directly injected, under fluoroscopic guidance, into the joint articulation. Subsequent MRI is performed using T1-weighted fat-suppressed sequences. Postarthrography imaging capitalizes on the general premise that leakage of the injected MR contrast agent into joint fluid creates distention of the articulation, while at the same time filling cartilaginous defects and providing high contrast between it and cartilage. As a result, this allows optimal visualization of the articular surface contour, improving detection of surface abnormalities, fissuring, and tears. Also, MRA is useful for the evaluation of various cartilage repair procedures.

When compared to other MR techniques, MRA has significant disadvantages. It is an invasive procedure that carries with it all the inherently associated risk factors of such a procedure. Furthermore, it is more time-consuming than most MRI techniques. Similar to other conventional MR techniques, MRA is insensitive in depicting the earliest structural changes of associated with grade 1 chondral lesions.

Computed Tomographic Arthrography

Similarly to MRA, CTA involves the intraarticular injection of an iodine-based contrast agent under fluoroscopic guidance, with subsequent imaging using dual detector spiral scanners (Table 2.3). Articular cartilage represents a structure of low attenuation that is outlined by subchondral bone plate on one end and the contrast media on the other. In a study investigating cartilage defects within cadaveric knees,

lesions observed upon gross examination were detected on CTA with a sensitivity of 80% and specificity of 88%. The MR results were similar, with a sensitivity and specificity of 83% and 80%, respectively.[83] The advantages of CT over MRI include its superior spatial resolution, as well as its availability for patients unable to undergo MRI studies (claustrophobic patients, patients with pacemakers, etc.). Similarly to MRA, CTA offers enhanced contrast between cartilage and joint fluid, accentuating filling defects. Disadvantages include its invasive nature and associated risks, as well as its relative poor soft tissue contrast, which precludes evaluation of intrinsic cartilage lesions. Similar to MRA, CTA is insensitive to early structural changes that precede morphologic defects (grade 1 lesions) and to changes within deeper layers of cartilage in which no surface abnormalities exist, thus relegating its evaluation of cartilage to tissue loss.

Volume Measurements

Several studies have reported the use of 3D reconstruction as a means of articular cartilage quantification and have determined that cartilage volumes can be determined with high accuracy with MRI in large articulations. This process is limited by the fact that global cartilage volume is measured rather than the cartilage defect in isolation. Cartilage thickness maps can combat these difficulties, but are difficult to obtain due to the small thickness of articular cartilage and the unavoidable mis-registration. Despite this, measurements of cartilage thickness, topographic maps, and volume analysis can be performed but require more facile and reproducible technique before becoming widely clinically applicable.[14,84]

T2 Mapping

Mapping of physiologic parameters with MRI has emerged as a promising means for the quantitative assessment of cartilage structure and function in both the normal and pathologic states. Unlike conventional MRI methods, mapping techniques are sensitive to specific changes in structural and biochemical composition of cartilage, thus enabling detection of the earliest chondral abnormalities. T2 mapping has emerged as a widely used technique in the evaluation of early compositional changes within the extracellular matrix (Table 2.3; Figs. 2.4 and 2.5).

It is proposed that collagen fatigue and breakdown are one of the earliest events in the cascade events leading to the development of OA.[36,85] These events lead to a loss of the tightly packed configuration of the ECM and subsequent increase in cartilage water.[86] An increase in water content leads to increased compressibility of the matrix, with the majority of the load placed upon the solid components of the ECM. Over time, such increased stress leads to structural fatigue and fragmentation of the solid components of the ECM,[87] culminating in visible changes such as partial-thickness defects (fissuring,

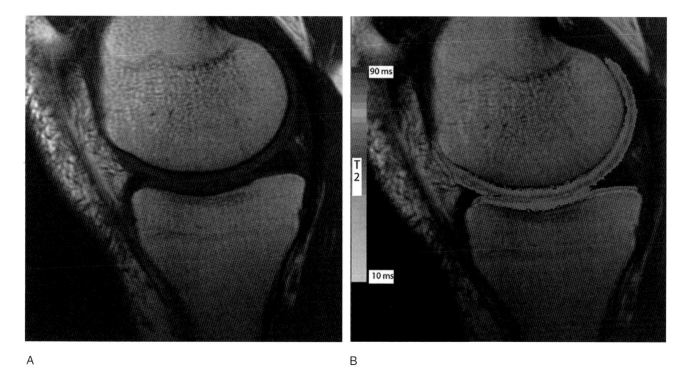

A   B

Fig. 2.4. Sagittal MR image and T2 map from a healthy volunteer. (A) Sagittal MR image shows the normal appearance of the medial femorotibial compartment articular cartilage. (B) T2 relaxation times have been superimposed on the corresponding articular surfaces (with grayscale display) and show that normal values range from 20 to 70 msec, with higher values located closer to the superficial cartilage surface.

fraying, and fibrillation) and full-thickness defects (Figs. 2.4 and 2.5). These changes result in accompanying changes in T2 values. The T2 of articular cartilage has been shown to be sensitive parameter for the evaluation of early abnormalities within articular cartilage.[88] The disruption of the structural framework of collagen and the subsequent loss of tissue anisotropy result in an increase in cartilage T2 values, a phenomenon observed in human osteoarthritic specimens.[88–90] In addition, increases in T2 values have been observed with increases in water content within human osteoarthritic specimens,[91–94] as well as with increases in water mobility that occur with the loss of the structural framework of collagen.[95] Of note, increases in T2 within the transitional zone have been associated with aging.[94]

T2 mapping capitalizes on the above-mentioned changes in T2 that occur in OA (Fig. 2.4). By measuring the spatial distribution of T2, itself a function of the intrinsic water content of articular cartilage, T2 mapping detects areas with changes in water content corresponding to areas of cartilage damage.[96] Most commonly, a multiecho SE technique is used, acquiring four to 12 images with echo time (TE) values ranging from 10 to 100 ms. A standard survey of the entire region in question is performed, with particular attention to areas of chondral abnormality. An image of the T2 is generated, with an accompanying color or gray scale map representing relaxation times. The T1 and T2 relaxation times are quantified on a pixel basis, assigned a value, and if desired, assigned a color to provide a visual assessment of the region of interest. T2 values are then obtained for regions with chondral abnormalities and compared with values obtained from the T2 map, with marked difference in values signifying abnormalities in chondral structure. Minimum inter-echo spacing must be used to evaluate articular cartilage, given the rapid rate of T2 decay in the radial zone.[88] This means of analysis provides an objective way to evaluate changes in signal intensity, and is more practical for evaluation of focal cartilage defects than volumetric analysis. However, it requires high-resolution imaging capabilities in the form of high field strength magnets or local gradient coils, and also requires significant imaging time and postprocess imaging at present depending on the MR scanner and platform used.[97]

High Field Strength Imaging

To date, the vast majority of conventional MRI of the musculoskeletal system in the clinical setting has been performed at 1.5 tesla (T) and lower, with higher field strength systems reserved for research purposes. High field strength MRI, mainly 3-T systems, are becoming an ever-prevalent entity in evaluating musculoskeletal abnormalities within the clinical setting, especially those associated with chondral abnormalities (Fig. 2.5).

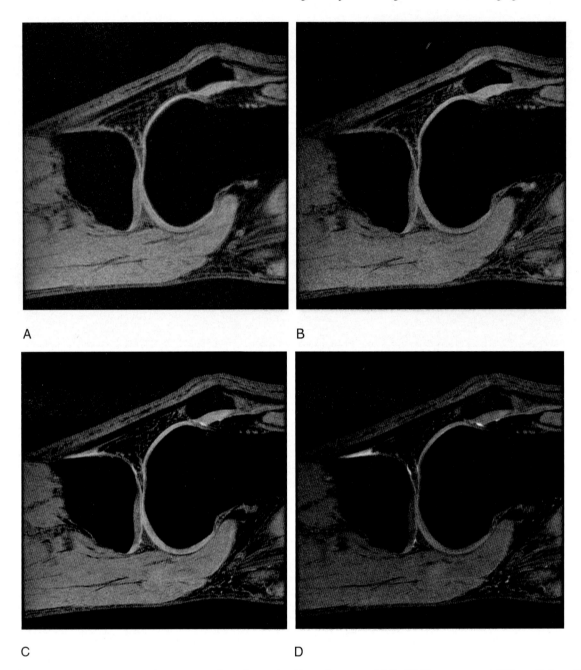

FIG. 2.5. High field strength imaging of articular cartilage from a healthy volunteer at 3.0 T. (A) Fat-suppressed (FS) spoiled gradient echo (SPGR) image. (B) Iterative decomposition of water and fat with Echo Asymmetry and Least squares (IDEAL) SPGR image. (C) IDEAL gradient echo (GRE) image with bright joint fluid. (D) IDEAL GRE image with a higher flip angle, increasing fluid to cartilage contrast.

Such growing interest can be attributed to the afforded increase in SNR, the increase in spatial resolution, and the shorter imaging acquisition time provided by higher strength magnetic imaging systems. However, the SNR benefit at 3.0 T can often be limited by various factors, including field-dependent changes in tissue relaxation times and chemical shift differences that exist between fat and water.[98] In addition, imaging of articular cartilage at higher field strengths introduces variability in T1 and T2 relaxation times.[98,99] In general, a slight increase of 10% to 15% in T1 relaxation times and a slight decrease of 10% to 15% in T2 relaxation times of articular cartilage have been shown with 3.0-T systems in comparison to 1.5-T systems.[98,99] These differences ultimately affect the selection of appropriate parameters, repetition time (TR) and TE, required to ensure optimal image contrast.[98]

Novel Magnetic Resonance Imaging Techniques

While conventional MRI techniques are excellent for the detection of high-grade chondral lesions, they provide limited information regarding biochemical and structural changes associated with the earliest chondral degeneration (grade 1 lesions).[60] This has prompted development of numerous novel MRI techniques that focus on these early changes. Inevitably, it is these techniques that offer the greatest promise for better understanding the pathogenesis of OA and advancing the development of chondroprotective therapies to treat and prevent progression of osteoarthritis. While several novel techniques exist, this discussion focuses on driven equilibrium Fourier transfer (DEFT) imaging, diffusion-weighted imaging (DWI), delayed gadolinium-enhanced MRI of cartilage (dGEMRIC)/contrast-enhanced imaging, and ultrashort TE (UTE) imaging (Table 2.4).

Driven Equilibrium Fourier Transform Imaging

In the past, DEFT imaging had been used as a method of signal enhancement in spectroscopy (Table 2.4).[100] Its application in cartilage imaging relies on its ability to produce image contrast that is a function of proton density, echo time, repetition time, and the intrinsic T1/T2 ratio of a given tissue.[51] Unlike T2W SE sequences, which produce contrast by attenuating cartilage signal, DEFT produces contrast by enhancing signal tissues with long T1 relaxation times, such as synovial fluid. It accomplishes this by using a 90-degree pulse to return magnetization to the z-axis after data acquisition.[80] This results in a high signal intensity of synovial fluid and an intermediate signal intensity of articular cartilage. Bone is dark and fat is suppressed, allowing for excellent contrast of cartilage from surrounding tissues (Fig. 2.6).

In addition, DEFT has a high SNR, preserving cartilage signal and enabling visualization of the structural elements of cartilage by requiring echo time to be as short as possible.[51] The benefit of DEFT is that is provides high contrast without loss of cartilage signal.

Diffusion-Weighted Imaging

Diffusion-weighted imaging in the assessment of cartilage is based on the premise that inherently avascular structure relies on diffusion for transport of nutrients and waste (Table 2.4). It is also presumed that this process is altered in the early stages of degradation, where overall morphology is grossly intact and changes that occur affect the concentrations and orientations of the macromolecular components of articular cartilage (Fig. 2.7).

Diffusion-weighted imaging has been shown to be sensitive to early cartilage degeneration in in-vitro experiments.[101,102] Preliminary work has shown that diffusion maps of water strongly reflect the spatial heterogeneity of cartilage. Moreover, extensive studies of diffusion in cartilage under a variety of circumstances with several small solutes, as well as water, have helped to establish the effect of the macromolecular environment on diffusion.

Diffusion measurements involve the application of diffusion-sensitizing gradients that cause phase accrual in the spins of tissues that is reduced to zero if spins are stationary. However, water undergoing diffusion accrues a random amount of phase; thus, it does not refocus. As a result there is loss of tissue undergoing diffusion. The amount of diffusion weighting applied is a function of the diffusion-sensitizing gradients and is expressed as the b-value.[80] And while MRI obtained with diffusion-weighted imaging enables the local measurement of diffusion coefficients, it also enables the construction of a map—the apparent diffusion coefficient (ADC) map—that demonstrates the amount of diffusion taken place, thus revealing spatial distribution of diffusion differences (Fig. 2.7).[54,80]

Diffusion-weighted imaging has several limitations. First, it increases the TE and makes the sequence sensitive to motion. This a major concern in tissues with short T2 relaxation times, such as cartilage, where the TE must be short to start with in order to maximize cartilage signal. Single-shot techniques have been used, but they have low SNR and spatial resolution.

TABLE 2.4. Summary of selected advanced MR imaging techniques for cartilage evaluation.

MR technique	Morphology	Matrix	Proteoglycan	Deep calcified layer	Advantages	Disadvantages
Driven equilibrium Fourier transform (DEFT)	+	+/−	−	−	High signal-to-noise ratio; high contrast without loss of cartilage signal	Experimental
Diffusion-weighted imaging (DWI)	+	+	−	−	Potential detailed matrix evaluation	Sensitivity to motion; requires very high field strength; experimental
Delayed gadolinium-enhanced MRI of cartilage (dGEMRIC)	+	−	+	−	Detailed proteoglycan evaluation	Time-consuming; invasive (minimally)
Ultrashort TE (UTE)	+	−	−	+	Evaluation of deepest zones; TE values 80 ms	Limited availability; experimental

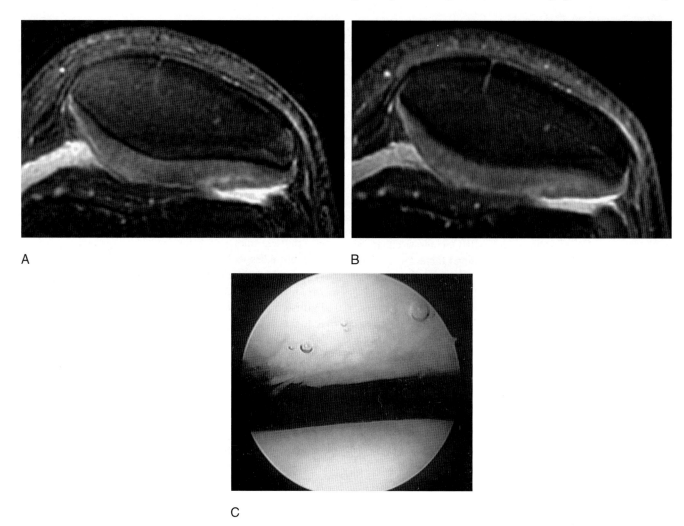

A   B

C

Fig. 2.6. A 3D driven equilibrium Fourier transfer (DEFT) imaging of a cartilage fissure. Images were done with a 3-inch surface coil for additional detail. (A) A 3D-DEFT image showing a fissure (arrow) in the lateral patella facet. (B) T2 fast spin echo (FSE) image showing the same fissure but not as clearly. (C) Arthroscopy, showing patella cartilage at the top and cartilage fissure. 3D-DEFT showed a greater extent of the fissure in this case.

Multiple acquisition techniques have also been used, improving SNR and resolution. However, sensitivity to motion continues to be a major factor.[103] Increases in the available gradient strength on clinical systems will be required to fully evaluate the clinical utility of this imaging sequence.[104]

Contrast-Enhanced Imaging (Delayed Gadolinium-Enhanced MRI of Cartilage)

Delayed $Gd(DTPA)^{2-}$-enhanced MRI (dGEMRIC), another biochemical evaluation of cartilage, is a technique that was developed to monitor the distribution of glycosaminoglycans (GAGs) and was validated biochemically and histologically in bovine and human cartilage (Table 2.4).[104–106] This technique uses the anionic contrast agent gadopentetate dimeglumine (Magnevist; Berlex Laboratories, Wayne, NJ), which, upon injection into the body, becomes negatively charged. The basis for the MR technique is that the GAGs are negatively charged,

and when depleted leave a net positive charge within the cartilage. If given time to penetrate the cartilage tissue, the anionic molecule $Gd(DTPA)^{2-}$ will distribute inversely to the concentration of the negatively charged GAGs, collecting in regions of GAG depletion (Figs. 2.8 and 2.9).

The general protocol for dGEMRIC is based on pilot clinical studies of the knee and hip in volunteers.[104,105] Gadopentetate dimeglumine (Magnevist) at a dose of 0.2 mM/kg (0.4 mL/kg) (double dose) is injected in a single bolus through an antecubital vein. Immediately after injection, the lower extremity is exercised for 10 minutes, theoretically increasing the delivery of contrast to the joint. An MRI is done 2 hours after the initial intravenous injection, allowing for penetration of contrast into the cartilage. The imaging protocol includes acquisition of inversion recovery (IR) turbo-spin-echo T1-weighted images with varying inversions times (25, 75, 180, 350, 650, 1100, and 1680 ms). T1 maps are subsequently generated that render images with T1 values ranging from 50 to 1500 ms. In general,

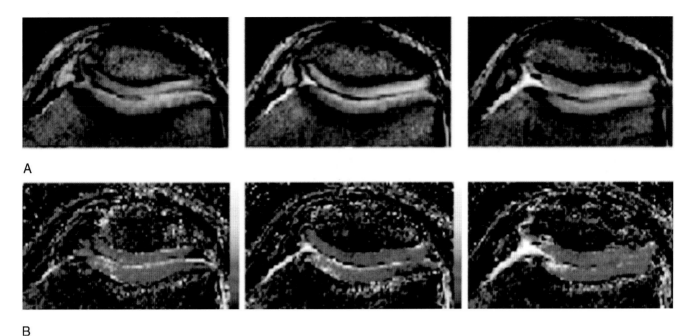

FIG. 2.7. Three-dimensional balanced steady-state free-precession diffusion-weighted imaging. (A) Proton density images. (B) Heat scale maps of the diffusion coefficient. The b values correspond to the degree of diffusion weighting. Diffusion imaging gives a sense of translational water mobility within the articular cartilage. The diffusion coefficients measured in normal cartilage are about $0.00145\,mm^2/s$, which correspond to similar values in the literature. (From Miller KL, Hargreaves BA, Gold GE, et al. Magn Res Med 2004;51:394–398, with permission.).

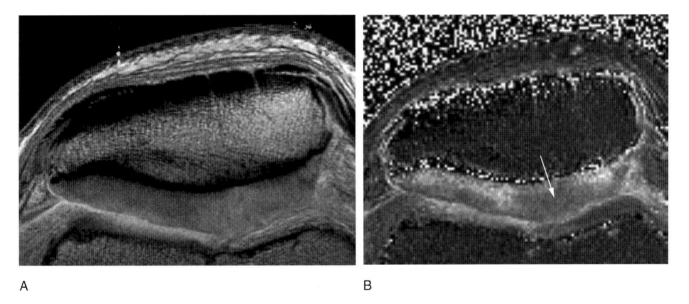

FIG. 2.8. Axial images of the knee in a patient with knee pain. (A) Proton density image. (B) Delayed T1 map after gadolinium injection demonstrates lower signal in a focal area of the patella cartilage relative to the other articular cartilage surfaces. This may represent depletion of glycosaminoglycan (GAG) in this region.

diseased cartilage demonstrates lower dGEMRIC T1 values (Figs. 2.8 and 2.9).

While this imaging technique is not widely used as a clinical application, it has shown great promise as a noninvasive means to assess GAG content within cartilage. It is difficult to implement clinically due to the timing of the contrast injection and ultimate delay in MRI.

Ultrashort TE Sequences

Although the exact pathogenesis of OA is poorly understood, it is believed that the formation of focal cartilage lesions represents the earliest event in the cascade of events that ultimately culminate in detectable chondral deformities. However, debate and uncertainty exist as to which zone is affected by these earliest

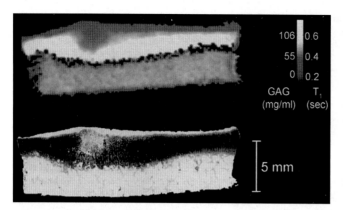

FIG. 2.9. Quantitative evaluation of glycosaminoglycan content in cartilage with delayed gadolinium-enhanced imaging. Top: Delayed gadolinium-enhanced image maps T1 to glycosaminoglycan (GAG) content and shows a focal area of low GAG concentration. Bottom: Photograph of the specimen after staining with toluidine blue shows a focal area of cartilage damage. (From Kramer et al.,[72] with permission.).

more superficial zones.[107–110] Furthermore, it has been established that lesions in the deeper layers can result from single impaction injury, all while leaving the superficial cartilage intact.[111]

Though much MRI research has focused on the evaluation of articular cartilage, to date only the superficial and middle zones of articular cartilage have been accessible with clinical MRI. The deeper layers, the radial zone and the zone of deep calcified cartilage, have been inaccessible to MRI evaluation, due mainly to the technical constraints of both conventional and novel MRI sequences to detect signal in the short T2 range present in these zones.

As discussed earlier, cartilage displays a zonal variation in mean T2, ranging from 30 to 40 ms in superficial layers, to 3 to 4 ms in its deepest layers (Fig. 2.1). However, ultrashort TE (UTE) sequences have, for the first time, enabled visualization of the morphologic features of these zones (Table 2.4). With TEs 20 to 50 times shorter than the 8 to 10 ms of conventional FSE studies, UTE sequences allow excellent depiction and evaluation of tissues with short T2 relaxation components (Fig. 2.10).

By providing a means of evaluating short T2 relaxation components in articular cartilage, predominating in the deep and calcified layers, all the basic structural components of the tissue can now be qualitatively and quantitatively assessed in a noninvasive manner with MRI. Images are optimized through coil selection, acquisition techniques, and subtraction techniques to improve SNR and contrast-to-noise ratios within cartilage. This information can be coupled with existing MR techniques to provide a global assessment of these zones, presenting new opportunities to assess pathogenesis, patterns

changes. Until recently, emphasis has been placed on chondral lesions involving the superficial most layers, as evidenced by accompanying gross morphologic changes and tissue loss or structural changes. More recently, however, the concept that abnormalities in the biochemical and structural components of the deeper radial and calcified layers of cartilage play a greater role in the pathogenesis of OA has gained momentum in the scientific literature. This concept suggests that lesions in the radial and calcified layers of cartilage serve to destabilize the foundation of the tissue, ultimately resulting in degeneration of the

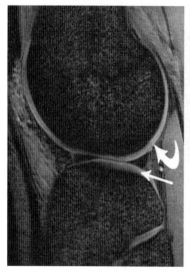

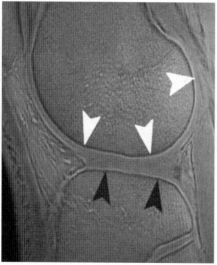

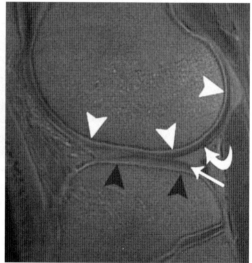

A   B   C

FIG. 2.10. Ultrashort echo time (UTE) MRI of the knee acquired at 3 T with (A) first image (TE = 8 μs), (B) second image (14 ms), and (C) difference image (first image minus second image). The calcified layer of cartilage is identified by its bright signal intensity just superficial to the subchondral bone in the femur (white arrowheads A). The more superficial layers of the femoral (curved arrow) and tibial (straight arrow) cartilage can be seen on the second image. (B) The difference image shows a more extensive high signal layer than for the radial zone (in A), which includes both the calcified layer and the deep radial zone. Compact subchondral bone appears black (black arrows, B and C).

of cartilage injury, and degeneration that lead to OA. Moreover, recent data suggest that the integrity of the deep layer of cartilage may afford prognostic information with regard to the effectiveness of different cartilage repair techniques.

Magnetic Resonance Imaging of Articular Cartilage Repair Techniques

Postsurgical imaging of articular cartilage is increasing in importance as a variety of different palliative surgical techniques have become available for the repair of chondral defects. As mentioned earlier, articular cartilage is a relatively avascular tissue with a limited capacity for repair, as well as an inherent inability to regenerate. As a result, damage or degeneration of articular cartilage is an irreversible process that may lead to a host of clinical symptomology, as well as considerably impact quality of life. Oftentimes, surgical intervention is indicated.

Current therapies can be categorized into two broad groups: palliative therapies dealing with treatment of symptoms without surgical intervention, and those focused on surgical repair of cartilaginous abnormalities. The former includes removal of loose bodies and osteophytes, replacement arthroplasty, and lavaging of the joint.[112] And while these treatments provide pain relief and slow the progression of cartilaginous defects, they fail to restore the structural integrity of cartilage. Surgical repair of cartilaginous abnormalities, which is the focus of the ensuing discussion, can be further subdivided into two categories: local stimulation and autologous transplantation of cartilage.[113] And while much has been written regarding these entities, to date no randomized studies comparing them has been reported.

Local Stimulation (Abrasion Arthroplasty, Microfracture, and Subchondral Drilling)

Local stimulation techniques are often performed as the primary repair procedure of cartilaginous defects, given the fact that they involve minimal instrumentation and can be performed concurrently with arthroscopy.[113] The three most commonly performed techniques that fall into this category are abrasion arthroplasty, microfracture, and subchondral drilling.[113]

Local stimulation techniques are modeled on the principle that full-thickness defects have a greater propensity for healing than do partial lesions. The reason is that unlike partial-thickness lesions, full-thickness defects extend into the subchondral bone, allowing for the extravasation of pluripotent stem cells, growth factors, and other proteins that are vital for mounting a repair response and for tissue remodeling.[113] Repair tissues have been shown to be composed of hyaline and fibrocartilage.[114] Thus, the penetration of subchondral bone underlying chondral defects is a key component performed in all local stimulation techniques. However, the manner in which the subchondral bone is penetrated varies. A burr is used in abrasion arthroplasty, a drill in subchondral drilling, and an awl or pick in microfracture to make multiple penetrations that are 3 to 4mm apart and measure about 4mm in depth.[15,115,116]

In general, local stimulation techniques are recommended for cartilaginous lesions smaller than 4cm^2, although they have been reported to treat defects as large as 10cm^2.[113]

Within the first few months following microfracture repair, repair tissue of intermediate intensity can be seen on MRI. This tissue is generally thinner than the adjacent healthy articular cartilage. In addition, surgically related edema-like patterns are commonly seen around the defect. With time, the signal intensity of repair tissue approaches, or becomes similar to, that of the native healthy cartilage, signifying increased repair tissue with complete filling of the defect.

The main limitation of local stimulation techniques is that the repair tissue does not have the same structure and durability as that of healthy hyaline cartilage. Abnormally low concentrations of type II collagen have been shown to be present, instead replaced by type I collagen, which is often not found in cartilage. In addition, repair tissue also has reduced proteoglycan content.[15,117,118]

Autologous Transplantation of Cartilage

The two technique of autologous transplantation of cartilage are autologous osteochondral transplantation (AOT) and autologous chondrocyte implantation (ACI). Both techniques have been advocated, due to their potential for formation of hyaline and hyaline-like repair tissue.[113]

Autologous Osteochondral Transplantation

Autologous osteochondral transplantation is a technique in which osteochondral plugs, harvested from non—weight-bearing or minimal weight-bearing regions of the articulation are used to fill osteochondral defects. Autologous osteochondral transplantation is also referred to as MosaicPlasty (Acufex, Smith & Nephew, Andover, MA), osteochondral autograft transfer system (OATS, Anthrex, Naples, FL), soft delivery system (SDS, Sulzermedica), and the Consistent Osteochondral Repair (COR) system (Mitek, Raynham, MA).[119,120] Such variety in nomenclature is reflective of the diverse array of instruments used in performing this procedure. The major objective of AOT is threefold: (1) to replace the defect with normal cartilage; (2) to approximate the interface of the graft with that of native bone, creating a congruent surface that will preserve joint mechanics; and (3) to achieve incorporation of the graft with underlying bone.

Plugs are most commonly taken from the intercondylar notch or the superior edge of the lateral or medial femoral condyles at the level of the patellofemoral joint. Prior to implantation, the chondral defect itself is debrided down to viable subchondral bone. Next, bone plugs are transplanted into the defect in a perpendicular fashion to the articular surface, with careful attention to maintaining congruent transition points between the cartilage surface and the subchondral interface.[113] And while a congruent cartilage-to-cartilage interface is often achieved, an incongruent bone-to-bone interface occurs between that of native and transplanted cartilage.[113] This has been attributed to the fact that grafts are often harvested from regions of the knee joint where the articular cartilage is thinner when compared to the recipient site.[113] Furthermore, curettage or abrasion arthroplasty is performed in the interstices between plugs, providing stimulation that results in an eventual filling of these spaces by a fibrocartilaginous-like repair tissue. Compared to adjacent native articular cartilage, this demonstrates increased T2 signal on FSE images and decreased signal intensity on 3D fat-suppressed SPGR sequences.[113]

Histologic confirmation of such repair tissue, as well as of viable hyaline grafts, has been reported.[114,121,122] Furthermore, AOT has been shown to increase defect fill from 90% to 100%.[113]

Magnetic resonance imaging provides accurate assessment of postsurgical changes, including graft positioning, graft incorporation, donor-site morbidity, and surface incongruities between repair tissue and adjacent native articular cartilage.[113] Surface incongruities are often designated as either protuberant or depressed. Magnetic resonance imaging not only facilitates visualization of these irregularities, but also provides valuable information regarding their cause, including graft displacement, gross graft motion, graft subsidence, and improper positioning of grafts.[113] Of note, surface irregularities have been shown to decrease over time on serial MR studies, most likely a result of filling defects by fibrocartilaginous-like repair tissue mentioned previously.[123] Loosening of graft placement is indicated by graft migration or displacement, as well as fluid surrounding the graft on T2W FSE images.[51]

In addition, signal characteristics of both the osseous and cartilaginous portion of the graft can be evaluated using MRI, enabling better assessment of postsurgical cartilaginous degeneration. Variability in the signal intensity of the graft implants has been noted in the postoperative period. Generally at 5 months posttransplantation, fatty marrow signal intensity is present to a variable degree within the central portion of the graft, and by 12 months the entire graft should demonstrate fatty marrow. The presence of contrast enhancement can indicate an intact vascular supply to the graft, although enhancement may not occur in the grafts for up to 4 weeks postsurgery. In studies to date, routine clinical MRI protocols have been used for postoperative evaluation that were composed of T2-weighted fat-suppressed fast spin echo, and T1-weighted spin echo sequences in various imaging planes.[51,124]

Variation in signal intensity is also seen within the donor site. In general, the donor site is initially either left empty or filled in with material from the recipient site. Over time, it fills with cancellous bone and fibrocartilaginous-like repair tissue.[123] During the early postoperative period, the donor site demonstrates low T1 and high T2 signal intensity compared to adjacent fatty marrow, as well as defects within its overlying cartilage and adjacent edematous bone marrow changes.[113] At 6 to 9 months postoperatively, there is filling of the donor-site defect with fibrocartilaginous-like repair tissue. Furthermore, the donor site returns to its normal fatty marrow-like signal intensity.[113]

Indications for AOT include focal osteochondral defects with a diameter of 1 to 4 cm².[114,123] Contraindications include age greater than 50, lesions larger than 8 cm², and diffuse cartilaginous defects (as typically seen in advanced OA, inflammatory arthritis, and postseptic arthritis).[114] The outcome of the procedure primarily depends on the position, orientation, and number of osteochondral plugs.[113]

Autologous osteochondral transplantation has many limitations. First, donor-site morbidity has been reported in approximately 3% of patients.[114] Second, the number of bone plugs that can be used is limited by the availability and morbidity of donor sites. Third, harvesting of plugs leads to irregularities of the tidemark, and in turn subsequent irregularities of the bone–cartilage interface. Finally, AOT is technically difficult procedure, require expertise training.

Autologous Chondrocyte Implantation

Autologous chondrocyte implantation is a two-stage cell-based surgical approach to the treatment of articular cartilage defects. The first stage involves diagnostic arthroscopic assessment of the joint and harvesting of about 200 to 300 mg of health articular cartilage for cell culture. As with AOT, specimens are harvested from non–weight-bearing sites within the joint. Cells are extracted from specimens using sophisticated enzymatic digestion methods and are subsequently cultured for 4 weeks until approximately 12 million cells are available for implantation.

During the second stage, a second open arthrotomy is performed in which the cartilaginous defect is debrided down to subchondral bone, with additional removal of any loose cartilage fragments from the margins of the defect. Of note, penetration of the subchondral bone plate, as in local stimulation techniques, is avoided.

Periosteum is harvested and trimmed to match the debrided cartilage defect. The periosteum is sewn over the cartilage defect and made water-tight with fibrin glue, leaving one free corner through which the cultured cell suspension is injected. After the cell suspension is injected, a final stitch is placed and the injection sight is sealed.

Histologic investigations have shown that the repair site maturation occurs through several phases.[125] The proliferative phase, accounting for the first 6 weeks, involves multiplication of the transplanted cells, resulting in filling of the defect with soft tissue. In the transition phase (between 7 and 26 weeks), there is production of collagen and proteoglycans, resulting in stiffening of the ECM. In the final or remodeling phase, there is further maturation of the ECM, in which the repair tissue becomes similar to that of the adjacent healthy articular cartilage.[113,125] Furthermore, in a mean follow-up approximately 4 years after ACI, biopsy specimens obtained from the repair site showed hyaline-like repair tissue in 75% to 80% of cases.[126,127] Of clinical relevance, the postsurgical MRI findings parallel the above-mentioned histologic changes. Thus, an overall appreciation of the mentioned histologic processes can assist in better understanding the MRI findings.

Magnetic resonance imaging of autologous chondrocyte grafts has proven particularly useful for evaluating the signal of the repair tissue, the degree of defect fill, the integration of the repair cartilage to the subchondral plate, as well as the status of the subchondral bone plate and bone marrow. Common imaging protocols incorporate primarily proton density and intermediate-weighted FSE sequences. Gradient echo sequences introduce excessive susceptibility artifact on the surface of the graft, interfering with graft evaluation. Utilization of arthrographic techniques has also been discussed, particularly for the differentiation between heterogeneous signal intensity within the graft repair cartilage and delamination defects or separation of the graft from the underlying bone.

The signal intensity of the graft repair tissue and underlying bone after ACI can be heterogeneous and variable, changing as the repair tissue matures.[15,128,129] The implications of the changes in signal intensity are currently not known. In the first month after surgery, the tissue repair demonstrates intermediate signal intensity on T1W SE and proton-density images, and increased signal intensity that is only faintly different from that of joint fluid on fluid sensitive sequences. In addition, the periosteal cover can be identified as a separate layer on the surface of the repair site, which often extends above the level of the articular surface. Linear fluid-like signal within the graft or at its junction with subchondral bone usually indicates a tear of the periosteal cover or poor integration of the graft. However, over time the signal intensity of the repair tissue comes to approximate that of articular cartilage, stabilizing at about 12 to 18 months postsurgery. The morphology of the repair tissue should mimic that of the native articular cartilage in its thickness and contour. It should restore the articular surface, filling the cartilage defect. The margins of the graft should be continuous with the adjacent native cartilage, as repair tissue integrates with native cartilage. However, the graft–cartilage interface, too, is variable and heterogeneous in appearance over time.[113]

In the first few months postsurgery, portions of this interface appear similar to fluid, falsely simulating a fissure.[113] However, unlike a true fissure, this fluid-like line runs orthogonally to the articular surface and does not extend between the repair tissue and bone interface. With the maturation of the graft–cartilage interface over time, this interface comes to demonstrate a dark band, or is discernible altogether, further distinguishing it from the findings of a true fissure. As for the subchondral bone plate beneath the graft, it may appear slightly irregular or smooth, and usually remains so over time. On MRI, an edema-like signal within the bone marrow, subjacent to or deep beneath the repair site, is expected in the early postoperative period. A decrease in marrow signal is observed over the next few months, with a normal appearance expected by 1 year. Persistence of abnormal bone marrow signal beyond 1 year is bothersome, and may indicate possible postoperative complications such as periosteal hypertrophy (discussed below) and poor integration of the repair tissue. However, often a thin line of edema-like signal may indefinitely remain beneath the subchondral bone subjacent to the graft site.

Several complications are encountered in ACI repair techniques. These can be categorized as either being related to the actual surgical procedure itself or as being related to the ACI repair tissue. By far, the most common arthrotomy-related complication is the formation intraarticular adhesions, occur-

ring in approximately 5% of patients.[130] Adhesions usually present as with knee stiffness and nonspecific knee pain. The diagnosis can be made clinically without the need for imaging. The most common symptoms include the sudden onset of painful catching or knee locking.[125] However, MRI of this subset of patients provides the radiologist with the advantage of being able to exclude graft failure as a possible cause of symptoms. On MRI, adhesions appear as thickenings of the joint capsule or focal bands of tissue within the infrapatellar fat pad that demonstrate lower signal intensity than that of fat on T1W SE and proton density images, and higher signal intensity than fat on fat-saturated proton density images.

A second complication is delamination of the repair tissue. Most commonly occurring within 6 months of surgery, delaminating defects can involve the complete separation of the entire graft from the defect site, termed a complete delamination, or can involve partial separation, termed partial delamination. Partial delamination usually occurs in a marginal fashion, involving the ACI-native cartilage junction.[125] Repair tissue may become displaced, leaving behind an empty fluid-filled defect within the graft detected on MRI. The displaced repair tissue appears as an intraarticular body within the joint. Partial delaminated graft tissue can also remain in place and produce a tissue flap seen on MRI.[113] Abnormal linear signal intensity has been reported at the base of the ACI graft, between it and the subjacent subchondral bone plate, representing fluid-like signal of the immature ACI graft tissue. However, it may be difficult to differentiate this from a delaminating defect. Magnetic resonance arthrography facilitates distinguishing these defects, given that the repair tissue is darker than fluid. Thus, it is important to express the degree of filling on MRI with respect to the linear depth and percent of volume of the defect.

Another complication of ACI is hypertrophy of the periosteal cover, occurring in up to 20% to 25% of patients. On MRI, this fibrous overgrowth of the periosteal cover appears as a thickening of the repair tissue with protrusion above the level of the articular contour.[130] It is commonly encountered between the third and seventh postoperative months. The clinical presentation is that of catching. In addition, the hypertrophic tissue can extend over the adjacent surface of cartilage, resulting in an observed overlapping flap of tissue seen on MRI, or it can grow into the intercondylar notch and interfere with the anterior cruciate ligament (ACL) when the ACI site is close to the intercondylar notch. The latter situation can be confused with the focal fibrosis seen in a cyclops lesion post-ACL reconstruction.[125,129] Treatment of symptomatic periosteal hypertrophy is arthroscopic chondroplasty and removal of overlapping fibrous tissue.[130]

Finally, failure of the ACI graft can occur. This is often due to poor bone integration, graft delamination, poor tissue quality, or degeneration of the repair tissue.[130] On MRI, the findings of repair tissue degeneration are similar to those of native cartilage degeneration. Fissures and partial- or full-thickness tears may be present, as well as edematous marrow signal or cyst formation in the underlying subchondral bone.[113,131]

B. Orthopedic Perspective: Clinical Applications of Magnetic Resonance Imaging of Articular Cartilage Pathology

Michael J. Angel, Nicholas A. Sgaglione, and Steve Sharon

Advances in musculoskeletal imaging technology have evolved significantly as novel articular cartilage surgical techniques have been introduced. The application of MRI has made possible the identification of focal hyaline cartilage pathology with extraordinary detail. Its application has begun to play an integral role in the decision-making process for precise diagnosis, treatment, and outcomes assessment. Traditional plain roentgenogram images have limited the interpretation of articular cartilage pathology to the evaluation of joint space narrowing, subchondral bone irregularities, and bone perimeter hypertrophy. Magnetic resonance imaging is able to evaluate the articular cartilage with precise detail, and while arthroscopy remains the standard for cartilage evaluation, the accuracy of MRI and its potential for improvement is invaluable.

Articular cartilage has limited potential for spontaneous repair following injury. Furthermore, injuries to the articular cartilage can subsequently lead to the development of osteoarthritis and degenerative joint disease. Approximately 75% of people over the age of 75 have osteoarthritis of the knee.[132] As our population ages and remains increasingly active, it is important to ensure a comprehensive approach to diagnosing and treating articular cartilage.

More recently, advances have been realized in the area of articular cartilage biosurgery and resurfacing. Established treatment methods such as arthroscopic debridement and drilling have been augmented or replaced by techniques such as arthroscopic marrow stimulation, osteochondral autograft and allograft tissue transplantation, ACI, and the use of bioresorbable synthetic scaffolds to repair or replace osteochondral defects.

This section reviews the clinical approach to articular cartilage pathology and treatment and the role MRI can play in that treatment algorithm. The use of MRI to evaluate articular cartilage injuries is discussed, including presentation, clinical detection and natural history of articular cartilage injuries, and how MRI may affect decision making pre- and postoperatively. Future trends in the field of articular cartilage repair and outcomes analysis as it relates to noninvasive imaging are also reviewed.

Magnetic Resonance Imaging and Articular Cartilage

Magnetic resonance imaging has emerged as the method of choice in noninvasive imaging and evaluation of articular cartilage defects. Magnetic resonance imaging of the musculoskeletal system has improved with the introduction of more advanced imaging software and stronger, more powerful imaging equipment that is able to reduce imaging time while increasing resolution and contrast. There is, however, wide variability in the imaging acquisition techniques used to evaluate articular cartilage, which is partly due to different imaging equipment used in different centers. Variability also arises from different techniques in which MRI manufacturers acquire data as well as the imaging sequence preference of radiologists performing examinations, including field strength characteristics, extremity coil selection, and positioning.

The most widely used imaging techniques for evaluation of articular cartilage have been the T1 fat-suppressed 3D spoiled gradient echo and T2-weighted fast spin echo technique.[133,134] Other techniques employ a moderate TE and relative long TR-weighted sequence with increased phase encoding and number of excitations (NEX), with a smaller field of view allowing for higher resolution, which enables greater contrast between tissues with different water content.[135] Fat-suppression techniques refer to the process of improving imaging contrast by darkening fat on MRI; however, it is associated with resolution reduction, which potentially could reduce diagnostic precision.

Recent studies have shown significant accuracy associated with the use of high-resolution modified echo time FSE sequence techniques to evaluate and predict lesion site, size, and depth.[136] Disler et al.[134] showed that the use of a fat-suppressed 3D spoiled gradient-echo sequence has a sensitivity of 86%, specificity of 97%, and accuracy of 91% for detection of cartilage lesions in the knee. Similar results have been proven using alternative techniques with a sensitivity of 87%, specificity of 94%, and accuracy of 92% with high field strength FSE images.[136]

Definition and categorization of MRI interpretation have been increasingly improved. The radiologist may report articular cartilage damage in a descriptive (i.e., heterogeneous, fissured, and thinned) or systematic manner. Brown and Potter et al.[135] define a detailed categorical evaluation of articular cartilage based on morphology, tissue volume, congruence, and integrity. Morphology is reported as depressed, flush, or proud; volume filling is categorized and quantified as good (67–100% fill), moderate (34–66% fill), or poor (0–33% fill); the native cartilage-repaired/damaged cartilage interface is evaluated for gaps that are categorized as small (≤ 2 mm) or large (>2 mm); subchondral marrow edema is described as mild (<1 cm^2), moderate (1 to 3 cm^2), and severe (>3 cm^2); and the presence or absence of osseous overgrowth is described.[135] The radiologist's ability to accurately describe articular cartilage damage on MRI broadens its role for diagnostic as well as perioperative evaluation by clinicians.

Incidence and Relevance

Articular cartilage damage occurs either acutely from a significant injury or chronically from repetitive overload and imbalance. It is common in patients of all ages and activity levels. An evaluation of 31,000 knee arthroscopies over a 4-year period determined that 63% of all patients who undergo knee arthroscopy for pain have some level of articular cartilage damage.[137] Similarly, Hjelle et al.,[138] in a prospective study of 1000 knee arthroscopies performed in a population of patients with a median age of 39 (range 13 to 96 years), found chondral or osteochondral lesions in 61% of all patients. Focal defects were found in 19% of patients and were most often noted in the medial femoral condyle and patella. Of the patients found to have articular cartilage lesions, 61% related their symptoms to a specific traumatic event.

Accurate clinical assessment of articular cartilage pathology and precise determination of surgical indications and significance of intraarticular defects identified during arthroscopic examination have not been completely optimized. In many cases, chondral lesions present in association with other confounding clinical pathology including ligamentous patholaxity, meniscus tears, patella instability, and malalignment. An assessment of 378 ACL-deficient knees showed articular cartilage lesions in 157 (42%) cases.[139] More extensive articular cartilage damage was noted in patients found to have a concomitant meniscal tear. In addition, it is difficult to determine if the injury to the cartilage resulted from the trauma, which caused the ligament damage, or if the cartilage lesion is from degeneration secondary to ligamentous instability. Patella instability is also commonly associated with chondral pathology. A review of 39 knees arthroscopically evaluated following acute lateral patella dislocations revealed a 95% (37 of 39) incidence of articular cartilage injuries with all 37 knees having defects noted on the patella surface, most often in the medial facet of the patella.[140] Twelve of the 37 knees (32%) had cartilage damage to the lateral femoral condyle as well. Aroen et al.[141] studied 993 patients undergoing knee arthroscopy for pain and found that 66% of all patients had damage to the articular cartilage, while only 70 (7%) had isolated cartilage lesions without associated pathology.

In an attempt to define the clinical significance of cartilage lesions with associated pathology, Drongowski et al.[142] studied patients with an articular cartilage injury or meniscus tear in ACL-deficient knees. Of 99 patients, almost 60% had associated chondral pathology. While patients with an associated meniscus tear reported no loss of function, patients with hyaline cartilage injuries subjectively reported decreased ability to run. This study suggests that operative intervention may be indicated when chondral pathology is found in association with ACL tears. However, no consensus has been reached and a study by Shelbourne et al.[143] reported on 6- to 8-year follow-up of 101 patients with a chondral defect following ACL reconstruction in which the chondral defect was not treated (Fig. 2.11). A statistically significant difference was noted in the subjective scores in those patients

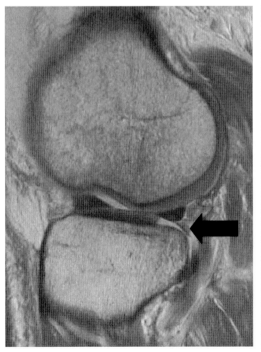 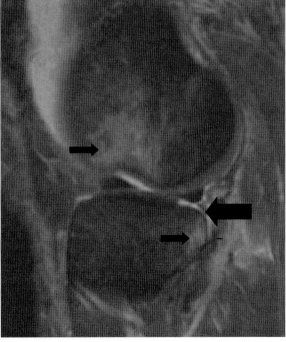

A   B

FIG. 2.11. (A) Sagittal proton density MRI. (B) Sagittal proton density fat suppressed sequence status post anterior cruciate ligament rupture with characteristic bone confusions (small arrows) and discrete defect at the posterior lateral tibial plateau (large arrows).

with chondral defects at approximately 6 years; however, both groups report excellent overall function clinically when followed for 12 years.

Natural History of Articular Cartilage Pathology

In general, there are three types of cartilage tissue: hyaline (articular), elastic (nose and ear), and fibrocartilage (meniscus, wrist triangular fibrocartilage complex, and the glenoid and acetabular labrum). Articular cartilage is commonly found lining diarthrodial joints, and it is approximately 2 to 4 mm in thickness, with the thicker areas usually found at the periphery of concave surfaces (medial tibial plateau) and the center of convex surfaces (patella). The function of articular cartilage is to provide load transmission via a low-friction articular surface. Its function is highly dependent on its structural composition and organization. Articular cartilage is avascular and aneural, consisting primarily of an extensive extracellular matrix that makes up 99% of its dry weight composition, while the remaining 1% is made up of chondrocytes.[144] The function of the chondrocytes is to produce, maintain, and subtend the extracellular matrix. They are metabolically active, increasing function in response to mechanical joint pressures. The matrix is mainly composed of water, making up 60% to 80% of its weight with collagen (95% type II, 5% types IV, VI, IX, X, and XI), and proteoglycan aggregates making up the remaining portion of the matrix.[145] The components of articular cartilage maintain a dynamic state of dependence to regulate the hydration and nutrition that subsequently affect loading, viscoelastic properties, and the coefficient of friction across the joint.

Ultrastructurally, hyaline cartilage is organized as four zones, each with different collagen orientation, cellular shape, profile, and matrix composition.[146] The *tangential* zone is the most superficial zone and contains collagen-oriented parallel to the joint surface and flattened chondrocytes. It is covered superficially by the lamina splendens, a thin electron-dense layer, approximately 0.5 μm, thick that provides structural protection. The second or *transitional* zone contains collagen oriented obliquely with spherical chondrocytes. The *radial* zone lies deep to the transitional zone, and its fibers and chondrocytes align perpendicular to the joint surface. The tidemark serves as demarcation between the noncalcified deep radial zone and the calcified cartilage. The collagen fibers of the radial zone cross the tidemark to anchor into the zone of calcified cartilage.

Focal articular cartilage lesions respond to injury differently depending on the lesion depth.[144–146] A chondral (superficial) lesion whether partial or full thickness (not penetrating the subchondral plate) often responds to injury either without a repair response or with incomplete repair. A full-thickness injury is likely to undergo a disordered repair response. An osteochondral lesion by definition penetrates the subchondral plate, which can result in an inflammatory response with release of bone marrow constituents as well as cytokines or proinflammatory mediators that can contribute to a healing or attempted repair. An MRI may be used effectively to differentiate between chondral and osteochondral defects.

Osteochondritis Dissecans Versus Osteochondral Fracture Versus Osteoarthritis

In many clinical studies, cases of osteochondritis dissecans (OCD), osteochondral fracture (OCF), and osteoarthritis (OA) may be combined and reported on, although the pathoetiology, presentation, natural history, and treatment options vastly differ. Osteoarthritis typically presents in the older patient (>60 years old). It tends to be chronic and progressive with symptoms of swelling, warmth, or stiffness. Patients with either OCD or OCF tend to be younger, typically presenting in the second or third decades with a history of trauma and mechanical symptoms such as catching and locking.

Osteochondral fractures typically present with more fragmentation and perimeter irregularity than osteochondritis dissecans (Fig. 2.12). Forty percent to 50% of the time, OCF occurs over the medial femoral condyle or medial patella facet.[147,148] It may present in a manner similar to other knee pathology. Terry et al.[148] reviewed the symptomatology of 18 patients found with isolated chondral fractures; 17 of them presented with a clinical exam consistent with a meniscus tear. Therefore, when a patient undergoes a "negative" arthroscopy for meniscus-related symptoms following trauma, a chondral fracture may be suspected and should be considered.

The term *osteochondritis dissecans* (OCD) refers to a focal region of subchondral bone necrosis with overlying osteochondral separation and detachment[149] (Fig. 2.13). Osteochondritis dissecans is most commonly noted over the lateral aspect of the medial femoral condyle of the knee, accounting for 75% of cases. The patella makes up approximately 15% of cases, with the remainder noted in the weight-bearing surfaces of the medial and lateral femoral condyles.[147] The most significant symptomatic presentation is associated with fragment detachment and resultant loose body formation.

Another traumatic pathologic entity often reported in association with ACL tears is an osseous contusion or bone bruise. This is a traumatic injury to the subchondral bone and overlying articular cartilage and is associated with marrow edema and retention of normal bony architecture. Plain roentgenograms are often negative, but on MRI marrow edema is commonly found, particularly over the medial aspect of the lateral femoral condyle and the posterior third of the lateral tibial plateau[150] (Fig. 2.14). The approach to an isolated osseous contusion consists of symptomatic treatment and activity restriction. In general, a favorable prognosis is noted; however, the presence of a concurrent underlying injury to the ligaments, meniscus, and cartilage

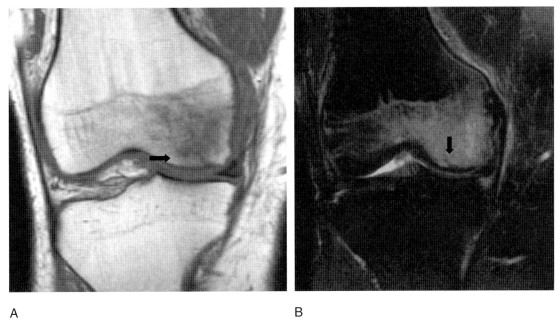

A   B

FIG. 2.12. (A) Coronal T1-weighted sequence of subchondral fracture (arrow) of medial femoral condyle. (B) Coronal T2 fat-saturated weighted sequence of bone contusion and subchondral fracture (arrow) of the medial femoral condyle.

must be considered. The long-term natural history of osseous contusions is yet to be clearly defined, particularly as more compelling biochemical mechanisms of articular cartilage degradation are elucidated.

Osteoarthritis is a chronic and progressive condition that is associated with a multifactorial etiology. Factors such as trauma, obesity, malnutrition, metabolic disorders, and genetics may play a role. An MRI of the arthritic knee demonstrates joint

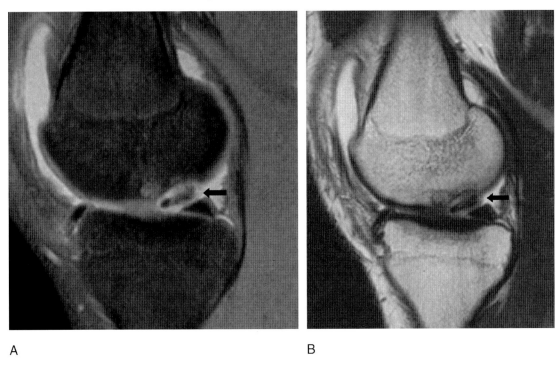

A   B

FIG. 2.13. (A) Sagittal proton density fat-suppressed sequence of osteochondritis dissecans lesion of the medial femoral condyle (arrow). (B) Sagittal T2-weighted sequence of osteochondritis dissecans lesion of the medial femoral condyle (arrow).

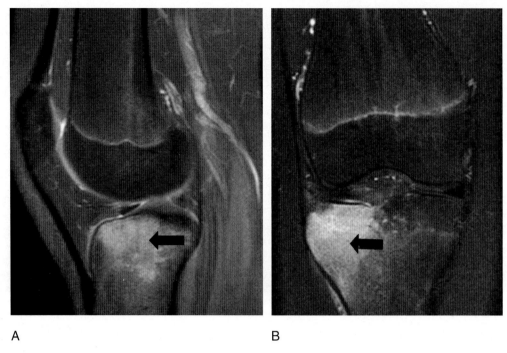

A   B

FIG. 2.14. MRI. (A) Sagittal proton density fat-suppressed sequence and (B) Coronal proton density fat-suppressed sequence demonstrating a bone contusion with the lateral tibial plateau (arrows).

space narrowing, articular cartilage degeneration, hypertrophic osteophytes subchondral sclerosis, and edema (Fig. 2.15). Osteoarthritis is often found in association with injuries such as meniscal and ligament pathology, which is likely representative of a joint degenerative process rather than injury or trauma.[151]

Classification

Classification of chondral pathology can be based on radiography, histology, clinical exam, or direct visualization during arthroscopy. An effective grading and assessment system should be easy to use, comprehensive, have good

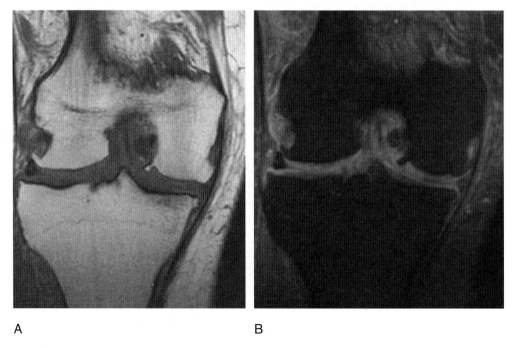

A   B

FIG. 2.15. (A) Coronal T1-weighted sequence of generalized osteoarthritis of the knee. (B) Coronal proton density fat-suppressed sequence of generalized osteoarthritis of the knee.

inter/intraobserver reliability, and diagnostic and prognostic significance and correlation. The standard for grading articular cartilage integrity has been intraoperative arthroscopic assessment. The most widely used visual classification system for chondral lesions is the Outerbridge classification system (Table 2.5; see also Table 2.2).[152] The original Outerbridge classification system was described to identify the extent of chondral wear associated with chondromalacia patellae and noted at arthrotomy. Defects were measured with calipers and described as follows: grade I, cartilage with softening and swelling; grade II, fragmentation and fissuring in an area half an inch or less in diameter; grade III, same as grade II but an area more than half an inch in diameter; and grade IV, erosion of cartilage down to bone.[153] The modified classification was described by Insall: grade I, softening; grade II, fissuring; grade III, fibrillation; and grade IV, exposed subchondral bone (without reference to defect size).[154]

The Noyes and Stabler grading system is also based on the visual inspection of the lesion during arthroscopy. The grading assesses four components: the articular surface, the depth, the diameter, and location of the lesion. This more comprehensive classification system has been shown to be applicable for use in chondral lesions.[155] Bauer and Jackson[156] classified articular cartilage lesions based on a more descriptive variability of damage patterns. Type I is a linear pattern. Type II is stellate. Type III is described as a flap. Type IV is described as a crater. Type V is represented by fibrillation. Type VI is indicative of subchondral bone exposure. Hunt et al.[157] described a new method of classification that assesses lesions based on location as well as depth and size, while taking into account the overall function, chronicity, and involvement of other structures. In this classification, the femur and tibia are divided into ten zones and the patella into six zones. The lesions are recorded diagrammatically based on intraoperative arthroscopic evaluation. Associated meniscus and ligament pathology are recorded on the same diagrams. Overall, Hunt et al. demonstrated good interobserver reliability and an accurate overall assessment of articular cartilage lesions.

Clinical patient evaluation may include subjective and objective findings as well as functional assessment tools. Measures that were initially described to assess ligament injury or osteoarthritis are currently being applied to chondral pathology including the Lysholm knee score, the Western Ontario and McMaster Universities Osteoarthritis Index (WOMAC), and the Knee Injury and Osteoarthritis Outcome Score (KOOS).[158] The Lysholm knee score is a subjective assessment of function measuring eight domains: limping, locking, stair climbing,

pain, support, instability, swelling, and squatting. A score of 0 to 100 is calculated based on the individual scores in each domain; a higher score means higher function. The Lysholm score has been validated for use as an effective assessment tool for chondral pathology in the knee.[159]

The WOMAC score is applicable to arthritis pathology of both the knee and hip. The index is designed to measure the dimensions of pain, disability, and joint stiffness. It is a self-administered 24-question assessment associated with numerous studies supporting its reliability and validity in multiple different languages and cultures.[160] The KOOS is a measure that was introduced based on the WOMAC score. This is a self-administered assessment of five categories: pain, symptoms, activities of daily living, sport/recreation function, and knee-related quality of life. This measure has proven reliable and reproducible in evaluation of patients with knee pathology and is being applied to articular cartilage lesions in an acute as well as chronic setting.[161] The Cincinnati Knee Rating System is a functional assessment based on six abilities essential for the participation in sports: walking; climbing stairs; squatting/kneeling; straight running; jumping/landing; and hard twists, cuts, or pivots.[158]

In 1998, the International Cartilage Repair Society (ICRS) established a grading system of articular cartilage injuries based on the assessment of the lesion architecture, size, depth, precise location, and a description of the opposing surface extent of the lesion[157] (Fig. 2.16). The ICRS Cartilage Injury Evaluation Package is a two-part evaluation completed by the patient as well as the surgeon.[162] The patient completes the International Knee Documentation Committee (IKDC) subjective knee evaluation form as part of the overall packet. It is scored from 0 to 100; a higher score means higher function. The surgeon's evaluation consists of seven domains: effusion, passive motion deficit, ligament examination, compartment findings, harvest site pathology, x-ray findings, and functional testing. The first three receive scores while the remaining domains are used qualitatively in the perioperative setting. These measures are used in conjunction with documentation of surgical methodology and histologic grading.

Clinical Examination

Knee chondral pathology may be initially diagnosed on history and physical exam in the patient who presents with mechanical symptoms including catching, locking, and crepitus. Patients with significant isolated chondral defects, however, may also present with less focal knee pain and recurrent effusions. The clinician must have a high index of suspicion in this patient to precisely diagnose a chondral defect. On examination, flexion of the joint may cause tenderness in the weight-bearing portion overlying the defect. Pain elicited at 30 degrees of flexion corresponds with the tibial spine coming into contact with the lateral aspect of the medial femoral condyle as is typical in OCD and OCF lesions. Wilson's sign is described as pain elicited on examination by internally rotating the tibia during knee extension between 30 and 90 degrees and subsequent relief with external rotation.

TABLE 2.5. Outerbridge classification.

Grade	Description
0	Normal cartilage
I	Softening and swelling
II	Partial-thickness defect, fissures less than 1.5-cm diameter
III	Fissures that reach subchondral bone, diameter greater than 1.5 cm
IV	Exposed subchondral bone

ICRS Grade 0 – Normal

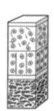

ICRS Grade I – Nearly Normal

A   B

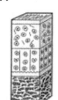 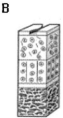

Superficial lesions. Soft indentation (A) and/or superficial fissures and cracks (B)

ICRS Grade II – Abnormal

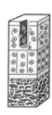

Lesions extending down to <50% of cartilage depth

ICRS Grade III– Severely Abnormal

A   B   C   D

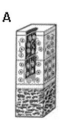 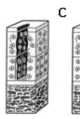 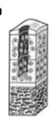

Cartilage defects extending down >50% of cartilage depth (A) as well as down to calcified layer (B) and down to but not through the subchondral bone (C). Blisters are included in this Grade (D)

ICRS Grade IV – Severely Abnormal

A   B

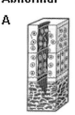 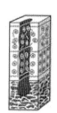

A

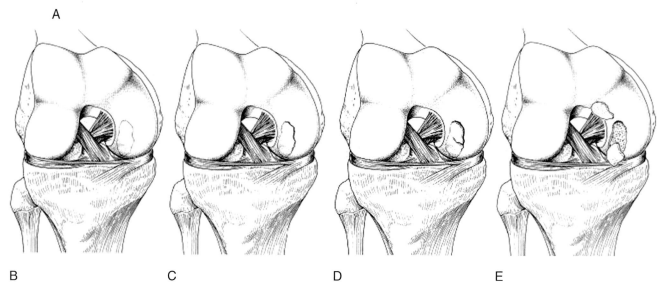

B   C   D   E

FIG. 2.16. (A) International Cartilage Repair Society (ICRS) classification systems for articular cartilage and osteochondritis dissecans (OCD). (B) ICRS OCD I: stable, continuity; softened area covered by intact cartilage. (C) ICRS OCD II: partial discontinuity, stable on probing. (D) ICRS OCD III: complete discontinuity, "dead in situ," not dislocated. (E) ICRS OCD IV: dislocated fragment, loose within the bed or empty defect. (From Brittberg,[162] with permission of ICRS.).

At this position of internal rotation, the tibial eminence comes in contact with the OCD lesion in the medial femoral condyle, resulting in a positive pain response.[163]

The clinician must consider articular cartilage pathology as well as the possibility of an osteochondral fracture in cases of trauma and an acutely painful knee particularly if a hemarthrosis is present. Hardaker et al.[164] evaluated 132 acutely injured knees associated with hemarthrosis. They found 8% of all patients had an isolated osteochondral fracture and 16% of all patients who presented with ACL tears had associated hyaline cartilage damage. An injury that transmits axial and rotational force to the knee joint (e.g., planting/twisting injury as occurs with an ACL tear) can result in a chondral injury. In addition, following direct trauma to the anterior knee area, patellofemoral joint (dashboard knee) injury is commonly associated with chondral impaction. In general, osteochondral fractures in the knee are noted to occur in approximately 4% of all trauma.[148] These patients with chondral impaction injury may be overlooked since plain radiographs may not usually define the true extent of the injury.

Treatment Options

Current treatment options include operative as well as nonoperative methods. Nonoperative treatment options for articular defects include the use of steroid injections, antiinflammatory medications, and bracing. In addition, physical therapy may be prescribed for conditioning and inflammation reduction. The biosurgical treatment options for articular cartilage defects have been rapidly evolving. Operative treatments include marrow stimulation, osteochondral autograft transplantation (OAT), osteochondral allograft transplantation, ACI, and more recently the use of bioresorbable synthetic scaffolds. Many investigators have attempted to enhance the healing of articular cartilage by drilling, abrading, or microfracturing the subchondral bone. Chondral injury that does not penetrate the underlying subchondral bone has resulted in an unpredictable or absent healing response, while those defects that involve violation of the subchondral bone may result in a fibrous tissue healing scar repair response characterized by proliferation of type I collagen.[165–167] By perforating the subchondral plate, marrow stimulation can release marrow elements and increase exposure to inflammatory cells, mesenchymal stem cells, and cytokines that are effective in spontaneous repair.[168] A recent prospective study by Mithoefer et al.[169] showed significant functional improvement in the use of microfracture in 48 patients with isolated full-thickness articular cartilage defects. Clinical evaluation at an average follow-up of 48 months resulted in 67% of patients reporting good to excellent results, with 25% reporting fair and 8% poor. The defects were also evaluated by assessment of defect filling on MRI; good defect filling was found in 54% of patients, with moderate fill in 29% and poor fill in 17%. The authors found that defect fill on MRI corresponded to functional scores with improved function in

those with higher fill grade. Images are provided below as a demonstration of the use of MRI in the evaluation of healing after microfracture (Fig. 2.17).

Osteochondral autograft transplantation is a method for transferring cylindrical plugs of native hyaline tissue including the underlying bone tissue from a less loaded region of the knee to the symptomatic lesion site via arthrotomy or arthroscopically. There are a number of proprietary systems available such as MosaicPlasty (Smith and Nephew, Andover, MA), OATS (Osteochondral Autograft Transfer System, Arthrex, Naples, FL) and COR (Consistent Osteochondral Repair, Depuy Mitek, Raynham, MA). The technique has been shown to result in transfer of viable hyaline tissue that can be securely press-fit into the defect and provides a predictable source of zoned hyaline-like tissue using a relatively less invasive method with a shorter term healing site profile[170,171] (Fig. 2.18). Several studies have reported good results, with 79% to 92% of patients (depending on the treated defect site) reporting clinical improvement at intermediate–term follow–up.[172–174]

Gudas et al.[175] compared osteochondral autograft transplantation with microfracture in a randomized prospective clinical trial in 57 athletes. Over a 3-year period, 96% of patients undergoing the OAT procedure had good or excellent results compared to 52% of patients undergoing microfracture; 93% of OAT patients returned to preinjury athletics at a mean of 6 months compared to 52% of microfracture patients. The use of autograft offers a technique with no risk of rejection or disease transmission. The disadvantages include size limitations in transplanting osteochondral autograft to adequately fill large defects, raising concern over donor-site morbidity.[176] In addition, the technique can be challenging, and technical errors may lead to suboptimal results.[177] Figure 2.19 displays an MRI of a failed OATS procedure. Osteochondral allograft transplantation is a technique that can be used as a salvage procedure for resurfacing larger lesions without concern for donor-site morbidity. The osteochondral allografts can be obtained fresh or cryopreserved and are sized and shaped to match the defect in the recipient.

Gross et al.[178] reported on a 95% 5-year survival (85% at 10 years) of fresh femoral condylar allograft in 60 patients. They also showed a 95% 5-year, 80% 10-year, and 65% 15-year survival rate in 65 patients who received fresh tibial plateau allograft. Jamali et al.[179] demonstrated improvement in pain, function, and range of motion, and a lower risk of progression to arthritis in 18 patients receiving fresh osteochondral allografts in treatment of patellofemoral joint defects.

Until recently, few studies compared osteochondral allograft to autograft in treatment of articular cartilage pathology. Glenn et al.[180] demonstrated that osteochondral autograft and allograft transplants performed on the medial femoral condyles of 18 canine models did not significantly differ in gross, histologic, biomechanical, radiographic or MRI evaluation at 3 or 6 months. The use of allograft would alleviate the problem of donor-site morbidity often found in osteochondral autograft transplantation, and therefore larger grafts may be

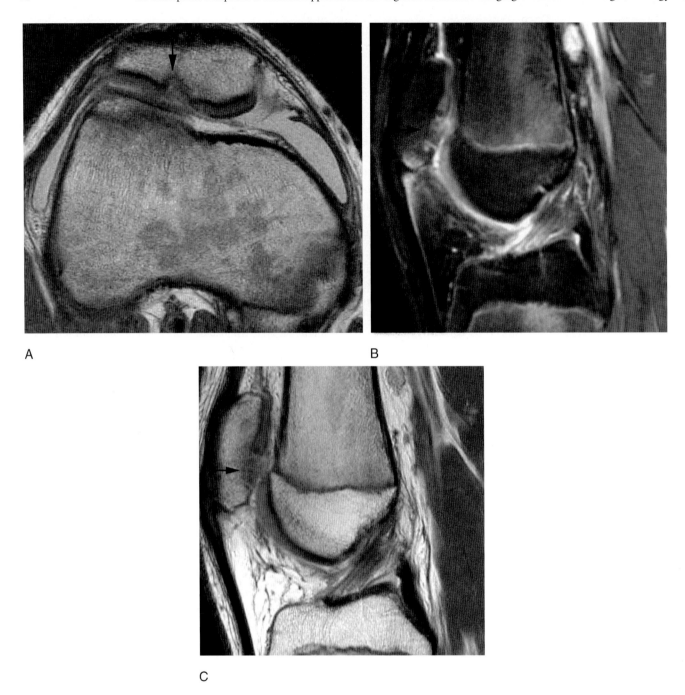

FIG. 2.17. (A) Axial proton density MRI, (B) Sagittal proton density fat suppressed MRI and (C) Sagittal proton density MRI of a 15 year old male after microfracture of a patella chondral defect. Note the presence of fibrocartilage (arrow) filling the defect.

used (Fig. 2.20). However, osteochondral allograft transplantation is associated with certain disadvantages, including the potential for disease transmission, graft rejection, cost issues, and procurement limitations.

Autologous chondrocyte implantation is a cell-based technique in which autologous chondrocytes are harvested arthroscopically, then cultured and expanded ex vivo for several weeks, and then implanted beneath a periosteal patch via arthrotomy during a second surgery (Carticel, Genzyme

Corp., Cambridge, MA). Autologous chondrocyte implantation has been reported to result in hyaline–like tissue with durable clinical and biomechanical results noted in 84% of cases and survivorship at extended follow–up.[181–184] Postoperatively, a successful result will show incorporation of the newly implanted tissue, a flush surface, good volume filling, and mild edema (Fig. 2.21). A more recent study, however, found that at 2-year follow-up in patients treated with ACI who underwent follow-up second-look tissue biopsies, only

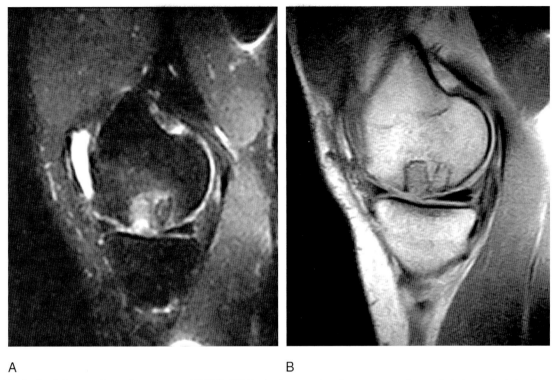

FIG. 2.18. (A) Sagittal short-tau inversion recovery (STIR). (B) Sagittal proton density sequences demonstrate transplanted autogenous osteochondral plugs within the medial femoral condyle at 5 months postoperatively.

39% of the treated defects were noted to be filled with hyaline cartilage, while 43% were noted to be filled with fibrocartilage and 18% with no healing tissue response at all. These histologic results were noted to be similar in a controlled comparison treatment study group that underwent microfracture, and both patient cohorts (at 2-year follow–up) had similar clinical outcomes.[185] In this study, only two of 40 ACI patients experienced graft failure compared to one microfracture patient; however, arthroscopic debridement was performed in 10 of 40 (25%) ACI patients for tissue hypertrophy compared to only four (10%) in the microfracture group.[185] Failure of ACI is evident on MRI by intense marrow edema, bony overgrowth,

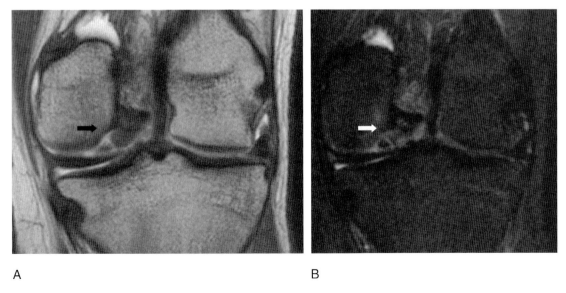

FIG. 2.19. (A) Coronal T1-weighted post sequence and (B) Coronal STIR sequence pre–intraarticular contrast (MR arthrogram) transplant (arrow) of an OCD lesion of medial femoral condyle.

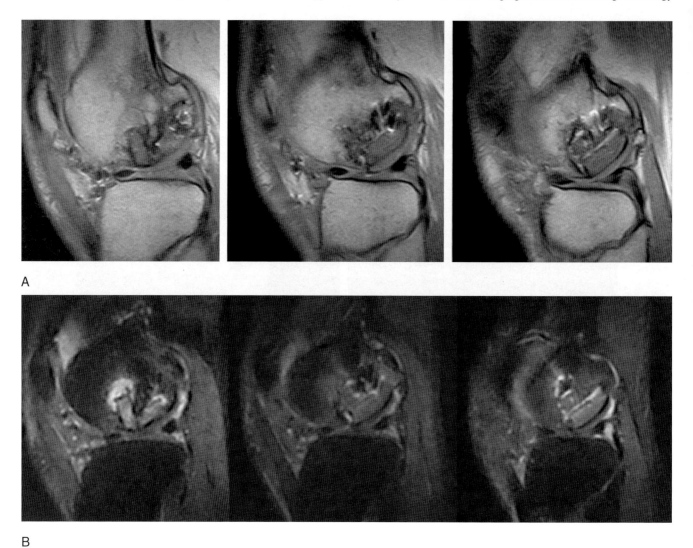

A

B

FIG. 2.20. (A) Sagittal proton density (PD)-weighted sequences and (B) Sagittal STIR weighted sequences status post–osteochondral allograft transplant of focal lateral femoral condyle osteonecrosis.

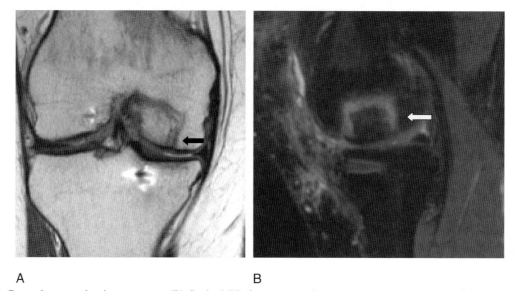

A   B

FIG. 2.21. (A) Coronal proton density sequence. (B) Sagittal PD fat suppressed sequence status post–successful osteochondral allograft (arrow) of the medial femoral condyle.

periosteal hypertrophy including a depressed or disrupted periosteal graft, and a fissured or gapped interface between the repair tissue and native tissue.

More recently, synthetic bioresorbable scaffolds have been introduced to treat osteochondral defects in the knee. Multiple scaffold designs have been cited in the literature.[186–189] A bioresorbable synthetic scaffold design that we have had success with is the TruFit Bone Graft Substitute Plugs (Osteobiologics, San Antonio, TX). These bioresorbable constructs are highly porous and are composed of a polylactide glycolide copolymer and calcium sulfate base. These cylindrical implants are effective in filling osteochondral defects and have been used as an adjunct for microfracture to augment a more congruent surface. Figure 2.22 shows an MRI of a knee following repair of an articular cartilage lesion with a bioresorbable synthetic scaffold.

The advent of new technology and molecular medicine in orthopedics continues to introduce the possibility of new surgical treatment options. Gene-modified therapy and tissue engineering hold great promise; they have the ability through gene transfer to deliver a therapeutic protein to a target cell or tissue in order to induce cells or tissue to engage in repair or regeneration and amplify healing. Various approaches may be taken using human recombinant gene models.[190–195] One approach includes the selection and transduction (or transfection) of a candidate gene that selectively codes for expression of a specific therapeutic protein that would hypothetically contribute to articular cartilage repair or regeneration by acting on chondroprogenitor cells. Once the gene has transduced the target cell, it would then function as a source of the therapeutic protein or bioactive factors, which upon their release would result in a higher quality structural repair tissue.

Another future trend on the horizon includes the application of anabolic factors to enhance repair. Basic science investigation has been reported on methods to introduce bioactive peptides onto scaffolds. Biologic materials that are being investigated include bone morphogenic protein (BMP) 2 and 7 and platelet-rich plasma. Through the use of gene therapy, the precise identification, delivery, and enhancement of growth factors and cytokines such as insulin-like growth factor-I (IGF-I), platelet-derived growth factor (PDGF), and transforming growth factor-β (TGF-β) have been associated with promising laboratory results. With the use of gene-modified tissue engineering, the future seems to point toward a more biologically based treatment approach.

Clinical Application of Roentgenograms and Magnetic Resonance Imaging

The use of radiographic images is an integral part of the clinical approach to evaluate articular cartilage pathology. However, plain radiographs remain limited and are not sensitive enough to be used for evaluation of certain articular cartilage lesions. A recent study by Wright et al.[196] demonstrated in 349 patients presenting with knee pain that standing anteroposterior and 45-degree posteroanterior x-rays both have reduced sensitivity in detecting grade I or II type articular cartilage lesions when evaluated arthroscopically. Magnetic resonance imaging has a more

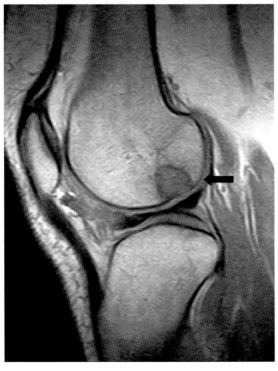 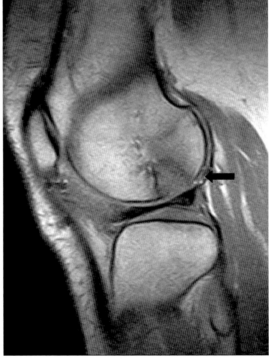

A B

FIG. 2.22. (A,B) Sagittal PD-weighted sequence after successful postoperative resorbable copolymer scaffold placement (arrows).

precise application in evaluation and detection of articular cartilage. Conventional MR sequences depict normal articular cartilage as a homogeneous intermediate signal intensity, whereas high-resolution MR can be used to assess the individual layers of the cartilage and structural abnormalities. Understanding and accurately interpreting the appearance of articular cartilage on MRI on different imaging sequences requires an understanding of the zones of articular cartilage. For articular cartilage lesions in particular, higher field–strength scanners (1.5 T or newly clinically available 3.0 T) are necessary, whereas the in-office 0.2-T scanners are not yet reliable.[134] It is important that the orthopedist communicate clinically correlative information with the musculoskeletal radiologist, as articular cartilage lesions are likely to be overlooked on traditional MRI sequences, whereas cartilage specific sequences are more sensitive.[134] Magnetic resonance imaging can be extremely useful to the orthopedist in accurately depicting the location of the lesion, as well as the size, depth, stability, and character of the lesion, and play a role in therapeutic decision making and surgical planning.

More recently, studies have shown that MRI may also be a valuable tool to evaluate the integrity of treated articular lesions postoperatively. It is not only being used as means to identify and classify the lesion itself, but also has been shown to successfully evaluate the lesions following surgical intervention and validate the repair.[135] Information following surgical intervention may differ depending on the procedure performed. The use of MRI to evaluate defects following microfracture is based on assessment of surface morphology as well as fill defect and subchondral marrow edema.[197,198] Early in the postoperative period, marrow edema may be prevalent, and hyperintense signal changes are evident that dissipate over time.

Following osteochondral autograft, the surgeon is most concerned with evaluation of the incorporation of the transplanted plugs, the nature of the bone, the defect fill, and any associated cyst, clefts, or fluid dissection identifying morphologic changes. High-resolution FSE proton density and fat-suppressed 3D SPGR sequences have proven effective in assessing vascularity, identifying repair tissue, and assessing the plugs relationship to surrounding articular cartilage and bone. However, fat-suppressed 3D SPGR sequences have the potential disadvantage of increased artifact susceptibility related to metallic debris.[197–199] Magnetic resonance imaging may also be applicable following autologous chondrocyte implantation, providing evaluation of the surface contour of the repair, the volume of defect filling, integration of repair tissue, and periosteal graft.[197,200] While the ability to evaluate the morphologic changes of the repair is quite valuable to the surgeon, the functional importance of signal changes, specifically associated with marrow edema, is still to be determined.

Algorithm

Clinical practice guidelines are useful to determine who should be treated nonoperatively and who should be treated surgically (Table 2.6). Strict use of indications in clinical practice may

TABLE 2.6. Surgical indications to repair articular cartilage lesions.

1. Acute traumatic lesions ≥1 cm^2 in diameter
2. Focal nondegenerative lesions and cases without history of gout, rheumatoid disease, sepsis, and systemic disease
3. Distal femoral condyle and trochlea lesions
4. Symptomatic grade IV lesions and grade 2, 3 and 4 OCD lesions (ICRS classification)
5. Associated lesions in active patients undergoing associated procedures (ACL, high tibial osteotomy, or meniscal allograft replacement)
6. Aligned, stable, and meniscal intact knee
7. Symptomatic patients after a failed prior cartilage resurfacing procedure
8. Body mass index less than 25 to 30
9. Rehabilitation compliance

not always be helpful, in that many clinical case scenarios do not precisely fit the model. Nonetheless, indication guidelines may serve as a reference from which an organized approach can be employed. One clinical approach to the patient with an articular cartilage lesion that considers both the lesion quality and patient profile is described in Table 2.7. The clinical guideline takes into account patient preferences, functional assessment and goals, history, physical exam, diagnostics, lesion definition, and rehabilitation compliance. Figure 2.23 is an algorithm that we use in conjunction with the patient profile described above.

Clinical Summary

The clinical approach to focal articular cartilage defects starts with precise assessment of symptoms and diagnosis, sorting out associated pathology, and determining whether all abnormalities should be treated at the index procedure or in stages. Nonoperative measures are always considered and carried out prior to surgery and concurrent with treatment counseling regarding various risks versus benefits, potential complications, prognosis, and outcomes, as well as natural history. Lesion size as determined on MRI or at the time of arthroscopic assessment is important; most symptomatic lesions over 100 mm^2 are appropriate for operative intervention.[201–203] Perimeter integrity and lesion containment are also important to consider, as a shouldered focal lesion may be associated with different rim stress loading profiles than less contained defects.[203]

Extremity mechanical axis alignment, physiologic and chronologic age, body mass index, and the potential presentation of early focal degenerative joint disease without history of correlative trauma should be taken into account. Site is a consideration, as certain patellofemoral lesions may have a different symptomatic presentation than femoral condylar lesions. Other factors include whether the patient is attempting to return to high-impact sports, work, or functional activities. Decision making regarding surgical options

TABLE 2.7. Clinical patient profile practice guideline for surgical treatment of focal articular cartilage lesions in the knee.

A. PATIENT PREFERENCES
  1. FUNCTIONAL RATING
    Manual labor/high-impact activities/competitive sport goals
    YES: TREAT; NO: MONITOR
  2. DEFINED SYMPTOMATOLOGY
    Symptomatic/pain/effusion/mechanical complaints
    YES: TREAT; NO: MONITOR
  3. REHABILITATION COMPLIANCE
    Patient acceptance of recovery time
    YES: TREAT; NO: MONITOR
B. HISTORY ANALYSIS
  1. TRAUMATIC
    Acute defined traumatic lesion versus degenerative lesion
    YES: TREAT; NO: MONITOR
  2. FAILED PRIOR PROCEDURE FOR FOCAL LESION (no prior associated complications)
    Failed debridement, marrow stimulation, osteochondral transfer, ACI
    YES: TREAT; NO: MONITOR
C. PHYSICAL EXAMINATION
  1. WEIGHT AND CONCOMITANT PATHOLOGY
    Body mass index less than 25 to 30/mechanical axis not within affected compartment/ligament stability/ipsilateral meniscus more than two thirds intact
    YES: TREAT; NO: MONITOR AND/OR CORRECT
  2. AGE-ASSOCIATED MEDICAL CONDITIONS
    <55 years/no significant associated medical history including infections, collagen vascular or metabolic disorders
    YES: TREAT; NO: MONITOR
D. DIAGNOSTICS/LESION DEFINITION
  1. PREOPERATIVE IMAGING DEFINES LESION
    Symptoms and radiographic diagnostic studies are correlated
    YES: TREAT; NO: MONITOR
  2. LESION PATTERN
    Focal pattern defined versus diffuse, degenerative and/or bipolar lesions
    YES: TREAT; NO: MONITOR
  3. LESION SITE
    Weight-bearing sites, condyle >trochlea >patellar >plateau
    YES: TREAT; NO: MONITOR

Source: Sgaglione and Abrutyn,[147] with permission.

is dependent on patient goals, expectations, compliance with rehabilitation, tolerance, expectation, and perception of methodology and prognosis. Finally, surgeon preference will be shaped by experience, the patient's comorbidities, and in certain cases reimbursement and regulatory issues. By and large, most procedures at this time have limited controlled comparison data to support clear-cut advantages of one method over another. It is therefore essential to consider a multitude of factors when reviewing treatments. There are many treatment options that the orthopedist may employ in treating articular cartilage lesions and most often more than one technique may be acceptable for any given lesion (Fig. 2.24).

Future of Magnetic Resonance Imaging and Articular Cartilage

There has been extremely rapid growth in the field of radiology, particularly with the technologic advances in MRI. Magnetic resonance imaging manufacturers are consistently introducing faster and stronger imaging equipment, allowing the radiologist to achieve better image quality, with higher image contrast and resolution, while decreasing acquisition time and reducing the probability of artifact related to patient motion. Manufacturers have recently introduced the 3.0-T MRI; however, these units are not readily available to most community-based orthopedic surgeons. Higher field strength will provide more detailed evaluation of articular cartilage based on a greater signal-to-noise ratio, keeping other variables equal. However, clinical observations have revealed that due to the intrinsic properties of articular cartilage, most notably increased T1 relaxation time, and relative increase in chemical shift artifact, improvement in image quality has been limited. Another new device, joint specific radiofrequency coils, is not yet widely available to operate with high field strength imaging systems, further limiting our potential to increase image quality.

As MRI technologies improve, clinical applications, access, and overall acceptance is likely to follow. It is reasonable to predict that in the near future, routine MRI of articular cartilage injuries will improve in detail and will become as

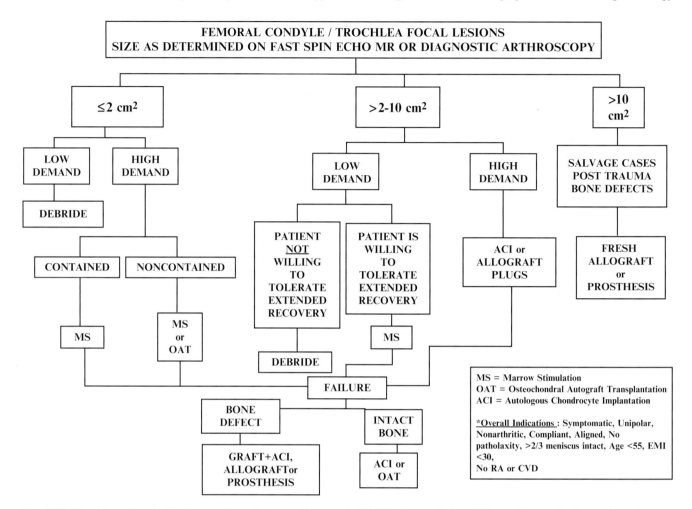

FIG. 2.23. Algorithm of surgical indications for articular cartilage repair. BMI, body mass index; CVD, cardiovascular disease; RA, rheumatoid arthritis. (From Sgaglione and Abrutyn,[147] with permission.).

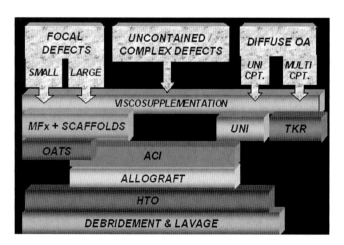

FIG. 2.24. Illustration of surgical possibilities for articular cartilage damage. ACI, autologous chondrocyte implantation; CPT, compartment; HTO, high tibial osteotomy; MFx, microfracture; OA, osteoarthritis; OAT, osteochondral autograft transplantation; TKR, total knee replacement.

integral a part of the postoperative assessment as it is for the preoperative diagnosis.

Newer molecular imaging techniques are being used to target the biochemical and structural properties of articular cartilage, such as dGEMRIC and T2 mapping, which are based on the extracellular matrix contents, electrical interaction between contrast agents and negatively charged proteoglycans, and type II collagen stratification.[204–206] The technique of dGEMRIC relies on an intravenous contrast-based MRI technique based on the premise that negatively charged proteoglycans are altered and reduced following articular cartilage degeneration, leaving a more positively charged joint surface; negatively charged gadolinium contrast should theoretically adhere to the sites of pathology. After a delay, T1-weighted measurements are performed, taking advantage of the T1-weighted properties of gadolinium, the contrast agent. Unfortunately, a limitation of this technique is that we cannot be certain that the distribution of contrast within the depleted cartilage tissue is solely based on these electrical charge interactions. Injured tissue typically receives increased blood flow and contrast enhancement may be multifactorial.

Another promising imaging technique, referred to as T2 mapping, evaluates articular cartilage structure quantitatively based on the relative T2 relaxation times, which differ based on collagen orientation, zone stratification, water content, and patient age. This method potentially allows for a numerical as well as visual (using digital color maps) determination of structural integrity of chondral surfaces. T2 values are lower in the deep zone of articular cartilage where collagen orientation is perpendicular to the subchondral bone. In the transitional zone, T2 values increase potentially due to change in structure and collagen orientation, which tends to be more random. T2 values are highest in the superficial zone, where collagen orientation is parallel to the surface. Another variable to consider is the orientation of fibers relative to the orientation of the magnetic field (B0). As the distance from B0 increases, TR values increase up to a certain threshold (approximately 55 degrees), commonly referred to as the magic angle effect. Increasing T2 values also correspond to areas of cartilage degeneration and injury, and researchers are applying this method of evaluating articular cartilage, which includes visual colored "maps" corresponding to areas of degeneration and injury.[207] Comparison with normal studies allows us to numerically define the extent of degeneration/injury.

Another developing technique is the use of sodium rather than hydrogen as a potential method in evaluating proteoglycan content. It also functions based on the charge characteristics. Wheaton et al.[208] demonstrated the ability to assess proteoglycan depletion in knee articular cartilage of pig models with reliable results. However, this technique does require more sophisticated MRI equipment, takes longer, and has lower signal-to-noise ratio.[199,209] These new applications allow us to detect changes in the structural integrity of articular cartilage, which to this point we have extrapolated based on MRI appearance. They all represent evolving and potentially significantly more accurate and precise methods to diagnose and define articular cartilage pathology, tissue repair response, and clinically correlative validation of symptoms, outcomes, and lesion resurfacing.[136,190,205,210]

Conclusion

The treatment of articular cartilage pathology continues to be an area of great interest and attention in orthopedic surgery. Evolving clinical approaches and surgical techniques have heightened the need to more precisely define treatment indications and better assess postoperative healing. The use of articular cartilage–specific MRI will continue to play a role in the decision making regarding these lesions. Radiographic evaluation with the use of MRI continues to improve exponentially, and with finer detail being achieved, MRI is quickly becoming the gold standard in evaluation of articular cartilage defects.

References

1. Cooper C. Occupational activity and the risk of osteoarthritis. J Rheumatol 1995;43:10–12.
2. Cova M, Toffanin R. MR microscopy of hyaline cartilage: current status. Eur Radiol 2002;12:814–823.
3. Felson DT. Epidemiology of hip and knee osteoarthritis. Epidemiol Rev 1998;10:1–28.
4. Felson DT, Zhang Y, Hannan MT, et al. The incidence and natural history of knee osteoarthritis in the elderly. The Framingham Osteoarthritis Study: the effects of specific medical conditions on the functional limitations of elders in the Framingham Study. Arthritis Rheum 1995;38(10):1500–1505.
5. Buckwalter JA, Saltzman C, Brown T. The impact of osteoarthritis: implications for research. Clin Orthop Rel Res 2004;427(suppl): S6–15.
6. Guccione AA, Felson DT, Anderson JJ, et al. The effects of specific medical conditions on the functional limitations of elders in the Framingham Study. Am J Public Health 1994;84(3):351–358.
7. Felson DT, Lawrence RC, Dieppe PA, et al. Osteoarthritis: new insights. Part 1: the disease and its risk factors. Ann Intern Med 2000;133(8):635–646.
8. Felson DT. The course of osteoarthritis and factors that affect it. Rheum Dis Clin North Am 1993;19:607–633.
9. Chan WP, Lang P, Stevens MP, et al. Osteoarthritis of the knee: comparison of radiography, CT, and MR imaging to assess extent and severity. AJR 1991;157:799–806.
10. Fife RS, Brandt KD, Braunstein EM, et al. Relationship between arthroscopic evidence of cartilage damage and radiographic evidence of joint space narrowing in early osteoarthritis of the knee. Arthritis Rheum 1991;34:377–382.
11. Armstrong CG, Mow VC. Variations in the intrinsic mechanical properties of human articular cartilage with age, degeneration, and water content. J Bone Joint Surg [Am] 1982;64:88–94.
12. Wojtys E, Wilson M, Buckwalter K, Braunstein E, Martel W. Magnetic resonance imaging of knee hyaline cartilage and intraarticular pathology. Am J Sports Med 1987;15: 455–463.
13. Peterfy CG, van Dijke CF, Janzen DL, et al. Quantification of articular cartilage in the knee with pulsed saturation transfer subtraction and fat-suppressed MR imaging: optimization and validation. Radiology 1994;192:485–491.
14. Hoch DH, Grodzinsky AJ, Koob TJ, Albert ML, Eyre DR. Early changes in material properties of rabbit articular cartilage after meniscectomy. J Orthop Res 1983;1:4–12.
15. Buckwalter JA, Mow VC. Cartilage repair in osteoarthritis. In: Moskowitz RW, Howell DS, Goldberg VM, Mankin HJ, eds. Osteoarthritis, Diagnosis and Medical/Surgical Management, 2nd ed. Philadelphia: Saunders, 1992:71–107.
16. Hayes CW, Balkissoon AA. Magnetic resonance imaging of the musculoskeletal system. II. The hip. Clin Orthop 1996;322:297–309.
17. Fritz RC, Steinbach LS. Magnetic Resonance imaging of the musculoskeletal system. III. The elbow. Clin Orthop 1996;324:321–339.
18. Siegel S, White LM, Brahme S. Magnetic resonance imaging of the musculoskeletal system. V. The wrist. Clin Orthop 1996;332:281–300.
19. Crotty JM, Monu JU, Pope TJ. Magnetic resonance imaging of the musculoskeletal system. IV. The knee. Clin Orthop 1996;330:288–303.

20. Oxner KG. Magnetic resonance imaging of the musculoskeletal system. VI. The shoulder. Clin Orthop 1997;334:354–373.

21. Haygood TM. Magnetic resonance imaging of the musculoskeletal system: VII. The ankle. Clin Orthop 1997;336:318–336.

22. Ruwe PA, Wright J, Randal RL, Lynch JK, Jokl P, McCarthy S. Can MR imaging effectively replace diagnostic radiology? Radiology 1992;183:335–339.

23. Winalski CS, Palmer WE, Rosenthal DI, Weissman BN. Magnetic resonance imaging of rheumatoid arthritis. Radiol Clin North Am 1996;34:243–258.

24. Palmer WE, Rosenthal DI, Schoenberg OI, et al. Quantification of inflammation in the wrist with gadolinium-enhanced MR imaging and PET with 2–[F-18]-fluoro-2–deoxy-D-glucose. Radiology 1995;196;647–655.

25. Akeson WH, Amiel DA, Gershuni DH. Articular cartilage physiology and metabolism. In: Resnick D, ed. Diagnosis of Bone and Joint Disorders, 3rd ed. Philadelphia: Saunders, 1995:769–790.

26. Resnick D. Articular anatomy and histology. In: Resnick D, ed. Diagnosis of Bone and Joint Disorders, 4th ed. Philadelphia: Saunders, 2002:688–707.

27. Ghadially FN. Structure and function of articular cartilage. Clin Rheum Dis 1981;7:3.

28. Pearle AD, Warren RF, Rodeo SA. Basic science of articular cartilage and osteoarthritis. Clin Sports Med 2005;24:1–12.

29. Goodwin DW. Visualization of the macroscopic structure of hyaline cartilage with MR imaging. Semin Musculoskel Radiol 2001;5(4):305–312.

30. Trattnig S. Overuse of hyaline cartilage and imaging. Eur J Radiol 1997;25:188–198.

31. Buckwalter JA, Mankin HG. Articular cartilage. I. tissue design and chondrocyte matrix interactions. J Bone Joint Surg [Am] 1997;79:600–611.

32. Imhof H, Nobauer-Huhmann IM, Krestan C, et al. MRI of cartilage. Eur Radiol 2002;12:2781–2793.

33. Morris NP, Keene DR, Horton WA. Morphology and chemical composition of connective tissue: cartilage. In: Royce PM, Steinmann B, eds. Connective Tissue and Its Heritable Disorders. Molecular, Genetic, and Medical Aspects. New York: Wiley-Liss, 2002:41–65.

34. Mankin HJ, Brandt KD. Biochemistry and metabolism of articular cartilage in osteoarthritis. In: Moskowitz RW, Howell DS, Goldberg VM, Mankin HJ, eds. Osteoarthritis, 2nd ed. Philadelphia: Saunders, 1992:109–154.

35. Mankin HJ, Mow VC, Buckwalter JA, Iannotti JP, Ratcliffe A. Articular cartilage structure, composition, and function. In: Buckwalter JA, Einhorn TA, Simon SR, eds. Orthopedic Basic Science: Biology and Biomechanics of the Musculoskeletal System. Rosemont, IL: American Academy of Orthopedic Surgeons, 1999:444–470.

36. Maroudas AI. Balanced between swelling pressure and collagen tension in normal and degenerate cartilage. Nature 1976;260(5554):808–809.

37. Soltz MA, Ateshian GA. Interstitial fluid pressurization during confined compression cyclical loading of articular cartilage. Ann Biomed Eng 2000;28(2):150–9.

38. McCauley TR, Disler DG. MR imaging of articular cartilage. Radiology 1998;209(3):629–640.

39. Mayne R, Brewton RG. New members of the collagen superfamily. Curr Opin Cell Biol 1993;5:883–890.

40. Mow VC, Proctor CS, Kelly MA. Biomechanics of articular cartilage. In: Nordin M, Frankel VH, eds. Basic Biomechanics of the Musculoskeletal System. Philadelphia: Lea & Febiger, 1989:31–57.

41. Clarke IC. Articular cartilage: a review and scanning electron microscopy study 1. The interterritorial fibrillar architecture. J Bone Joint Surg 1971;53B:732–750.

42. Maroudas A, Muir A, Wingham J. The correlation of fixed negative charge with glycosaminoglycan content of human articular cartilage. Biochem Biophys Acta 1969;177:492–500.

43. Paul PK, Jasani MK, Sebok D, Rakhit A, Dunton AW, Douglas FL. Variation in MR signal intensity across normal human knee cartilage. J Magn Reson Imaging Eng 1993;3:569–574.

44. Modl JM, Sether LA, Haughton VM, Kneeland JB. Articular cartilage: correlation of histologic zones with signal intensity at MR imaging. Radiology 1991;181:853–855.

45. Redler I, Mow VC, Zimmy ML, et al. The ultrastructure and biomechanical significance of the tidemark of articular cartilage. Clin Orthop Rel Res 1975;112:357–362.

46. Green WT Jr, Martin GN, Eanes ED, et al. Microradiographic study of the calcified layer of articular cartilage. Arch Pathol 1970;90:151.

47. Fawns HT, Landells JW. Histochemical studies of rheumatic conditions; observations on the fine structures of the matrix of normal bone and cartilage. Ann Rheum Dis 1953;12:105.

48. Oegema TR, Thompson RC. Histopathology and pathobiochemistry of the cartilage-bone interface in osteoarthritis. In: Kuettner KE, Goldberg V, eds. Osteoarthritic Disorders. New York: Raven Press, 1995:205–217.

49. Disler DG, McCauley TR, Holmes TJ, Cousins JP. Articular cartilage volume in the knee: semiautomated determination from three-dimensional reformations of MR images. Radiology 1996;198:855–859.

50. Peterfy CG, van Dijke CF, Lu Y, et al. Quantification of the volume of articular cartilage in the metacarpophalangeal joints of the hand: accuracy and precision of three-dimensional MR imaging. AJR 1995;165:371–375.

51. Mohana-Borges A, Resnick D, Chung CB. Magnetic resonance imaging of knee instability. Semin Musculoskeletal Radiol 2005;9(1);17–33.

52. Disler DG, McCauley TR, Kelman CG, et al. Fat-suppressed three-dimensional spoiled gradient-echo MR imaging of hyaline cartilage defects in the knee: comparison with standard MR imaging and arthroscopy. AJR 1996;167:127–132.

53. Daenen BR, Ferrara MA, Marcelis S, Dondelinger RF. Evaluation of patellar cartilage surface lesions: comparison of CT arthrography and fat-suppressed FLASH 3D MR imaging. Eur Radiol 1998;8:981–985.

54. Bredella MA, Tirman PF, Peterfy CG, et al. Accuracy of T2–weighted fast spin-echo MR imaging with fat saturation in detecting cartilage defects in the knee: comparison with arthroscopy in 130 patients. AJR 1999;172:1073–1080.

55. Suh JS, Lee SH, Jeong EK, Kim DJ. Magnetic resonance imaging of articular cartilage. Eur Radiol 2001;11:2015–2025.

56. Sonin AH, Pensy RA, Mulligan ME, Hatem S. Grading articular cartilage of the knee using fast spin-echo proton density-weighted MR imaging without fat suppression. AJR 2002;179:1159–1166.

57. Mohr A, Priebe M, Taouli B, Grimm J, Heller M, Brossmann J. Selective water excitation for faster MR imaging of articular cartilage defects: initial cartilage results. Eur Radiol 2003;12:686–689.

58. Noyes FR, Stabler CL. A system for grading articular cartilage lesions at arthroscopy. Am J Sports Med 1989;17(4):505–513.

59. Outerbridge RE. The etiology of chondromalacia patellae. J Bone Joint Surg Br 1961;43B:752–757.

60. Hayes CW, Sawyer RW, Conway WF: Patellar cartilage lesions: in vitro detection and staging with MR imaging and pathologic correlation. Radiology 1990;176:479–483.

61. Karvonen RL, Negendank WG, Fraser SM, Mayes MD, An T, Fernandez-Madrid F. Articular cartilage defects of the knee: correlation between magnetic resonance imaging and gross pathology. Ann Rheum Dis 1990;49(9):672–675.

62. Chandnani VP, Ho C, Chu P, Trudell D, Resnick D. Knee hyaline cartilage evaluated with MR imaging: a cadaveric study involving multiple imaging sequences and intraarticular injection of gadolinium and saline solution. Radiology 1991;178:557–561.

63. Wolff SD, Chesnick S, Frank JA, Lim KO, Balaban RS. Magnetization transfer contrast: MR imaging of the knee. Radiology 1991;179:623–628.

64. Brown SM, Schneider E, Song S, et al. Saturation transfer: a new technique to detect articular cartilage defects in the knee. In: Book of Abstracts. Berkeley, CA: Society of Magnetic Resonance in Medicine, 1992:324(abst).

65. Recht MP, Resnick D. MR imaging of articular cartilage: current status and future directions. AJR 1994;163:283–290.

66. Kramer J, Stiglbauer R, Engel A, Prayer L, Imhof H. MR contrast arthrography (MRA) in osteochondrosis dissecans. J Comput Assist Tomogr 1992;16:254–260.

67. McCauley TR, Moses M, Kier R, Lynch JK, Barton JW, Jokl P. MR diagnosis of tears of anterior cruciate ligament of the knee: importance of ancillary findings. AJR 1994;162:115–119.

68. Recht MP, Kramer J, Marcelis S, et al. Abnormalities of articular cartilage in the knee: analysis of available MR techniques. Radiology 1993;187:473–478.

69. Gagliardi JA, Chung EM, Chandnani VP, et al. Detection and staging of chondromalacia patellae: relative efficacies of conventional MR imaging, MR arthrography, and CT arthrography. AJR 1994;163:629–636.

70. Handelberg F, Shahabpour M, Casteleyn PP. Chondral lesions of the patella evaluated with computed tomography, magnetic resonance imaging, and arthroscopy. Arthroscopy 1990;6:24–29.

71. Weiss C, Mirow S. An ultrastructural study of osteoarthritis changes articular change of human knees. J Bone Joint Surg Am 1972;54–A95.

72. Kramer J, Recht MP, Imhof H, Engel A. MR contrast arthrography (MRA) in assessment of cartilage lesions. J Comput Assist Tomogr 1994;18:218–224.

73. Fry ME, Jacoby RK, Hutton CV, et al. High-resolution magnetic resonance imaging of the interphalangeal joints of the hand. Skeletal Radiol 1991;20:273–277.

74. Recht MP, Piraino DW, Paletta GA, et al. Accuracy of fat-suppressed three-dimensional spoiled gradient-echo FLASH MR imaging in the detection of patellofemoral articular cartilage abnormalities. Radiology 1996;198:209–212.

75. Potter HG, Linklater JM, Allen AA, et al. Magnetic resonance imaging of articular cartilage in the knee. An evaluation of use of fast-spin-echo imaging. J Bone Joint Surg Am 1998;80:1276–1284.

76. Disler DG, McCauley TR, Wirth CR, et al. Detection of knee hyaline cartilage defects using fat-suppressed three-dimensional spoiled gradient-echo MR imaging: comparison with standard MR imaging and correlation with arthroscopy. AJR 1995;165:377–382.

77. Winalski CS, Gupta KB. Magnetic resonance imaging of focal articular cartilage lesions. Topics Magn Reson Imaging 2003;14(2):131–144.

78. Disler DG, Peters TL, Muscoreil SJ, et al. Fat-suppressed spoiled GRASS imaging of knee hyaline cartilage: technique optimization and comparison with conventional MR imaging. AJR 1994;163:887–892.

79. Kawahara Y, Uetani M, Nakahara N, et al. Fast spin-echo MR of the articular cartilage in the osteoarthritic knee. Correlation of MR and arthroscopic findings. Acta Radiol 1998;39:120–125.

80. Gold GE, Hargreaves BA, Reeder SB, Vasanawala SS, Beaulieu C. Controversies in protocol selection in the imaging of articular cartilage. Semin Musculoskeletal Imaging 2005;9(2):161–172.

81. Erickson SJ, Waldschmidt JG, Czervionke LF, et al. Hyaline cartilage: Truncation artifact as a cause of trilaminar appearance with fat-suppressed three-dimensional spoiled gradient-recalled sequences. Radiology 1996;201:260–264.

82. Gylys-Morin VM, Hajek PC, Sartoris DJ, Resnick D. Articular cartilage defects: detectability in cadaver knees with MR. AJR 1987;148:1153–1157.

83. Vande Berg BC, Lecouvet FE, Poilvache P, et al. Assessment of knee cartilage in cadavers with dual-detector spiral CT arthrography and MR imaging. Radiology 2002;222:430–436.

84. Pilch L, Stewart C, Gordon D, et al. Assessment of cartilage volume in the femorotibial joint with magnetic resonance imaging and 3D computer reconstruction. J Rheumatol 1994;21:2307–2321.

85. Maroudas A, Venn M. Chemical composition and swelling of normal and osteoarthrotic femoral head cartilage. II. Swelling. Ann Rheum Dis 1977;36:399–406.

86. Venn M. Chemical composition and swelling of normal and osteoarthritic femoral head cartilage. Ann Rheum Dis 1977;36:121–129.

87. Mow VC, Zhu W, Ratcliffe A. Structure and function of articular cartilage and meniscus. In: Mow VC, Hayes HC, eds. Basic Orthopedic Biomechanics. New York: Raven Press, 1991:143–189.

88. Mosher TJ, Dardzinski BJ. Cartilage MRI T2 relaxation time mapping: overview and applications. Semin Musculoskeletal Radiology 2004;8(4):355–368.

89. Mori Y, Kubo M, Okumo H, Kuroki Y. A scanning electron microscopic study of the degenerative cartilage in patellar chondropathy. Arthroscopy 193;9:247–264.

90. Muir H, Bullough P, Maroudas A. The distribution of collagen in human articular cartilage with some of its physiological implications. J Bone Joint Surg Br 1970;52:554–563.

91. Lusse S, Knauss R, Werner A, Grunder W, Arnold K. Action of compression andcatios on the proton and deuterium relaxation in cartilage. Magn Reson Med 1995;33:483–489.

92. Dardzinski BJ, Mosher TJ, Li S, Van Slyke MA, Smith MB. Spatial variation of T2 in human cartilage. Radiology 1997;205:546–550.

93. Xia Y. Heterogeneity of cartilage laminae in MR imaging. J Magn Reson Imaging 2000;11:686–693.

94. Mosher TJ, Dardzinski BJ, Smith MB. Human articular cartilage: influence of aging and early symptomatic degeneration on the spatial variation of T2—preliminary findings at 3T. Radiology 2000;214:259–266.

95. Packer KJ. The dynamics of water in heterogeneous systems. Philos Trans R Soc Lond B Biol Sci 1977;278:59–87.

96. Gold GE, Thedens DR, Pauly JM, et al. MR imaging of articular cartilage of the knee: new methods using ultrashort TEs. AJR 1998;170:1223–1226.

97. Frank LR, Wong EC, Luh WM, Ahn JM, Resnick D. Articular cartilage in the knee: mapping of the physiologic parameters at MR imaging with a local gradient coil—preliminary results. Radiology 1999;210:241–246.

98. Gold GE, Han E, Stainsby J, Wright G, Brittain J, Beaulieu C. Musculoskeletal MRI at 3.0 T: relaxation times and image contrast. AJR 2003;183:343–351.

99. Duewell SH, Ceckler TL, Ong K, et al. Musculoskeletal MR imaging at 4 T and 1.5 T: comparison of relaxation times and image contrast. Radiology 1995;196:551–555.

100. Becker ED, Farrar TC. Driven equilibrium Fourier transform spectroscopy. A new method for nuclear magnetic resonance signal enhancement. J Am Chem Soc 1969;91:7784–7785.

101. Kneeland JB. MRI probes biophysical structure of cartilage. Diagn Imaging (San Franc) 1996;18:36–40.

102. Xia Y, Farquhar T, Burton-Wurster N, Lust G. Origin of cartilage laminae in MRI. J Magn Reson Imaging 1997;887–894.

103. Stevens KJBF, Hishioka H, Steines D, Genovese M, Lang PK. Contrast-enhanced MRI measurement of GAG concentrations in articular cartilage of knees with early osteoarthritis. In: Proceedings of the Radiology Society of North America. Chicago: Radiological Society of North America, 2001:275.

104. Bashir A, Gray ML, Boutin RD and Burstein D. Glycosaminoglycan in articular cartilage: in vivo assessment with delayed Gd(DTPA)(2-)-enhanced MR imaging. Radiology 1997;205:551–558.

105. Bashir A, Gray ML, Burnstein D. Gd-DTPA2—as a measure of cartilage degradation. Magn Reson Med 1996;36:665–673.

106. Allen RG, Burnstein D, Gray ML. Monitoring glycosaminoglycan replenishment in cartilage explants with gadolinium-enhanced magnetic resonance imaging. J Orthop Res 1999;17:430–436.

107. Burr DB. Anatomy and physiology of the mineralized tissues: role in the pathogenesis of osteoarthrosis. Osteoarthritis Cartilage 2004;12(suppl A):S20–30.

108. Martel-Pelletier J. Pathophysiology of osteoarthritis. Osteoarthritis Cartilage 2004;12(suppl A):S31–33.

109. Muir P, McCarthy J, Radtke CL, et al. Role of endochondral ossification of articular cartilage and functional adaptation of the subchondral plate in the development of fatigue microcracking of joints. Bone 2005.

110. Squires GR, Okouneff S, Ionescu M, Poole AR. The pathobiology of focal lesion development in aging human articular cartilage and molecular matrix changes characteristic of osteoarthritis. Arthritis Rheum 2003;48(5):1261–70.

111. Donohue JM, Buss D, Oegema TR Jr, Thompson RC Jr. The effects of indirect blunt trauma on adult canine articular cartilage. J Bone Joint Surg Am, 1983;65(7):948–57.

112. Jackson RW. The role of arthroscopy in diagnosis and management of osteoarthritis. In: Moskowitz RW, Howell DS, Goldberg VM, Mankin HJ, eds. Osteoarthritis, 2nd ed. Philadelphia: Saunders, 1992:527–534.

113. Recht MP, Goodwin DW, Winalski CS, White LM. MRI of articular cartilage: revisiting current status and future directions. AJR 2005;185:899–914,

114. Hangody L, Rathonyi GK, Duska Z, Vasarhelyi G, Fules P, Modis L. Autologous osteochondral mosaicplasty: surgical technique. J Bone Joint Surg Am 2004;86(suppl):65–72.

115. Pridie KH, Gordon G. A method of resurfacing osteoarthritic knee joints. J Bone Joint Surg Br 1959;41:618–619.

116. Steadman J, Rodkey W, Singleton S, Briggs K. Microfracture technique for full-thickness chondral defects: technique and clinical results. Oper Tech Orthop 1997;7:300–304.

117. Howell DS, Altman RD. Cartilage repair and conservation in osteoarthritis. Rheum Dis Clin North Am 1993;19:713–724.

118. Bert JM. Role of abrasion arthroplasty and debridement in the management of osteoarthritis of the knee. Rheum Dis Clin North Am 1993;19:725–739.

119. Berlet CG, Mascia A, Miniaci A. Treatment of unstable osteochondritis dissecans lesions of the knee using autogenous osteochondral grafts (mosaicplasty). Arthroscopy 1999;15:312–316.

120. Duchow J, Hess T, Kohn D. Primary stability of press-fit-implanted osteochondral grafts: influence of graft size, repeated insertion, and harvesting technique. Am J Sports Med 2000;28:24–27.

121. Hangody L, Kish G, Karpati Z, Eberhardt R. Osteochondral plugs: autogenous osteochondral mosaicplasty for the treatment of focal chondral and osteochondral articular defects. Oper Tech Orthop 1997;7:312–322.

122. Pearce SG, Hurtig MB, Clarnette R, Kalra M, Cowan B, Miniaci A. An investigation of 2 techniques for optimizing joint surface congruency using multiple cylindrical osteochondral autografts. Arthroscopy 2001;17:50–55.

123. Recht M, White LM, Winalwski CS, et al. MR imaging of cartilage repair procedures. Skeletal Radiol 2003;32:185–200.

124. Sanders TG, Mentzer KD, Miller MD, Morrison WB, Campbell SE, Penrod BJ. Autogenous osteochondral "plug" transfer for the treatment of focal chondral defects: postoperative MR appearance with clinical correlation. Skeletal Radiol 2001;30:570–78.

125. Minas T, Peterson L. Advanced techniques in autologous chondrocyte transplantation. Clin Sports Med 1999;18:13–44.

126. Peterson L, Minas T, Brittberg M, Nilsson A, Sjogren-Jansson E, Lindahl A. Two- to 9–year outcome after autologous chondrocyte transplantation of the knee. Clin Orthop 2000;374:212–234.

127. Peterson L, Brittberg M, Kiviranta I, Akerlund EL, Lindahl A. Autologous chondrocyte transplantation: biomechanics and long-term durability. Am J Sports Med 2002;30:2–12.

128. Alparslan L, Winalski CS, Boutin RD, Minas T. Postoperative magnetic resonance imaging of articular cartilage repair. Semin Msuculoskel Radiol 2001;5(4):345–363.

129. Alparslan L, Minas T, Winalski CS. Magnetic resonance imaging of autologous chondrocyte implantation. Semin Ultrasound CT MR 2001;22:341–351.

130. Minas T. Autologous chondrocyte implantation for focal chondral defects of the knee. Clin Orthop 2001;391S:349–361.

131. Azer N, Winalski CS, Minas T. Magnetic resonance imaging for surgical planning and postoperative assessment in early osteoarthritis. Radiol Clin North Am 2004;42:43–60.

132. Lawrence RC, Hochberg MC, Kelsey JL, et al. Estimates of the prevalence of selected arthritic and musculoskeletal diseases in the United States. J Rheumatol 1989;16(4):427–441.

133. McCauley T, Disler D, Magnetic resonance imaging of articular cartilage of the knee. J Am Acad Orthop Surg 2001;9:2–8.

134. Disler DG, McCauley TR, Kelman CG, et al. Fat-suppressed three-dimensional spoiled gradient-echo MR imaging of hyaline cartilage defects in the knee: comparison with standard MR imaging and arthroscopy. Am J Roentgenol 1996;167:127–132.

135. Brown WE, Potter HG, Marx RG, et al. Magnetic resonance imaging appearance of cartilage repair in the knee. Clin Orthop Rel Res 2004;422:214–223.

136. Potter H, Linklater J, Answorth A. Magnetic resonance imaging of articular cartilage in the knee: an evaluation with use of fast-spin-echo imaging. J Bone Joint Surg Am 1998;80:1276–1284.

137. Curl WW, Krome J, Gordon ES, et al. Cartilage injuries: a review of 31,516 knee arthroscopies. Arthroscopy 1997;13:456–460.

138. Hjelle K, Solheim E, Strand T, et al. Articular cartilage defects in 1,000 knee arthroscopies. Arthroscopy 2002;18:730–734.

139. Maffulli N, Binfield P, King J. Articular cartilage lesions in the symptomatic anterior cruciate ligament-deficient knee. Arthroscopy 2003;19:685–690.

140. Nomura E, Motoyasu I, Makoto K. Chondral and osteochondral injuries associated with acute patellar dislocation. Arthroscopy 2003;19:717–721.

141. Aroen A, Loken S, Heir S. Articular cartilage lesions in 993 consecutive knee arthroscopies. Am J Sports Med 2004;32:211–215.

142. Drongowski R, Coran A. Wojtys E. Predictive values of meniscal and chondral injuries in conservatively treated anterior cruciate ligament injuries. Arthroscopy 1994;10:97–102.

143. Shelbourne KD, Jari S, Gray T. Outcome of untreated traumatic articular cartilage defects of the knee. J Bone Joint Surg Am 2003;85(2):8.

144. Alford JW, Cole B. Cartilage restoration. Part I. Am J Sports Med 2005;33:295–306.

145. Newman A. Current Concepts: articular cartilage repair. Am J Sports Med 1998;26: 309–324.

146. Buckwalter JA, Mankin HJ. Instructional Course Lectures, The AAOS-articular cartilage. Part I: tissue design and chondrocytes-matrix interactions. J Bone Joint Surg Am 1997;79:600–611.

147. Sgaglione N, Abrutyn D. Update on the treatment of osteochondral fractures and osteochondritis dissecans of the knee. Sports Med Arthrosc Rev 2003;11:222–235.

148. Terry GC, Flandry F, Van Manen JW, et al. Isolated chondral fractures of the knee. Clin Orthop Rel Res 1988;234:170–177.

149. Williams JS Jr, Bush-Joseph CA, Bach BR Jr. Osteochondritis dissecans of the knee. Am J Knee Surg 1998;11:221–232.

150. Graf BK, Cook DA, De Smet AA. "Bone bruises" on magnetic resonance imaging evaluation of anterior cruciate ligament injuries. Am J Sports Med 1993;21:220–223.

151. Hunter DJ, Zhang YQ, Niu JB, et al. The association of meniscal pathologic changes with cartilage loss in symptomatic knee osteoarthritis. Arthritis Rheum 2006;54:795–801.

152. Cameron ML, Briggs KK, Steadman JR, Reproducibility and reliability of the Outerbridge classification for grading chondral lesions of the knee arthroscopically. Am J Sports Med 2003;31:83–86.

153. Outerbridge RE. The etiology of chondromalacia patella. J Bone Joint Surg 1961;43B:752–757.

154. Insall J, Falvo K, Wise D. Chondromalacia patellae. A prospective study. J Bone Joint Surg Am 1976;58:1–8.

155. Noyes FR, Stabler CL. A system for grading articular cartilage lesions at arthroscopy. Am J Sports Med 1989;17(4):505–513.

156. Bauer M, Jackson RW. Chondral lesions of the femoral condyles: a system of arthroscopic classification. Arthroscopy 1988;4:97–102.

157. Hunt N, Sanchez-Ballester J, Pandit R, et al. Chondral lesions of the knee: a new localization method and correlation with associated pathology. Arthroscopy 2001;17:481–490.

158. Marx RG, Jones EC, Allen AA, et al. Reliability, validity, and responsiveness of four knee outcome scales for athletic patients. J Bone Joint Surg Am 2001;83:1459–1469.

159. Kocher M, Steadman JR, Briggs K. Reliability, validity, and responsiveness of the Lysholm knee scale for vari-

ous chondral disorders of the knee. J Bone Joint Surg Am 2004;86:1139–114.

160. McConnell S, Kolopack P, Davis AM. The western Ontario and McMaster universities osteoarthritis Index (WOMAC): a review of its utility and measurement properties. Arthritis Rheum 2001;45:453–456.

161. Roos E, Roos, H, Lohmander L, et al. Knee injury and osteoarthritis outcome score (KOOS)—development of a self-administered outcome measure. J Orthop Sports Phys Ther 1998;28:88–96.

162. Brittberg M. ICRS clinical cartilage injury evaluation system. Third ICRS Meeting, April 28, 2000.

163. Wilson JN. A diagnostic sign in osteochondritis dissecans of the knee. J Bone Joint Surg Am 1967;49:477–480.

164. Hardaker W, Garrett W, Bassett F. Evaluation of acute traumatic hemarthrosis of the knee joint. South Med J 1990;83:640–644.

165. Guilak F, Fermor B, Keefe F. The role of biomechanics and inflammation in cartilage injury and repair. Clin Orthop Rel Res 2004;423:17–26.

166. O'Driscoll S. The healing and regeneration of articular cartilage. J Bone Joint Surg Am 1998;80:1795–1807.

167. Vachon A, Bronlage L, Gabel A, et al. Evaluation of the repair process of cartilage defects of the equines third carpal bone with and without subchondral bone perforation. Am J Vet Res 1986;4:2637–2645.

168. Kim HKW, Moran ME, Salter RB. The potential for regeneration of articular cartilage in defects created by chondral shaving and subchondral abrasion. An experimental investigation in rabbits. J Bone Joint Surg Am 1991;73:1301–1315.

169. Mithoefer K, Williams R, Warren R, et al. The microfracture technique for the treatment of articular cartilage lesions in the knee: a prospective cohort study. J Bone Joint Surg Am 2005;87:1911–1920.

170. Hangody L, Fules P. Autologous osteochondral mosaicplasty for the treatment of full thickness defects of weight–bearing joints; ten years of experimental and clinical experience. J Bone Joint Surg Am 2003;85:25–32.

171. Barber A, Chow J. Arthroscopic osteochondral transplantation: histologic results. Arthroscopy 2001;17:832–835.

172. Chow JC, Hantes M, Houle JB. Arthroscopic autogenous osteochondral transplantation for treating knee cartilage defects: a 2 to 5 year follow–up study. Arthroscopy 2004;20:681–690.

173. Horas U, Pelinkovic D, Aigner T. Autologous chondrocyte implantation and osteochondral cylinder transplantation in cartilage repair of the knee joint: a prospective comparative trial. J Bone Joint Surg Am 2003;85:185–192.

174. Evans P, Miniaci A, Hurtig M. Manual punch versus power harvesting of osteochondral grafts. Arthroscopy 2004;20:306–310.

175. Gudas R, Stankevicius E, Monastyreckiene E, et al. Osteochondral autologous transplantation versus microfracture for the treatment of articular cartilage defects in the knee joint in athletes. Knee Surg Sports Traumatol Arthrosc 2006.

176. Duchow J, Hess T, Kohn D. Primary stability of press–fit implanted osteochondral grafts. Am J Sports Med 2000;28:24–27.

177. LaPrade RF, Botker JC. Donor-site morbidity after osteochondral autograft transfer procedures. Arthroscopy 2004;20:69–73.

178. Gross A, Shasha N, Aubin P. Long-term follow-up of the use of fresh osteochondral allografts for the posttraumatic knee defects. Clin Orthop Rel Res 2005;435:79–87.

179. Jamali A, Emmerson B, Chung C, et al. Fresh osteochondral allografts. Clin Orthop Rel Res 2005;437:176–185.

180. Glenn E, McCarty E, Potter H. Comparison of fresh osteochondral autografts and allografts: a canine model. Am J Sports Med 2006;34(7):1084–1093.

181. Sgaglione N, Miniaci A, Gillogly S, Carter T. Update on advanced surgical techniques in the treatment of traumatic focal articular cartilage lesions of the knee. Arthroscopy 2002;18:9–32.

182. Peterson L, Brittberg M, Kiviranta I, et al. Autologous chondrocyte transplantation; biomechanics and long-term durability. Am J Sports Med 2002;30:2–12.

183. Peterson L, Minas T, Brittberg M, Lindahl A. Treatment of osteochondritis dissecans of the knee with autologous chondrocyte transplantation. J Bone Joint Surg Am 2003;85:17–24.

184. Minas T, Peterson L. Advanced techniques in autologous chondrocyte transplantation. Clin Sports Med 1999;18:13–44.

185. Knutsen G, Engbretsen L, Ludvigsen T. Autologous chondrocyte implantation compared with microfracture in the knee: a randomized trial. J Bone Joint Surg Am 2004;86:455–464.

186. Kang HJ, Han C, Kang E, et al. An experimental intraarticular implantation of woven carbon fiber pad into osteochondral defect of the femoral condyle in rabbit. Yonsei Med J 1991;32:108–116.

187. Minnus RJ, Flynn M. Intraarticular implant of filamentous carbon fiber in the experimental animal. J Bioeng 1978;2:279–286.

188. Minnus RJ, Muckle DS, Donkin JE. The repair of osteochondral defects in osteoarthritic rabbit knees by the use of carbon fiber. Biomaterials 1982;3:81–86.

189. Robinson D, Efrat M, Mendes D, et al. Implants composed of carbon fiber mesh and bone-marrow derived chondrocyte-enriched cultures for joint surface reconstruction. Bull Hosp Joint Dis 1993;53:75–82.

190. Sgaglione N. The future of cartilage restoration. J Knee Surg 2004;17:235–243.

191. Bruder S. Current and emerging technologies in orthopaedic tissue engineering. Clin Ortho Rel Res 1999;376:S406–409.

192. Grande D, Mason J, Dines D. Stem cells as platforms for delivery of genes to enhance cartilage grafts. J Bone Joint Surg Am 2003;85:111–116

193. Hannallah D, Peterson B, Lieberman JR, et al. Gene therapy in orthopaedic surgery. Instr Course Lect 2003;2:70–76.

194. Jackson D, Scheer M, Simon T. Tissue engineering principles in orthopaedic surgery. Clin Orthop Rel Res 2001;9:37–52.

195. Muschler GF, Nakamoto C, Griffith LG. Engineering principles of clinical-cell based tissue engineering. J Bone Joint Surg Am 2004;86:1541–1558.

196. Wright R, Boyce RH, Michener T. Radiographs are not useful in detecting arthroscopically confirmed mild chondral damage. Clin Orthop Rel Res 2006;442:245–251.

197. Recht M, Bobic V, Burstein D, Magnetic resonance imaging of articular cartilage. Clin Orth Rel Res 2001;391:S379–396.

198. Alparslan L, Winalski CS, Boutin R. Postoperative magnetic resonance imaging of articular cartilage repair. Semin Musculoskeletal Radiol 2001;5:345–363.

199. Chung C, Frank L, Resnick D. Cartilage imaging techniques: current clinical application and state of the art imaging. Clin Orthop Rel Res 2001;391:S370–378.

200. Winalski CS, Mina T. Evaluation of chondral injuries by magnetic resonance imaging: repair assessments. Oper Tech Sports Med 2000;8:108–119.

201. Guettler JH, Demetropoulos CK, Yang, KH, et al. Osteochondral defects in the human knee: Influence of defect size on cartilage rim stress and load redistribution to surrounding cartilage. Am J Sports Med 2004;32:1451–1458.

202. Brittberg M, Lindahl A, Nilsson A, et al. Treatment of deep cartilage defects in the knee with autologous chondrocyte transplantation. N Engl J Med 1994;331:889–895.

203. Minas T, Nehrer S. Current concepts in the treatment of articular cartilage defects. Orthopedics 1997;20:525–538.

204. Bashir A, Gray, MI, Boutin RD, et al. Glycosaminoglycan in articular cartilage: in vivo assessment with delayed Gd(DTPA)2–enhanced MR imaging, Radiology 1997;205:551–558.

205. Burstein D, Gray M. Potential of molecular imaging of cartilage, Sport Med Arthrosc Rev 2003;11:182–191.

206. Mosher TJ, Dardzinski BJ, Smith MB. Human articular cartilage: influence of aging and early symptomatic degeneration on the spatial variation of T2—preliminary findings at 3 T. Radiology 2000;214:259–266.

207. Mosher T, Smith H, Collins C, et al. Change in knee cartilage T2 at MR imaging after running: a feasibility study. Radiology 2005;234:245–249.

208. Wheaton AJ, Borthakur A, Dodge GR. Sodium magnetic resonance imaging of proteoglycan depletion in an in vivo model of osteoarthritis. Acad Radiol 2004;11:21–28.

209. Insko EK, Reddy R, Leigh JS. High resolution, short echo time sodium imaging of articular cartilage. J Magn Reson Imaging 1997;7:1056–1059.

210. Burstein D, Gray M. New MRI techniques for imaging cartilage. J Bone Joint Surg Am 2003;85:70–77.

3
Bone

A. Radiologic Perspective: Patterns of Bone Marrow Edema Based on Mechanism of Injury

Sailaja Yadavalli and Donald Resnick

Today magnetic resonance imaging (MRI) of the knee is widely used after an acute traumatic event to assess for soft tissue injuries and occult fractures.[1–4] Complex injuries of the knee are rarely due to complete disruption of a single ligament without either microscopic or macroscopic changes in one or more of the supporting structures. Bone marrow edema is also frequently encountered with these injuries. The pattern of ligamentous disruption and bone marrow edema depends on the type and direction of force causing the injury.[5–7] This chapter discusses the various patterns of bone contusion and correlates each to a specific mechanism of injury. A thorough understanding of this relationship is important, as it is a valuable predictor of associated soft tissue injuries.

Restraints to Joint Motion

The muscles, ligaments, tendons, and menisci around the knee are the main stabilizers of the joint.[8] The supporting structures around the knee provide primary and secondary resistance against the forces acting on the joint. Primary resistance to anterior and posterior tibial translation is provided by the anterior and posterior cruciate ligaments, respectively. The lateral collateral ligamentous complex is the primary resistor of a varus force, whereas the medial collateral ligament acts to resist motion when a valgus force is applied. In the case of hyperextension forces, the posterior cruciate ligament acts as the main restraint. With the femur in a fixed position, the primary resistance to forces that cause internal and external rotation of the tibia is provided by the lateral and medial collateral ligaments, respectively. In addition, depending on the type and magnitude of the applied force, other supporting structures may come into play as secondary resistors. The primary and secondary resistors to stress exerted on the knee joint are detailed in Table 3.1.

Pathogenesis of Knee Injury

The types of forces applied to the knee that cause injury are divided into external (or direct) and internal (or indirect).

As the name suggests an external force originates outside the patient and is a factor of the environment in which the injury occurs (i.e., environmental force). External forces acting on the knee may take the form of a direct blow or an impact when the knee strikes a hard and unyielding object. The location, direction, and magnitude of the external force and the position of the knee at the time of application of the stress are the main determinants of the pattern of injury that occurs. External forces may be applied above, at, or below the knee joint. Internal forces refer to a bone striking against bone during a traumatic event. It is important to note that external and internal forces need not occur in conjunction with each other for a complex injury to occur. Thus, during an injury, external forces alone, internal forces alone, or both types of forces may occur. These forces can cause hyperextension, axial loading, translation, angulation, or rotation of the tibia with respect to the femur. The type of injury also depends on whether the knee is in flexion or extension at the time the force is applied and the degree to which it is bent. Injuries to the knee due either to one type of force alone or to a combination of both direct and indirect forces can be seen in accidents and sports that involve a quick change of direction of motion, or a significant amount of contact between players, or falls. Examples of such sports include soccer, American football, skiing, and ice hockey.

Injuries to bones can range from gross fractures to trabecular microfractures manifest as bone bruises. In the case of environmental forces acting on the knee, associated soft tissue edema may also be present and can be seen on MRI in the acute stage. However, bone marrow edema is known to last over a long period, ranging from weeks to years in some rare instances. The internal forces can be classified into three types: (1) those that cause impaction due to axial loading, (2) shear forces that occur with rotational motion of the joint, and (3) tensile forces that cause avulsion type injuries. Axial loading can result in wedge or subchondral fractures or cartilage defects. Bone bruising is worst with impaction type injuries and usually affects a large area (Fig. 3.1A).[9] It is least prominent and more focal with avulsion of ligaments or tendons. Most often no bone marrow

TABLE 3.1. Primary and secondary restraints to knee joint motion with their relation to applied stress.

Motion	Primary restraint	Secondary restraint
Anterior translation	Anterior cruciate ligament	Major: medial collateral ligament
		Minor: lateral collateral ligament, posterior capsule
Posterior translation	Posterior cruciate ligament	Minor: medial collateral ligament
Varus (medial to lateral)	Lateral collateral ligament	Major: posterior capsule
		Minor: anterior and posterior cruciate ligaments
Valgus (lateral to medial)	Medial collateral ligament	Minor: anterior and posterior cruciate ligaments
Internal rotation (with fixed femur)	Lateral collateral ligament, popliteus	Major: anterior cruciate ligament
		Minor: posterior capsule
External rotation (with fixed femur)	Medial collateral ligament	Major: posterior cruciate ligament
		Minor: posterior capsule
Hyperextension	Posterior cruciate ligament	Major: anterior cruciate ligament, posterior capsule

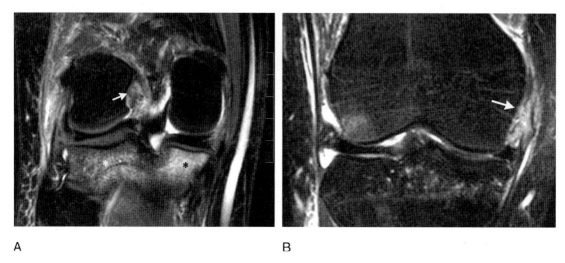

A   B

FIG. 3.1. Patterns of bone marrow edema with impaction and distraction. (A,B) Coronal fat-suppressed intermediate-weighted (repetition time/echo time [TR/TE], 5200/55) turbo spin echo magnetic resonance imaging (MRI) in a 28-year-old woman with anterior cruciate ligament tear (white arrow in A) show extensive bone marrow edema in the lateral tibial plateau (white asterisk) and medial tibial plateau (black asterisk) due to impaction type injury. In contrast, no bone marrow edema is seen in the medial femoral condyle with avulsion of the medial collateral ligament (white arrow in B) at its femoral attachment.

edema is seen with distraction type injuries (Fig. 3.1B). These last injuries are therefore easily overlooked during interpretation of an MRI examination.[9]

Patterns of Bone Marrow Edema Classified by Mechanism of Injury

To establish a relationship between the pattern of bone marrow edema seen on magnetic resonance (MR) studies and the mechanism of injury, one should keep in mind that multiple forces are in play on a joint in motion at the time of injury, and imaging is accomplished later when the knee is usually in extension and static. This section discusses various scenarios causing knee injuries and the associated bone contusion patterns.

External Varus or Valgus Injuries

Pure varus or valgus forces (Fig. 3.2) are environmental stresses that cause impaction-type injury at the site of entry with associated focal bone marrow edema and a distraction type of injury on the opposite side of the joint. In essence these are coup-contrecoup types of injuries. Contrecoup injury may also result in a mild impaction on the opposite side of the applied force as the knee reduces after the initial, coup phase of the injury. The bone marrow edema associated with the contrecoup impaction forces is typically not as extensive as that caused by the primary force.

Pure varus stress acts in a medial to lateral direction (Fig. 3.3). The resulting osseous injury on the medial side is variable, ranging from minor bone contusion to fracture (Fig. 3.3B). With a varus external force, tensile forces act on the lateral aspect of the knee and the lateral ligaments are at risk.

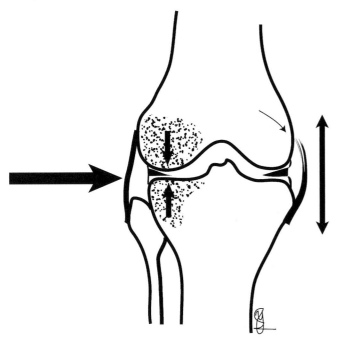

FIG. 3.2. Valgus force illustration shows an external valgus force (large straight arrow) applied to the lateral aspect of the knee. The lateral femoral condyle strikes the lateral tibial plateau (short straight arrows) resulting in bone contusion along the impacting surfaces (shaded regions). Distraction forces act on the opposite side (double arrow) with avulsion of the medial collateral ligament (curved arrow) at its femoral attachment. (Courtesy of Sailaja Yadavalli, MD, PhD.).

Bone marrow edema may be seen on the lateral side (Fig. 3.3) as the knee assumes a valgus alignment during the contrecoup portion of the injury. A pure varus injury is rare due to the inherent protection of the medial aspect of the knee by the other extremity.

A pure valgus injury may be seen in what is known as a clip injury in American football, in which a player's helmet hits the lateral aspect of another player's knee with the knee in mild degree of flexion.[10] Bone contusion due to direct blow is seen in the lateral femoral condyle (Fig. 3.4) and lateral tibial plateau. Edema may be seen in the medial femoral condyle or medial tibial plateau, or in both, due to a contrecoup type of impaction and at the attachments of the medial collateral ligament due to avulsion.[11–15] The ligament itself may suffer a mild partial or a complete tear (Fig. 3.4). Bone injuries on the entry side of force may have a wide spectrum with minimal bruising to severe fractures. If internal forces come into play, with axial loading, significant fractures such as wedge or depression fractures of the tibial plateau may result. In the absence of an obvious wedge fracture it is important to look for subtle osteochondral injuries associated with the bone marrow edema.

Hyperextension Injuries

These injuries result when an environmental force is applied to the anterior aspect of the knee with the joint in a fully extended position. Examples include a pedestrian being hit by a car bumper and a helmet hitting a player along the anterior aspect of the joint with the knee in a locked position. This type of injury causes contiguous areas of bone marrow edema, with the anterior aspect of the femoral condyle striking the anterior aspect of the tibial plateau. These are also known as "kissing" contusions. The force exits through the posterior aspect of the joint and, depending on the severity of the force, tears of the posterior cruciate ligament and posterior capsule will result.[16,17] In extreme cases, after tearing of the posterior cruciate ligament and capsule, posterior tibial translation and dislocation may also occur. In these cases special attention should be given to evaluation of the posterior neurovascular structures.[18]

With the knee in hyperextension a varus force causes bone bruising in the anteromedial region (Fig. 3.5) and the exiting force disrupts supporting structures in the posterolateral aspect of the joint.[19] A valgus force with the knee fully extended results in bone injury to the anterolateral aspect (Fig. 3.6), and tensile forces cause soft tissue injury in the posteromedial corner of the joint. A close inspection for chondral and subchondral fractures is essential (Fig. 3.6). These are severely debilitating injuries, as the structures in the posteromedial and posterolateral corners are the major resistors to rotational motion.

Hyperflexion Injuries

With the knee in flexion the posterior aspect of the femoral condyle comes in contact with the tibial plateau. When the knee is imaged in extension, the regions of bone marrow edema in the femoral condyle and the tibial plateau are not contiguous. The exact location of bone contusion in the femoral condyle depends on the degree of flexion at the time of injury (Fig. 3.7). The pattern of soft tissue injury depends on whether an external force is acting at the same time, the magnitude of the force, and the existence of any component of rotation.

An example of hyperflexion injury is when the dashboard strikes the anterior aspect of the proximal tibia with the knee in a flexed position during a head-on collision, also know as a dashboard injury (Fig. 3.8). The magnitude of the applied force is usually quite significant, and extensive bone marrow edema is seen in the anterior tibial plateau. The impact causes the tibia to translate posteriorly and the first ligament to fail is the primary resistor to posterior translation, namely the posterior cruciate ligament (Fig. 3.8).[20,21] With the knee in a flexed position, the patellar tendon is taut and an avulsion injury at the inferior pole of the patella may also be seen (Fig. 3.8C). As the force exits along the posterior aspect of the femorotibial joint, disruption of posterior capsule may also result (Fig. 3.8C). If the point of contact is higher, osteochondral injuries or fractures of the patella may also occur. In general, the anterior cruciate ligament is not injured, as it is lax with the knee in flexion (Fig. 3.8D). With extreme forces, posterior dislocation of the tibia causes rupture of multiple ligaments and tendons.

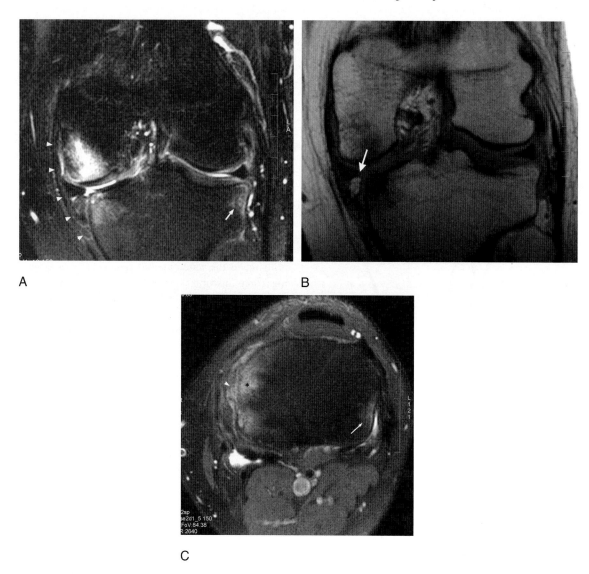

Fɪɢ. 3.3. Pure varus injury. External force applied to the medial side of the knee, either to the femur or the tibia or both, results in a pure varus type injury as seen in this 24-year-old man who was struck by a car 1 month prior to the MRI. (A) Coronal fat-suppressed intermediate-weighted (TR/TE, 5600/52) turbo spin echo MRI shows bone marrow edema in the medial femoral condyle and medial tibial plateau along the site of impact (arrowheads). Mild bone marrow edema in the lateral tibial plateau (arrow) is due to contrecoup type injury. (B) Coronal proton density (TR/TE, 1100/12) spin echo MR image shows a fracture of the medial tibial plateau with a slightly displaced fragment (arrow). This illustrates the importance of non–fat-suppressed images in the detection of fractures that may be easily overlooked on the fluid sensitive sequences. (C) Axial fat-suppressed intermediate-weighted (TR/TE, 2640/50) turbo spin echo MRI shows bone marrow (asterisk) and associated soft tissue edema (arrowhead) to be broad-based with focal edema in the posterior aspect of lateral tibial plateau (arrow).

Rotational Instability

The vertical axis of the knee normally passes near the center of the joint (Fig. 3.9). To understand rotational instability the tibial plateau is divided into four quadrants (Fig. 3.9). With disruption of any of the supporting ligaments, the axis of the knee shifts along the anterior to posterior line, the medial to lateral line, or into one of the four quadrants.[22,23] Shift along a straight line leads to medial, lateral, anterior, or posterior instability. Alternatively, rotational, or combined instability is the result of movement of the axis into one of the quadrants. These are also known as pivot shift injuries. Rotational injuries, with the knee in some degree of flexion, are an important cause of anterior cruciate ligament rupture. By convention these combined type of injuries are described as rotation of the tibia with respect to a fixed femur, even though many of these occur with the foot planted firmly, that is, with a fixed tibia and a rotating femur.

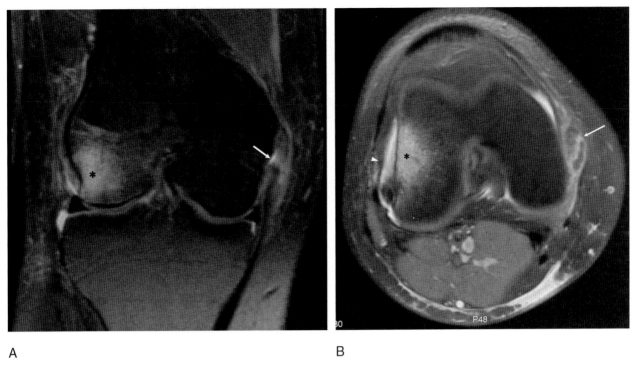

A   B

Fig. 3.4. Pure valgus injury. External forces when applied to the lateral aspect of the knee can cause pure valgus injury as seen in this 22-year-old woman who was kicked while playing soccer. (A) Bone contusion is seen in the lateral femoral condyle (asterisk) in this coronal fat-suppressed intermediate-weighted (TR/TE, 2800/45) turbo spin echo MRI. Avulsion of the medial collateral ligament (arrow) at its femoral attachment is noted, compatible with a distraction type injury. (B) Axial fat-suppressed proton density (TR/TE, 3100/15) turbo spin echo MRI shows broad-based bone marrow edema in the lateral femoral condyle (asterisk) with subjacent soft tissue edema (arrowhead) at the site of impaction. The medial collateral ligament is split and thickened (arrow).

Anteromedial Rotary Instability (AMRI)

An important mechanism of rupture of the anterior cruciate ligament (Fig. 3.10) is a valgus force applied to a mildly flexed knee with external rotation of the tibia. With the disruption of this important restraint the tibia translates anteriorly and the posterior portion of the lateral tibial plateau comes in contact with the midportion of the lateral femoral condyle, resulting in bone marrow edema or osteochondral injuries in noncontiguous regions of the femur and the tibia (Fig. 3.10).[24–32] This is an impaction or shear type injury related to the anterior cruciate ligament tear.

Tensile forces on the opposite side of the knee lead to avulsion of the medial collateral ligament (Fig. 3.10C). Bone marrow edema associated with failure of medial collateral ligament may be minimal to none. In addition, tensile forces in the posteromedial corner can lead to avulsion-type injuries of the semimembranosus tendon (Fig. 3.11) with subjacent bone marrow edema in the posterior aspect of medial tibial plateau.[33,34] Furthermore, as the knee reduces from the initial phase of injury due to valgus stress, with the tibia externally rotated on the femur, the midportion of the medial femoral condyle may come into contact with the posterior lip of the medial tibial plateau due to a contrecoup mechanism (Fig. 3.12).[35] The resulting bone contusion on the medial side is usually not as extensive, as most of the axial loading occurs during the coup portion of injury. In rare cases, the injury may be severe enough to cause subchondral fractures. More often contusion is seen in the posterior lip of the medial tibial plateau, and osseous abnormality in the medial femoral condyle is variable in severity and location.

Anteromedial rotary instability is characteristic of the O'Donoghue's triad of injuries, consisting of tears of the anterior cruciate ligament, medial collateral ligament, and medial meniscus. However, studies have shown that lateral meniscal tears are in fact more common with this mechanism of injury.[36] It is important to note that both menisci are at risk, and a careful search should be made for meniscal injuries.

Anterolateral Rotary Instability (ALRI)

A varus force applied to a mildly flexed knee with the tibia in internal rotation can also lead to anterior cruciate ligament tear (Fig. 3.13A). In this scenario the tibia is allowed to translate anteriorly with impaction of the lateral femoral condyle with the posterolateral tibial plateau. The characteristic bone marrow edema pattern associated with anterior cruciate ligament tears is seen on the lateral side. However, tensile forces act on the lateral side due to the varus external force, leading to disruption of the lateral supporting structures, including those in

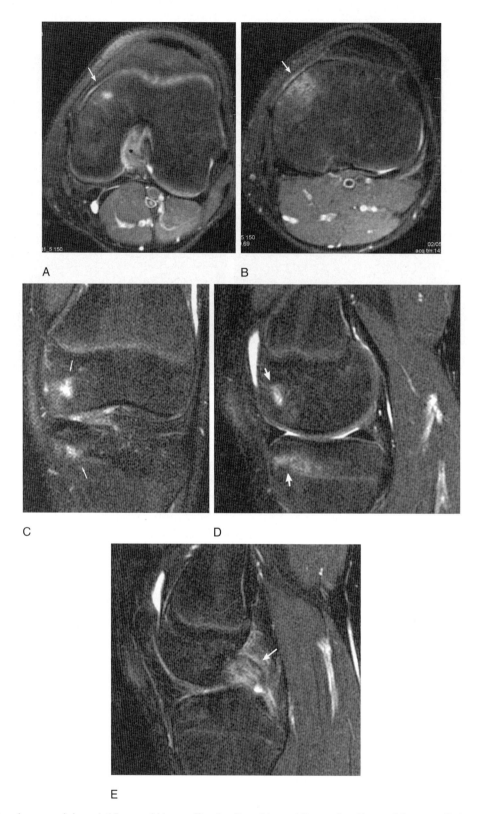

FIG. 3.5. Hyperextension varus injury. A 15-year-old boy suffered a direct blow while running. External force applied to a hyperextended or "locked" knee on the medial aspect produces contiguous areas of bone contusion (A,B) seen on axial fat-suppressed intermediate-weighted (TR/TE, 2700/50) turbo spin echo MRI. Bone marrow edema is seen in the anteromedial aspect of the femoral condyle (arrow in A) and tibial plateau (arrow in B) due to impaction. These may be severe enough to cause fractures. The posterior cruciate ligament is often torn (asterisk in A) with severe hyperextension injuries. Coronal fat-suppressed intermediate-weighted (TR/TE, 5870/55) turbo spin echo MRI (C)) and sagittal fat-suppressed intermediate-weighted (TR/TE, 4530/55) turbo spin echo MRI (D) show that the regions that came in contact (arrows) are contiguous. (E) Sagittal fat-suppressed intermediate-weighted (TR/TE, 4530/55) turbo spin echo MRI shows rupture of the posterior cruciate ligament. A significant exit force may result in distraction injury in the posterolateral corner, not seen in this patient.

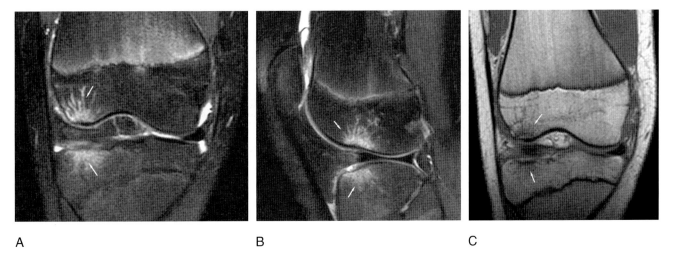

FIG. 3.6. Hyperextension valgus injury. External force applied to the anterolateral aspect of a hyperextended knee results in "kissing" contusions as seen in this 14-year-old basketball player. Contiguous areas of bone marrow edema (arrows) are seen in the lateral femoral condyle and lateral tibial plateau along the articular surfaces in coronal fat-suppressed intermediate-weighted (TR/TE, 4570/55) turbo spin echo (A) and sagittal fat-suppressed intermediate-weighted (TR/TE, 3320/66) turbo spin echo (B) MRI. (C) Coronal proton density (TR/TE, 900/12) spin echo MRI shows horizontal low signal (arrows), which represents microfractures in the lateral femoral condyle and tibial plateau. The posterior cruciate ligament may be disrupted in hyperextension injuries. It was intact in this patient.

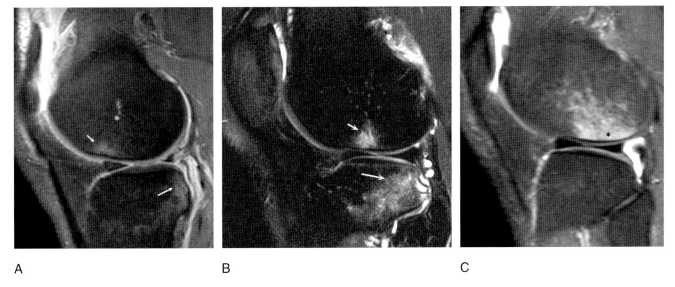

FIG. 3.7. Relationship between bone marrow edema and degree of flexion. (A,B) Three patients with anterior cruciate ligament tears have the typical bone marrow edema pattern associated with it in the lateral femoral condyle (short arrows) and the posterior aspect of the lateral tibial plateau (long arrows). Location of bone contusion in the lateral femoral condyle depends on the degree of flexion of the knee at the time of injury. (A) In this 26-year-old man, the knee was in minimal flexion at injury with contusion resulting in the anterior aspect of the lateral femoral condyle (short arrow) as seen on this sagittal fat-suppressed proton density (TR/TE, 3810/14) turbo spin echo MRI. (B) During injury the knee was in a moderate degree of flexion in this 25-year-old man with bone marrow edema in the midportion of the lateral femoral condyle (short arrow) as seen on the sagittal fat-suppressed intermediate-weighted (TR/TE, 3440/66) turbo spin echo MRI. (C) Sagittal fat-suppressed intermediate-weighted (TR/TE, 4600/43) turbo spin echo MRI in this 28-year-old woman shows bone marrow edema in the posterior portion of the lateral femoral condyle (asterisk). This pattern of injury corresponds to significant flexion of the knee at injury.

the posterolateral corner (Fig. 3.13B). Recognizing loss of stabilizing structures in the posterolateral corner is essential, as it is a major cause of rotary instability resulting in severe disability. The posterior capsule, which is a secondary restraint, may also rupture with significant injury (Fig. 3.13C). Segond

(Fig. 3.13) and fibular avulsion fractures are associated with this type of injury.[37–39] Indeed, the Segond fracture with an anterior cruciate ligament tear is the prototype of an injury leading to anterolateral rotary instability. Both the medial and lateral menisci are at risk for injury.

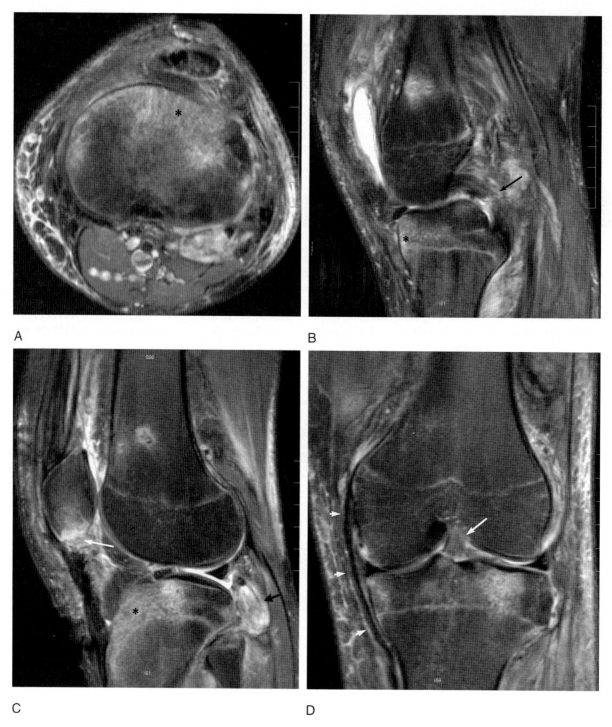

FIG. 3.8. Hyperflexion injury—dashboard injury. This 23-year-old man was involved in a high-speed head-on motor vehicle collision and suffered multiple injuries including knee trauma and left hip fracture-dislocation. Typically this type of injury occurs when an anterior force is applied to the flexed knee, resulting in posterior tibial translation, the classic example being the dashboard injury as in this patient. (A) Axial fat-suppressed intermediate-weighted (TR/TE, 3200/54) turbo spin echo MRI shows bone marrow edema along the anterior aspect of the tibia (asterisk). (B) The primary restraint to posterior tibial translation is the posterior cruciate ligament, which is disrupted (arrow) as seen in the sagittal fat-suppressed intermediate-weighted (TR/TE, 4000/54) turbo spin echo MRI. Bone contusion is again seen in the anterior aspect of the tibia (asterisk). (C) Other associated injuries often include patellar contusion or avulsion of patellar tendon at the inferior pole of the patella (white arrow) and rupture of the posterior capsule (black arrow). Edema in the proximal tibia can be quite extensive (asterisk). (D) With the knee in flexed position the anterior cruciate ligament is lax and is usually not ruptured with a dashboard type injury unless there is dislocation of the femorotibial joint, as the anterior cruciate ligament is a restraint to anterior tibial translation. As seen on this coronal fat-suppressed intermediate-weighted (TR/TE, 3200/54) turbo spin echo MRI, the anterior cruciate ligament (long arrow) and the medial collateral ligament (short arrows) are intact.

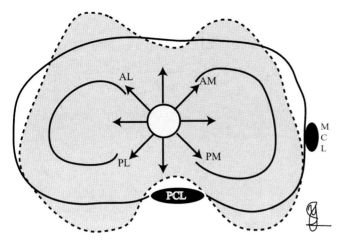

FIG. 3.9. Direction of instability. The vertical axis of the knee is usually through the center of the joint. With failure of a single ligament the axis may translate along anterior to posterior or medial to lateral lines, causing the tibia (white) to shift with respect to the femur (gray). With failure of more than one ligament the axis may shift into any one of the four quadrants: (1) anterolateral (AL), (2) anteromedial (AM), (3) posterolateral (PL), or (4) posteromedial (PM). A shift into one of the quadrants will result in rotational instability. PCL, posterior cruciate ligament. MCL, medial collateral ligament. (Courtesy of Sailaja Yadavalli, MD., PhD.).

Posterolateral Rotary Instability (PLRI)

This type of instability is seen with hyperextension, varus stress, and external rotation of the tibia. The posterior cruciate ligament is believed to remain intact and acts as the axis of rotation. Injury is predominantly to the lateral collateral ligamentous complex and the smaller supporting structures in the posterolateral corner, including the arcuate ligament. Bone marrow edema is seen in the anterior aspect of medial femoral condyle and anteromedial tibial plateau.

Posteromedial Rotary Instability (PMRI)

This mechanism of injury is attributed to valgus stress with hyperextension and internal rotation of the tibia. Bone marrow edema is seen on the anterolateral aspects of the femoral condyle and the tibial plateau (Fig. 3.14). The medial supporting structures, posteromedial capsule, posterior cruciate ligament, and possibly the anterior cruciate ligament are injured (Fig. 3.14).

Combined Rotational Instability

Multiligamentous injury with involvement of both lateral and medial supporting structures and rupture of the anterior cruciate ligament may be seen with combined anteromedial and anterolateral rotational instability.

Lateral Patellar Dislocation

Lateral patellar dislocation is seen with valgus force on a flexed knee and internal rotation of the femur on a fixed tibia. Although this is similar to anteromedial rotational instability, it is usually categorized separately to describe lateral patellar dislocation. Typically the patella dislocates laterally with the medial aspect of the patella striking the anterior aspect of the lateral femoral condyle. The degree of injury may be variable (Fig. 3.15). The resulting bone

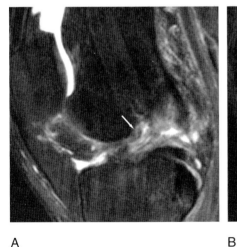
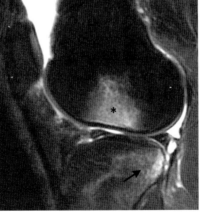
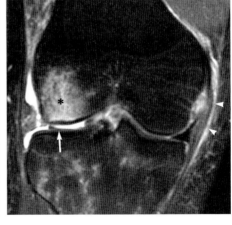

A   B   C

FIG. 3.10. Anteromedial rotary instability (AMRI). A 39-year-old man injured his knee while playing basketball. (A,B) Sagittal fat-suppressed intermediate-weighted (TR/TE, 3020/62) turbo spin echo MRI shows anterior cruciate ligament rupture (white arrow in A) and the associated bone marrow edema pattern in the lateral tibial plateau (black arrow in B) and lateral femoral condyle (asterisk in B) due to impaction injury by internal forces. (C) Coronal fat-suppressed intermediate-weighted (TR/TE, 3800/52) turbo spin echo MRI shows partial tear of the medial collateral ligament (arrowheads) due to tensile forces. In addition, note the lateral meniscal tear (white arrow) and the bone marrow edema in the lateral femoral condyle (asterisk). Patient also had a medial meniscal tear (not shown here). All findings were confirmed at surgery.

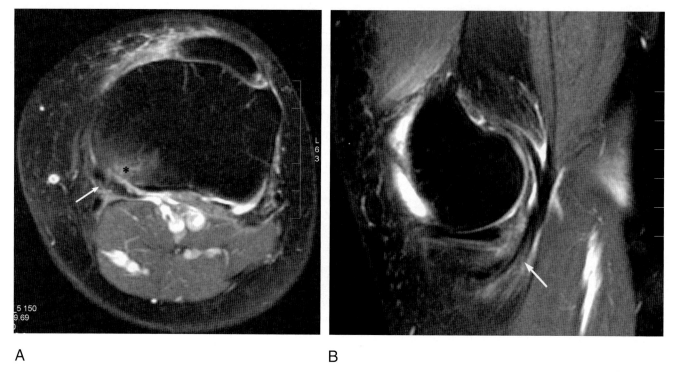

A   B

FIG. 3.11. Semimembranosus injury. This 49-year-old woman presented with knee pain after a twisting injury. Rupture of the anterior cruciate ligament was seen (not shown here). Tensile forces on the medial side of the joint can cause avulsion of the semimembranosus tendon in addition to tears of the medial collateral ligament. Axial (TR/TE, 2700/50) (A) and sagittal (TR/TE, 4000/52) (B) fat-suppressed intermediate-weighted turbo spin echo MRIs show soft tissue edema in the posteromedial corner and a partial tear of semimembranosus tendon (arrow). Associated bone marrow edema is more focal (asterisk in A) as seen with avulsion injuries.

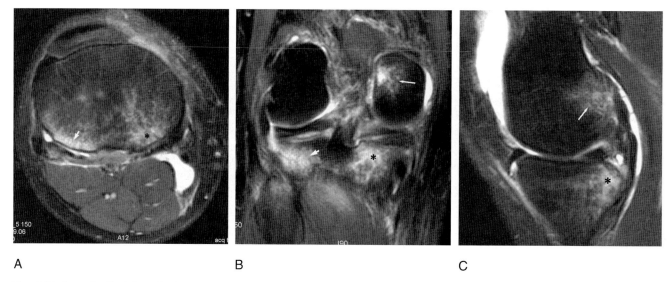

A   B   C

FIG. 3.12. Posterior lip injury. In the same patient as in Figure 3.10, bone marrow edema is seen on the medial aspect of the knee due to countercoup injury that occurs as the knee is reducing following anterior cruciate ligament disruption. Axial (TR/TE, 2570/52) (A), coronal (TR/TE, 3800/52) (B), and sagittal (TR/TE, 3020/62) (C) fat-suppressed intermediate-weighted turbo spin echo MRIs show bone contusion in the posterior lip of the medial femoral condyle (asterisk). Bone bruising in the medial femoral condyle (long arrow in B and C) is seen away from the articular surface compatible with the flexed position of the knee at time of injury. Bone contusion is seen in the lateral tibial plateau (short arrow in A and B) from the initial phase of injury.

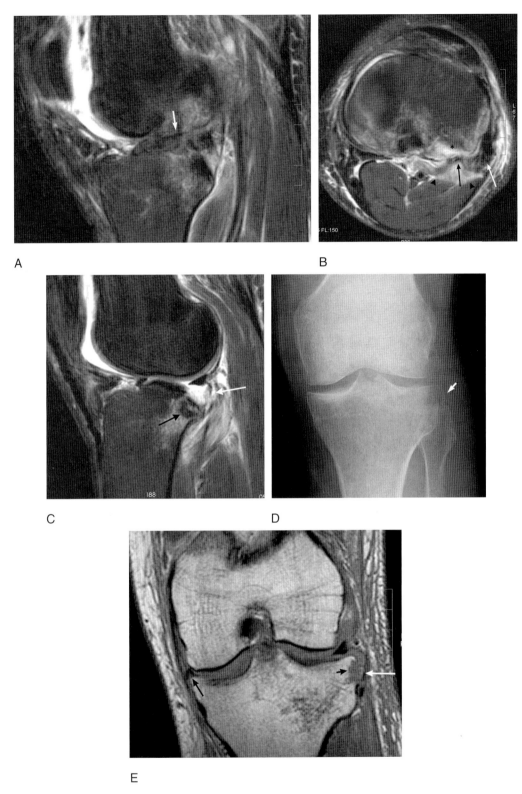

FIG. 3.13. Anterolateral rotary instability (ALRI). A 49-year-old man suffered a twisting injury to his knee when his motorcycle slid under a truck. (A) Sagittal fat-suppressed intermediate-weighted (TR/TE, 4000/55) turbo spin echo MRI shows anterior cruciate ligament tear (arrow). (B) Axial fat-suppressed intermediate-weighted (TR/TE, 2640/47) turbo spin echo MRI shows distraction injury in the posterolateral corner with extensive soft tissue edema (arrowheads). The conjoined portion of the fibular collateral ligament and biceps femoris tendon has a partial tear (white arrow). The popliteus tendon is also attenuated, compatible with a partial tear (black arrow). (C) Sagittal fat-suppressed intermediate-weighted (TR/TE, 4000/55) turbo spin echo MRI shows rupture of the posterior capsule (white arrow). A depressed fracture of the posterior aspect of lateral tibial plateau (black arrow) is also seen. (D) A small ossific density (arrow) along the lateral tibial plateau, easily seen on this radiograph, represents a Segond fracture. (E) The Segond fracture avulsed fragment (white arrow) is not as easily discernible on this coronal (TR/TE, 1200/12) proton density spin echo MRI. The donor site of the avulsed fragment is more readily apparent (short black arrow). Also note the medial meniscal tear (long black arrow).

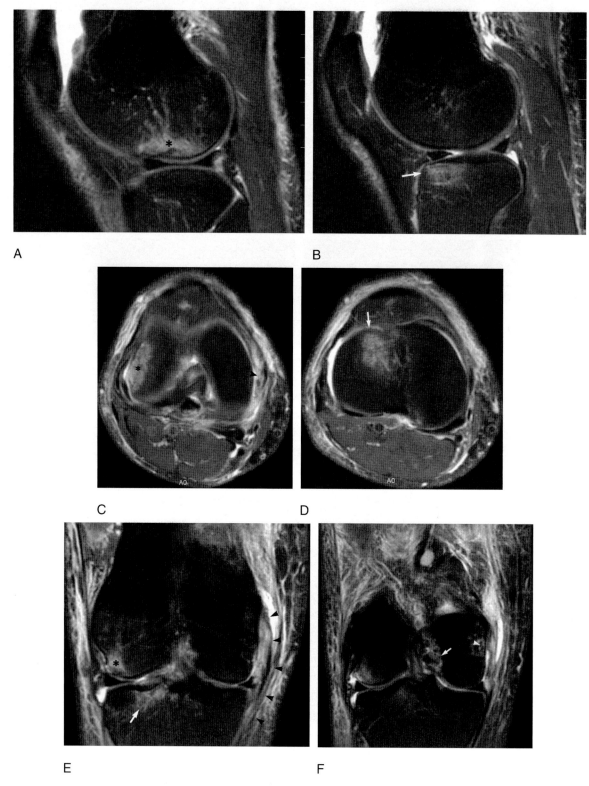

Fig. 3.14. Posteromedial rotary instability (PMRI). A 43-year-old man who presented for evaluation of medial collateral ligament and posterior cruciate ligament injury. Sagittal (TR/TE, 3450/62) (A,B), axial (TR/TE, 2660/49) (C,D), and coronal (TR/TE, 3550/52) (E,F) fat-suppressed intermediate-weighted turbo spin echo MR images are shown here. Bone marrow edema along the weight-bearing surface of the lateral femoral condyle is seen (asterisk in A, C, and E) and in the anterior aspect of the lateral tibial plateau (short white arrow in B, D, and E). The posterior cruciate ligament (short arrow in F) was torn. Tensile forces on the medial side resulted in rupture of the medial collateral ligament (arrowheads in C, E, and F). The anterior cruciate ligament was intact in this patient. These findings suggest that the mechanism of injury is related to posteromedial rotary instability.

marrow edema pattern in this injury involves the infero-medial aspect of the patella and the anterolateral aspect of the femoral condyle.[40] This pattern should be distinguished from the edema seen with anterior cruciate ligament rupture, in which the contusion is seen in the midportion to posterior aspect of the femoral condyle and from hyperextension injuries with valgus forces, where a "kissing" contusion is seen in the anterior aspect of tibial plateau. The medial aspect of the patella may fracture (Fig. 3.15A). A search for chondral defects or osteochondral injuries along the patella and the trochlear groove is extremely important

(Fig. 3.15E).[41,42] Soft tissue injuries include possible disruption of the medial retinaculum (Fig. 3.15C) and medial patellofemoral ligament, the avulsion of which may cause edema in the adductor tubercle of the femur.[43–49] Patella alta and a shallow trochlear groove are predisposing factors for patellar dislocation.

Direct Trauma

With direct trauma, injury to the osseous structures of the knee and the soft tissues between the site of impact and the bone

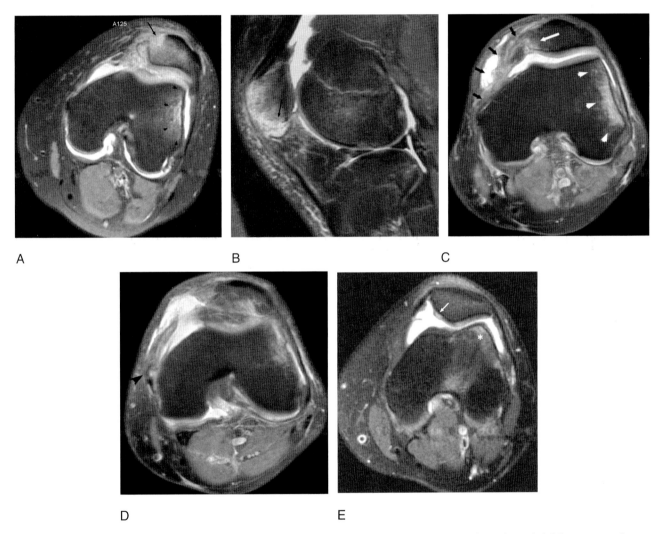

A   B   C

D   E

FIG. 3.15. Patellar dislocation. Pattern of injury with lateral patellar dislocation in three patients are shown here. Axial fat-suppressed proton density (TR/TE, 2800/14) turbo spin echo MRI (A) and sagittal fat-suppressed intermediate-weighted (TR/TE, 5260/43) turbo spin echo MRI (B) show an avulsion fracture of the inferomedial aspect of the patella (arrow) with associated bone marrow edema in this 13-year-old girl who twisted her knee. Bone contusion is seen in the axial image in the lateral femoral condyle (arrowheads). (C,D) Axial fat-suppressed proton density MRIs in another patient with lateral patellar dislocation show more severe injury to the soft tissues with disruption of the medial retinaculum (black arrows in C) and a tear at the junction of the medial retinaculum and the medial collateral ligament (black arrowhead in D). Bone marrow edema is seen in the medial aspect of the patella (white arrow in C), and lateral femoral condyle (white arrowheads in C). (E) Sometimes the findings of patellar dislocation may be more subtle as seen in this 35-year-old woman who presented for MRI with history of knee injury. Axial fat-suppressed intermediate-weighted (TR/TE, 2570/52) turbo spin echo MRI shows the typical bone bruise in the lateral femoral condyle (asterisk), but only a focal cartilage defect (arrow) is seen along the medial facet of the patella.

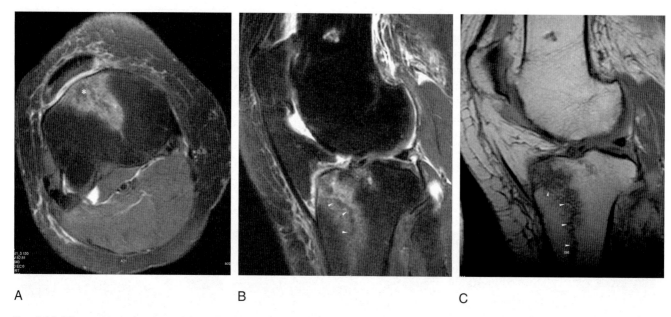

FIG. 3.16. Direct trauma. An external force applied to any part of the knee may result in injury only to the soft tissues and underlying bone at the site of impact. Most commonly this occurs with a fall on knee. These classic findings are seen in this 46-year-old woman who tripped and fell on her bent knee while walking her dogs. (A) Axial fat-suppressed intermediate-weighted (TR/TE, 2640/50) turbo spin echo MRI shows significant bone contusion along the anterior aspect of the tibia (asterisk). Sagittal fat-suppressed intermediate-weighted (TR/TE, 4300/55) turbo spin echo MRI (B) and sagittal proton density (TR/TE, 1100/12) spin echo MRI (C) show a curvilinear low signal (arrowheads) compatible with a nondisplaced fracture that was occult on radiographs.

may result. A large area of contusion is typically seen with no other injuries. A fall onto the knee is an example of this type of injury with patellar and trochlear contusion (Fig. 3.16). Direct trauma can result in fractures, especially of the patella. Some of the fractures may be occult on radiographs and readily seen on MRI (Fig. 3.16).

Meniscal Injury

Traumatic meniscal injuries are usually attributed to a single event. The menisci are at greatest risk with rotational injuries with the knee in the flexed or extended position (see Fig. 3.10C).[50] Meniscal injuries that occur with the knee in extension are often associated with ligamentous injuries and tibial plateau fractures. With significant axial loading, the hoop stress mechanism of the meniscus may fail, resulting in tears. Thus when fractures associated with axial loading are seen, a search for meniscal injuries is essential (Fig. 3.17). Meniscal injuries may be present in the absence of any ligamentous injury as in the patient in Figure 3.17.

Osteochondral Lesions

A variety of abnormalities may cause irregularity or fragmentation along the articular surface with associated bone marrow edema. Earlier in the chapter we discussed the presence of subchondral fractures with acute injuries due to axial loading or shear stresses.

Osteochondritis dissecans is an entity often seen in the skeletally immature and young adults.[51–57] The etiology of this lesion is controversial, and many causes ranging from genetic predisposition to trauma have been proposed. Currently it is widely believed that the injury is likely due to repetitive trauma.[55,57] This is supported by the fact that although earlier studies reported a preponderance of this lesion among boys, more recently, with increasing participation of girls in sports, and with children participating at younger ages, the gender gap has narrowed and the age of onset has decreased.[57] The lesion is perhaps initialized by a traumatic event that causes a subchondral fracture that progresses to fragmentation and eventually becomes symptomatic. The most common location is along the posterolateral aspect of the medial femoral condyle (Fig. 3.18).

The differential diagnosis for osteochondral lesions includes spontaneous osteonecrosis of the knee, which is seen in the elderly and is characterized by acute onset of pain.[58] The lesion is most commonly seen along the weight-bearing surface of the medial femoral condyle and may have associated bone marrow edema and cystic changes deep to the lesion (Fig. 3.19). Bone infarcts can extend to the articular surface and result in subchondral collapse (Fig. 3.20) and bone marrow edema.[59] Nontraumatic causes of bone marrow edema are numerous and include infection, arthritides, and tumor. These are most often easily distinguished from traumatic causes by the associated soft tissue changes or lesions.[60]

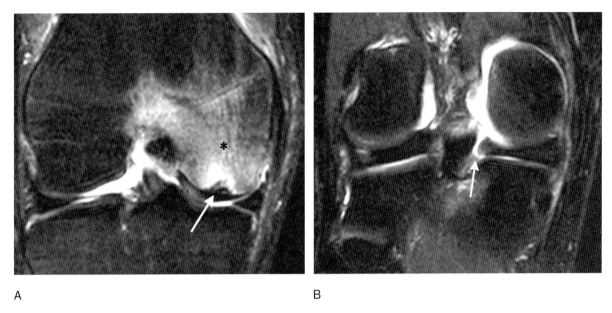

A   B

FIG. 3.17. Medial meniscal tear. Two coronal fat-suppressed intermediate-weighted turbo spin echo MRIs of a 50-year-old man who was hit on the medial side of his knee are shown here. Extensive bone marrow edema is seen in the medial femoral condyle (asterisk in A) with a subchondral fracture (arrow in A), suggesting that there was a component of axial loading at time of injury. A search revealed a radial tear of the posterior horn of the medial meniscus (arrow in B). The patient had no ligamentous injury.

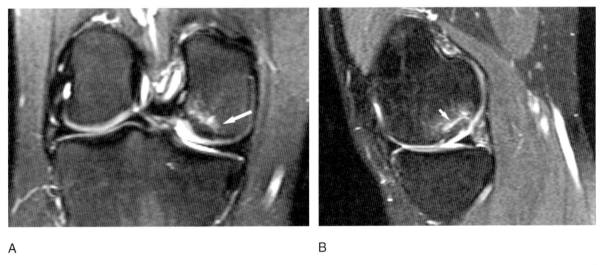

A   B

FIG. 3.18. Osteochondritis dissecans. A 16-year-old girl with a history of a meniscal tear presented for MRI for persistent pain. (A) Coronal fat-suppressed intermediate-weighted (TR/TE, 4250/54) turbo spin echo MRI shows an osteochondral lesion (arrow) along the inner aspect of the medial femoral condyle with mild associated bone marrow edema and minimal cystic changes. (B) Sagittal fat-suppressed intermediate-weighted (TR/TE, 3900/54) turbo spin echo MRI shows the lesion along the posterior aspect of the medial femoral condyle (arrow). Curvilinear high signal is seen between the fragment and the donor site, suggesting that this might be an unstable lesion, confirmed at surgery.

Conclusion

A pattern of bone marrow edema seen on an MR study may be thought of as a fingerprint left behind, implicating a particular mechanism of injury. This in turn provides clues to the associated soft tissue injuries. Understanding this relationship enables radiologists to increase their accuracy in the detection of subtle ligamentous, tendinous, or meniscal injuries. Usually a distinction can be made between injuries caused by external or internal forces. Internal forces are more apt to lead to chondral or osteochondral lesions and subchondral marrow edema. Tensile forces and external forces are rarely responsible for injuries along or extending to the articular surfaces. Subchondral injuries are more often seen with shear stress or impaction forces.

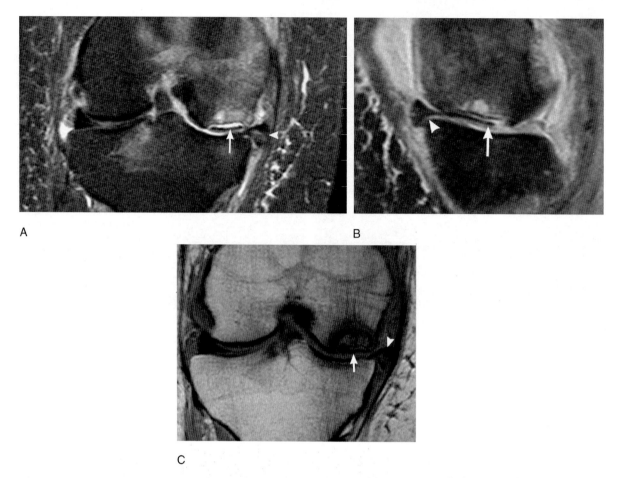

Fig. 3.19. Spontaneous osteonecrosis of the knee. A 61-year-old woman with knee pain presented for MRI to evaluate for avascular necrosis. Coronal fat-suppressed intermediate-weighted (TR/TE, 5720/26) (A), sagittal fat-suppressed proton density (TR/TE, 3810/14) (B), and coronal proton density (TR/TE, 1360/16) (C) turbo spin echo MRIs show an osteochondral fragment (arrow) along the weight-bearing surface of the medial femoral condyle. Subjacent cystic changes are seen along with extensive bone marrow edema. Severe osteoarthrosis of the medial compartment is also seen with cartilage loss, joint space narrowing, and medial meniscal degeneration and extrusion (arrowhead).

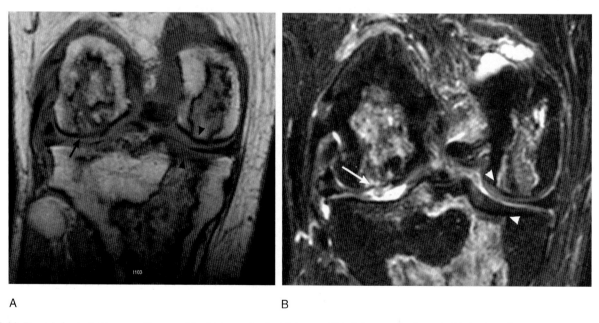

Fig. 3.20. Bone infarct. A 44-year-old man with a history of spinal injury and hip injury on ipsilateral side had persistent knee pain. Coronal proton density (A) and coronal fat-suppressed intermediate-weighted turbo spin echo (B) images show large areas of bone infarcts in the femoral condyles and proximal tibia. The infarct extends to the articular surface with collapse of subchondral bone and loss of cartilage along the lateral femoral condyle (arrow). On the medial side the infarcts extend to the articular surface. However, the cartilage appears intact (arrowheads). The high signal on fluid sensitive sequences with well-defined margins is typical of bone infarcts.

B. Orthopedic Perspective: Bone Injuries in Sports Medicine

Catherine Robertson, Ryan Serrano, and Robert A. Pedowitz

Although soft tissue injuries are the focus of most sports medicine practitioners, a number of bony lesions may occur in the athlete. While most will be detected on radiographs eventually, advanced imaging techniques such as MRI may result in earlier diagnosis, show a more detailed anatomic picture, and simplify treatment decisions.

Stress Fractures

Stress fractures are overuse injuries commonly seen in the athlete, with an incidence approaching 20% in high-risk groups.[61,62] Because their clinical presentation may be confusing or nonspecific, imaging may prove the key to rapid diagnosis or confirmation of diagnosis. Most of these injuries will heal with a period of protected weight bearing; however, certain high-risk stress fractures require operative fixation to promote healing and avoid potentially devastating complications.

Biology and Etiology

Bone undergoes a constant cycle of reabsorption and regeneration. When bone is challenged with repetitive, submaximal loading, a stress reaction will lead to physiologic and mechanical changes. Physiologically, there is not only a failure of bony synthesis but also an increase in osteoclast activity. Mechanically, there is a decrease in ultimate strength, leading to an increased risk of microfracture. With continued stress, mechanical failure may occur through these microfracture sites, resulting in a stress fracture.[63]

Although stress fractures generally occur via this biologic pathway, the anatomic location of the fracture and patient characteristics also play important roles. Stress fractures tend to occur at relatively hypovascular sites in the bone, a factor that also predisposes to slow healing.[61] Additionally, muscle attachment at a specific anatomic site may lead to a localized area of high bone stress.[64] Finally, stress fractures predominate in the lower extremities, which experience much higher stresses than the upper extremities. Patient characteristics also influence the development of stress fractures. These injuries are ten times more common in women military recruits, perhaps related to hormonal and nutritional deficiencies.[62,65] Lower bone density for any reason is also a risk factor as are less common metabolic bone diseases and collagen disorders[61,66] (Table 3.2).

Presentation and Physical Examination

Stress fractures classically present with the insidious onset of pain after an increase in activity—for example, in athletes who suddenly ramp up their training or in new recruits in basic training. Pain is generally worse with activity and improved or even absent with rest. Symptoms often occur at a specific and well-localized anatomic site but may be vague—for example, a long-distance runner with medial knee pain attributable to the hip. The history should include specifics of the training regimen and any recent changes in activity. Sports that involve high-stress activities such as running and jumping result in a higher incidence of stress fracture[63] (Table 3.3). In women, the presence of the female athlete triad (eating disorder, amenorrhea, and osteoporosis) predisposes to stress fractures, which may fail to heal or recur unless the underlying metabolic disorder is corrected.[65] A focused patient history by an attentive clinician is important in making the diagnosis of stress fracture, as physical exam findings are often nonspecific.

Superficial stress fractures may be point tender, while deeper structures may simply be irritable with motion. Swelling or a palpable periosteal reaction may also be present, again at superficial sites only. Knowledge of the common anatomic

TABLE 3.2. Risk factors for stress fractures.

- Female
- Nutritional deficiencies
- Osteopenia
- Endurance sports
- Collagen disorders
- Metabolic disorders
- Hormonal imbalance in women and men
- Sleep disorders
- Female athlete triad

TABLE 3.3. Associations of stress fracture location and sport.

Anatomic site	Sport
Femoral neck	Long distance running
Tibia	Jumping sports
2nd Metatarsal base	Dancing, gymnastics
5th Metatarsal	Basketball
Humerus, ulna	Throwing sports
Ribs	Golf, rowing

sites of stress fracture, discussed below, may also guide diagnosis. Differential diagnosis differs somewhat by anatomic site but may include soft tissue strain (muscle, tendon, or ligament), bone bruise, periostitis, tendonitis, and bursitis.

Imaging

Imaging of a suspected stress fracture may include radiography, bone scan, computed tomography (CT), or MRI. Radiographs are the first-line study as they are readily available in the physician's office and may show a subtle fracture line, cortical lucency, or periosteal reaction. Chronic stress fractures or nonunions are characterized by intramedullary sclerosis or cystic changes, related to bony remodeling. However, a negative radiograph in no way rules out the presence of a stress fracture. The radiographic changes of a stress fracture are generally not present on plain radiographs for at least 2 to 3 weeks and will never become easily visualized in up to 55% of cases.[67,68] Accordingly, further imaging modalities are frequently employed, especially when the diagnosis is in doubt or in high-level or professional athletes who require a rapid diagnosis and return to play.

Magnetic resonance imaging and bone scan are the most commonly used secondary means of imaging for suspected stress fractures. On bone scan, a stress fracture is seen as a discrete area of increased uptake on all phases of a technetium-99 m diphosphonate bone scan. These fractures may be differentiated from soft tissue injuries, which do not show high intensity in the third (delayed) phase of the bone scan. With healing of a stress fracture, the bone scan slowly reverts to normal in a phase-by-phase manner that lags far behind clinical improvement.[61,67]

Bone scan is the more traditional modality for imaging stress fractures; however, MRI has gained predominance as its availability and affordability have increased. Magnetic resonance imaging also possesses a number of inherent advantages. Bone scans show high sensitivity, approximately 90% but a specificity of only 50%, with high intensity frequently seen at asymptomatic sites.[61] Conversely, MRI shows both high sensitivity and specificity in the diagnosis of stress fractures, 90% and nearly 100%, respectively, in the tibia.[69] Bone scans typically image the entire body, which can be an advantage if there are multiple areas of interest or if stress reaction is suspected. However, this lack of anatomic specificity can be a disadvantage in imaging sites such as the foot, where small bones may become indistinguishable from one another. Magnetic resonance imaging can easily distinguish between anatomic sites but may not allow for whole-body imaging. Another advantage of MRI is that it does not carry the radiation exposure of bone scans, approximately 3 mSv.[69] Finally, unlike bone scans, which demonstrates healing that lags behind the actual stress fracture healing, MRI may be used to both diagnose and predict the healing of stress fractures. Arendt and Griffiths[70] have proposed a classification of stress fractures using bone scan and MRI data to predict time to healing (Table 3.4). Because MRI findings are more specific, the predicted healing time using MRI data is potentially more accurate. Their classification uses the following sequences for MRI evaluation: first, short-tau inversion recovery (STIR) images are most sensitive and show early intramedullary edema; T2 images then show edema and may show a fracture line; and T1 images finally may show a low-signal fracture line.[70]

Treatment: General Principles

Determining a treatment plan for a specific stress fracture requires assessment of several factors, including anatomic location, mechanical location, displacement, and chronicity. Treatment by specific anatomic site is detailed below, but certain anatomic sites, for example the femoral neck and anterior tibia, have shown historically lower healing rates and higher complication rates with nonoperative treatment. The mechanical location of the stress fracture should also be noted, as fractures on the tension side of the bone tend to widen and have a lower rate of healing when compared with compression-side fractures. Displaced fractures similarly have a lower healing rate compared with nondisplaced fractures. Finally, a stress

TABLE 3.4. Arendt and Griffiths classification of stress fracture.

	X-ray	Bone scan	MRI	Treatment
Grade 1	Normal	Poorly defined ↑ activity	Positive STIR image	3 weeks rest
Grade 2	Normal	More intense but poorly defined	Positive STIR plus positive T2	3–6 weeks rest
Grade 3	Discrete line	Sharply defined area of ↑ activity	Positive T1 and T2, but without definite cortical break	12–16 weeks rest
	Discrete periosteal reaction			
Grade 4	Fracture or periosteal reaction	More intense transcortical localized uptake	Positive T1 and T2 fracture line	16+ weeks rest

STIR, short-time inversion recovery.
Source: Arendt and Griffiths,[70] with permission.

fracture that is chronic based on the patient history or radiographic changes (cystic changes or intramedullary sclerosis) is less likely to heal by nonoperative means.[61]

Stress fractures that are stable and nondisplaced generally heal with a period of unloading and a careful return to activity. The patient is first placed on protected weight bearing for several weeks, with a gradual increase in loading as the patient becomes pain free. Immobilization with a cast or functional brace is important during this period, and the use of the brace may continue as activity is resumed. Training may then recommence with short-duration, low-impact activities (biking, swimming), which are slowly increased in duration and then intensity based on patient tolerance. If pain recurs, training should be immediately curtailed with lower level activity beginning after several days of rest.[61] Another nonoperative modality that has shown promise for treatment of recalcitrant stress fractures is electrical bone stimulation, although no randomized controlled trials are available.[71] Pulsed ultrasound has also been employed with some success in promoting bony union; however, a recent randomized controlled trial of tibial stress fractures showed no improvement.[72] Higher risk sites or recalcitrant stress fractures may require operative fixation or bone grafting due to their increased rates of nonunion and other complications.[61]

The second tenet of treatment for stress fractures is the identification and correction of predisposing factors. This includes a careful review of the training regimen and diet. In women with the female athlete triad, resumption of menses via decreased training or use of hormone replacement, usually oral contraceptives, will improve healing potential. Dual-energy x-ray absorptiometry (DEXA) scans at baseline and during treatment may be used to track bone mineral density in this patient group.[65] Finally, patients with metabolic disorders may benefit from consultation with an endocrinologist.

Specific Stress Fractures and Their Treatment

Femoral Neck

A missed stress fracture of the femoral neck that displaces often results in long-term morbidity in the young athlete. For this reason, the clinician must maintain a high level of suspicion, consider early MRI for definitive diagnosis, and pursue an aggressive treatment plan when this diagnosis is suspected. The most common presentation of a femoral neck stress fracture is activity-related groin pain in a high-level athlete, such as a long-distance runner. Symptoms, however, may be vague, and imaging of the hip should be considered in high-risk patients with knee pain (possibly referred) without another attributable cause. The location of the stress fracture, compression or tension side, largely determines treatment (Fig. 3.21). Compression-side fractures of the femoral neck start at the inferior cortex and rarely displace. They may be treated nonoperatively with protected weight bearing and close follow-up, but must be pinned if they progress or become complete. Patient compliance with weight-bearing restrictions should also be monitored closely. Tension-side fractures start at the superior cortex and tend to displace with stress (Fig. 3.21).[73]

Although several case series have successfully used prolonged bed rest to treat tension-side femoral neck fractures, most authors advocate internal fixation to avoid completion of the fracture or displacement, with its high rate of complication.[73,74] Regardless of the treatment modality, stress fractures must be protected until clinical and radiographic healing

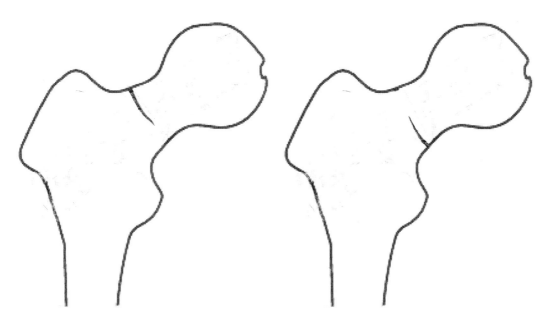

FIG. 3.21. Femoral neck stress fracture patterns. Stress fractures of the femoral neck may occur on the tension (A) or compression (B) side. Location of the fracture largely determines stability and therefore treatment.

occurs. If a stress fracture of the femoral neck becomes complete and displaces, expedited open reduction with anatomic alignment and internal fixation is required. Complications of a displaced femoral neck fracture include malunion, nonunion, and avascular necrosis, resulting from a disruption in blood supply to the femoral head.[73] Specifically, Johansson et al.[75] found a complication rate of 60% in patients with displaced femoral neck stress fractures in spite of appropriate treatment. Also, in this study, no elite athlete returned to the same level of play, reflecting the seriousness of these injuries.

Tibia

The tibial shaft is the most common anatomic site of stress fractures, accounting for 20% to 75% of stress fractures in athletes[61] (Fig. 3.22). Tibial stress fractures generally present with activity-related pain and tenderness on exam. Other potential diagnoses include periostitis and exertional compartment syndrome, which may be clearly differentiated on imaging studies. Two types of tibial stress fracture have been identified: the more common posteromedial compression variety, and the less common but higher risk anterior tension fracture. Activity modification reliably leads to union in the stable, posteromedial fractures, and supplemental use of a pneumatic brace may reduce healing time.[76] Conversely, anterior, midshaft fractures show a higher rate of nonunion, likely due to their tension-side location and relative hypovascularity. The dreaded "black line" on a plain radiograph heralds nonunion at this site. The anterior tibial stress fracture takes a minimum of 4 to 6 months to heal despite protected weight

bearing. If a widening of the anterior cortical disruption on x-ray does occur, the likelihood of healing is low, and placement of an intramedullary nail may be considered. Early fixation is also an option in a competitive athlete.[61,77,78]

Foot and Ankle Sites

Stress fractures in the foot and ankle represent approximately 25% of cases.[61] In general, they are not easily seen on standard radiographs, due to oblique fracture lines, or on bone scan, due to the close proximity of a number of small bones. An MRI should be considered if a stress fracture is suspected, as early lesions without a radiographically apparent fracture line are more responsive to nonoperative treatment.

Stress fractures in the metatarsals represent approximately 10% of the whole, with fractures of the second and third metatarsal neck predominating.[61,66] Stress fractures of the fifth metatarsal are less common but more problematic because of their slow healing and high refracture rate (Fig. 3.23). These occur in jumping and sprinting athletes, for example basketball players, in the proximal metatarsal shaft, just distal to the tuberosity. Physical exam reveals point tenderness and pain with foot inversion. An early lesion (radiographically negative, MRI positive) may be treated with protected weight bearing and a functional brace while advanced lesions (symptoms >3 weeks or radiographically positive) are more likely to respond to prolonged casting or internal fixation with a compression screw. In an established nonunion, the fracture site should be curettaged prior to fixation with consideration of bone grafting.[61,79] Another metatarsal site of stress fractures

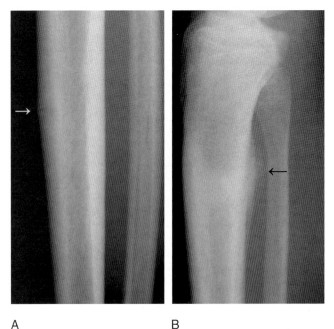

A   B

FIG. 3.22. Tibial shaft stress fractures. Stress fractures of the tibia generally occur by two patterns: (A) the high-risk anterior shaft fracture, and (white arrow) (B) the relatively benign posteromedial fracture (black arrow).

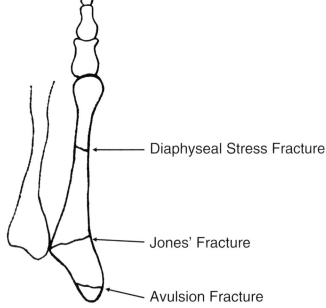

FIG. 3.23. The three common locations of fractures of the fifth metatarsal, with stress fractures generally occurring in the proximal diaphysis.

in athletes is the second metatarsal base in dancers. Although these will heal reliably with activity modification and a non–weight-bearing interval, high-demand athletes may benefit from surgical fixation.[79,80]

In the ankle, the distal fibula and medial malleolus may incur stress fracture related to repetitive impingement on the talus. Fibular stress fractures are low risk and heal reliably with activity modification, while medial malleolus fractures are considered high risk. Magnetic resonance imaging–positive, radiograph-negative medial malleolar fractures may be treated with bracing in lower-level athletes or casting and strict non–weight bearing in competitive athletes. Competitive athletes unable to wait the 4- to 5-month healing time or patients with radiographically positive lesions should undergo internal fixation with malleolar screws.

Navicular stress fractures occur in the sagittal plane in the midlateral portion of the bone, an area of high stress and poor vascularity. This lesion is frequently missed on radiographs due to its orientation and is best imaged by MRI as bone scan has poor specificity for differentiating stress reaction from fracture at this site. Again, early lesions may be treated with casting and non–weight bearing, while chronic or displaced lesions should be stabilized surgically. Stress fractures of the sesamoids predominate on the medial side. These fractures may easily be confused with a bipartite sesamoid on radiographs (present in 5% to 30% of the population) but are reliably identified on bone scan or MRI. Again, early lesions may be treated conservatively, while chronic or recalcitrant lesions may be treated with bone grafting or excision, being careful to maintain the position of the flexor hallucis brevis to avoid late hallux valgus deformity. A final rare stress fracture in the foot occurs at the lateral process of the talus. This fracture may extend into the subtalar joint, resulting in sinus tarsi pain, and is poorly identified on radiographs. Casting and non–weight bearing for at least 6 weeks is necessary for healing.[61]

Stress Fractures of the Upper Extremity

Stress fractures in the upper extremity represent a small minority, approximately 5% to 15% depending on the study.[61,81] As stress fractures are a response to overuse, athletes who use their arms to throw, swing, or bear weight (gymnasts, weight lifters) are the most commonly affected. Stress fractures in every bone from the shoulder girdle to the distal phalanx have been reported; however, injuries of the ulna, olecranon, and humerus are the best studied. Ulnar shaft stress fractures occur in the thin middle third in throwers and racquet sports players, are low risk, and heal well with activity modification. Stress fractures of the olecranon occur predominately in baseball pitchers, likely related to repeated impaction on the olecranon fossa or increased stress at the triceps insertion. While olecranon tip fractures heal poorly and are best treated with excision or operative fixation, mid-olecranon fractures heal with rest and avoidance of throwing in 6 to 8 weeks. Stress fractures of the humerus likely occur related to high stresses created by the

deltoid, biceps, and triceps, and are most commonly seen as spiral fractures of the middle to distal shaft. Operative treatment is often indicated in completed or displaced fractures.[81]

Discussion

Stress fractures are overuse injuries of bone that present with localized, activity-related pain. They are generally slow to resolve, and secondary patient characteristics should be addressed to optimize healing. The early use of MRI in radiographically negative patients may improve treatment by allowing early immobilization and potentially avoiding surgical treatment. Treatment differs by site based on the risk of displacement, the nonunion rate, and the usual time to healing. Nonoperative treatment of stable fractures includes a period of activity modification and protected weight bearing followed by a slow return to activity. Higher risk fractures may be treated nonsurgically if identified early or with internal fixation in compression if diagnosed late or in high-demand athletes.

Bone Bruises and Subchondral Fractures

The bone bruise is a common finding on MRI after traumatic injury, particularly of the knee. It is less a diagnosis to be sought but rather an MRI finding that must be interpreted by the clinician with regard to its clinical significance and treatment required, if any. The bone bruise has traditionally been seen as a secondary marker of ligamentous injury but may have some significance as an isolated clinical entity or as a prognostic indicator.

In the literature, a number of synonymous terms have been used for bone bruise, including bone contusion and occult bone lesion. Regardless of the term used, the entity described is actually a spectrum of injuries to subchondral bone seen on MRI but not on plain radiography. Histologic changes have been correlated with these MRI findings confirming that bone bruises may represent bony edema, hemorrhage, or in cases of higher energy trauma, microfracture of the trabeculae.[82] A number of classification systems have been described in the radiology literature seeking to separate the benign from the clinically important, with variable success. The most commonly used are the Vellet and the Mink and Deutsch.[2,83] For the orthopedic practitioner, the more important distinction is between a simple bone bruise and a subchondral fracture (by definition, displacement of 2 mm) extending into cartilage or a depressed osteochondral lesion, both of which reliably indicate chondral injury.[83]

Common Patterns

As the bone bruise is a bony response to loading during trauma, its location is a reliable radiographic indicator of the mechanism of injury and associated injuries, most commonly ligamentous. The bony findings are generally anatomically opposite to their ligamentous counterparts as the area of compression (bony injury) is distant from the area of tension (ligamentous injury) (Table 3.5).[84,85]

The pattern of bone bruising after anterior cruciate ligament (ACL) injury is well described as a bone bruise centrally in the lateral femoral condyle and posterior on the lateral tibial plateau (Fig. 3.24). A contrecoup bruise on the posterior lip of the medial tibial plateau may also occur and is associated with medial meniscus tear in some studies.[85] The usual mechanism of the ACL tear occurs by an axial and valgus load to the knee with relative external rotation of the tibia. The anteriorization of the tibia during ACL disruption results in the posterior lesion on the tibia. This pattern of bone bruising has a sensitivity of 80% to 90% and a specificity of approximately 90% for the ACL tear, making it a helpful marker in cases where the ACL is not well imaged or disrupted but nondisplaced.[86] Conversely, a lack of bony bruising may be an indicator of a lower energy injury or partial tear.[87] In adolescents, this ACL pattern of bone bruising may be seen without ligament tear, perhaps due to increased ligamentous laxity. Finally, a bone bruise in ACL injury is associated with prolonged effusions and pain and a longer time to normalization of range of motion.[88]

The pattern of bone bruises in posterior cruciate ligament (PCL) injury is not as anatomically reliable, but a bone bruise is seen in more than 80% of these ligament disruptions.[89] This may be because a number of mechanisms may result in PCL tear, including a dashboard-type injury and hyperextension, or because PCL injuries have a high association with other injuries in the knee, including a tear of the meniscus and collateral structures. The most common pattern is an anterior bone bruise on the tibia, sometimes associated with a bruise of the posterior patella. Bone bruises may also occur after injury to the menisci and collateral ligaments but at lower rates, approximately 50% to 60%.[90] In accordance with biomechanical principles, bone bruises occur anatomically distant from the site of collateral ligament injury, for example in the lateral knee after a medial collateral ligament (MCL) tear. However, bone bruises may also occur at the site of soft tissue injury, such as near a meniscal tear or at the bony avulsion site of a ligament. These principles may also be applied to injuries of the ankle, where bone bruises may be seen in areas of impaction after a sprain or at the site of an avulsion injury.

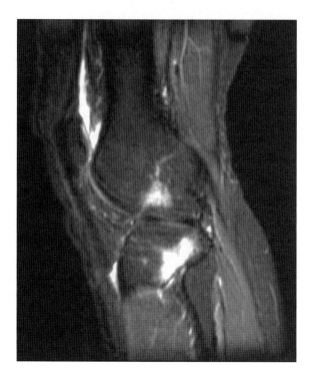

FIG. 3.24. After anterior cruciate ligament injury, characteristic bone bruises in the lateral femoral condyle and posterior tibial plateau are commonly seen.

Isolated Bone Bruise

A single study by Wright et al.[91] describes the outcomes of isolated bone bruises in the knee, emphasizing their common association with other injuries. In this study of only 23 patients, 21 returned to preinjury activity after an average of 3.2 months with Lysholm scores of 90 points. Outcome was not correlated to the Vellet classification of the lesion on the injury MRI, and follow-up MRI was not done.

Clinical Significance and Treatment

After a diagnosis of bone bruise is made, the clinician must decide whether treatment is required and whether any short- or long-term sequelae are implied.[92] The MRI signal changes of bone bruises resolve over time in almost all cases, though the time to resolution varies from months to 1 to 2 years.[93] The more important determination is of associated chondral injury (Fig. 3.25). Evidence of an osteochondral fracture or depression is highly correlated with chondral damage.[83] This may be due to direct damage to chondrocytes from blunt trauma or by increased stress on the cartilage after damage to the subchondral bone. However, the literature does not clearly support long-term cartilaginous deficiency resulting from simple bone bruises. Rates of 10% to 70% of chondral injuries after bone bruise have been noted on follow-up MRI or arthroscopy, including softening or fissuring, but few good studies exist.[84] If a chondral injury is noted, it tends to persist on

TABLE 3.5. Ligament injuries and associated bone bruise patterns.

ACL	Central in lateral femoral condyle and posterior on lateral tibial plateau
PCL	Variable
	Anterior tibia, chondral surface of patella
Collateral ligaments	Compartment opposite to ligament tear
Meniscal tear	Tibial surface underlying tear

ACL, anterior cruciate ligament; PCL, posterior cruciate ligament.

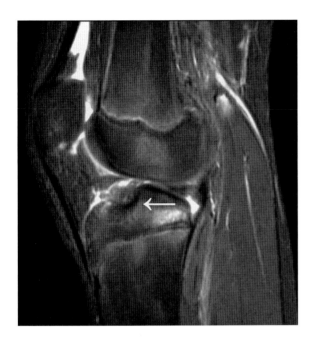

FIG. 3.25. Chondral injury may be seen as depression or fracture of the articular surface (arrow) associated with a bone bruise.

imaging but may or may not be symptomatic.[92] Thus, a change in weight-bearing status or follow-up MRI is generally not recommended after a simple bone bruise is noted. Equally, in our experience, interpretation of these lesions as a bone bruise or subchondral fracture does not alter diagnosis, though the literature on this subject is limited.

Discussion

A bone bruise is an impaction injury of the subchondral bone occurring after trauma. Its location may suggest an associated pattern of ligamentous injury and a higher energy injury. Bone bruises with associated osteochondral fracture or depression have a high rate of persistent chondral damage, while simple bone bruises are more likely to resolve with time.

Avulsion Fractures

Avulsion fractures are a group of sports injuries characterized by failure of bone at a bone–soft tissue interface. A small fleck of bone on the initial radiograph often serves as a clue to the diagnosis, but advanced imaging can be helpful to clarify anatomy and guide treatment. Avulsion fractures may be better understood by separating injuries based on skeletal maturity.

Pediatric/Adolescent Avulsion Fractures

In adolescents and children, these injuries occur at apophyses or secondary growth centers that are not yet fused. A forceful contraction of muscle at its origin results in disruption of the apophyseal cartilage, essentially a Salter-Harris fracture.

These injuries most commonly occur in the pelvis and knee and present with the sudden onset of localized pain or even a pop heard or felt during exertion. Young athletes involved in sprinting, kicking, and hurdles are at highest risk. Physical examination may reveal tenderness or swelling at the site of injury, subtle weakness of the involved muscle group, and pain with resisted activation of that muscle. Initial radiographs may show a fleck of displaced bone or may appear normal if the fracture is nondisplaced or the area not fully calcified. In these cases, further imaging may be considered. A CT scan best evaluates the fracture fragment with regard to size and amount of displacement. An MRI is useful when the diagnosis is unclear, to better evaluate the soft tissues and cartilage, and to differentiate from muscle strains and contusions. A number of common avulsion fractures in adolescents are presented in Table 3.6.[93]

Once the diagnosis of avulsion fracture is made, treatment is generally nonoperative. Patients are restricted from athletic activities and placed on protected weight bearing. A return to activity is not recommended until early callus is seen on follow-up radiographs, usually at 3 to 4 weeks. Weight bearing and a regimented muscular rehabilitation program are then initiated. To prevent reinjury, return to sports should be delayed until muscular strength and radiographic healing are noted, usually at the 3- to 4-month mark. Surgical treatment by internal fixation may be considered if conservative treatment fails, in highly displaced fractures, or in high-level athletes to limit convalescence. While asymptomatic nonunions may be treated conservatively, symptomatic nonunions often require surgical fixation, especially when displaced. A displaced avulsion fracture, whether acute or chronic, may not be chronically painful but may lead to a loss of force if the muscle heals in a shortened position. Another complication of avulsion fractures is the development of a painful exostosis due to abundant callus formation. An exostosis is more likely to occur in displaced fractures and may be resected if it causes pain or mechanical symptoms.

A second group of pediatric avulsion fractures occur at ligament insertions. Two examples of this are pediatric tibial

TABLE 3.6. Anatomy of adolescent avulsion fracture.

Origin	Muscle	Comments
Ischial tuberosity	Hamstring (all three possible)	Most common Associated with hurdles
ASIS	Sartorius, tensor fascia lata	Associated with sprinting, baseball
AIIS	Straight head of rectus femoris	
Greater trochanter	Gluteus medius	
Lesser trochanter	Iliopsoas	
Iliac crest	Internal and external obliques	
Patella, superior pole	Quadriceps	Chronic or acute
Distal femur	Medial gastrocnemius	May be acute or chronic

AIIS, anterior inferior iliac spine; ASIS, anterior superior iliac spine.

spine fractures and medial epicondyle apophysitis, or little league elbow. In the child, the tibial spine may fracture before the ACL is torn. If the spine is not yet ossified, this will not be readily differentiated on radiographs and may require an MRI for diagnosis. This distinction is important because a chondral fragment of the tibial spine may be repaired primarily while a ligament failure must be reconstructed.[94] Similarly, medial epicondyle apophysitis occurs when the apophyseal cartilage instead of the ulnar collateral ligament (UCL) fails after repeated stress of the elbow. Although this is more often a chronic condition, pitchers may present with an acute injury, concerning for avulsion fracture or ligament injury. Moreover, many of these children have delayed closure of the involved growth plate, further confusing diagnosis. An MRI will identify whether the UCL is in continuity and may detect loose chondral bodies associated with this condition. Though conservative, symptomatic treatment is preferred, the epicondyle may be fixed with a compression screw, and the ligament repaired as needed.[95] Finally, there may be an increased risk of avulsion fracture at sites of apophysitis, for example at the patellar tendon insertion in Osgood-Schlatter disease.[94]

Avulsion Fractures in Adults

In adults, avulsion fractures occur at the attachment point on bone of ligaments, tendons, or muscles. In most cases, the fleck of bone seen on plain radiographs is simply a marker of injury and will not alter treatment. For example, small avulsion fragments may be seen after ankle sprain, indicating lateral ligament injury, or after finger hyperextension, indicating volar plate injury. Other common avulsion injuries include those related to the collateral ligaments of the knee and the base of the fifth metatarsal. In rare cases, a large or displaced avulsion fragment will require surgical fixation in order to heal. In these cases, CT may be helpful to detail the bony anatomy and displacement or MRI to further examine soft tissues.[96]

An avulsion fracture may also act as a marker for other injuries. For example, the Segond fracture is an avulsion fracture of the lateral tibial plateau found in as many as 90% of ACL injuries (Fig. 3.26). The less common medial Segond injury is associated with PCL tears. These are helpful indicators on plain radiographs, which may assist diagnosis or lead to further imaging.[94]

Discussion

Avulsion fractures occur at soft tissue–bone interfaces when bone is the failing tissue. More often avulsion fractures may be viewed as a marker of soft tissue injury and treated accordingly. However, when diagnosis is unclear, avulsion fragments are large or displaced, or conservative treatment fails, advanced imaging and surgical treatment may be indicated.

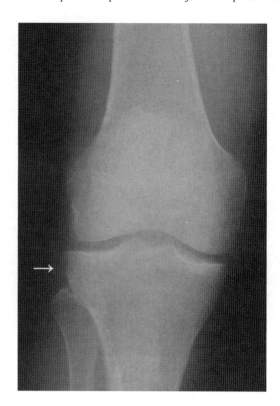

FIG. 3.26. Segond fracture of the lateral tibial plateau (arrow).

Osteonecrosis/Avascular Necrosis (AVN)

Osteonecrosis literally means "death of bone." It occurs via a wide range of etiologies in a diverse group of patients but with a common end, necrosis of bone, leading to pain and dysfunction. Although sports medicine practitioners are not usually the primary care provider in cases of osteonecrosis, they may treat patients with AVN as it generally occurs in the active 20 to 50 age group. Osteonecrosis, or avascular necrosis, also occurs after trauma, a common etiology in the athletic population.

Background

Osteonecrosis results from a disruption of the blood supply to bone. Mankin[97] characterized these vascular insults as mechanical vascular interruption, thrombosis and embolism, injury to or pressure on a vessel wall, or venous occlusion. Thus, osteonecrosis is more a description of disease that may result from a number of insults rather than a specific disease entity. The subchondral bone is most affected because sinusoids make an about face turn at the bone–cartilage interface, resulting in a heightened sensitivity to embolism or thrombosis.

A number of risk factors predispose to vascular compromise and are listed in Table 3.7, while 10% to 20% of cases are idiopathic. Risk factors occurring in the sports population are trauma, use of corticosteroids, alcohol abuse, and diving exposure, but as the athletic population expands, renal transplant recipients, HIV-positive individuals on antiretroviral

TABLE 3.7. Risk factors for osteonecrosis.

- Trauma
- High-dose corticosteroid use
- Alcohol abuse (>400 mL/day)
- Coagulopathies
- High lipid states
- Radiation treatment
- Sickle cell disease
- Caisson disease/diving
- Chemotherapy
- Antiretroviral therapy

therapy, and patients with metabolic disorders may join this group. Traumatic causes include any event that may compromise the vascular supply to a bone, for example after hip dislocation or talus fracture. High-dose corticosteroid use is also a risk factor by an unclear mechanism; however, occasional intraarticular steroid injections do not increase risk. Identification of risk factors is important because MRI is generally warranted in a symptomatic patient with normal radiographs and because discontinuation of the offending agent may prevent disease progression.[98,99]

The presentation of osteonecrosis is often vague, with nonspecific pain as the most common complaint. The clinician should emphasize the identification of risk factors in the initial interview, as the physical exam is often equally vague. Pain with range of motion and loss of terminal motion are most commonly encountered. Disease in the lower extremities is often more symptomatic and may present earlier, perhaps due to the increased stress borne by these joints.

Radiographs are the first line of imaging in avascular necrosis and will be normal in early disease. In atraumatic cases, bilateral radiographs should be obtained and will be positive in 40% to 80% of cases in the hip.[100] If the collapse and sclerosis of osteonecrosis are seen on initial radiographs, no further imaging is needed. However, if radiographs are normal in an at-risk patient, an MRI is warranted. Even early in the disease, MRI details the size and location of the lesion and is approximately 90% sensitive for identifying osteonecrosis, compared with 70% to 80% for bone scan.[101] Also, most of the classification systems used to guide treatment use MRI data in the early stages. Finally, MRI may be used to track resolution of disease in certain syndromes, for example in Kienböck's disease of the lunate.[102]

Although specific classification systems exist for most anatomic classifications, most generally follow the example of the Ficat system for the femoral head: in stage I, radiographs are normal; in stage II, sclerotic or cystic changes are seen without collapse or fragmentation; in stage III, early subchondral collapse or fracture is seen; and in stage IV, severe collapse is seen.[98] Though treatment is site specific, early disease (stages I and II) may respond to decompression or bone grafting while late disease generally requires arthroplasty or arthrodesis. Of course, radiographs do not necessarily correlate with symptoms, while treatment should be dictated by

symptoms. Also, as the natural course, in terms of symptoms at least, is variable, surgical treatment should be limited to symptomatic patients.[98]

Specific Syndromes of Avascular Necrosis

Femoral Head

Osteonecrosis of the femoral head occurs in 10,000 to 20,000 patients per year, most often in middle-aged men. Its natural history is poor, with progression of disease and femoral head collapse occurring in greater than 80% of cases. Protected weight bearing has proved ineffective for managing disease, but may be considered in minimally symptomatic or medically ill patients. Core decompression with or without bone grafting may be tried early in disease, but studies vary widely as to its success, with rates of 80% to 95% in Ficat stage I and 20% to 75% in stage II. Vascularized fibular bone grafting is another newer technique that has been used with variable success in patients with early to moderate disease.[103] After collapse occurs, arthroplasty is the standard treatment for intractable pain, though resurfacing of the femoral head shows promise and potentially preserves bone in young patients.[99]

Spontaneous Osteonecrosis of the Knee

Spontaneous osteonecrosis of the knee (SONK) is an idiopathic condition occurring in older patients, more often women. Patients present with sudden onset of knee pain and often report a minor precipitating injury. On exam, there is tenderness over the affected area, usually the medial femoral condyle, a small effusion, and relatively preserved range of motion.

First-line imaging is again the radiograph, which will be negative early in the course of disease. Lesions involving greater than 50% of the condyle tend to progress and have a worse prognosis. If radiographs are negative, a bone scan or MRI is the preferred second-line study and confirms the diagnosis of osteonecrosis (Fig. 3.27). Bone scan shows static-phase uptake limited to the condyle, as opposed to the diffuse pattern of osteoarthritis. Although MRI is probably more commonly obtained in these patients, especially if SONK is not suspected, it may be negative early in disease. This may result in unsuccessful arthroscopic treatment, as degenerative meniscal tears are common in this age group. This has led to speculation regarding a causative relationship between arthroscopy and SONK; however, misdiagnosis or overuse after arthroscopy is also a possible cause.[104]

In the acute phase (6 to 8 weeks), pain due to SONK may be severe and is often worse at night. Protected weight bearing should be implemented and the patient followed symptomatically. Another option is the use of an unloader brace. Early lesions may resolve spontaneously with time. Although traditionally definitive treatment has been deferred until symptoms and the radiologic lesion stabilize, early percutaneous drilling to decompress the lesion has shown some promise.[105] If nonsurgical treatment fails, osteotomy or unicompartmental or total

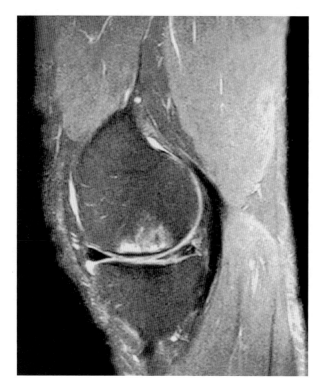

FIG. 3.27. MRI showing spontaneous osteonecrosis of the knee (SONK). Findings include a meniscal tear, loss of articular cartilage, and marrow edema.

knee arthroplasty is usually required. Osteochondral allografting has also been successful in 70% of patients at 10 years.[106]

Talus

Osteonecrosis of the talus is of interest to the sports practitioner as it predominately occurs in younger patients after talar neck fracture. Osteonecrosis complicates at least 40% of Hawkins stage II talar neck fractures (fracture with subluxation of the subtalar joint) and 90% of type III fracture (fracture with displacement of the talar body). After fracture, the Hawkins sign (subchondral osteopenia) may show revascularization at 6 to 8 weeks, but full revascularization can take 36 months. Magnetic resonance imaging may be used if diagnosis is in doubt, but is not needed if collapse has occurred. In patients with intractable pain despite bracing and antiinflammatories, arthrodesis is the gold standard surgical treatment. Arthroplasty is also available but not appropriate in young, active patients. Fresh osteochondral allografting is another new treatment modality for young patients but has been performed in only a small group of patients (Fig. 3.28).[107,108]

Discussion

Osteonecrosis of bone generally occurs in a young population and can cause significant morbidity unless diagnosed early. The clinician should consider the diagnosis in at-risk patients, even

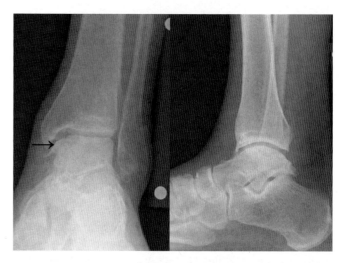

A

B

FIG. 3.28. Osteochondral allografting has shown promise for treating posttraumatic osteonecrosis of the talus. These radiographs show allograft replacement of a localized necrosis in the articular surface of the talus (arrows). (A) Preoperative. (B) Postoperative.

with nonspecific symptoms (Table 3.8). An MRI is helpful to make the diagnosis and define the lesions when radiographs are negative. Early diagnosis is important, as joint-preserving procedures will not be successful in later stages.

Other Lesions

A number of other bony lesions may be identified on MRI, from rare but morbid conditions like malignant tumors to common entities like osteoarthritis.

Table 3.8. Other sites of osteonecrosis.*

Anatomic site	Eponym	Comments
Metatarsal head, 2nd 3rd	Freiberg's	Occurs in adolescent girls Generally responds to symptomatic treatment
Navicular	Kohler's	Occurs in young males Usually resolves spontaneously
Lunate	Kienbock's	Usually occurs in a one-vessel lunate Associated with repetitive trauma
Scaphoid	Preiser's	Commonly occurs after fracture Rarely spontaneous
Capitellum	Panner's	Occurs in young males Usually resolves spontaneously
Proximal humerus	Hass's	Similar to avascular necrosis (AVN) of the hip though generally less symptomatic

*The precise cause of some of these lesions and their relationship to osteonecrosis are debated

Tumor

Tumors of bone are rare, and a full discussion of this topic is beyond the scope of this chapter. In the young, athletic population, however, osteoid osteoma is one of the more common primary bone tumors. It classically presents in young men with pain about the knee at night that is relieved by aspirin. Osteoid osteoma may be seen on plain radiographs as sclerosis or a nidus but is better localized on CT or the highly sensitive bone scan. An MRI will show a variable appearance of the lesion and surrounding edema. Osteoid osteoma may be treated with radiofrequency ablation or curettage. Conversely, enchondromas are frequently and well seen on MRI but rarely require treatment. Enchondromas are islands of mature hyaline cartilage within bone that are benign and rarely symptomatic. However, if multiple enchondromas are seen, further workup should be initiated because of the high rate of malignant transformation in Ollier's and Mafucci's syndromes.[109]

Infection

Magnetic resonance imaging is highly sensitive in identifying osteomyelitis and has a negative predictive value of 95%. However, the marrow edema seen in osteomyelitis may be nonspecific and may be confused with other inflammatory conditions.[109]

Arthritis

Osteoarthritis is a common finding in the aging athlete. It is most reliably imaged on plain radiographs. Magnetic resonance imaging is a sensitive tool for detecting the diffuse changes of bone, cartilage, and meniscus seen in osteoarthritis but is not routinely used. However, MRI may be considered if an injury occurs in the setting of arthritis, and soft tissue injury is suspected.

Metabolic Disorders

Metabolic disorders such as rickets, osteomalacia, and Paget's disease, show characteristic changes on plain radiographs such that MRI is generally not the first-line imaging modality.

Conclusion

While bone may be overlooked as simply the mechanical framework of the body, it is, in reality, a dynamic and responsive tissue. Accordingly, injuries to bone are common in the athlete and must be treated and rehabilitated with both mechanical and physiologic means. While severe or chronic injuries to bone are often seen on the radiograph, early and subtle injuries often require advanced imaging techniques for accurate diagnosis and early treatment.

References

1. Yao L, Lee JK. Occult intraosseous fractures: detection with MR imaging. Radiology 1988;167:835–838.
2. Mink JH, Deutsch AL. Occult cartilage and bone injuries of the knee: detection, classification and assessment with MR imaging. Radiology 1989;170:823–829.
3. Kapelov SR, Teresi LM, Bradley WG, et al. Bone contusion of the knee: increased lesion detection with fast spin-echo MR imaging with spectroscopic fat saturation. Radiology 1993;189:901–904.
4. Berger PE, Ofstein RA, Jackson DW, et al. MRI demonstration of radiographically occult fractures: what have we been missing? Radiographics 1989;9(3):407–436.
5. Lynch TCP, Crues JV, Morgan FW, et al. Bone abnormalities of the knee: prevalence and significance at MR imaging. Radiology 1989;171:761–766.
6. Hayes CW, Brigido M, Jamadar DA, Propeck T. Mechanism-based pattern approach to classification of complex injuries of the knee depicted at MR imaging. Radiographics 2000;20:S121–S134.
7. Sanders TG, Medynski MA, Feller JF et al. Bone contusion patterns of knee at MR imaging: footprint of the mechanism of injury. Radiographics 2000;20:S135–S151.
8. Hayes CW, Conway WF. Normal anatomy and magnetic resonance appearance of the knee. Top Magn Reson Imaging 1993;5:207–227.
9. Palmer WE, Levine SM, Dupuy DE. Knee and shoulder fractures: association of fracture detection and marrow edema on MR images with mechanism of injury. Radiology 1997;204:395–401.
10. Derscheid GL, Garrick JG. Medial collateral ligament injuries in football: non-operative management of grade I and grade II sprains. Am J Sports Med 1981;9:365–368.
11. Fetto JF, Marshall JL. Medial collateral ligament injuries of the knee: a rationale for treatment. Clin Orthop 1978;132:206–218.
12. Holden DL, Eggert AW, Butler JE. The non-operative treatment of grade I and II medial collateral ligament injuries to the knee. Am J Sports Med 1983;11:340–344.
13. Ellsasser JC, Reynolds FC, Omohundro JR. The non-operative treatment of collateral ligament injuries of the knee in professional

football players: an analysis of seventy-four injuries treated non-operatively and twenty-four injuries treated surgically. J Bone Joint Surg Am 1974;56:1185–1190.

14. Schweitzer ME, Tran D, Deely DM, Hume EL. Medial collateral ligament injuries: evaluation of multiple signs, prevalence and location of associated bone bruises, and assessment with MR imaging. Radiology 1995;194:825–829.

15. Gravin GJ, Munk PL, Vellet AD. Tears of the medial collateral ligament: magnetic resonance imaging findings and associated injuries. Can Assoc Radiol J 1993;44:199–204.

16. Sonin AH, Fitzgerald SW, Hoff FL, et al. MR imaging of the posterior cruciate ligament: normal, abnormal and associated injury patterns. Radiographics 1995;15:551–561.

17. Sonin AH, Fitzgerald SW, Friedman H, et al. Posterior cruciate ligament injury: MR imaging diagnosis and patterns of injury. Radiology 1994;190:455–458.

18. Hoover NW. Injuries of the popliteal artery associated with fractures and dislocations. Surg Clin North Am 1961;41:1099–1112.

19. Miller TT, Gladden P. Straron RB, Henry JH, Feldman F. Posterolateral stabilizers of the knee: anatomy and injuries assessed with MR imaging. AJR Am J Roentgenol 1997;169:1641–1647.

20. Yu JS, Goodwing D, Salonen D, et al. Complete dislocation of the knee: spectrum of associated soft-tissue injuries depicted by MR imaging. AJR Am J Roentgenol 1995;164:135–139.

21. Twaddle BC, Hunter JC, Chapman JR, et al. MRI in acute knee dislocation: a prospective study of clinical, MRI and surgical findings. J Bone Joint Surg Br 1996;78:573–579.

22. Hughston JC, Andrews JR, Cross MJ, Moschi A. Classification of knee ligament instabilities. Part I. The medial compartment and cruciate ligaments. J Bone Joint Surg Am 1976;58(2):159–172.

23. Hughston JC, Andrews JR, Cross MJ, Moschi A. Classification of knee ligament instabilities. Part II. The lateral compartment. J Bone Joint Surg Am 1976;58(2):173–179.

24. Rosen MA, Jackson DW, Berger PE. Occult osseous lesions documented by magnetic resonance imaging associated with anterior cruciate ligament ruptures. Arthroscopy 1991;7:45–51.

25. Kaplan PA, Walker CW, Kilcoyne RF, et al. Occult fracture patterns of the knee associated with anterior cruciate ligament tears: assessment with MR imaging. Radiology 1992;183:835–838.

26. Murphy BJ, Smith RL, Uribe JW, et al. Bone signal abnormalities in the posterolateral tibia and lateral femoral condyle in complete tears of the anterior cruciate ligament: a specific sign? Radiology 1992;182:221–224.

27. Remer EM, Fitzgerald SW, Friedman H, et al. Anterior cruciate ligament injury: MR imaging diagnosis and patterns of injury. Radiographics 1992;12:901–915.

28. Cobby MJ, Schweitzer ME, Resnick D. The deep lateral femoral notch: an indirect sign of a torn anterior cruciate ligament. Radiology 1992;184:855–858.

29. Graf BK, Cook DA, De Smet AA, Keene JS. "Bone bruises" on magnetic resonance imaging evaluation of anterior cruciate ligament injuries. Am J Sports Med 1993;21:220–223.

30. Tung GA, Davis LM, Wiggins ME, et al. Tears of the anterior cruciate ligament: primary and secondary signs at MR imaging. Radiology 1993;188:661–667.

31. Robertson PL, Schweitzer ME, Bartolozzi AR, Ugoni A. Anterior cruciate ligament tears: evaluation of multiple signs with MR imaging. Radiology 1994;193:829–834.

32. Gentili A, Seeger LL, Yao L, Do HM. Anterior cruciate ligament tear: indirect signs at MR imaging. Radiology 1994;193:835–840.

33. Chan KK, Resnick D, Goodwin, Seeger LL. Posteromedial tibial plateau injury including avulsion fracture of the semimembranosus tendon insertion site: ancillary sign of anterior cruciate ligament tear at MR imaging. Radiology 1999;211:754–758.

34. Yao L, Lee JK. Avulsion of the posteromedial tibial plateau by the semimembranosus tendon: diagnosis with MR imaging. Radiology 1999;172:513–514.

35. Kaplan PA, Gehl RH, Dussault RG, Anderson MW, Diduch DR. Bone contusions of the posterior lip of the medial tibial plateau (contrecoup injury) and associated internal derangement of the knee at MR imaging. Radiology 1999;211:747–753.

36. Shelbourne KD, Nitz PA. The O'Donoghue triad revisited. Combined knee injuries involving anterior cruciate and medial collateral ligament tears. Am J Sports Med 1991;19(5): 474–477.

37. Dietz GW, Wilcox DM, Montgomery JB. Segond tibial condyle fracture: lateral capsular ligament avulsion. Radiology 1986;159:467–469.

38. Weber WN, Neumann CH, Braakos JA, et al. Lateral tibial rim (Segond) fractures: MR imaging characteristics. Radiology 1991;180:731–734.

39. Stallenberg B, Genevois PA, Sintzoff SA Jr, et al. Fracture of the posterior aspect of the lateral tibial plateau: radiographic sign of anterior cruciate ligament tear. Radiology 1993;187:821–825.

40. Kirsch MD, Fitzgerald SW, Friedman H, Rogers LF. Transient lateral patellar dislocation: diagnosis with MR imaging. AJR Am J Roentgenol 1993;161:109–113.

41. Rorabeck CH, Bobechko WP. Acute dislocation of the patella with osteochondral fracture: a review of eighteen cases. J Bone Joint Surg Br 1976;58:237–240.

42. Sanders TG, Paruchuri NB, Zlatkin MB. MRI of osteochondral defects of the lateral femoral condyle: incidence and pattern of injury after transient lateral dislocation of the patella. AJR Am J Roentgenol 2006;187(5):1332–1337.

43. Starok M, Lenchikl L, Trudell D, Resnick D. Normal patellar retinaculum: MR and sonographic imaging with cadaveric correlation. AJR Am J Roentgenol 1997;168:1493–1499.

44. Sallay PI, Poggi J, Speer KP, Garrett WE. Acute dislocation of the patella: a correlative pathoanatomic study. Am J Sports Med 1996;24:52–60.

45. Feller JA, Feagin JA Jr, Garrett WE. The medial patellofemoral ligament revisited: an anatomical study. Arthroscopy 1993;1:184–186.

46. Conlan T, Grath WP Jr, Lemons JE. Evaluation of the medial soft-tissue restraints of the extensor mechanism of the knee. J Bone Joint Surg Am 1993;75682–693.

47. Hautamaa PV, Fithian DC, Kaufmann KR, et al. Medial soft tissue restraints in lateral patellar instability and repair. Clin Orthop 1998;349:174–182.

48. Spritzer CE, Courneya DL, Burk DL Jr, et al. Medial retinacular complex injury in acute patellar dislocation. AJR Am J Roentgenol 1997;168:117–112.

49. Hunter SC, Marascalco R, Hughston JC. Disruption of the vastus medialis obliquus with medial knee ligament injuries. Am J Sports Med 1983;11:427–431.

50. Zanetti M, Pfirrman CW, Schmid MR, et al. Patients with suspected meniscal tears: prevalence of abnormalities seen on MRI of 100 symptomatic and 100 contralateral asymptomatic knees. AJR Am J Roentgenol 2003;81(3):635–641.

51. McCauley TR. MR imaging of chondral and osteochondral injuries of the knee. Radiol Clin North Am 2002;40(5):1095–1107.
52. Hinshaw MH, Tuite MJ, De Smet AA. "Dem bones": osteochondral injuries of the knee. Magn Reson Imaging Clin North Am 2000;8(2):335–348.
53. O'Connor MA, Palaniappan M, Khan N, Bruce CE. Osteochondritis dissecans of the knee in children. A comparison of MRI and arthroscopic findings. J Bone Joint Surg Br 2002;84(2):258–262.
54. De Smet AA, Ilahi OA, Graf BK. Untreated osteochondritis dissecans of the femoral condyles: prediction of patient outcome using radiographic and MR findings. Skeletal Radiol 1997;26:463–467.
55. Crawford DC, Safran MR. Osteochondritis dissecans of the knee. J Am Acad Orthop Surg 2006;14:90–100.
56. De Smet AA, Fisher DR, Graf BK, Lange RH. Osteochondritis dissecans of the knee: value of MR imaging in determining lesion stability and the presence of articular cartilage defects. AJR Am J Roentgenol 1990;155(3):549–553.
57. Kocher MS, Tucker R, Ganley TJ, Flynn JM. Management of osteochondritis dissecans of the knee. Current concepts review. Am J Sports Med 2006;34: 1181–1191.
58. Gil HC, Levine SM, Zoga AC. MRI findings in the subchondral bone marrow: a discussion of conditions including transient osteoporosis, transient bone marrow edema syndrome, SONK, and shifting bone marrow edema of the knee. Semin Musculoskelet Radiol 2006;10:177–186.
59. Lecouvet FE, Malghem J, Maldague BE, Vande Berg BC. MR imaging of epiphyseal lesions of the knee: current concepts, challenges, and controversies. Radiol Clin North Am 2005;43(4):655–672.
60. Beltran J, Shankman S. Magnetic resonance imaging of bone marrow disorders of the knee. Magn Reson Imaging Clin North Am 1994;2(3):463–473.
61. Boden BP, Osbahr DC. High-risk stress fractures: evaluation and treatment. J Am Acad Orthop Surg 2000;8:344–53.
62. Synder RA, Koester MC, Dunn WR. Epidemiology of stress fractures. Clin Sports Med 2006;25:37–52.
63. Pepper M, Akuthota V, McMarty EC. The pathophysiology of stress fractures. Clin Sports Med 2006;25:1–16.
64. Stanitski CL, McMaster JH, Scranton PE. On the nature of stress fractures. Am J Sports Med 1978;6:391–6.
65. Brunet M. Female athlete triad. Clin Sports Med 2005;21:623–36.
66. Bennell KL, Malcolm SA, Thomas SA, et al. Risk factors for stress fractures in track and filed athletes. A twelve-month prospective study. Am J Sports Med 1996;24:810–18.
67. Sofka CM. Imaging of stress fractures. Clin Sports Med 2006;25:53–62.
68. Greaney RB, Gerber FH, Laughlin RL, et al. Distribution and natural history of stress fractures in U.S. marine recruits. Radiology 1983;146:339–46.
69. Gaeta M, Minutoli F, Scribano E, et al. CT and MR imaging findings in athletes with early tibial stress injuries: comparison with bone scintigraphy findings and emphasis on cortical abnormalities. Radiology 2005;235:553–61.
70. Arendt EA, Griffiths HJ. The use of MR imaging in the assessment and clinical management of stress reactions of bone in high-performance athletes. Clin Sports Med 1997;16:291–306.
71. Rettig AC, Shelbourne KD, McCarroll JR, Bisesi M, Watts J. The natural history and treatment of delayed union stress fractures of the anterior cortex of the tibia. Am J Sports Med 1988;16:250–55.
72. Rue JP, Armstrong DW, Frassica FJ, Deafenbaugh M, Wilckens JH. The effect of pulsed ultrasound in the treatment of tibial stress fractures. Orthopedics 2004;27:1192–5.
73. Shin AY, Gillingham BL. Fatigue fractures of the femoral neck in athletes. J Am Acad Orthop Surg 1997;5:293–302.
74. Fullerton LR, Snowdy HA. Femoral neck stress fractures. Am J Sports Med 1998;16:365–77.
75. Johansson C, Ekenman I, Tornkvist H, Eriksson E. Stress fractures of the femoral neck in athletes: the consequences of a delay in diagnosis. Am J Sports Med 1990;18:524–28.
76. Swenson EJ, DeHaven KE, Sebastianelli WJ, Hanks G, Kalenak A, Lynch JM. The effect of a pneumatic leg brace on return to play in athletes with tibial stress fractures. Am J Sports Med 1997;25:322–28.
77. Young AJ, McAllister DR. Evaluation and treatment of tibial stress fractures. Clin Sports Med 2006;25:117–28.
78. Chang PS, Harris RM. Intramedullary nailing for chronic tibial stress fractures: a review of five cases. Am J Sports Med 1996;24:688–92.
79. Fetzer GB, Wright RW. Metatarsal shaft fractures and fractures of the proximal fifth metatarsal. Clin Sports Med 2005;25:139–150.
80. Muscolo L, Migues A, Slullitel G, Costa-Paz M. Stress fracture nonunion at the base of the second metatarsal in a ballet dancer: a case report. Am J Sports Med 2004;32:1535–37.
81. Jones GL. Upper extremity stress fractures. Clin Sports Med 2006;25:159–74.
82. Ryu KM, Jin W, Ko YT. Bone bruises: MR characteristics and histological correlation in the young pig. J Clin Imaging 200;24:371–80.
83. Vellet AD, Marks PH, Fowler PJ, Muntro TG. Occult post-traumatic osteochondral lesions of the knee: prevalence, classification, and short-term sequelae evaluated with MR imaging. Radiology 1991;28:545–60.
84. Boks SS, Vroebindeweij D, Koes BW, Myriam-Hunink MG, Bierma-Zeinstra SM. Follow-up of occult bone lesions detect at MR imaging. Radiology 2006;238:853–62.
85. Mandalia M, Fogg AJB, Chari R, Murray J, Beale A, Henson JHL. Bone bruising of the knee. Clin Radiol 2005;60:627–36.
86. Lee JK, Yo L, Phelps CT, Wirth CR, Czajka J, Lozman J. Anterior cruciate ligament tears: MR imaging compared with arthroscopy and clinical tests. Radiology 1988;166:861–4.
87. Zeiss J, Paley K, Murray K. Comparison of bone contusion seen my MRIT in partial and complete tears of the anterior cruciate ligament. J Comput Assist Tomogr 1995;19:773–6.
88. Johnson DL, Bealle DP, Brand JC, Nyland J, Caborn DNM. The effect of a geographic lateral bone bruise on knee inflammation after acute anterior cruciate ligament rupture. Am J Sports Med 2000;28:152–4.
89. Mair SD, Schlegel TF, Gill TJ, Hawkins RJ, Steadman JR. Incidence and location of bone bruises after acute posterior cruciate ligament injury. Am J Sports Med 2004;32:1681–87.
90. Kaplan PA, Gehl RH, Dussault RG, Anderson MW, Diduch DR. Bone contusions of the posterior lip of the medial tibial plateau (contrecoup injury) and associated internal

derangements of the knee at MR imaging. Radiology 1989;211:747–53.

91. Wright RW, Phaneuf MA, Limbird TJ, Spindler KP. Clinical outcome of isolated subcortical trabecular fractures (bone bruise) detected on magnetic resonance imaging in knees. Am J Sports Med 2000;28:663–7.

92. Faber K, Dill J, Thain L. Intermediate follow-up of occult osteochondral lesions following ACL reconstruction. Arthroscopy 1996;12:370–71.

93. Mora SA, Mandelbaum BR, Byrd JWT. Hip and pelvis. In: Garrick JG, ed. Orthopaedic Knowledge Update: Sports Medicine 3. Rosemont, IL: American Academy of Orthopaedic Surgery, 2004:139–42.

94. Mellado JM, Ramos A, Salvado E, Camins A, Calmet J, Sauri A. Avulsion fractures and chronic avulsion injuries of the knee: role of MR imaging. Eur Radiol 2002;12:2463–73.

95. Tuite MJ, Kijowski R. Sports-related injuries of the elbow: an approach to MRI interpretation. Clin Sports Med 2006;25:387–408.

96. Morrison WB. Magnetic resonance imaging of sports injuries of the ankle. Topics MR Imaging 2003;14:179–98.

97. Mankin HJ. Nontraumatic necrosis of bone (osteonecrosis). N Engl J Med 1992;326:1473–9.

98. Lavernia CJ, Sierra RJ, Grieco FR. Osteonecrosis of the femoral head. J Am Acad Orthop 1999;7:250–61.

99. Cushner MA, Friedman RJ. Osteonecrosis of the humeral head. J Am Acad Orthop 1997;5:339–46.

100. Mont MA, Hungerford DS. Non-traumatic avascular necrosis of the femoral head. J Bone Joint Surg Am 1995;77:459–74.

101. Kokubo T, Takatori Y, Ninomiya S, Nakamura T, Kamogawa M. Magnetic resonance imaging and scintigraphy of avascular necrosis of the femoral head. Prediction of subsequent segmental collapse. Clin Orthop Rel Res 1992;277:54–60.

102. Allan CH, Joshi A, Lichtman DM. Kienbock's disease: diagnosis and treatment. J Am Acad Ortho 2001;9:128–36.

103. Marciniak D, Furey C, Shaffer JW. Osteonecrosis of the femoral head. A study of 101 hips treated with vascularized fibular grafting. J Bone Joint Surg Am 2005;87:742–47.

104. Ecker ML, Lotke PA. Spontaneous osteonecrosis of the knee. J Am Acad Ortho 1994;2:173–78.

105. Marulanda G, Seyler TM, Sheikh NH, Mont MA. Percutaneous drilling for the treatment of secondary osteonecrosis of the knee. J Bone Joint Surg Br 2006;88:740–46.

106. Jamali AA, Emmerson BC, Chung C, Convery FR, Bugbee WD. Fresh osteochondral allografts. Clin Orthop Rel Res 2005;437:176–85.

107. Fortin PT, Balazsy JE. Talus fractures: evaluation and treatment. J Am Acad Orthop 2001;9:114–27.

108. Meehan R, McFarlin S, Bugbee W, Brage M. Fresh ankle osteochondral allograft transplantation for tibiotalar joint arthritis. Foot Ankle Int 2005;26:793–802.

109. Canale T. Campbell's Operative Orthopaedics, 10th ed. St. Louis: Mosby, 2003.

4
Spine

A. Radiologic Perspective: Imaging of the Spine in Sports Medicine

Mini N. Pathria

Diagnostic imaging plays an increasingly important role in the detection, management, and follow-up of spinal disorders. The use of a wide range of imaging modalities such as routine radiography and scintigraphy, as well as newer imaging modalities such as computed tomography (CT) and magnetic resonance imaging (MRI) allow accurate diagnosis of a broad range of osseous, articular, and soft tissue abnormalities in the spine. This chapter presents a broad overview of the appropriate use of these modalities in relation to an accurate workup of degenerative conditions, neoplastic disease, infection, and spinal trauma, and discusses the indications for and the role of diagnostic imaging for specific disorders of the spine related to sports medicine, with special emphasis on MRI assessment. The MRI appearance of a number of common sports related disorders of the spine is discussed and illustrated. While diagnostic imaging accurately depicts the anatomy of a multitude of disorders involving the spine, it must be emphasized that the findings from imaging studies must be interpreted in conjunction with clinical and laboratory findings for accurate diagnosis and optimal patient management.

Overview of Imaging Modalities

Imaging modalities are categorized into two groups based on whether or not they employ ionizing radiation to form an image. The commonly used modalities that employ ionizing radiation are radiography, conventional tomography, CT, myelography, and scintigraphy. Magnetic resonance imaging and ultrasound do not require the use of ionizing radiation to form an image.

Conventional Radiography

Conventional radiography is the initial screening examination for the spine due to its ability to visualize osseous structures with high spatial resolution, relatively low cost, and widespread availability.[1] The ability to visualize compact cortical bone is excellent, but the trabecular bone is more difficult to

evaluate. Bone lesions producing disruption of the vertebral cortex, such as fractures and neoplasms destroying the vertebral borders, are relatively easily visualized. Bone loss limited to trabecular bone from tumor, osteoporosis, or infection is less easily seen. The presence of metal is not a limiting factor for radiography as it is for many advanced imaging techniques, allowing assessment of the postoperative spine safely and without artifact. Assessment of the soft tissues, however, is limited due to the poor contrast resolution of radiography. Conventional radiographs are helpful for identifying soft tissue gas or radiopaque foreign bodies, but are very limited for detailed assessment of soft tissue lesions other than gross swelling and large masses.

While standard radiographs are a static form of imaging, dynamic fluoroscopy and stress radiography are commonly employed to assess spinal alignment, motion, and stability. Radiographs can be obtained at the extremes of the voluntary range of motion or during manual application of distraction or angular stress. These stressed views may demonstrate malalignment or abnormal motion due to instability when no abnormalities are seen in the neutral position.

Conventional and Computed Tomography

Tomographic imaging methods allow imaging of a selected predetermined plane section of a solid object. Conventional tomography is an obsolete radiographic technique whereby synchronous motion of the film and x-ray tube produced blurring of objects outside the selected focal plane. Conventional tomography was widely used in the past for assessment of spinal injury and spinal fusion but is no longer widely employed, having been virtually replaced by CT.

Computed tomography is an ionizing radiographic technique whereby the body is visualized as a series of stacked slices, decreasing tissue overlap and affording higher contrast resolution as compared to conventional radiography. The technique has excellent spatial resolution and is excellent for assessment of the osseous structures. Metallic objects produce extensive artifact and limit the use of this technique in patients with orthopedic instrumentation or metallic foreign bodies. While CT images are typically acquired in the axial plane, the data are easily manipulated to allow for planar and three-dimensional reconstructed images. Reformatted planar and three-dimensional images generated from the CT data are valuable for enhancing visualization of abnormalities and for rendering complicated spatial information in easily understandable planes.[2]

In sports medicine imaging, CT is an important adjunct to radiographs, particularly in areas of complex skeletal anatomy such as the spine and pelvis. It is particularly well suited for the assessment of spinal injury, and for identification of posterior arch stress injuries, identifying acute fracture lines, detecting retropulsed bone fragments narrowing the spinal canal, and assessing spinal alignment (Fig. 4.1). Recent advances in CT, such as the advent of rapid imaging using helical CT, have decreased the imaging time significantly, allowing CT to be used as rapid and efficient screening tool in the acutely injured patient.[3] Due to advances in imaging technology and concerns about legal liability for missed injuries, CT is rapidly replacing radiography as the preferred imaging modality for screening of the injured spine, largely due to its higher sensitivity for osseous injury.[4]

Myelography

Myelography is an invasive technique that involves the injection of iodinated contrast material, or less frequently air, into the subarachnoid space within the spinal canal via a cervical or lumbar puncture. Complications of the technique include headache, leakage of cerebrospinal fluid, contrast reaction, infection, and, rarely, herniation of cranial contents due to spinal canal depressurization in patients with elevated intracranial pressure. Myelography has largely been replaced by MRI for assessment of the contents of the spinal canal. Myelography is still considered the gold standard for accurate diagnosis of arachnoiditis, delineation of subarachnoid cysts, assessment of spinal block, and the diagnosis of traumatic nerve root avulsion. Currently, the technique is typically combined with a planar imaging techniques such as CT.[5]

Scintigraphy

Three-phase bone scanning with technetium-99 M–labeled diphosphonate compounds plays an important role in sports medicine imaging.[6] In the spine, scintigraphy is used most often to survey the skeleton for metastatic disease, to identify stress injuries, and for the early diagnosis of spinal infection. While anatomic spatial resolution is limited on bone scans, scintigraphic activity correlates with functional bone turnover, affording much higher sensitivity for stress-related injury to the bone than conventional imaging techniques.[6] Scintigraphic techniques are particularly helpful for early diagnosis and assessment of the metabolic activity and clinical significance of radiographically evident spondylitic defects.[7] Single photon emission computed tomography (SPECT) images afford

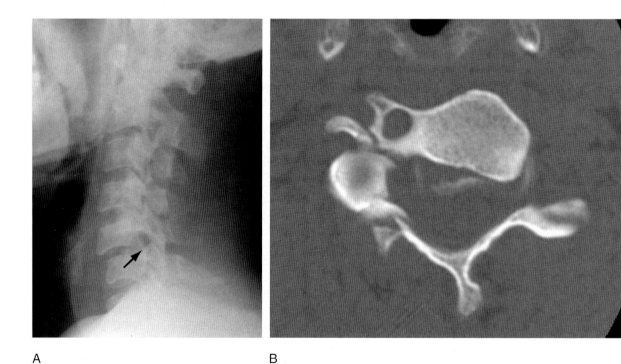

A   B

FIG. 4.1. Spine fracture. (A) Lateral radiograph of the cervical spine shows anterolisthesis of C5 relative to C6 (arrow) with rotation and malalignment of the facet joints at this level. (B) The injury is better characterized on the axial computed tomography (CT) image obtained at the bottom of C5. The CT shows multiple fractures with rotation of the C5 body toward the left.

improved spatial localization of areas of uptake and are particularly useful for assessing the posterior vertebral arch (Fig. 4.2); SPECT images illustrate stress changes in the posterior arch, particularly in the area of the pars interarticularis, prior to the development of radiographic abnormality.[8]

Magnetic Resonance Imaging

Magnetic resonance imaging has an increasingly important role in the assessment of spinal disorders due to its high sensitivity and accuracy for detecting anatomic abnormalities involving the osseous and soft tissue structures of the spine. The technique is noninvasive and does not employ ionizing radiation, leading to high patient acceptance. Magnetic resonance imaging is multiplanar and provides excellent contrast and spatial resolution. Due to advances in coil design and imaging times, MRI can evaluate long segments of the spine, allowing visualization of a broad anatomic region at one sitting. The major disadvantages of MRI include relatively high cost (although the cost has dropped considerably in the last decade), long examination times requiring a cooperative patient who can hold still, somewhat limited availability, and numerous contraindications related to implanted metallic materials. Absolute contraindications for MRI include implanted pacemakers, cardiac valve replacements, implanted electrical devices, intraocular metallic bodies, and intracranial aneurysm clips.[9] While implanted orthopedic devices are not a contraindication to the study, the extreme sensitivity of this technique to implanted metal often results in imaging artifacts that render the exam uninterpretable.

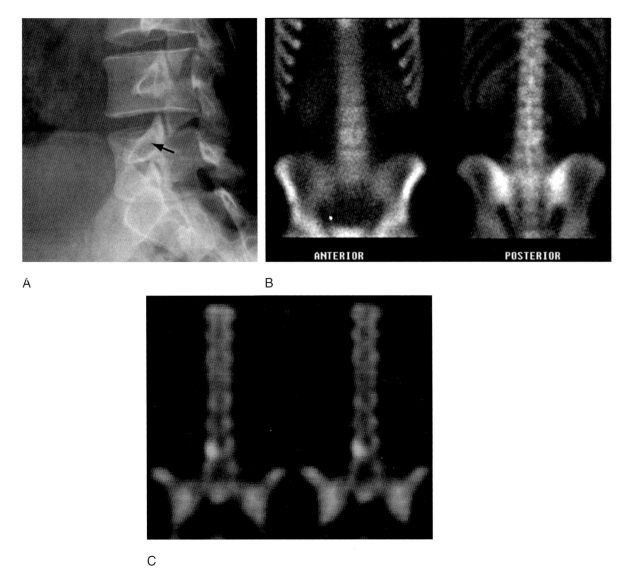

A   B

C

FIG. 4.2. Stress fracture of pars. (A) The oblique lumbar radiograph shows a questionable area of lucency in the anterior pars interarticularis of L4 (arrow), but no definite fracture line is visible. (B) The conventional bone scan appears normal. (C) The single photon emission computed tomography (SPECT) image shows abnormal uptake in the area of the right L4 pars corresponding to the stress fracture.

The soft tissue contrast resolution of MRI is far superior to other modalities. Normal bone marrow in adults is high signal intensity on both T1 and T2 images owing to the predominance of fat. The intervertebral disk, which is low signal on T1 images and increases to intermediate high signal on T2 images, is well seen and easily distinguished from adjacent tissues. The spinal ligaments and cortical bone are low signal on all imaging sequences. While mineralized trabecular bone is not as well seen as with CT, the medullary changes associated with the osseous pathology render MRI more sensitive than CT for bone trauma, osteomyelitis, and marrow replacement processes.

Degenerative Diseases of the Spine

Degenerative disease of the spine represents the most common cause of spine symptoms in the general population. The syndromes associated with degenerative conditions involving the spine range from the acute back pain syndrome that resolves spontaneously over a period of days to weeks, to chronic debilitating back pain that interferes with the patient's long-term well-being and functional ability.

Acute Back Pain Syndrome

The acute back pain syndrome is a common and expensive health care problem in our society. Approximately 2% of all adults visit a doctor because of back pain annually, and 60% to 80% of adults develop severe incapacitating low back pain at some time in their life. Among athletes, the incidence of acute back pain is even higher, presumably due to overuse and injury of the spine in this population.[10] The cause of the majority of acute back pain episodes remains unclear. Regardless of the exact cause, the vast majority of patients with acute back pain syndrome resolve spontaneously or with conservative therapy. Muscle strains, ligament strain, facet capsule inflammation, tears of the annulus fibrosus, and disk herniation have all been proposed as etiologic factors.[10] While mechanical causes play a role in the syndrome, biochemical undoubtedly play a role. It has been noted that a pronounced inflammatory response to disk material is initiated in some patients.[11] This inflammatory response results in the liberation of phospholipase A, arachidonic acid, and other mediators of the prostaglandin pathway.[12] Antiinflammatory drugs are often successful in alleviating the symptoms of the degenerative disk condition without altering the underlying anatomic lesion.

The role of routine imaging in patients with acute back pain is controversial because of the relatively poor correlation between clinical symptoms and imaging findings in patients with acute back pain. There is general agreement that immediate imaging is not indicated unless the patient is at significant risk for fracture, infection, or neoplasia.[13] While numerous imaging guidelines have been proposed, all of which vary in their details, the general recommendations related to the acute back pain syndrome advocate conservative management for 4 to 7 weeks prior to any diagnostic imaging, unless the patient meets criteria for earlier radiographic evaluation.[14] Suggested appropriateness criteria for early imaging include neurologic deficit, suspected fracture due to severe trauma or underlying osteoporosis, suspected infection, history of malignancy, prior radiation therapy, and postoperative back pain.

Chronic Degenerative Disorders of the Spine

Degenerative changes in the spine are a common finding and increase in frequency with aging. Some of the numerous degenerative conditions that affect the spine include disk dehydration, thinning and herniation, degenerative tears of the annulus, osteophyte formation, facet osteoarthritis, and bony proliferation. Inconsistencies in terminology, poor correlation between imaging findings and clinical symptoms, and limited impact on patient outcome have led to confusion and controversy about the value of imaging in patients with degenerative conditions involving the spine. It must be understood that in the typical patient with low back due to degenerative disease, early imaging does not appear to have a significant effect on treatment and outcome.[15]

In order for imaging to play a useful role in patients with degenerative spinal disease, accurate communication using a common and consistent terminology is essential. Terms used by radiologists and surgeons to describe degenerative diseases of the spine include *spondylosis deformans, intervertebral osteochondrosis, osteoarthrosis, osteoarthritis, diffuse idiopathic skeletal hyperostosis, enthesopathy, degenerative spondylosis, disk desiccation, disk degeneration, disk herniation, annular fissure, annular tear,* and numerous other terms that may not be applied consistently or precisely. As a result, the North American Spine Society (NASS), in conjunction with the American Society of Spine Radiology and the American Society of Neuroradiology, has developed a consistent terminology that can be used for describing degenerative abnormalities of the spine.[16]

The NASS terminology avoids the use of the nebulous term *disk herniation* and describes lesions of the disk according to the appearance of the disk and annulus on MRI.[16] The earliest finding of disk degeneration is dehydration, which is manifest as loss of signal of the nuclear material on T2-weighted sequences. A generalized bulge refers to the disk's protruding circumferentially 3 mm or more beyond the bone margin due to weakening of annular fibers. A disk protrusion is a focal but broad-based projection of disk material into the spinal canal. The hallmark of a disk protrusion is that it is wider in the coronal plane than in the sagittal plane. A bulge or protrusion may be associated with focal area of high signal in the annular fibers representing an annular tear. These forms of degenerative disk disease are commonly seen in the asymptomatic population.[17] A disk extrusion has a narrow pedicle and is elongated in the sagittal plane (Fig. 4.3).

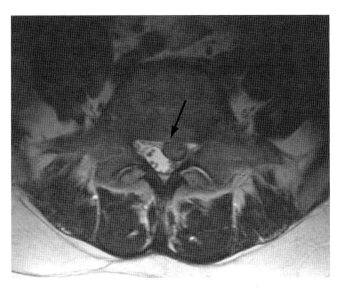

FIG. 4.3. Disk extrusion. An axial T2-weighted MRI at the L5-S1 level shows a large left paracentral disk extrusion (arrow) displacing the thecal sac.

The most advanced form of disk pathology is a sequestered disk, in which the displaced disk fragment has lost its attachment to the parent disk. Utilizing the NASS terminology, Jensen et al.[17] assessed the spinal MRI findings in 98 asymptomatic adults who had never experienced back pain or radiculopathy. Only 36% of these asymptomatic individuals had a completely normal MRI examination, 52% of patients had at least one bulging disk, and 27% had at least one disk protrusion. Schmorl nodes (19%), annular defects (14%), facet joint osteoarthrosis (8%), and spondylolysis (7%) were also common (Fig. 4.4). This landmark study showed that the only findings that are infrequent in asymptomatic individuals are the presence of a frank disk extrusion or sequestration. Studies utilizing conventional radiography had previously shown that there is little difference between symptomatic and asymptomatic individuals in the frequency of spinal anatomic lesions such as disk space narrowing, osteophyte formation, and spondylolysis.[18] The finding that MRI also failed to distinguish between symptomatic and asymptomatic individuals has led to further questions regarding the usefulness of imaging in patients with degenerative disorders of the spine.

Acute Spine Injury

Annually, up to 10,000 patients in the United States survive a spinal cord injury, the majority of which are caused by motor vehicle accidents and falls.[1] Approximately 10% of these serious injuries are athletic, occurring during a variety of contact and individual sports.[19] The exact incidence of spinal injury due to sports is difficult to assess due to underreporting of minor injuries such as sprain and strain. Fortunately, few athletes sustain serious traumatic injury to the spine, and the incidence of

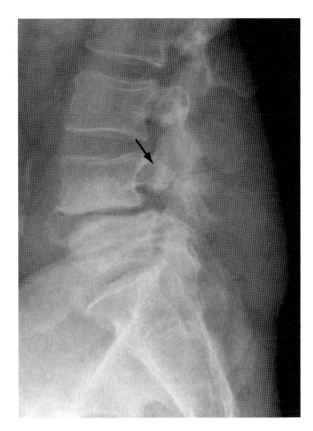

FIG. 4.4. Degenerative arthritis. A lateral radiograph of the lumbar spine shows numerous abnormalities. There are pars defects at L4 (arrow) with anterolisthesis at the L4-L5 level. There is severe degenerative disease at L4-L5, producing disk space narrowing, endplate sclerosis, and osteophytes. Moderate degenerative changes are also present at L5-S1.

serious trauma has decreased with improvements in training and equipment and due to the banning of dangerous maneuvers such as spear-tackling in football.[20] The majority of spinal injuries related to sports are transient myofascial syndromes produced by nonspecific soft tissue injury. These soft tissue syndromes resolve spontaneously over a period of several weeks. The exact pathophysiology of many posttraumatic soft tissue injuries, such as cervical "whiplash" from rapid acceleration-deceleration, remains unclear. These nonspecific soft tissue pain syndromes do not have any imaging correlates, so routine imaging for minor spinal injury is not productive. Paraspinal soft tissue injury in the form of muscle tear or muscle hematoma can be visualized with CT or MRI, but such morphologic abnormalities are rare in the spinal region (Fig. 4.5).

Imaging the Acutely Injured Spine

Imaging is reserved for patients with major trauma, neurologic deficit, or significant risk factors for spinal injury. Radiography, CT, and MRI are all useful for assessment of the injured spine. Early identification and accurate imaging characterization of spinal trauma is critical for determining appropriate management and preventing further morbidity or mortality.

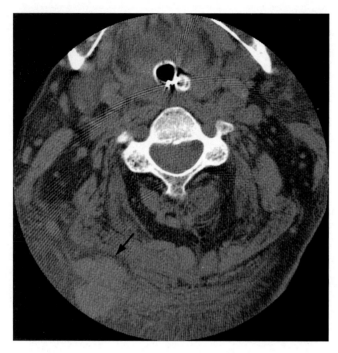

Fig. 4.5. Hematoma. An axial CT examination of the neck in a patient who sustained direct blunt trauma shows a high attenuation hematoma (arrow) in the right posterior soft tissues.

Initial evaluation of the traumatized spine begins with conventional radiography. Radiographic assessment of the cervical spine typically consists of an odontoid view, an anteroposterior (AP) view, a lateral view, and a swimmer's view of the cervicothoracic junction if this region is inadequately visualized on the lateral projection. The thoracic and lumbar regions are assessed with AP and lateral projections. The radiographic examination should be evaluated for soft tissue swelling, indicating acute trauma; alignment of the osseous structures, which allows for an indirect assessment of ligament integrity; and disruption of bony contours, indicating fracture. While radiographs are a reasonable screening examination and show the majority of significant spinal injuries, advanced imaging with CT and MRI is more accurate and often necessary for adequate assessment of spinal injury.[1] Because of its higher sensitivity for spinal injury, most institutions currently rely on rapid CT for initial screening of the severely injured patient. Whether CT should be used for screening in all patients with spinal injury, including patients with low impact trauma with a low risk of injury, remains controversial.[4] Magnetic resonance imaging is useful in patients sustaining traumatic neurologic injury unexplained by CT due to its ability to directly visualize the nerve roots and spinal cord with this modality.[21]

Acute spinal trauma is categorized by the location of the injury, its presumed mechanism and by the presence or absence of instability.[1] The most common locations of injury are the lower cervical and thoracolumbar regions, and the most common mechanisms of spinal trauma are flexion and axial loading. The topic of acute spinal injury is extensive and beyond the scope of this chapter; a brief review of the imaging finds of common spinal injuries is presented.

Craniocervical Trauma

The craniocervical junction includes the occipital condyles, as well as the C1 and C2 vertebral bodies, which have distinctive anatomy as compared to the remaining vertebrae. This region of the spine is often difficult to assess radiographically due to the complexity of its anatomy and the relatively subtle nature of fractures in this region.[22] Injuries of the upper cervical vertebrae are often associated with cranial and facial trauma.[1] The craniocervical junction is particularly vulnerable to injury in children under the age of 10 due to incomplete ossification, ligamentous laxity, weak neck muscles, and a relatively large head.[23]

Fractures of the occipital condyles are typically unilateral and are markers of high-impact trauma.[24] The only radiographic finding in such fractures is prevertebral edema; the fracture is notoriously difficult to see on radiographs and is seen best with CT.[22] Craniocervical dissociation is a rare injury that is almost always fatal at the time of the injury. The mechanism of injury is typically a severe distractive force resulting in anterior and superior displacement of the cranium relative to the superior articular facets of C1.[22] Radiographic findings include distraction and anterior displacement of the anterior rim of the foramen magnum (basion) in relation to the dens, widening of the occipitoatlantal articulations, and an abnormal Power's ratio.[25]

Atlantoaxial instability refers to abnormal alignment between C1 and C2. There are several forms of instability at this joint, the most common being anterior displacement of C1 relative to C2 due to incompetence of the transverse ligament. Less common forms of malalignment include inferior, posterior, superior, and rotary malalignment. Traumatic atlantoaxial rotary fixation (AARF) is a poorly understood form of atlantoaxial malalignment in which the ring of C1 becomes fixed in rotation relative to C2, resulting in a rigid torticollis deformity.[1] The odontoid view shows persistent asymmetry in the sizes of the C1 lateral masses and in the distance between the dens and the lateral masses of C2. Rotary fixation may be due to trauma, but is more commonly associated with retropharyngeal and upper respiratory tract infection.

Traumatic atlantoaxial instability is most commonly due to a tear of the transverse ligament or avulsion of the tubercle to which it attaches to the lateral mass of C1. This injury can be quite subtle on neutral radiographs and may be apparent only when the patient flexes the spine.[22] Flexion results in anterior translation of C1 relative to C2, with widening of the space between the posterior margin of the C1 vertebral body and the anterior margin of the dens. While transverse ligament incompetence is frequently traumatic, there are numerous congenital and inflammatory disorders that can disrupt the ligament. Common atraumatic causes of atlantoaxial instability include rheumatoid arthritis and other inflammatory arthropathies,

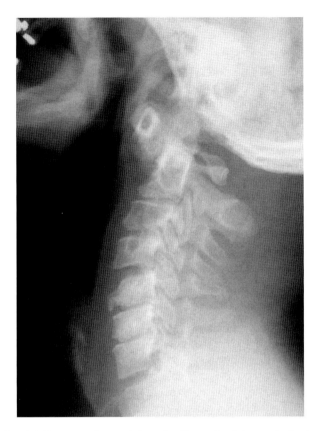

FIG. 4.6. Down syndrome. A lateral radiograph of the cervical spine in a patient with Down syndrome demonstrates congenital hypoplasia of the posterior arch of C1 and marked widening of the atlantoaxial joint. Degenerative changes are present in the lower cervical spine.

infection, osseous anomalies, and congenital laxity or deficiency of the transverse ligament. The most common congenital etiology is Down syndrome; atlantoaxial instability is estimated to be present in 10% to 40% of patients with the disorder, but it is rarely symptomatic.[26] An atlantoaxial distance of greater than 4.5 mm on lateral flexion and extension radiographs has been recommended as the criterion for atlantoaxial instability[27] (Fig. 4.6). During the 1980s, the National Special Olympics Committee and the American Academy of Pediatrics recommended that sports participation be restricted for individuals meeting this criterion, though the need for such restriction remains controversial.[28] The American Academy of Pediatrics no longer recommends routine radiography prior to sports participation, but instead recommends careful neurologic evaluation in children with Down syndrome prior to participation in sports, particularly sports that result in hyperextension of the spine.[28]

The most common fractures seen at the C1 level include the relatively benign isolated fracture of the posterior arch produced by hyperextension, and the more significant Jefferson injury, which involves both anterior and posterior arches of the atlas. Isolated fractures of the posterior arch may be unilateral or bilateral and are well seen on lateral radiographs and CT. Unilateral fractures are typically undisplaced, whereas bilateral fractures show superior displacement of the posterior fragment. The clinical course of these fractures is benign, though some patients experience severe occipital neuralgia related to the proximity of the occipital nerve to the fracture line.[1] The Jefferson fracture of C1 is an axial loading injury resulting in both anterior and posterior arch fractures, creating a sagittal defect in the vertebra that allows peripheral extrusion of the fracture fragments. The Jefferson fracture may be unilateral or bilateral. The odontoid projection shows characteristic lateral displacement of the lateral masses of C1 with respect to the lateral masses of C2. While the fracture lines may not be directly visualized on routine radiographs, CT clearly demonstrates the pattern of osseous failure.

The most common fractures at the C2 level are fractures of the base of the odontoid process and traumatic spondylolisthesis (hangman's fracture).[22] Odontoid fractures are subdivided into three types. The rarest form is the type 1 fracture, in which the fracture line occurs obliquely in the upper dens. Type 2 fractures are transverse fractures involving the base of the dens, whereas type 3 injuries extend into the C2 vertebral body.[1] Fractures of the odontoid are frequently overlooked due to the undisplaced nature of many such injuries and difficulty obtaining high-quality open-mouth radiographs.[22] Fracture displacement, if present, results in disruption and step-off of the posterior vertebral margin of C2, and malalignment of spinolaminar line at the C1-C2 level. Since odontoid fractures are frequently transversely oriented, thin sections and reconstructions are recommended for adequate CT assessment. Traumatic spondylolisthesis of C2, also referred to as a hangman's fracture, is typically caused by hyperextension. In this injury, there are bilateral fractures of the pars interarticularis of C2 that develop immediately anterior to the inferior articular facets. Approximately 20% of such injuries extend into the C2 vertebral body; vertebral canal disruption may also be present with resultant vascular injury. On radiographs, the fracture typically results in kyphosis and anterior displacement of the body of C2 relative to C3, with retropulsion of the posterior arch of C2.

Lower Cervical Spine Trauma

The lower cervical spine is the most common location for nonfatal vertebral fractures in adults. Injuries in the lower cervical spine are categorized according to their presumed mechanism.[29] The most common mechanisms of injury are hyperextension or hyperflexion, either alone or combined with rotation. Axial loading, lateral bending, and shearing mechanism account for the remainder of lower cervical injuries.

Flexion injuries to the spine are the most common form of lower injury; these injuries are typically related to a blow on the posterior skull or indirect injury resulting in flexion and compression of the cervical region. Stable injuries associated with flexion include minor compression fractures of the superior endplate of the vertebral body and the "clay shoveler's" fracture of the spinous process. The latter fracture is an avulsion fracture that develops most commonly at the C7 and T1 levels. Unstable flexion injuries include the flexion teardrop fracture and bilateral facet lock. The teardrop fracture refers to an avulsed triangular piece of bone arising from the antero-inferior vertebral body in association with posterior ligament injury and malalignment of the spine.[30] This fracture may be difficult to distinguish from the classic burst fracture caused by axial loading as the two injuries are closely related.[1] Bilateral facet lock is due to massive posterior ligament injury and is easily recognized on the lateral view owing to anterior vertebral displacement of the superior vertebra; the displacement is typically greater than 50% of vertebral body width (Fig. 4.7).

The most difficult flexion injury to identify radiographically is flexion instability related to injury limited to the posterior soft tissues. In the majority of cases of posterior ligament disruption, there is no fracture and the use of cervical collars and spasm at the time of injury can mask malalignment and angular deformity (Fig. 4.8). If present, radiographic findings indicating significant damage to the posterior ligaments, include widening of the interspinous space, widening of the facet joint, focal kyphotic angulation, and greater than 3 mm of anterior vertebral translation.[31] In severe injuries, the initial lateral film may show these findings, but mild injuries frequently require

delayed flexion radiographs for detection. Computed tomography is typically normal unless the injury is severe.

The diagnosis of isolated ligament injury is made most effectively with MRI.[32] The normal ligaments appear as thin well-defined linear bands of low signal intensity. Torn ligaments appear thickened, irregular, or disrupted on T1-weighted images, and show high signal within their substance on the T2-weighted images.[33] Adjacent soft tissue swelling and hemorrhage are present in the acute phase of the injury. Assessment of the spinal ligaments is hampered significantly by patient scoliosis and obliquity of position.

Flexion combined with rotation results in the unilateral facet lock injury. This dislocation can be difficult to identify on radiographs as the degree of vertebral displacement may be minimal. Findings on radiographs include focal rotation at the site of injury, narrowing of the spinolaminar distance, and mild anterolisthesis of the superior vertebra.[29] The most specific finding is the presence of an abnormal reversal of the relationship of the involved facets with anterior displacement of the inferior articulating facet of the cranial vertebra relative to the superior articulating facet of the lower vertebra. Computed tomography shows the displacement well and enables assessment of the foraminal stenosis commonly associated with this injury.[34] On axial images, CT shows a "naked" facet and the abnormal reversed position of the dislocated facet

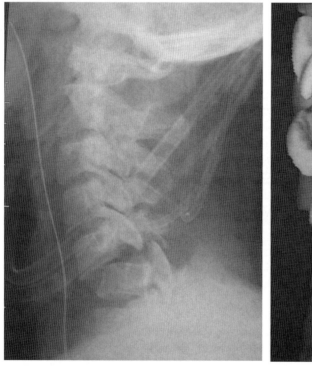
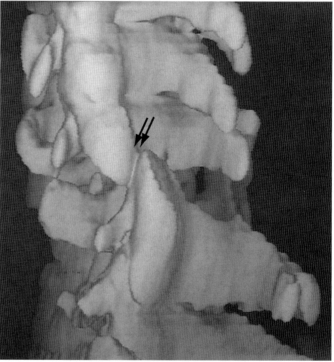

A   B

FIG. 4.7. Bilateral facet lock. (A) The lateral cervical radiograph shows anterior displacement of C5 relative to C6 of greater than half the width of the vertebral body. There is severe kyphosis and facet malalignment at the injured level. (B) The reconstructed 3D CT image shows facet malalignment (arrow) with the C5 facet dislocated anterior to the C6 facet.

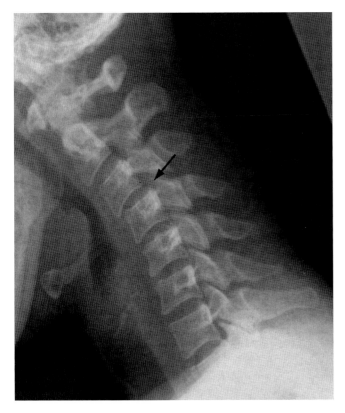

FIG. 4.8. Hyperflexion injury. A lateral radiograph of the cervical spine obtained in flexion shows subtle abnormalities at the C3-C4 level consistent with flexion injury to the posterior ligaments. There is 2 mm of anterolisthesis, as well as widening of the C3-C4 interspinous distance, widening of the posterior aspect of the C3-C4 facet joints (arrow), and a mild kyphotic deformity at the injured level.

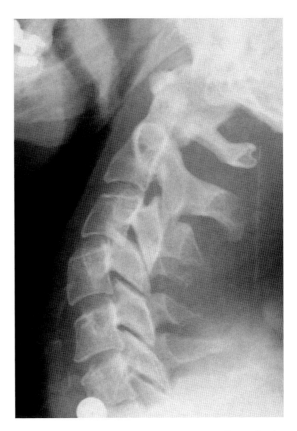

FIG. 4.9. Hyperextension injury. The lateral radiograph shows a hyperlordotic deformity at the C3-C4 level. There is widening of the anterior disk and anterior aspect of the facet joints, as well as retrolisthesis of the C3 vertebral body.

joint, though these findings are easier to appreciate on the sagittal reconstructed images.

Hyperextension of the lower cervical spine produces a wide spectrum of osseous and soft tissue spinal injuries. These injuries typically develop due to an abrupt deceleration related to motor vehicle accidents or from impaction injury of the craniofacial region. The hyperextended position narrows the spinal canal, and patients can sustain severe neurologic damage with a paucity of radiographic findings.[35] Lower cervical injuries produced by hyperextension include the extension teardrop fracture, hyperextension dislocation, and hyperextension sprain. The extension teardrop fracture is a triangular avulsion fracture originating from the anteroinferior corner of one of the upper cervical vertebrae. In the absence of malalignment and angulation, this type of fracture typically has a benign clinical presentation and outcome.

Hyperextension dislocation results from a more severe force that causes injury to the anterior longitudinal ligament and then disrupts the disk, anulus fibrosus, or bony attachments of the annulus to such a degree that vertebral retrolisthesis can develop.[36] Prevertebral hematoma is generally present following an injury of this type. Thin linear avulsion fractures arising from the endplate are seen in a small minority of patients.

Retrolisthesis may be minimal despite significant ligament injury.[37] In patients with degenerative disease, distinction of acute from chronic retrolisthesis is difficult, but listhesis greater than 3 mm is suggestive of trauma, particularly if there is disk widening or an associated lordotic deformity (Fig. 4.9). Disk space widening may be apparent only on extension views after the patient is placed in skeletal traction.[37]

Significant neurologic injury can occur in the hyperextended spine in the absence of ligament damage or frank vertebral displacement.[38] In this injury, referred to as hyperextension sprain, the spinal cord is compressed between the posterior vertebral body or posterior osteophytes and the infolded ligamenta flava, resulting in cord damage.[38] The typical clinical presentation is either transient neuropraxia or central cord syndrome caused by hemorrhage in the central gray matter.[39] Neurologic deficit related to hyperextension sprain develops most frequently in the elderly patient with degenerative changes. In young patients, congenital spinal stenosis significantly increases the risk of spinal cord injury following a hyperextension injury. Spinal canal stenosis can be detected radiographically by measuring the sagittal diameter of the spinal canal or by measuring the ratio of the diameter of the spinal canal to the width of the vertebral body.[40] The latter method is more accurate because it is not as affected by film magnification or body habitus.[40] Other than showing degenerative changes or stenosis, radiographs in patients with hyperextension sprain are typically normal or show only mild prevertebral soft tissue swelling. Computed tomography is also insensitive for detection of ligament and cord injury. Magnetic resonance imaging is the optimal method for evaluating the spine in such patients. Prevertebral hematoma, disruption of the anterior longitudinal ligament, anulus fibrosus, and intervertebral disk, as well as the presence or absence of cord compression or hemorrhage can all be visualized directly with MRI[41] (Fig. 4.10).

Prior to MRI, assessment of the spinal cord was limited to detecting gross compression or transaction. Magnetic resonance imaging allows direct assessment of the cord substance itself. Spinal cord transection and laceration are irreversible lesions of the cord that show anatomic discontinuity and disruption of the cord substance on T2-weighted images (Fig. 4.11). Contusions are hemorrhagic lesions of the cord that have a variable prognosis, depending on their size and signal characteristics. Macroscopic cord hemorrhage results in signal inhomogeneity of the cord substance on T1-weighted sequences and is associated with a poor prognosis.[42] A better prognosis is seen in patients with cord "edema," a form of mild contusion. In this pattern, the cord may be enlarged focally, shows normal signal on T1-weighted sequences and demonstrates signal abnormalities only on T2-weighted sequences.[32] The area of contusion is seen as a linear or spindle-shaped focus of hyperintense signal within the cord substance. Edema extending over multiple spinal segments has a worse prognosis than short regions of signal abnormality.

Upper Thoracic Spine Trauma

The upper thoracic spine is relatively rigid because of the large size of the vertebral facets and the support provided by the ring formed by the spine, sternum, and rib cage.[43] Though fractures and fracture-dislocations in the upper thoracic spine are not common, they exhibit a disproportionate risk of neurologic injury due to the relatively small size of the spinal canal in this anatomic area.[44] Upper thoracic fracture-dislocations are severe injuries related to major trauma that are associated with a very high incidence of severe neurologic deficit. Fracture-dislocations are easily recognized on radiographs due to the extensive bone fragmentation and vertebral displacement typically present in these injuries.[44] Recent advances in CT technology enable the assessment of long segments of the

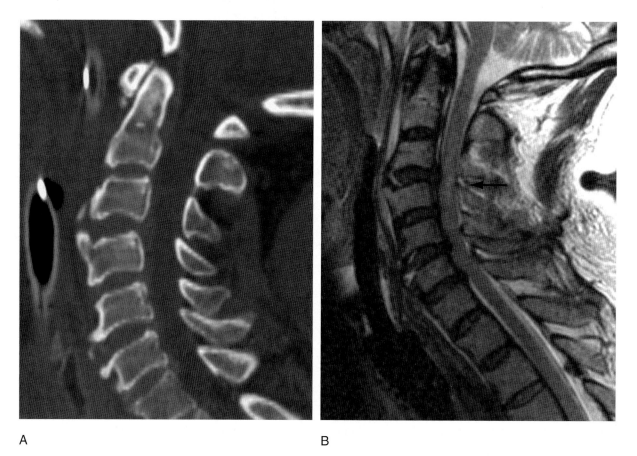

A   B

FIG. 4.10. Cord contusion. (A) The sagittal CT image shows extensive degenerative disease with osteophytes and multifocal disk protrusions. (B) The corresponding T2-weighted MRI shows compression of the cervical cord and mild high signal (arrow) within the cord substance due to contusion. Note the edema in the anterior prevertebral soft tissues.

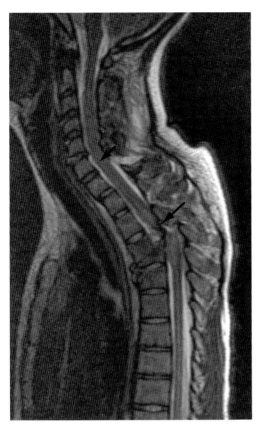

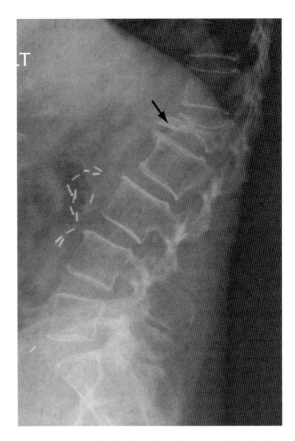

FIG. 4.11. Cord transaction. A T2-weighted sagittal MRI of the cervical and upper thoracic spine shows a fracture-dislocation involving T3-T5, with transection of the thoracic cord (arrow) at the level of the injury. Note the thickening and abnormal signal in the damaged cord adjacent to the transaction. Ligament damage with disruption of the ligamenta flava is present in the lower cervical region (arrowhead).

FIG. 4.12. Osteoporosis. The lateral radiograph of the lumbar spine in a 68-year-old woman shows diffuse osteopenia. There is a severe compression fracture of the L1 vertebral body (arrow) with loss of height of the anterior and posterior vertebral body.

spine rapidly and efficiently in patients with complex thoracic injury.[45] Magnetic resonance plays a complementary role for evaluation of the osseous injury, but is preferred for evaluating the spinal canal and spinal cord.

The majority of fractures encountered in the T1 to T10 region are compression fractures related to diminished bone mass caused by osteoporosis.[46] On conventional radiographs, the most common appearance seen with osteoporotic fractures is vertebral body height loss of greater than 20% limited to the anterior vertebral body. Alternate radiographic patterns are concavity or compression of the central portions of the vertebral endplates, or less commonly, height loss limited to the posterior vertebral margin.[46] Due to the brittle nature of osteoporotic bone, many osteoporotic fractures develop height loss of both the anterior and posterior vertebral body with retropulsion of bone into the spinal canal, leading to neurologic compromise[47] (Fig. 4.12). In the severely osteopenic patient, mild fractures can be difficult to appreciate with conventional radiography. Minimally compressed fractures can also be difficult to appreciate on CT due to the lack of a clear-cut fracture line in the deformed bone. Magnetic resonance imaging is an excellent method for assessment of osteoporotic compression fractures. Acute fractures manifest bone edema replacing the normal fatty marrow signal on T1-weighted images. Magnetic resonance imaging is also helpful for distinguishing compression fractures related to osteoporosis from pathologic fractures.[48]

Thoracolumbar Trauma

After the lower cervical region, the most commonly injured region of the spine is the thoracolumbar junction. The most widely used classification for injuries at the thoracolumbar junction is the Denis classification, which divides the spine anatomically into three longitudinal columns.[49] The anterior column includes the anterior half of the vertebral body, the anterior half of the intervertebral disk, as well as the anterior longitudinal ligament. The middle column, which is functionally the most important for maintaining spinal stability, includes the posterior half of the vertebral body, the posterior half of the disk, and the posterior longitudinal ligament. The pedicles and all the osseous and ligaments structures posterior to them make up the posterior column.

The Denis classification subdivides injuries of the thoracolumbar region into minor and major variants. The minor category includes those injuries consisting of a single unilateral fracture limited to the posterior bony arch, such as an isolated laminar or transverse process fracture. Major injuries include compression fractures, burst fractures, seat-belt type injuries, and fracture-dislocations. These injuries are defined based on the number and patterns of columns involved.[1] Compression fractures are common injuries typically produced by flexion where the osseous disruption is limited to the anterior column. The burst fracture is a more severe injury caused by axial loading, with disruption of bone at both the anterior and middle columns, often resulting in retropulsion of bone fragments into the spinal canal. On radiographs, burst fractures can be distinguished from compression fractures by identifying the loss of height of the posterior vertebral margin or retropulsed bone fragments in the spinal canal. Burst fractures with associated posterior element fractures can result in widening of the interpedicular distance. The extent of osseous retropulsion is well seen with both CT and MRI, though MRI is preferred for direct visualization of the neural structures and for assessing the spinal ligaments.[33] Computed tomography is superior for mapping the fracture lines and for visualizing undisplaced fractures of the posterior vertebral body column. Seat-belt injuries are produced by hyperflexion of the spine, resulting in distraction injury of the posterior and middle columns. Such injuries produce posterior ligament injury and horizontal vertebral fractures, often resulting in a kyphotic deformity. Fracture-dislocations are the most severe injury, resulting in disruption of all three spinal columns, allowing translation and displacement of the injured vertebrae[49] (Fig. 4.13).

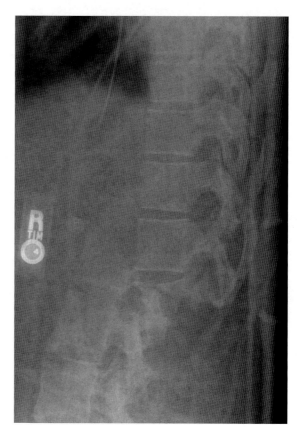

FIG. 4.13. Fracture-dislocation. A lateral radiograph of the thoracolumbar junction shows a complex fracture-dislocation centered at L2. There is malalignment of all the spinal columns and telescoping of the spine at the level of the injury.

Lower Lumbar Trauma

The lower lumbar spine includes the vertebra below L2. The same injuries that are found at the thoracolumbar region also occur in the lower lumbar spine, though with decreased frequency. This anatomic region is less mobile, deeper, and better protected by large overlying muscles and is therefore less commonly injured. The most common fractures seen following acute trauma to the lower lumbar spine are compression fractures, burst fractures, and fractures of the transverse processes. Compression fractures in the lower lumbar region tend to show more prominent central height loss of the endplate than the typical anterior height loss associated with thoracolumbar fractures. Burst fractures in the lower lumbar region show a similar pattern of preferential central height loss with a relative lack of kyphotic deformity.[50]

Transverse process fractures are common injuries related to lateral bending of the lumbar spine; multiple ipsilateral fractures are typically present.[51] There is also an increased incidence of transverse fractures of the lower lumbar vertebrae in patients with injury to the posterior pelvis, presumably due to avulsion by the iliolumbar ligaments.[52] Transverse process fractures are considered mechanically stable, though one must be aware that a small proportion are associated with psoas hemorrhage or injury to the genitourinary tract.[51] Fractures of the transverse processes may be difficult to identify on radiographs due to the presence of overlying bowel material and intestinal gas. They are frequently first identified on abdominal CT, a technique that also enables assessment of the adjacent retroperitoneal soft tissue structures.[51]

Chronic Repetitive Injury

Spondylysis and Spondylolisthesis

Spondylolisthesis is a form of spinal malalignment that refers to anterior slippage of the superior vertebral body relative to the inferior vertebral body. Wiltse and coworkers[53] have classified spondylolisthesis into dysplastic, isthmic, degenerative, traumatic, and pathologic types. The most common causes are degenerative due to osteoarthritis of the facet joints and isthmic due to defects of the pars interarticularis related to chronic fatigue fractures resulting from repeated trauma and stress. The sports most commonly associated with spondylolysis of the pars are gymnastics, diving, and contact sports such as football, hockey, soccer, and lacrosse.[54] Acute fractures of the pars interarticularis, which are far less common than chronic spondylolysis, are secondary to severe hyperextension trauma, and are typically undisplaced.[55] Pars interarticularis defects typically develop between the ages of 5 and 15 years.[53] Predisposing factors include male gender, positive family history, and the presence of developmental deficiency of the posterior vertebral arch.[56] The prevalence of pars interarticularis defects in adults is 2.3% and 10%, though the majority of these are not symptomatic.[56]

The lateral radiograph demonstrates the defect as an oblique lucent line coursing in a posterosuperior to anteroinferior direction through the pars interarticularis. In very early lesions without a clearly established fracture line, only osteopenia, narrowing, or elongation of the pars may be apparent. As the defect matures, sclerosis and fragmentation in the area of the defect become apparent.[57] Oblique radiographs are not usually necessary but can be helpful in equivocal cases. On oblique radiographs, the isthmic defect appears as a collar around the neck of the so-called Scottie dog of Lachapèle.[56] Oblique views are particularly helpful in patients with unilateral defects, as these rarely result in malalignment and are difficult to visualize on the lateral view due to the superimposition of the normal contralateral side. Unilateral spondylolysis produces reactive sclerosis and hypertrophy of the contralateral posterior arch[58] (Fig. 4.14). The bony sclerosis can simulate the appearance of an osteoid osteoma, although the absence of a nidus and the presence of dense homogeneous sclerosis favor reactive hypertrophy.

Spondylolisthesis due to spondylolysis occurs most frequently at the L5-S1 level. Over 90% of pars interarticularis defects that allow slippage occur at this level, with the remainder occurring mainly at L4-L5[59] (Fig. 4.15). By contrast, degenerative malalignment caused by facet osteoarthritis occurs at L4-L5 in 90% of cases.[59] Spondylolisthesis is graded according to the degree of malalignment. The grade of the slip increases with each quarter of the AP dimension of the lower vertebra that is uncovered. With severe slippage, secondary changes in the morphology of the vertebral body may be evident with exaggerated posterior wedging of superior vertebra and rounding of the superior margin of the inferior vertebra.[56]

Transaxial CT scans clearly demonstrate lytic defects of the pars interarticularis as disruptions in the vertebral ring just above the superior aspect of the apophyseal joints.[59] Pars interarticularis defects can be differentiated from facet joints by their more horizontal orientation and the presence of irregularity or fragmentation at the edges of the defect. Sagittal reformatted images more clearly demonstrate the course of the osseous defect and allow accurate quantification of the presence and degree of anterior displacement of the vertebral body. The combination of anterior vertebral displacement and posterior extrusion of the isolated posterior arch produces a characteristic elongated appearance of the AP diameter of the spinal canal[60] (Fig. 4.16).

Magnetic resonance imaging shows higher specificity for stress injuries of the pars interarticularis. Edema within the pedicle can be identified prior to the development of a frank defect, affording earlier detection.[60] The presence of bone edema results in increased signal within the marrow of the affected pars interarticularis on T2-weighted and short-tau

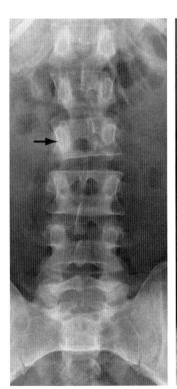
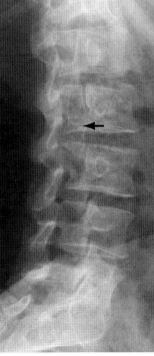

A   B

FIG. 4.14. Unilateral spondylolysis. (A) An anteroposterior (AP) radiograph of the lumbar spine shows sclerosis and hypertrophy of the right L2 pedicle (arrow). There is a mild scoliosis at this level and the L2 spinous process is deviated to the left. (B) The oblique radiograph shows a well-defined defect (arrow) through the left L2 pars interarticularis.

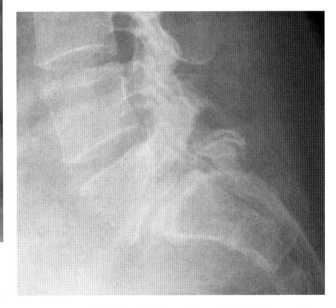

FIG. 4.15. Spondylolisthesis. A lateral view of the lumbosacral junction shows grade 2 anterolisthesis of L5 relative to the sacrum due to chronic bilateral pars defects. Note the degenerative changes at the L5-S1 disk space.

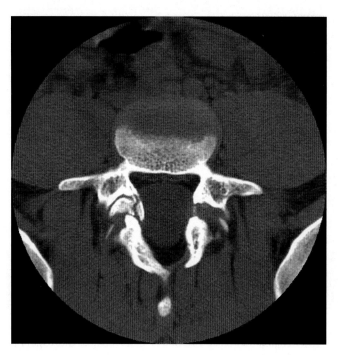

FIG. 4.16. Spondylolysis. An axial CT examination in a patient with bilateral L5 pars defects show the characteristic elongation of the spinal canal seen in this disorder due to anterior displacement of the vertebral body relative to the isolated posterior arch.

inversion recovery (STIR) images. Established pars interarticularis defects typically are of intermediate signal intensity on all pulse sequences, although their signal intensity is somewhat variable depending on the exact composition of the tissues within the defect.[60] Reactive alterations in the bone marrow within the adjacent pedicles, presumably due to altered biomechanics, may also be present.[60] Magnetic resonance is excellent for demonstrating associated spondylolisthesis, disk herniation, and foraminal stenosis associated with spondylolisthesis. The foraminal deformity can be detected on sagittal CT reformations but is easier to evaluate on sagittal MRI.[61] Obliteration of the fat surrounding the nerve root suggests nerve root entrapment within the narrowed foramen.[61]

Unlike the preceding imaging techniques, scintigraphy affords a functional assessment of metabolic activity in the region of the isthmus. In one study, Pennell et al.[62] noted that scintigraphy was positive in 73% of patients with pars sclerosis, whereas only 40% of patients with lytic defects and 17% of patients with well-established chronic defects had abnormal bone scans.[62] Single photon emission computed tomography is more sensitive for detection of stress injuries to the posterior vertebral arch than conventional bone scans.[63] In one series of 71 patients with abnormal SPECT images, only 32 had findings on planar scintigraphy[63] (Fig. 4.17). Discordance between radiography and scintigraphy occurs commonly because acute stress injuries of the pars interarticularis may not be apparent radiographically, and sites of long-standing spondylolysis may not be active metabolically.[7] Despite its ability to detect functional bone turnover, the correlation between clinical symptoms

and the pattern of radionuclide uptake in patients with spondylolysis is still poor, and clinical assessment is essential to determine the significance of spondylolysis.

Stress Fractures

While stress injuries of the pars interarticularis are common and well known, other sites within the spine are also vulnerable to stress fracture in the athlete, though the frequency of non–pars-related stress injuries is considerably lower.[64] Spinal stress fractures can involve the pedicle, lamina, spinous process, upper sacrum, and the ring apophysis. Increased scintigraphic activity is often the clue to the presence of these uncommon injuries, though anatomic injuries may also manifest abnormalities, particularly MRI. Stress fractures of the pedicle may be unilateral or bilateral. The most common etiology for stress fractures of the pedicle appears to be overload related to a unilateral spondylolysis involving the contralateral pars interarticularis.[65] Oblique fractures of the upper sacrum are typically seen in elite runners who present with low back pain and symptoms simulating sciatica.[66] Sacral fatigue fractures, like the more common insufficiency fracture of the sacrum associated with underlying osteoporosis, are well demonstrated on CT and MRI.

Injuries of the Ring Apophyses

The ring apophyses are thin growth centers at the superior and inferior endplates that are not fused with the vertebral body during childhood and adolescence. These ring apophyses serve as the attachment site of the longitudinal spinal ligaments and the intervertebral Sharpey's fibers.[67] Avulsions of the posterior apophyseal ring of the lumbar vertebrae are traumatic lesions that develop in children and adolescents. Acute and chronic injuries of the vertebral ring apophysis can take place in any region of the spine. Acute avulsions are most common in the cervical region, whereas chronic abnormalities with delayed presentation are more commonly seen in the thoracic and lumbar regions.[1] The limbus vertebra, which represents detachment of the anterior portion of the ring apophysis, is typically located at the anterosuperior endplate of one of the thoracolumbar vertebrae. This lesion is typically asymptomatic, though it may be seen in association with Scheuermann's disease. Posterior injuries are more likely to come to medical attention due to back and leg pain, paraspinal spasm, and signs of nerve entrapment.[68]

The detached limbus may be difficult to visualize on conventional radiographs, particularly those that are located posteriorly (Fig. 4.18). Findings on the lateral view include mild disk space narrowing, irregularity of the affected vertebral corner, and an irregular wedge-shaped ossific density displaced from the vertebral body.[68] On CT scans, the osseous fragment is clearly visualized, typically appearing as a well-corticated, rounded or arcuate bone fragment adjacent to a vertebral body defect that simulates a Schmorl node.[69] The fragment must be differentiated from calcified disk material and osteophytes. On sagittal MRI, the displaced bone fragment is less clearly defined and easily confused with an ossified disk-osteophyte complex.

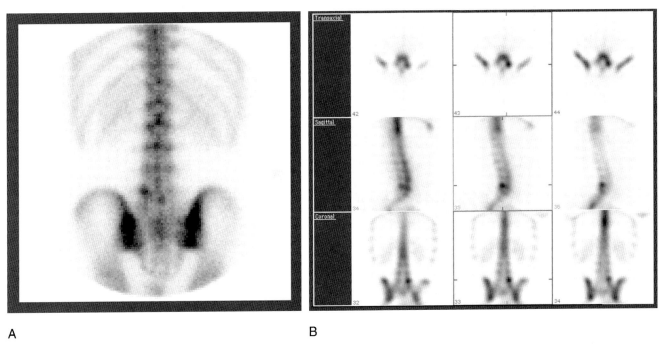

A   B

FIG. 4.17. Scintigraphy of pars defect. (A) Planar bone scan images from an adolescent female gymnast with back pain show no abnormality. (B) The SPECT images show uptake in the region of the left pars interarticularis due to a stress fracture.

Scheuermann's Disease and Schmorl Node

Scheuermann's disease, also referred to as juvenile kyphosis or Scheuermann's spondylodystrophy, is a common disorder of the spine affecting adolescents and young adults. Mild changes of Scheuermann's disease may be evident radiographically in 20% to 30% of adults, the majority of whom are asymptomatic and do not remember any traumatic event.[70] Symptomatic Scheuermann's disease is typically seen in adolescents, particularly in active adolescent boys, who present with mild to moderate pain that is relieved with rest. Scheuermann's disease typically affects the thoracic region, though lumbar involvement may be seen in association with thoracic disease, or less commonly, in an isolated fashion.

Although numerous theories have been advanced to explain Scheuermann's disease, the complete form of this disorder is most likely caused by repetitive traumatic stress to the growing spine.[71] Proponents of the posttraumatic theory believe that repetitive stress under high velocity on the immature spine, especially in the forward-bent posture utilized in sports such as elite skiing and ski jumpers, results in an osteochondrosis at the vertebral endplate.[72,73] Others believe that trauma plays a minor role in the development of this disorder, and that Scheuermann's disease simply represents one of the variant responses to standard degenerative disease of the disk that can occur in the immature spine.[74] Congenital factors may also play a role in the development of this disorder as familial clustering has been described.[75] Whatever the exact etiology, the abnormalities at the endplate ultimately reflect a unique form of premature degenerative disk disease.

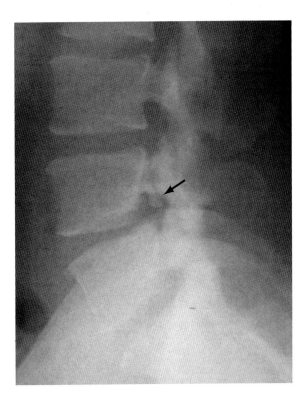

FIG. 4.18. Posterior limbus. The lateral radiograph shows a well-corticated bone fragment (arrow) within the spinal canal posterior to the inferior margin of the L4 vertebral body. There is loss of height of the L4-L5 disk and a defect at the posteroinferior corner of the L4 vertebral body. Note the loss of height of the posterior vertebral margin of L4.

The radiographic findings include disk space narrowing, endplate irregularity, multiple Schmorl nodes, and exaggerated anterior wedging of the vertebral bodies (Fig. 4.19). An increased incidence of limbus vertebrae is also found in this disorder.[74] Disk space narrowing tends to be of moderate degree and often involves multiple levels. In one study, it was noted that vertebral wedging in adolescents increased in frequency with their duration of competitive water-ski jumping, resulting in repetitive axial loading of the spine.[71] The degree of anterior height loss appears to correlate with the presence of back pain. In one study, elite adolescents skiers with greater than 18% anterior height loss were significantly more likely to be symptomatic than skiers with more minor anterior lesions.[73] In its complete form, the disorder results in a kyphotic deformity that extends over at least three vertebral bodies. On MRI, Scheuermann's disease demonstrates disk desiccation and dehydration, producing loss of disk signal on T2-weighted images, a generalized loss of disk height, and variable herniation of nuclear material into the annulus fibrosus or vertebral endplates.[74] The intraosseous herniations of diskal material are typically small and numerous, and affect multiple spinal segments.[74]

A Schmorl node develops when portions of the nucleus pulposus of the intervertebral disk become displaced into the vertebral body via a defect in the cartilaginous vertebral endplate. While Schmorl nodes are a constant feature of Scheuer-mann's disease, such intraosseous diskal herniations are more frequently identified as an isolated finding on spinal radiographs.[76] These intraosseous extensions of the disk are very common, found in 36% to 79% of cadaveric studies, and are typically asymptomatic. Over 80% of isolated Schmorl nodes are located between T7 and L2.[76] The etiology of the endplate defect is variable and often multifactorial. Congenital endplate deficiency, acute trauma, repetitive trauma, degenerative disease of the diskovertebral junction, metabolic disease with bone weakening, and neoplastic destruction of the endplate can all lead to mechanical failure of the endplate.

On radiographs, a Schmorl node is seen as a well-defined rounded lucent lesion with thin sclerotic borders located immediately adjacent to the vertebral endplate. The sclerotic margins are better visualized on CT, whereas MRI often shows contiguity with the disk and typically shows that the intraosseous material is isointense to normal disk. Magnetic resonance imaging may reveal evidence of vascularization and adjacent bone marrow edema in up to 10% of Schmorl's nodes, findings suggestive of biologic activity and possibly reflecting acute symptomatology.[77] The degree of inflammatory response can be dramatic and occasionally produce diagnostic difficulty distinguishing an inflamed Schmorl node from focal osteomyelitis (Fig. 4.20). Another potential source of diagnostic difficulty are large lesions referred to as "giant cystic Schmorl nodes."[78] Unlike classic Schmorl nodes, this giant form is not associated with Scheuermann's disease, preferentially involves the lower lumbar spine, and shows contrast enhancement.[78]

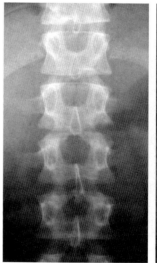 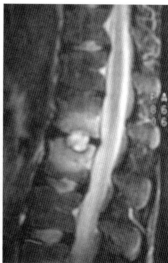

A   B

FIG. 4.20. Schmorl node. (A) An AP radiograph of a 15-year-old boy with back pain shows subtle irregularity of the inferior left endplate of L1. (B) The sagittal T2–weighted MRI examination shows a focal destructive lesion centered at the L1-L2 disk space, with edema in the adjacent vertebral body. Two biopsies of the area showed only disk material, with no findings of infection. The symptoms and MRI findings resolved spontaneously, consistent with an inflamed Schmorl node.

FIG. 4.19. Scheuermann disease. A lateral radiograph of the thoracolumbar junction in a young man reveals mild endplate irregularity, multiple Schmorl nodes and anterior wedging of the vertebral bodies.

Nontraumatic Disorders

While the majority of spinal pathology in sports medicine relates to degenerative disease and posttraumatic disorders, it must be kept in mind that athletes, like the rest of the population, can present with tumors, infection, rheumatologic disorders, and other nontraumatic etiologies of back pain.[79,80] Features that indicate that there may be a serious underlying disorder include systemic signs such as fever, neurologic deficit such as cauda equine syndrome, and significant features in the history such as intravenous drug use, HIV infection, unexplained weight loss, nonmechanical pain, night pain, or a history of prior malignancy.[10,81] In particular, back pain in young children should not be assumed to be related to athletic endeavors as children are more likely than adults to have a nontraumatic etiology for back pain and symptoms are relatively mild.[70] In the young child, warning features include the persistence of symptoms for greater than 4 weeks, interference with function, and systemic features such as fever, neurologic deficits, and new onset of scoliosis.[70]

Neoplastic Disease

The patient with a spinal neoplasm typically presents with nonmechanical local pain that is often worse at night, a pathologic fracture, or neurologic deficit. A history of previous malignancy is often present in patients with metastatic disease. Occasionally a spinal tumor is detected as an incidental finding in an asymptomatic patient; in this situation, the lesions are typically benign. Radiography, CT, MRI, and scintigraphy play complementary roles in the imaging evaluation of patients with spinal neoplasms. While it has been estimated that neoplasms account for less than 1% of all causes for low back pain, tumors still represent the most common serious systemic disorder affecting the spine.[81]

Metastatic disease represents more than 90% of all osseous neoplasms, and is largely a disease of adults and the elderly. In adults, the spine represents the largest reservoir of hematopoietic marrow in the body, and therefore is the most common site of skeletal metastasis. The most common primary neoplasms to metastasize to the spine include lung, breast, prostate, and kidney. Most patients with metastatic disease have disseminated disease, with multiple noncontiguous sites of involvement.

Conventional radiographs show poor sensitivity for lytic metastatic disease. It has been estimated that more than half the trabecular bone in a vertebra must be destroyed prior to the development of radiographic abnormalities. While the vertebral body is involved with equal or greater frequency than the posterior elements, bone destruction of the cortical posterior elements is easier to recognize on radiographs and CT.[82,83] Destruction of a pedicle or spinous process, which are composed largely of cortical bone, is the most apparent radiographic finding in patients with lytic metastases (Fig. 4.21). Sclerotic lesions, which are

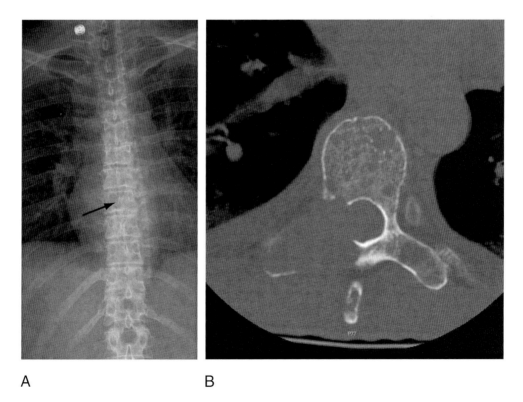

A   B

FIG. 4.21. Metastatic disease. (A) An AP radiograph of the thoracic spine shows destruction of the right pedicle (arrow) at the T8 vertebral level. (B) Axial CT at the T8 level shows a lytic lesion destroying the right pedicle, transverse process, and lamina. Smaller lytic lesions are also evident in the vertebral body.

particularly common in patients with prostate or breast cancer, are well seen on radiographs and CT. Computed tomography of metastatic disease typically shows eccentric destruction within the vertebra and a much higher frequency of posterior arch involvement than is typically seen with infection.[83] On T1-weighted MRI, metastases appear as focal areas of diminished signal loss within the marrow. The signal of metastases on the T2-weighted images is more variable, depending on the nature of the adjacent bony response. Lytic neoplasms show increased signal on T2-weighted sequences, whereas sclerotic lesions appear hypointense or isointense. Magnetic resonance is the optimal method for detecting soft tissue extension of the neoplasm producing compression on the neural structures.

Scintigraphy is traditionally used as the initial imaging test for the detection of metastatic disease in a patient with a known primary malignancy[84] (Fig. 4.22). Scintigraphy allows rapid whole-body screening, and is highly sensitive for bone metastasis, though it is clear that scintigraphy is less sensitive than MR, particularly for infiltrative or small lesions.[85]

Primary tumors of the spine are considerably less common than metastases, representing only 5% of all spinal neoplasms.[86] Accu-

rate diagnosis requires consideration of the patient's age, presenting symptoms, precise location, as well as the specific imaging and pathologic features of the lesion.[87] Multiple myeloma is the most common primary malignant neoplasm affecting the spine, typically presenting in the elderly patient as nonspecific bone pain or by development of a pathologic fracture. Multiple myeloma can present as a solitary lesion known as a plasmacytoma. Such solitary lesions frequently are large, with involvement of multiple contiguous vertebrae, similar to the appearance of spinal lymphoma and chordoma. Multiple myeloma is more commonly a diffuse disorder with multiple small lesions widely disseminated throughout the skeleton at the time of diagnosis. The diffuse form is notoriously difficult to identify with scintigraphy and conventional radiography due to the infiltrative nature of the disease and the paucity of reaction by the adjacent bone. Nonspecific diffuse osteopenia is often the only radiographic finding. As the lesions enlarge and coalesce, multiple well-defined foci of osteolysis become apparent. The MR appearance of myeloma is variable and depends on the pattern and degree of infiltration.[88] Mild disease produces only subtle marrow inhomogeneity and is difficult to detect (Fig. 4.23). It has been estimated that 20% to 25%

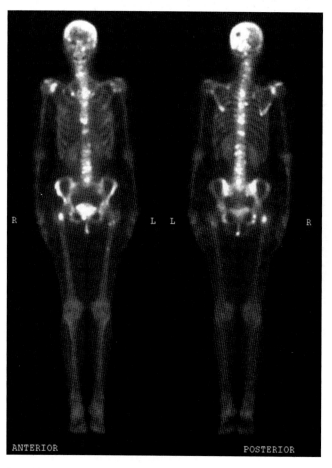

FIG. 4.22. Metastatic disease. Anterior and posterior projections from a bone scan in a patient with lung carcinoma demonstrate multiple foci of abnormal activity throughout the skull, spine, and axial skeleton consistent with widespread metastatic disease.

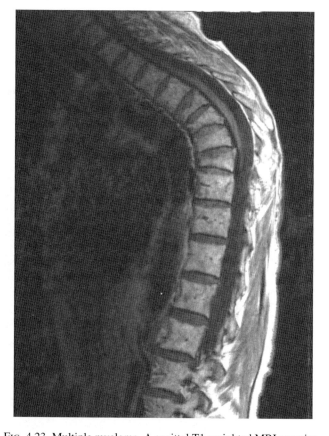

FIG. 4.23. Multiple myeloma. A sagittal T1-weighted MRI examination of the thoracic spine in an elderly patient with recently diagnosed multiple myeloma reveals multiple compression fractures in the upper thoracic spine with a kyphotic deformity. The underlying marrow shows subtle signal heterogeneity consistent with diffuse infiltration by multiple myeloma.

of cases of early myeloma may not be detected by MRI.[88] With more advanced disease, marrow replacement resulting in loss of marrow signal on T1-weighted images becomes apparent.

Common primary benign neoplasms of the skeleton include hemangioma, osteoid osteoma, osteoblastoma, aneurysmal bone cyst, and giant cell tumor.[86,87] Primary neoplasms typically do not involve the disk space and remain confined to the vertebral body and posterior arch. Hemangiomas are the most common benign spinal neoplasm, present in up to 5% of elderly patients. They are often an incidental imaging finding, as the majority of vertebral hemangioma are asymptomatic. Hemangiomas may involve the entire vertebral body or they may be round or oval focal lesions, involving the vertebral body. The radiographic findings of this lesion are distinctive. Conventional radiographs and CT demonstrate characteristic organized linear or stellate thickened trabeculae within the lesion, producing a classic "corduroy" appearance (Fig. 4.24). On MR, in contradistinction to other spinal neoplasms, mature hemangiomas are bright on T1-weighted sequences due to their high adipose content. In the younger patient with an immature hemangioma or in patients with aggressive hemangioma, the characteristic high signal on T1-weighted images may not be present.[89]

Osteoid osteoma of the spine is a painful lesion seen in adolescents and young adults. Osteoblastoma is a histologically related neoplasm that tends to be larger, less painful, and contain osseous matrix. In the spine, osteoid osteoma is most commonly located in the posterior elements, producing severe pain, classically worse at night, and a painful scoliosis. Scintigraphy shows intense uptake within the lesion, with milder uptake in the adjacent bone, which typically shows intense reactive sclerotic changes. Conventional radiographs often visualize the reactive sclerosis, but the actual nidus, which is often very small, may be difficult to visualize. Magnetic resonance can visualize the nidus and sclerosis, but the most prominent feature on MR is often the peritumoral edema in the bone and adjacent soft tissues.[90] Computed tomography remains the preferred method for identification and localization of the nidus of osteoid osteoma.[87]

Infection

Infection of the spine can be limited to the disk, limited to the vertebral body or posterior osseous elements, or, in its most common form, involve the osseous elements as well as the intervening disk and articulations. Isolated disk infection is rare, occurring as a limited infection in children presumably due to persistent disk vascularity in this age group. Isolated disk infection in adults is rare and is typically due to iatrogenic penetration of the disk at surgery. The childhood form of idiopathic diskitis originates within the disk itself, typically before the age of 10, with a peak incidence in the first 6 years of life.[91] The etiology of childhood diskitis is infectious in a minority of cases; only 25% of cases grow organisms on culture.[70] The etiology of the remainder of cases of childhood diskitis is postulated to be viral infection, autoimmune, or a nonspecific inflammatory reaction. Radiographic changes are mild and delayed, and scintigraphy and MR are more sensitive for diagnosis.

Infection of the spine is typically of hematogenous origin, developing initially in the anterior vertebral body, with subsequent destruction of the adjacent vertebral endplate and extension into the nearby disk. Once the disk is infected, the infection can erode the remaining endplate and extend into the adjacent vertebral body. The combination of disk infection and involvement of both adjacent vertebra is referred to as infectious spondylitis. The conventional radiographic findings of infectious spondylitis consist of soft tissue edema, narrowing of the involved disk space, indistinctness and erosion of the vertebral margins, and ultimately bone destruction (Fig. 4.25). These findings are delayed, and definite radiographic evidence of infection may not be present for weeks after the onset of symptoms. Scintigraphy offers much higher sensitivity but the presence of increased activity is nonspecific

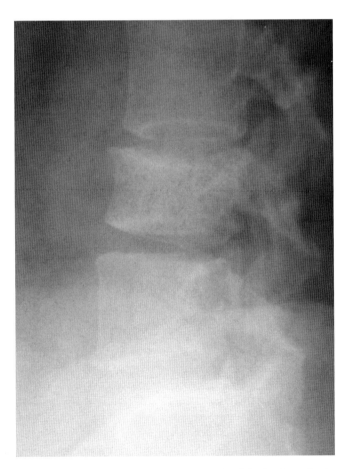

FIG. 4.24. Hemangioma. A lateral radiograph of the lumbar spine in a 28-year-old woman demonstrates a pathologic fracture of the superior endplate L4 vertebral body. The underlying vertebra is mildly sclerotic and shows prominent vertical trabeculae diagnostic of a hemangioma.

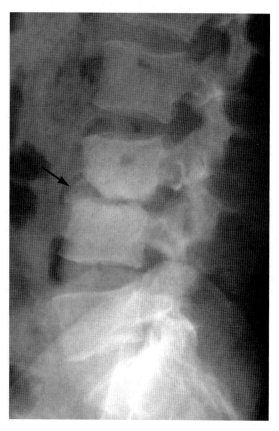

FIG. 4.25. Spinal infection. A lateral radiograph of the spine in an adult with spinal infection shows disk space narrowing and endplate erosions (arrow) at the L3-L4 level.

of its internal architecture, which is replaced by high signal intensity material within its substance on T2-weighted sequences. Disk height is variable, with a significant number of patients demonstrating preservation of disk height on MRI.[92] Paraspinal soft tissue inflammatory change is present early in the course of the disease and is a very sensitive indicator of spinal infection, seen in over 95% of patients with active infection.[92] Irregularity due to erosive changes at the endplates and frank vertebral destruction are seen with more advanced disease.[93]

Enhancement following intravenous gadolinium administration is avid. The contrast enhanced images are particularly useful for distinguishing inflammatory phlegmon from a frank abscess requiring drainage by noting a lack of enhancement within the central portions, indicating the liquefied components of an abscess. The presence of an epidural abscess is best assessed on enhanced MRI (Fig. 4.26). Such abscesses typically require drainage, particularly if they are large or compressing adjacent neural structures.[94] Large paraspinal abscesses, particularly in patients with a history of disease chronicity and slow progression, are suggestive of nonpyogenic infection due to tuberculosis or fungal infection.[95]

Noninfectious Inflammatory Disorders

Degeneration of the disk leads to alterations in the adjacent vertebral body, most commonly resulting in increased intraosseous fat adjacent to abnormal disk.[96] In approximately 4% of patients with noninfectious disk degeneration, the degenerative process itself results in a pattern of inflammatory-like edema in the adjacent endplates on MRI. Modic et al.[97] classified this pattern of endplate abnormality as type 1 endplate changes and suggested that the marrow alteration is a reactive inflammatory response to a relatively acute disk degeneration. The resultant alterations can be difficult to distinguish from infection. Type 1 endplate changes are not associated with the systemic features of infection and tend to resolve spontaneously over a period of a few months. In addition, MRI in patients with type 1 endplate changes demonstrates that the paraspinal soft tissues are normal, the marrow abnormalities are limited to the bone near the endplate, and the intranuclear cleft of the disk and the vertebral endplates are preserved (Fig. 4.27). In cases where infection cannot be excluded, aspiration of the involved disk and follow-up MRI may be necessary.

Rheumatoid arthritis is a common polyarticular inflammatory arthropathy that affects the spine in up to 50% of patients afflicted with the disease.[98] Hypertrophic synovial tissue results in the formation of aggressive pannus that can cause erosions of the odontoid, vertebral bodies, posterior elements, and ligaments, and damage the joints, resulting in instability and ultimately fusion.[98] Spinal rheumatoid arthritis is most commonly clinically symptomatic in the upper cervical spine, specifically at the atlantoaxial and craniocervical articulations. The most common manifestation of spinal rheumatoid arthritis is anterior instability at the atlantoaxial joint. Flexion-extension radiographs are essential for accurate assessment of the

and scintigraphy is unable to assess development of abscess requiring draining or compression of the spinal cord. Computed tomography is an excellent method for assessing endplate erosion and bone destruction, but these finding are a late feature of spinal infection.[91] Computed tomography is also useful for detecting small foci of intraosseous gas and sequestered bone, but these features are less commonly present in infections involving the spine as compared to the appendicular skeleton. Computed tomography is also limited in its ability to determine the degree of extension beyond the vertebra into the adjacent soft tissues and encroachment of the spinal canal.

Magnetic resonance imaging has replaced scintigraphy and CT as the definitive modality for the detection and evaluation of suspected spinal infection. It is more sensitive than conventional radiography and CT for early infection, and has been shown to have sensitivity, specificity, and accuracy of greater than 90% for diagnosis of infection.[91,92] At the same time, it provides detailed anatomic information about the paraspinal and spinal tissues and the adjacent thecal sac. The MRI findings of infection consist of diminished marrow signal in the affected vertebral bodies of the T1-weighted images, with increased signal on the T2-weighted images. The marrow alterations are more prominent on fat-suppressed T2-weighted images.[92] The disk typically enhances, and demonstrates disorganization

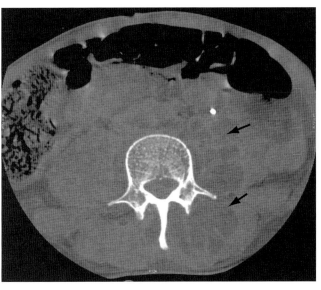

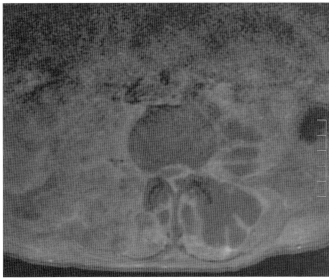

A   B

FIG. 4.26. Paraspinal abscess. An axial CT (A) and contrast-enhanced MRI (B) show a large left-sided paraspinal abscess in a patient with spinal infection with methicillin-resistant *Staphylococcus aureus*. The CT shows low signal fluid collections (arrows) accumulating within the left psoas muscle and left posterior paraspinal musculature. Note the absence of contrast enhancement in the center of the abscess on the MR study.

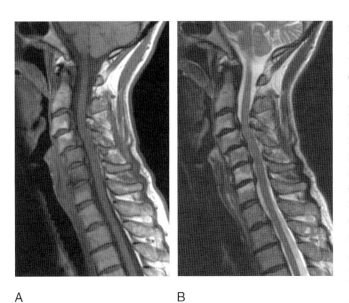

A   B

FIG. 4.27. Degenerative disease. Sagittal T1-weighted (A) and T2-weighted (B) MRIs of the spine demonstrate multilevel degenerative disease with disk dehydration, disk protrusions, and multiple levels of degenerative listhesis. On the T2 images, there is increased signal at the endplates adjacent to the disk degeneration due to inflammatory changes reactive to disk degeneration.

atlantoaxial joint, as abnormal widening of the joint is often seen only when the spine is flexed. Instability of the occipitoatlantal joints, cranial settling, and subaxial instability may also be present. Conventional radiographs and CT are useful for identifying erosive disease, which tends to predominate in

the region of the dens. Magnetic resonance imaging can better visualize the extent of soft tissue pannus, characterize if it is vascular or fibrotic, and accurately assess the degree of canal compression by tissue proliferation[99] (Fig. 4.28).

The seronegative spondyloarthropathies are a group of polyarthritides associated with the human leukocyte antigen (HLA) B27 that have a predilection for sacroiliac and spinal involvement. This group of inflammatory arthropathies includes ankylosing spondylitis, psoriatic arthritis, reactive arthritis (such as Reiter's syndrome), arthritis related to bowel disease, and undifferentiated forms.[100] The most common form is ankylosing spondylitis, which most commonly presents in young men. Symptoms include the gradual onset of stiffness and progressive low back and sacroiliac pain. A suggestive feature of these conditions is that the pain is frequently alleviated with exercise.[81] Radiographic changes of inflammatory sacroiliitis include widening of the joint due to marginal and central erosions, irregularity of the osseous margins, and paraarticular bone sclerosis (Fig. 4.29). With further disease progression, the sacroiliac joints narrow, and in some of these diseases, particularly ankylosing spondylitis, undergo osseous fusion. Both CT and MRI are more sensitive for early detection and characterization of erosive changes at the sacroiliac joints, vertebra, and paraspinal soft tissues.[100] Spinal involvement in the seronegative spondyloarthropathies takes the form of bony proliferation, either in the form of syndesmophytes, or in the development of frank ankylosis as is seen in patients with advanced ankylosing spondylitis. A well-recognized complication of ankylosing spondylitis is the development of a horizontal fracture through the fused spine, with subsequent formation of a pseudoarthrosis.

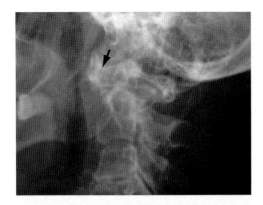

A

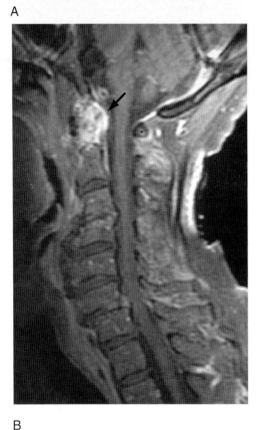

B

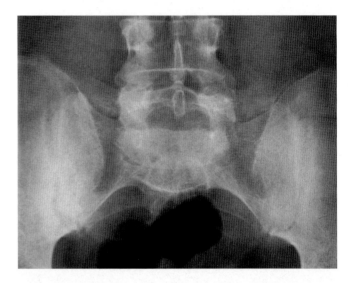

FIG. 4.29. Sacroiliitis. An AP radiograph of the sacroiliac joints in a male patient with ankylosing spondylitis shows bilateral symmetric erosion of the sacroiliac joints with adjacent sclerosis.

FIG. 4.28. Rheumatoid arthritis. (A) A lateral radiograph shows widening of the atlantoaxial joint (arrow) with anterior displacement of the C1 vertebra relative to C2. (B) The corresponding T1-weighted fat-suppressed sagittal MRI obtained following administration of intravenous contrast enhancement shows avid enhancement of pannus (arrow) at the C1-C2 joint.

Small amounts of asymptomatic crystal deposition in spinal ligaments and disk is a frequent finding, especially in the elderly. Symptomatic crystal-induced arthritis of the spine, however, is uncommon and frequently misdiagnosed as infection or neoplasm. Significant crystal deposition resulting in symptoms is generally seen in adults and the elderly. Deposition of urate crystal within the disk and paraspinal soft tissues in patients with advanced gout can cause erosions of the odontoid process and endplates of the vertebral bodies, as well as a destructive arthropathy of the facet joints.

Calcium pyrophosphate deposition disease (CPPD) produces crystal deposition in articular cartilage, hyaline cartilage, and, less commonly, in ligaments and tendons. In the spine, CPPD is seen most commonly in the annulus, the disk, and the transverse ligament at the atlantoaxial joint. Mass-like deposits of CPPD crystals in the atlantoaxial region can produce significant neural compression resulting in myelopathy and paraplegia.[101] Cystic and erosive changes in the adjacent bone, particularly at the base of the dens, increase the risk of fracture of the dens following even minor trauma.[102]

Calcium hydroxyapatite deposition disease (HADD) characteristically results in paraarticular intratendinous calcific deposits, particularly around the shoulder. In the spine, symptomatic HADD is seen most frequently in the tendon of the longus colli muscle. The calcification produces a painful, inflammatory tendinitis anterior to the C2 vertebral body, resulting in soft tissue swelling and local tissue inflammation.[103] The calcific deposit is best visualized on CT.

Spinal neuroarthropathy (Charcot spine) is an uncommon process leading to dissolution and disorganization of the spine. The most common etiologies are diabetes mellitus, prior spinal cord or central nervous system injury, syringomyelia, and tabes dorsalis.[104] The radiographic and CT appearance simulates that of bone destruction produced by infection. Magnetic resonance imaging shows variability in the signal characteristics of the involved region, and distinction from infection is frequently impossible.[105] Dialysis-induced spondyloarthropathy is also an uncommon disorder related due to amyloid deposition within the disk space.[106] Slowly progressive endplate erosion, disk space narrowing, and vertebral destruction that simulate infection are identified, often involving multiple disks. On MRI, the vertebral bodies also show normal marrow signal, except for minimal alterations adjacent to the erosions, and the adjacent soft tissues are normal.[107] T2-weighted images are particularly helpful as they show a paucity of high signal in the affected region.[106]

B. Orthopedic Perspective: The Spine in Sports

Douglas G. Chang, Choll W. Kim, and Steven R. Garfin

Neck and low back pain is common in the general population, as well as among athletes. Although a precise anatomic diagnosis is difficult to make in many patients, basic principles of management help the majority. Most patients recover in about 6 weeks.[108–110] Therefore, it is usually not necessary to perform imaging studies acutely, unless there is a history of injury. If patients do not improve within 4 weeks, imaging studies should be ordered, depending on the diagnostic suspicion.[111]

In several situations imaging studies should be ordered immediately. In less than 10% of patients with low back pain, a specific condition is suspected, such as a fracture related to trauma, nerve root compression, and acute spondylolysis. Also, there are several "red flags" in the medical history that warrant acute diagnostic evaluation and treatment.[112] These conditions are fracture, tumor, infection, cauda equina syndrome, and myelopathy.

However, other explanations for back pain should be kept in mind. These include inflammatory causes (rheumatoid arthritis, ankylosing spondylitis, etc.), medical causes (parathyroid disease, hemoglobinopathies), visceral causes (nephrolithiasis, prostatitis, pelvic inflammatory disease, pancreatitis), vascular causes (aortic aneurysm), psychological causes (depression, substance abuse behavior, psychosomatic disorders, individual personality response to pain and disability) and social causes or medicolegal issues (worker's compensation, legal case).

The majority of patients with low back pain do not present as a result of fracture, tumor, infection, or myelopathy. There is a less than 1% incidence of malignancy in patients presenting to busy multidisciplinary spine centers.[113] Patients without "red flags" or specific suspected conditions should be managed with 6 weeks of nonoperative care, including activity modification, medication, and exercise, and they should be provided with information regarding their condition. After these 6 weeks, patients without clinical improvement should be referred for diagnostic imaging.

Spinal problems, while individual, usually have a common approach in terms of natural history, evaluation, and management. This section describes the typical pain management approach in the cervical, thoracic, and lumbar regions, and discusses specific spinal disorders that require additional understanding. The goal of this section is to place MRI of the spine in sports within an overall context of clinical presentation, physical examination, and treatment.

Patient History

The history is taken to provide a clear determination of pain location, onset, character, radiation to the upper or lower extremities, aggravating and alleviating factors, associated sensorimotor symptoms, and previous treatments.[114] It is important to get a sense of how easily the pain is aggravated to determine the type and intensity of the treatment plan. A psychosocial history, including substance abuse, disability compensation, and mental health, also helps in planning treatment and estimating the prognosis.

Specific elements of the history may raise the suspicion for fracture, tumor, infection, cauda equina syndrome, or myelopathy. For a fracture, the associated elements are major trauma (motor vehicle accident, fall from a height), minor trauma, or strenuous lifting in an older or osteoporotic patient.

For a tumor or infectious condition, commonly associated findings are age greater than 50 or less than 20, cancer history, recent bacterial infection, intravenous drug use, tobacco use, constitutional symptoms (fever, chills, unexplained weight loss), immunosuppression (corticosteroid use, organ transplant recipient, human immunodeficiency infection), failure of bed rest to relieve pain at night, and pain that is worse in the supine position. Infectious etiologies that could present with back pain include osteomyelitis, diskitis, tuberculosis, abscess, and urinary tract infection. Tumor etiologies of back pain include metastasis, multiple myeloma, and lymphoma.

Cauda equina syndrome or myelopathy might be suspected with complaints of saddle anesthesia, recent onset of bowel or bladder dysfunction (particularly retention), gait disturbance, or progressively severe neurologic deficit in an extremity.[113]

Numbness in the arms or legs, particularly into the hand or below the knee, and weakness increase the likelihood of neurologic involvement. Involvement of the toes, calf, thigh, or buttocks is suggestive of a lumbosacral radiculopathy. Lower extremity pain with ambulation, which is eased by leaning forward onto a shopping cart, is suggestive of lumbar spinal stenosis. Pain with lumbar flexion may indicate a diskogenic etiology, while pain with extension may implicate the posterior spinal elements.

Pain characterized as lancinating in a dermatomal distribution to the fingers, forearm, upper arm, interscapular area, or shoulder is also suggestive of neurologic involvement, for example, a cervical radiculopathy. However, the history and physical exam of an acute cervical radiculopathy may be indistinguishable from an even more rare syndrome, a brachial plexus neuritis. Functional problems with fine manipulative tasks, handwriting, and lack of coordination may be suggestive of a cervical radiculopathy, but more commonly result from a peripheral problem such as carpal tunnel syndrome. Headaches often arise from a cervicogenic cause. Inflammatory pain may present with worsening in the morning with stiffness. A mechanical problem may present with worsening with use. Talking on the phone (lateral flexion) may compress the facet joints or the neural elements exiting through compressed neuroforamina. Symptoms of vertigo or light-headedness with cervical motion may suggest vertebral artery insufficiency. A smoking history with constitutional complaints may raise the specter of a Pancoast tumor.

In the thoracic spine, the patient may complain of pain around the shoulder blades, aggravated by rotation or lateral flexion. In cases of scoliosis, a cosmetic concern is often the presenting complaint. Particular attention should be paid to sensory symptoms, which might be consistent with a radiculopathy.

Physical Examination

Cervical Spine

Examination of the cervical spine begins with observation of posture and range of motion. Passive motion in flexion, extension, lateral bending, and side glance should be checked. Normal flexion range allows the chin to touch the chest, extension range allows the patient to view the ceiling directly above, side glance range allows the patient's chin to come almost in line with the shoulder, and normal lateral bending is about 45 degrees.[115] It is convenient to express range of motion in percent terms of normal, for example, "Cervical flexion was approximately 85% of normal." Mobility in the upper versus lower cervical segments can be evaluated more discretely with active maneuvers. The palpatory exam is important to distinguish irritation in the occiput, spinous processes, apophyseal joints, paraspinal muscles, levator scapulae, and the anterior/posterior triangles of the neck. Spurling's maneuver is a special neural provocative test. The cervical spine is extended with the head rotated toward the affected side and then the spine is axially loaded. A positive test is considered when there is reproduction of radicular symptoms.

The neurologic examination of the extremities is an important component in the evaluation of neck pain, as it is with back pain. The focus is on deep tendon reflexes and motor strength. The C5, C6, and C7 nerve roots mediate the deep tendon reflexes of the biceps, brachioradialis, and triceps tendons, respectively. Unfortunately, there is no good reflex to evaluate C8 or T1 function. Diminished reflexes may be seen in lower motor syndromes, and brisk reflexes may be seen in upper motor syndromes. Upper motor release signs can be elicited by the Hoffman's test (middle finger flick causes transient finger flexion). Motor testing involves deltoid (C5), elbow flexion

(C6), wrist extensors (C6), elbow extensors (C7), wrist flexors (C7), finger flexors (C8), and small finger abduction (T1). Coordination problems with finger-to-finger movements are a sensitive measure of central nervous system pathology.

Subjective sensory complaints are important,[116] but a formal sensory examination is often unreliable for a variety of reasons. These include patient comprehension, language skill, dermatomal variations in innervation, body habitus, age, or postsurgical nerve tract changes, and the lack of time and equipment to test the variety of peripheral nervous system tracts in a controlled fashion. One of the most important confounders to the sensory exam is the effect of pain on the patient's sensory perceptions. Furthermore, in the upper extremities, often there can be carpal or cubital tunnel syndromes that cause additional diagnostic confusion.

Usually, the most important information about the sensory system is not quantitative, but rather simply the patient's own qualitative history about where altered sensation is subjectively experienced.[116] Dermatomes according to the American Spinal Cord Injury Association (ASIA) conventions map the lateral antecubital fossa (C5), dorsal thumb (C6), dorsal middle finger (C7), dorsal small finger (C8), and medial antecubital fossa (T1) areas. If genuine concern exists for a peripheral neuropathy, formal electrodiagnostic testing is preferred[117] (Table 4.1).

A basic shoulder examination should be considered as well, because many shoulder pathologies involve radiation of pain to the neck and arm. Conversely, many neck pathologies involve pain around the shoulder that is not particularly provoked by the specific shoulder exam.

Thoracic Spine

Observation for scoliosis and kyphosis should be done initially. Then active movements in flexion, extension, rotation, as well as cervical motion should be noted. In cases of severe end-stage ankylosing spondylitis, there is loss of normal chest wall expansion (reduced to $<2\,cm$). Palpation of the paraspinal muscles and shoulder; percussion of the spinous processes; special tests of the cervical, lumbar spine, and shoulders; and a neurologic exam should be performed also.

Lumbar Spine

The physical examination of the patient with low back pain starts with a functional assessment. Global observation of the patient standing can reveal scoliosis, spinal tilt, asymmetri-

TABLE 4.1. Upper extremity physical examination of the spinal nerve roots.

Nerve root	Deep tendon reflex	Pin-prick sensation territory
C5-C6	Biceps tendon	Lateral aspect of antecubital fossa
C6	Brachioradialis tendon	Thumb
C7	Triceps tendon	Middle finger
C8	–	Little finger
T1	–	Medial side of antecubital fossa

cal muscle development, and the degree of lumbar lordosis. Increased lordosis may reflect spondylolisthesis or obesity. Decreased lordosis may reflect disk or vertebral body collapse. Lastly, functional biomechanical evaluation of the athlete includes an examination of sports specific skills, technique, and equipment.

Gait analysis can reveal muscle weakness and leg length discrepancies. For example, weakness of the gluteus medius-minimus (L4-S1 innervated muscles) can result in a pelvic drop or Trendelenburg gait. As another example, weakness in the L4-L5 innervated anterior tibialis muscle may result in a foot slap or drop after heel contact, or steppage gait, where the hip and knee are flexed to clear the foot during the swing phase of gait. A very weak gastrocnemius muscle limits the toe-off movement during gait, and may result in a shortened step length of the contralateral leg. The patient should be asked to perform ten one-legged toe raises to evaluate gastrocnemius strength. This S1-S2 innervated muscle normally supports the patient's total body weight and more (with jumping or running activities). As such, it defies isolated manual muscle testing by examiners providing resistance with their own hands. Lastly, patients with quadriceps weakness may walk with a back knee gait to lock their knees in extension. Additionally, they may not be able to accelerate through the swing phase without abnormal hip rotation.[115]

At times, functional testing provides a quick and global examination of the lower extremities that might complement, or supplant, individual manual muscle testing. Functional testing evaluates patients' leg strength against their body weight, but may be confounded by isolated knee, ankle, or foot pain. Also, the functional examination may detect a relative restriction or weakness in the kinetic chain, which may predispose injury in another segment.

Active spinal movement in flexion and extension reveals motion asymmetries, qualitative information about stiffness, pain and pain behaviors, and semiquantitative information about the range of motion that can be followed with serial examinations over time to evaluate interventions. If there is a concern about ankylosing spondylitis, the Schober's test may be performed.[115] Pain provoked by flexion and relieved by extension may point to disk pathology. Conversely, the pain provoked by extension and relieved by flexion may point to a diagnosis of lumbar spinal stenosis or apophyseal pathology. Active movement in combined extension, lateral flexion, and rotation to each side tends to provoke the apophyseal joint. However, there are large variations seen in the segmental motion parameters of the lumbosacral spine, with uncertainties introduced by measurement technique, radiographic image quality, anatomic degenerative changes, and patient effort.[118] These factors prevent an exact analysis. Therefore, there is limited useful information to be derived from so-called quantitative methods of measuring the lumbosacral spine's range of motion, and no valuable information is gained to help a clinician in the diagnosis of disease.[111,119,120]

A palpatory examination should be performed. This is performed most easily with the patient in the prone posi-tion. The degree of tenderness, accessory movement, and muscle tone can be evaluated in the various structures of the spinous processes, apophyseal joints and transverse processes, paraspinal muscles, gluteus medius, piriformis, sacroiliac joints, greater femoral trochanters, and iliotibial bands. Muscle pain may indicate spasm or trigger points. Spinous process pain may indicate degeneration, fracture, or infection.

Special maneuvers include the straight leg raise and other so-called neural tension tests such as the slump test or prone knee bend. A tension test is considered positive under four conditions: (1) it reproduces the patient's symptoms, (2) the test response is changeable with patient repositioning, (3) there are large side-to-side differences, or (4) there are differences from what is considered normal.[121] In terms of the straight leg raise, sciatic nerve stretch is said to be maximal between 30 and 70 degrees of hip flexion. Pain with straight leg raise above 70 degrees is most likely due to nonneurogenic causes, such as hamstring tightness.

Pathologies due to hip, knee, or sacroiliac joints can be evaluated with testing the hip's range of motion and the flexion, abduction, and external rotation (FABER) maneuver.[115] The FABER exam can also demonstrate iliotibial band/greater trochanteric bursitis problems. Trochanteric bursitis and iliotibial band problems frequently mimic a lumbosacral radiculopathy, particularly in women with a large Q angle at the knee. However, these entities may coexist because of L4-S1 hip muscle weakness. Suspicion for an iliotibial band syndrome and trochanteric bursitis can be further evaluated with the Ober test of range of motion, and also hip abduction strength testing. To this end, asking the patient to perform a one-legged squat is a good functional test. Pathology of the sacroiliac joint is relatively uncommon, but the joint can be further evaluated with pelvic compression testing.[115] To check for muscle atrophy, calf circumferences can be measured, with the expectation that normal side-to-side variation should be within 2 cm.

A neurologic examination of the lower extremities is important, with emphasis on reflexes and motor strength. The deep tendon reflex at the patellar tendon is mediated mainly through the L3 and L4 nerve roots, at the medial hamstring by the L5 nerve root, and at the Achilles tendon by S1. Diminished reflexes may be noted with lower motor neuron syndromes such as spinal stenosis or a herniated disk. Brisk reflexes may indicate an upper motor neuron pathology. Upper motor neuron release signs can be elicited by the Babinski, a test of long-tract spinal cord or brain involvement. Central nervous system pathology can express itself first in difficulties with toe-tap or foot-pat coordination. Muscle weakness is generally considered a reliable indicator of nerve compression. Manual muscle testing of the lower extremities involves hip flexion (L1, L2), knee extension (L3, L4), ankle dorsiflexion (L4, L5), extensor hallucis longus (L5), and big toe flexion (L5, S1). As mentioned earlier, the gastrocnemius-soleus complex defies manual motor testing and should be tested functionally (Table 4.2).

TABLE 4.2. Lower extremity motor examination of the spinal nerve roots.

Nerve root	Motor exam	Functional test
L3, L4	Extend knee	Squat down and rise
L4, L5	Dorsiflex ankle	Walk on heels
L5	Dorsiflex big toe	Walk on heels
S1	Plantarflex ankle	Walk on tip-toes (plantarflexed ankle)

TABLE 4.3. Lower extremity physical examination of the spinal nerve roots.

Nerve root	Deep tendon reflex	Pin-prick sensation territory
L3	Patellar tendon	Lateral thigh-medial femoral condyle
L4	Patellar tendon	Medial leg and medial ankle
L5	Medial hamstring	Lateral leg and dorsum of foot
S1	Achilles tendon	Sole of foot and lateral heel

Many myotomal maps have been published to describe the spinal nerve root innervation of peripheral muscles. The innervation of these muscles remains debatable, and there is considerable individual variation. Nevertheless, there is some consensus.[117]

The sensory exam in the lower extremities is not that reliable for a variety of reasons that were already mentioned. Again, the most important information about the sensory system is not quantitative but rather the patient's own qualitative history about where altered sensation is subjectively experienced.[116] Dermatomes according to the American Spinal Cord Injury Association (ASIA) conventions map medial (L4), dorsal (L5), and lateral (S1) aspects of the foot as well as medial knee (L3), thigh (L2), and groin (L1) areas (Table 4.3). If genuine concern exists for a peripheral neuropathy, formal electrodiagnostic testing is preferred.[117]

Investigations

Laboratory tests in the investigation of spine pain are somewhat nonspecific. However, they may be useful in a few circumstances: alkaline phosphatase (Paget's disease, osteomalacia), amylase (pancreatitis), complete blood count (malignancy), erythrocyte sedimentation rate (infection, malignancy, polymyalgia rheumatica), pregnancy test (ectopic pregnancy), rheumatoid factor/antinuclear antibodies (rheumatologic disease), and urinalysis (urinary tract infection, prostatitis, nephrolithiasis).

Diskography is performed by injecting dye or saline into the nucleus pulposus of the intervertebral disk. Concordant reproduction of the patient's pain is said to verify the disk as the source. However, false-positive results can be especially problematic in patients with chronic pain processes, emotional

distress, and litigation.[121] Furthermore, it is unclear to what extent patients may subjectively localize deep somatic pain generators from among the different individual spinal structures, especially when the patient is partially sedated for the procedure.

Electromyography (EMG) and nerve conduction studies may be useful to evaluate for signs of nerve irritation within the setting of an otherwise mild appearing MRI, or in cases of suspected peripheral nerve entrapment or polyneuropathy. The studies are also helpful in patients who may not be able to obtain an MRI (e.g., cardiac pacemaker). For a variety of reasons, the study has high specificity and low sensitivity within the setting of a radiculopathy. Therefore, electromyography cannot be used to exclude a radiculopathy with confidence.[117] Electromyography needle studies are usually performed at least 3 weeks after an injury. A good exam includes testing of the paraspinal muscles. The hallmark EMG findings in an acute radiculopathy are the presence of fibrillation potentials and positive sharp waves. Chronic radicular findings are noted after a few months of nerve root involvement. These involve more subtle interpretations of the muscle firing patterns, such as early recruitment and decreased interference pattern, which may also be influenced by patient pain, discomfort, and motivation levels during the test. Nerve conduction studies evaluate the peripheral nerves, which should not be affected in a radiculopathy. The late response, or H reflex, is a quantitative evaluation of the S1 deep tendon reflex arc. As such, an abnormal study might suggest a S1 radiculopathy.

Electrodiagnostic studies are useful in cervical spine disorders to evaluate the possibility of peripheral neuropathies such as carpal tunnel syndrome. This is important because of the "double crush" syndrome, which suggests that a proximal nerve injury (e.g., cervical spinal nerve root) may make it susceptible to a distal injury, and frequently the entities coexist. It is difficult to use an EMG study to evaluate high cervical lesions because of the lack of peripherally innervated muscles above the C5 spinal nerve root. Fortunately, most cervical radiculopathies involve the lower cervical spine, with 70% of cases involving the C7 nerve root and 20% to 25% of cases involving the C6 nerve root.[117]

Epidural and facet joint injections with local anesthetic and corticosteroid may provide both diagnostic and therapeutic roles in identifying a pain generator. However, the diagnostic information must be tempered by a possible placebo effect.[121] In general, there is decent scientific evidence to support the use of epidural steroid injections to treat low back pain with radicular features.[122–124] Interventional pain procedures to treat axial low back pain are controversial, and the supporting evidence remains little better than anecdotal.[110] However, in the cervical spine there is more substantial evidence to support interventional therapies to the facet joints.[125] The main problem is that most studies of radicular and axial low back pain treatments were not well designed. Many of the studies (which show no benefit of intervention) did not evaluate patients with

MRI or CT scanning to document the type or location of pathology, and a surprising number of studies did not utilize radiographic confirmation of needle placement and injection of medications properly into the epidural space.[124,126]

Imaging Evaluation

Experienced clinicians recognize that diagnostic imaging in low back pain has a high rate of asymptomatic incidental abnormalities, and symptomatic "negative" tests.[110] Imaging is one piece of the overall puzzle that must be viewed within the context of the history and physical examination.

X-ray imaging should be performed in patients who raise suspicion for sinister pathology, fracture (trauma, stress), or instability, as well as in patients unresponsive to treatment. It offers a global view of the spine, with information on the number of vertebrae, presence of transitional anatomy, spondylosis, spondylolisthesis, and facet joint anatomy. X-ray examination of the neck involves AP, lateral, and, sometimes, oblique views. A coned-down AP view of the odontoid is essential in the trauma series. A swimmer's view is a mandatory part of the trauma series if the C7 vertebral body is incompletely visualized on the lateral view. Lateral flexion and extension films are useful to evaluate cervical spine mobility.[127] In the thoracic spine, x-ray examination is helpful to evaluate for Scheuermann's kyphosis, fracture, or cases where a neoplastic disorder is suspected. Computed tomography and MRI are helpful in cases of fracture, neoplasm, or, rarely, in cases of thoracic intervertebral disk herniation. With the lumbosacral spine AP view, the whole pelvis can be included and this may give additional information about the hips and sacroiliac joints. Lateral flexion and extension views can be used to evaluate lumbar motion. Such studies have gross inaccuracies, and the concept of lumbar stability is a controversial topic. However, there is general consensus that more than 3 mm of sagittal translation may be abnormal.[111] It is usually the case that plain radiographs are unrewarding, and MRI may be a better initial study, particularly if malignancy or nerve irritation is suspected.[121]

Computed tomography scanning is most useful to evaluate traumatic fractures, facet joint arthropathy, a pars interarticularis defect, and spinal canal stenosis. It is increasingly supplanting the use of the trauma x-ray series for the evaluation of cervical spine injuries.[128] Depending on the software, it can be useful in patients with instrumented spinal fusions to assess the fusion continuity as well as metal placement. Computed tomography scans may be helpful, along with myelography, in the many patients who cannot be referred for an MRI due to claustrophobia or the presence of cardiac pacemakers, spinal stimulators, or pumps.

Magnetic resonance imaging is used to visualize the intervertebral disks and vertebral bodies. It is useful to evaluate sites of spinal canal and neuroforaminal stenosis. The use of STIR imaging or gadolinium contrast is suggested in patients who raise a suspicion of an infection or malignancy, or who have undergone previous operations on the spine. Magnetic resonance imaging has a high false-positive rate, with 15% to 30% of asymptomatic volunteers demonstrating cervical spine abnormalities.[129] In MRI of the lumbar spine, significant abnormalities have been shown in asymptomatic volunteers. In those over the age of 60, there was a 57% rate of abnormalities, including 37% who had a herniated nucleus pulposus. For volunteers younger than age 60, the false-positive rate approached 20%.[130] Conversely, there are instances where patients present with radicular pain but have a relatively benign-appearing spinal MRI. In these instances, an electrodiagnostic study can be valuable.[117] In summary, MRI provides important information, but it is one piece of the overall picture. Whether the observed pathology is responsible for the patient's pain, or the severity of the patient's pain, is a clinical decision.

Triple-phase bone scan may be helpful to evaluate infection, trauma, pathologic fracture, osteoarthritic degeneration, heterotopic ossification, or complex regional pain syndromes. Gamma radiation is emitted from a radioisotope tracer (e.g., technetium 99 m), which accumulates in areas of high bone turnover. The findings are highly sensitive, but poorly specific. Single photon emission computed tomography is another radionucleotide study that has application in the evaluation and management of spondylolysis.

Cervical Spine Pain

Presentation

Neck pain is about as common as low back pain. Population surveys yield a 15% point prevalence and a 15% to 60% one-year prevalence.[131] Lifetime prevalence of neck pain is similar to that of low back pain, about 70%. Certain occupations seem to have a higher risk of neck pain (miners, dentists, secretaries). The occurrence of neck pain after a motor vehicle accident ("whiplash" syndrome) seems to be increasing.

Natural History

The etiology of back pain is often nonspecific, and this is even more the case with the cervical spine.[132] In scientific studies, neck pain is often grouped together with shoulder region pain. Patients complain differently of neck pain, stiffness, or headache, or more generally of diffuse pain in the neck, shoulder, arm, or hand, with decreased endurance and limited hand function. The reason is that the muscles and nerves in these regions interact, and distinction is difficult. As with the low back, there are often important confounding psychosocial factors such as work status, legal cases, individual personality, and medical comorbidities. Therefore, it is difficult to find studies that comment on the natural history of neck pain.

Pathophysiology

Similar to the case of low back pain, it is convenient to think of neck pain in terms of pathological disk, bone, apophyscal joints, neural elements, ligaments and musculature. Again it is convenient to think of neck pain in terms of axial versus radicular pain. Sometimes this is an easy distinction, but often neck and shoulder pain coexist in a relatively small region and the distinction becomes more difficult. For example, in patients initially diagnosed with shoulder impingement syndrome, 5% had definite electrodiagnostic evidence for a C5/C6 cervical radiculopathy, and an additional 25% had "possible" electrodiagnostic evidence of a radiculopathy.[133] Often the clinician suspects a relative contribution from neck versus shoulder pathology, and treatment should involve both regions. The patient with neck pain often presents with little more than myofacial pain, muscle spasm, and a forward-stooped posture with rounded shoulders, tight pectoral muscles, shoulder movement restrictions, and forward carriage of the head. Acceleration/deceleration injuries, or so-called whiplash, may involve microtrauma to the paraspinal muscles and intervertebral ligaments (as in a sprain), or intervertebral disks. "Stingers" or "burners" are seen relatively frequently in American football players, but remain rather rare in players of other sports. They are characterized by transient upper extremity pain, paresthesias, and weakness. The presumed etiology is an injury either to the upper trunk of the brachial plexus or to cervical nerve roots. Acute cervical nerve root pain from an intervertebral disk should always be considered with pain radiating beyond the neck to the shoulder or distally.

Treatment

Management of neck pain is similar to that of low back pain, with medications, modalities, therapies, and interventions. Cervical orthoses have also been recommended.[108] The scientific evidence to support many such treatments is actually rather slim. This may be due to the difficulties in obtaining uniform diagnostic classifications among the patient groups, as well as large placebo effects, involved in the scientific studies. Because of inconsistent findings, it is not possible to determine the effect of either muscle relaxants or other drug therapies in the treatment of acute and chronic neck pain.[134,135] Other passive modalities may have mild benefit but in general show no significant treatment effect compared to placebo for vapocoolant sprays, laser therapy, infrared light, electromagnetic collars and necklaces, transcutaneous electrical nerve stimulation, acupuncture, traction by equipment, and the use of cervical orthoses. In acute and subacute neck pain, active physical therapy programs with mobilization, exercise, home training programs, and ergonomic education[136] do seem to provide benefit. Manual medicine techniques, within the context of other active exercise regimens, seem to provide benefit. Unfortunately, these benefits have not been as dramatic in studies of chronic neck pain patients.[134,137]

Manual medicine techniques to treat neck pain include joint mobilization, manual traction, massage therapy, neural stretching, and active exercise programs. Common soft tissue abnormalities found in the neck are shortened, tight muscles (especially trapezius, levator scapula, anterior scalenes), focal areas of increased tone, and areas of fascial thickening. Massage techniques are used to identify and eliminate areas of muscular tension and tenderness that impede mobility, compromise biomechanics, and create pain. Examples of techniques include transverse friction to the neck extensors with some slight neck rotatory motion, sustained myofacial tension to the sternocleidomastoid with ipsilateral neck rotation, and transverse friction applied to the levator scapulae.[108] There are several joint mobilization techniques. For the upper cervical spine, there are gentle axial traction, posteroanterior (PA) central pressure, and PA unilateral pressure applied over the apophyseal joints. For the lower cervical spine there are transverse pressure, gentle and controlled oscillating lateral flexion movements, and rotations. Exercise therapy is important and involves stretches, range-of-motion exercises, self-resisted strengthening exercises, and postural training such as chin retraction exercises.[138]

An athlete who has completed a rehabilitative plan for neck and back pain must show significant improvement before returning to play. There should be full strength, and the pain should be manageable without the requirement of analgesics or abnormal motion patterns. Additionally, the athlete should demonstrate good core strength, aerobic fitness, and the ability to perform sports-specific skills.[139]

Selected Cervical Spine Syndromes

The majority of cervical spine syndromes are nonspecific, myofascial in nature, with strains, sprains, abnormal posture, and muscle spasm. The management for these kinds of problems was previously described. Other cervical spine syndromes include cervical disk disease, disk herniations, and facet joint arthropathy. The management of these problems mirror the treatment used in the lumbosacral spine (discussed later). We will recap some of the notable differences.

For nonspecific neck pain, the use of muscle relaxant medications is not scientifically justified. For axial neck pain, the use of cervical traction and radiofrequency ablation procedures to the facet joints has a good scientific basis.[125,140] The use of intervertebral disk replacements in the cervical spine to treat degenerative disk disease is presently experimental. In the treatment of radicular cervical spine pain due to a herniated disk, the use of epidural steroid injections is supported.[139,141]

Stingers and Burners

Stingers and burners are upper extremity dysesthesias and weakness seen almost exclusively among American football players. Nearly half of college players report these symptoms during the course of a season.[139,142] The symptoms are transient, but typically are recurrent. The mechanism seems to involve a tackle where the tackling player's shoulder is depressed while the neck is laterally bent to the contralateral side. Stingers are thought to involve a traction injury to the upper trunk of the brachial plexus, but the exact etiology in unclear. Alternatively, recurrent symptoms have been seen in players with nerve root compression secondary to cervical disk disease narrowing the neural foramen. A high incidence of cervical spinal stenosis also has been found among players with recurrent symptoms.[108] Weakness is found in the C5-C6 distribution, and a player typically presents with his arm adducted after a blow or fall. Immediate burning and tingling down the arm to the thumb and index fingers often is felt. The differential includes a shoulder dislocation or cervical radiculopathy. When a stinger or burner occurs on the field, great care must be exercised to evaluate for a cervical spine or cord injury. Physical examination shows a full, pain-free range of neck motion without midline tenderness. Bony tenderness mandates radiographic examination. Neurologic dysfunction is self-limited and commonly involves the deltoid, supraspinatus, infraspinatus, and biceps (C5-C6) muscles. Pain resolves within minutes, with strength returning within 48 hours, although sometimes it takes a few weeks.[143]

A player with a brief, or momentary, stinger or burner may return to play immediately if the cervical spine range-of-motion is painless, there is normal strength, and the player is symptom free.[143] Usually symptoms subside over the course of minutes to days. If the player experiences a significant and sustained stinger, a cervical spine MRI should be performed to rule out a structural abnormality before the player returns to play. If there are persistent neurologic symptoms, the player should be withheld from athletic participation, and a complete workup with cervical spine imaging undertaken. This includes cervical spine trauma series radiographs and an MRI. If there is suspicion for an occult fracture, a CT or SPECT scan is helpful. An EMG can help determine the location of the injury, but pathologic changes are not present until about 21 days postinjury. Postinjury rehabilitation focuses on neck strengthening and stretching performed with the chest held out. Prevention is accomplished with shoulder pads that fit snugly to the chest and have a modified A-frame shape. Other restrictions on neck movement include the use of neck rolls outside the pads, or lifters inside the pads.[139,142]

Transient Quadriparesis, Cervical Cord Neuropraxia, Cord Concussion, or Burning Hand Syndrome

Known by these several names, this is a rare transient neurologic episode, thought to be of cervical spinal cord origin, without a visible structural abnormality seen on imaging. The occurrence is said to be about 7 per 100,000 football players.[142] In this syndrome, there are transient paresthesias (burning pain, tingling, or loss of sensation) in two or more limbs. In 80% of cases all four extremities are involved. Neck pain is usually not the chief complaint. Motor changes may or may not be present. They range from bilateral upper and lower extremity weakness to complete paralysis. Sensory disturbances include burning pain or sensory loss. The mechanism seems to involve brief stenosis of the spinal canal, caused by hyperflexion or hyperextension. Furthermore, biomechanical impact studies have shown that temporarily bulging disks can cause transient spinal canal stenosis when the spine is axially loaded.[144] Transient quadriplegia risk factors include cervical stenosis, kyphosis, congenital fusion, cervical instability, disk protrusion, or herniation. Vascular and metabolic etiologies may be involved.[143] The Torg ratio is defined as the width of the spinal canal divided by the width of a vertebral body, as seen on lateral radiographs. A value of less than 0.80 is indicative of cervical spinal stenosis. The ratio has high sensitivity (93%) when it is 0.80 or higher. However, a poor positive predictive value (0.2%) limits its use as a screening tool for athletic participation.

The prognosis is excellent. Recovery is usually within 15 minutes, but it can take up to 48 hours. After an episode of transient quadriparesis, the player should not continue to play that day, even if a full recovery occurs quickly. If the symptoms are momentary, a complete neurologic and radiographic evaluation must be done in a timely fashion. Repeat evaluations should be made if motor or sensory symptoms persist.[143] A fracture is suspected until proven otherwise if the patient has neck pain, significant stiffness, or pain with axial head compression. A cervical orthosis should be used if neurologic symptoms persist during the evaluation, and the patient should be transported to a medical facility. Players with MRI evidence of cord injury or spinal instability, or with more than 36 hours of neurologic symptoms, should not return to contact sports. After recovery, there is an overall high rate of transient quadriplegia recurrence (60%) after returning to football.[142] Many players choose not to return to contact football. A subset of football players is identified at high risk for a catastrophic cervical injury. These players have four factors: congenital stenosis (Torg ratio less than 0.8), straightening or reversal of the normal cervical lordosis, preexisting posttraumatic radiographic abnormalities, and a history of spear-tackling head-first techniques seen on videotape.[142] These players have "spear-tackler's" spine—an absolute contraindication to participation in collision sports.

Acceleration/Deceleration Injury

Acceleration/deceleration injuries with rapid flexion-extension, or so-called whiplash, represent a controversial syndrome. While commonly associated with motor vehicle accidents, this syndrome can also occur in sports when the cervical spine is suddenly flexed and extended by a collision with an opponent, or from contact with the ground. Nonradiating, axial neck pain is common, usually experienced over the course of 48 hours after the initially painless traumatic incident. The etiology is thought to be related to some combination of cervical muscle, ligamentous, or facet joint capsular injury with nonorganic overtones.[108,145,146] Physical examination often reveals areas of soft tissue tenderness, spasm, and a pain-limited range of motion. The neurologic examination and radiographic imaging studies are normal. Clinical experience suggests that ~1 week of soft cervical collar use acutely is particularly helpful. Nonsteroidal antiinflammatory drug (NSAID) use and local modalities have also been suggested. The use of manual therapies is approached with caution initially. Later, stretching exercises, gentle massage, and aerobic exercise are suggested.[135]

Down Syndrome and Cervical Spine Instability

Instability at the occiput–atlas (C1) joint is rare in occurrence and generally insignificant clinically (Fig. 4.30). However, instability at the atlas (C1)–axis (C2) junction is common among individuals with Down syndrome. The instability is seen in 10% to 30% of adolescent patients with Down syndrome.[147] About 15% of these patients are said to develop neurologic symptoms, sometimes with a catastrophic presentation. Usually the neurologic manifestations include easy fatigability, gait difficulties, decreased neck mobility, torticollis, incoordination, clumsiness, sensory deficits, spasticity, hyperreflexia, clonus, or other upper motor neuron signs. Atlantoaxial instability is defined radiographically when there is evidence of a 5-mm or greater interval between the atlas and dens of the axis. The suspected pathology is ligamentous laxity. About 7% of patients with normal radiographs initially

have been shown to progress with abnormal radiographs in 3 to 6 years. Conversely, about 20% of patients with abnormal radiographs initially had normal radiographs on follow-up.[148] It is important to keep the perspective that only 41 documented pediatric cases of symptomatic atlantoaxial instability with Down syndrome were described in the published literature prior to 1995.

Routine radiographic screening is controversial.[128,148] The Special Olympics requires all athletes with Down syndrome to have radiographs of the cervical spine. The Spine Care Foundation of Australia and American Academy of Pediatrics currently do not advise it, except in cases where there is persistent neck pain, cervical spine muscle spasm ("wry neck"), decreased stamina of recent onset, recent gait disturbance, or loss of previously controlled urination. In any case, a Down syndrome child with normal radiographs and neurologic examination has no restrictions. If there is progressive atlantoaxial instability or significant spondylosis with a normal neurologic exam, the patient should be restricted from neck-stressing sports. These are defined by the Special Olympics as gymnastics, diving, diving starts and the butterfly stroke in swimming, high jump, soccer, pentathlon, and certain warm-up exercises. Periodic follow-up examinations and radiographs are advised. If there is progressive instability with myelopathic features, then surgical stabilization should be considered, although there is a high complication rate associated with the procedure.[128,147]

Congenital Stenosis

Cervical spinal stenosis is a narrowing of the spinal canal. Acquired stenosis is caused by degenerative changes of the facet joints, ligaments, and intervertebral disks. Congenital

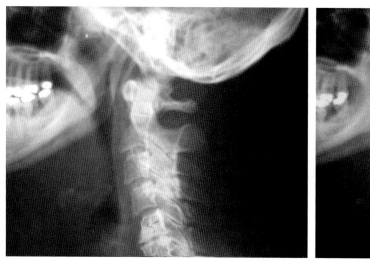
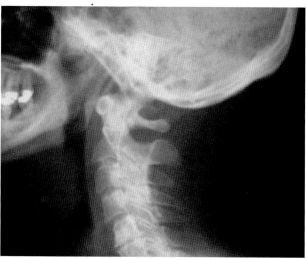

A   B

FIG. 4.30. (A,B) Cervical flexion and extension radiographs of a 41-year-old woman with Down syndrome. The patient had 2 years of neck pain with reduced range of motion, and numbness into her fingertips and toes. The radiographs demonstrated occiput-C1 instability and slight anterolisthesis of C3 on C4, and C4 on C5. There are also degenerative changes at C4-C5, C5-C6, and C3-C4. There is no evidence of C1-C2 instability. A complete workup was performed, and the patient was treated with a posterior occiput to C5 instrumented fusion.

stenosis affects individuals born with a smaller diameter canal than the general population. It is believed to predispose athletes to injury. The precise definition is debatable; therefore, prevalence data are difficult to estimate. The Torg ratio, mentioned previously, has gained some acceptance as a measurement criteria. This ratio of canal width to vertebral body width is said to be normal when greater than 0.8. One limitation is the susceptibility to overestimate narrowing in those athletes with large vertebral bodies. For example, about 50% of professional American football players have been shown to have abnormally small Torg ratios.[149] The other limitation is that only the spinal canal is considered, without concern for the spinal cord anatomy itself. Therefore, the Torg ratio should be considered a screening tool. Further radiographic assessment using MRI should be considered (Fig. 4.31). Another entity, Chiari type I hindbrain malformation, can cause functional cervical spinal stenosis. The cerebellar tonsils are caudally displaced in this condition, and transient quadriparesis in a football player with this entity has been reported.[149] Chiari I malformation with the presence of a spinal cord syrinx (fluid-filled cavity) is a well-described risk factor for spinal cord injury.

Cervical spinal stenosis has been suggested to be a risk factor for cervical cord neurapraxia, and associations with spinal cord injury have also been described.[139,149] Particular risk exists when there are high-velocity impacts combined with hyperextension. Biomechanical testing shows that significant transient cervical spinal canal stenosis occurs also with axial impact loads.[144] A handful of guidelines for return to play have been published, but not one of them is considered standard.

Criteria for Return to Play After Cervical Spine Injuries

There are a variety of opinions regarding the safe return to play guidelines for players with cervical spine injuries.[139,142,143,149,150] Clinical experience, and respect for the autonomous decision making by a well-informed athlete can modify these guidelines. However, individual return to play decisions should be medically based and take into account the mechanism of injury, prior history of neck injury, physical exam findings, and diagnostic imaging results. They should not be based on the player's desire to play, any sports contract provisions, or the opinions of the player's friends, family, teammates, coaches, or team owners (Table 4.4).

Thoracic Spine Pain

Pathophysiology

As with neck and low back pain, often it is not possible for the clinician to make a precise diagnosis of pain in the thoracic spine region. The most common problems are paraspinal or periscapular muscle strain, intervertebral joint syndromes (disk, apophyseal joints), and, in adolescents, scoliosis (often not associated with pain) and Scheuermann's kyphosis.

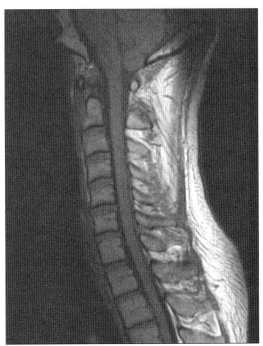
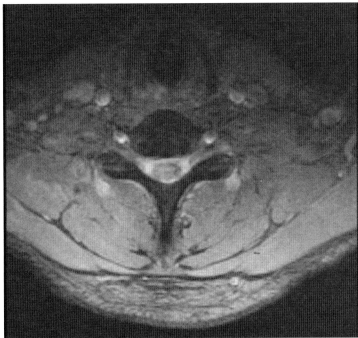

A   B

FIG. 4.31. Congenital cervical spine stenosis in a 28-year-old man. (A) Sagittal T1-weighted MRI of the cervical spine. (B) Axial T1 gradient echo MRI of the C6-C7 level.

TABLE 4.4. Return to play guidelines.

No contraindications to return to play:

Congenital: spina bifida occulta, type II Klippel-Feil congenital single level fusion (excluding the C0-C1 articulation), asymptomatic congenital stenosis (Torg ratio less than 0.8)
Fractures: healed stable C1 or C2 fracture with normal cervical range of motion, asymptomatic "clay shoveler's" (C7 spinous process) fracture
Degenerative: degenerative disk disease with only occasional neck stiffness and no change in baseline neurologic status
Postsurgical: healed one-level surgical fusion
Other: history of two resolved stingers

Relative contraindication to participation:

Congenital: an occipital-C1 assimilation
Postsurgical: healed two-level cervical fusion, healed single-level posterior fusion with lateral mass segmental fusion
Other: Three or more stingers in the same season, history of transient quadriplegia (with normal strength, pain-free range of cervical motion)

Absolute contraindications to participation:

MRI evidence: cervical spinal cord abnormality, Arnold-Chiari malformation, basilar invagination, evidence of residual cord encroachment following a healed stable subaxial spine fracture
X-ray evidence: C1-C2 hypermobility, evidence of spear-tackler's spine, ankylosing spondylitis, diffuse idiopathic skeletal hyperostosis (DISH), healed subaxial spine fracture with kyphotic sagittal plane or coronal plane abnormality
Computed tomography: fixed atlantoaxial (C1-C2) rotatory abnormality
Other radiographic findings: evidence of a distraction-extension cervical spine injury
Congenital: a multiple level Klippel-Feil deformity, odontoid agenesis
Degenerative: history of C1-C2 cervical fusion, symptomatic disk herniation
Postsurgical: three-level fusion, status post–cervical laminectomy
Soft tissue: asymptomatic ligamentous laxity
Other: more than two episodes of transient quadriplegia; cervical cord neuropraxia lasting more than 36 hours; clinical history or physical examination findings of cervical myelopathy; clinical or radiographic evidence of rheumatoid arthritis; after a cervical spine injury, the presence of persistent neck discomfort, decreased range of motion, or neurologic deficit

Prolapse of a thoracic intervertebral disk is rare in athletes, but when present is usually at T11-T12. However, a cervical radiculopathy can present with pain about the shoulder blades, and C7-T1 degenerative disk disease can present with pain at the base of the neck and upper shoulder. Rib fractures usually present as chest (not solely as thoracic spine) pain. In the elderly there is also concern for osteoporotic vertebral body compression fractures. Other medical causes such as cardiac pathology, gastrointestinal ulcer, or tumor (breast) should always be kept in mind.[108]

General Treatment

Stretching, manual medicine techniques, and correction of predisposing factors are the mainstay of treatment for thoracic spine pain. A light, backpack-like thoracolumbar orthosis is often well accepted by patients with osteoporotic vertebral body compression fracture, and may be used for Scheuermann's kyphosis as well.[151]

Selected Thoracic Spine Syndromes

Scheuermann's Kyphosis

Scheuermann's kyphosis is most commonly seen in skeletally immature adolescents, with an estimated 1% to 8% incidence. Water skiers and competitive swimmers are reported to have an increased incidence. There is a strong hereditary tendency, but the exact etiology is unknown. Diagnostic criteria are (1) thoracic kyphosis greater than 45 degrees (normal is 25 to 40

degrees), (2) wedging of greater than 5 degrees in three adjacent vertebrae, and (3) thoracolumbar kyphosis greater than 30 degrees (normal is straight). Associated conditions include the presence of Schmorl's nodes, spondylolysis of the L5 pars interarticularis, and scoliosis. Clinically, patients demonstrate an angular thoracic kyphosis that doesn't reverse with hyperextension, tight hamstrings, pain at the apex of the kyphosis, hyperlordosis of the cervical and lumbar spines, and low back pain. Neurologic deficits are uncommon. This condition is differentiated from "postural round back," where there is no wedging on radiographs, and the patients have a flexible round back. The diagnosis is made with radiographic verification. Pain usually subsides at the end of growth, but the natural history is controversial. Treatment is related to pain, deformity progression, and appearance. Curves of less than 50 degrees that are stable may be observed. An exercise program focuses on stretching of the back and hamstrings. Bracing to address the thoracic kyphosis may be useful in patients with pain. More severe curvatures of 50 to 60 degrees are treated with orthotics, worn around-the-clock for 1 year, followed by 2 years of nighttime bracing. Surgical correction appears successful in alleviating pain and is the only reliable method for cosmetic correction. However, surgery may also be associated with significant morbidity.[152]

Idiopathic Scoliosis

Idiopathic scoliosis is generally divided into three age groups. Infantile scoliosis occurs before age 3. Juvenile scoliosis occurs from ages 3 to 10. Idiopathic scoliosis occurs in adolescents, and represents 80% of cases. Certain sports have been associated with scoliosis, such as gymnastics, swimming, volleyball, ballet dancing, tennis, and javelin.[153] Repetitive loading patterns on immature bone are a contributing factor. Girls are at greater risk than boys. Hypoestrogenism is also a contributing factor. The prevalence of idiopathic scoliosis in the general population is said to be 2% to 3%, with a 10-fold higher incidence seen in rhythmic gymnasts. There is often a positive family history, but the pattern of inheritance is unclear. Back pain prevalence is significantly higher than in control populations.[154] The majority of idiopathic curvatures are right thoracic curves. There may be slow progression before age 10, but rapid after age 10. On radiographic exam, the level of the most rotated vertebra at the apex of the primary curve has an important prognostic value. Bracing is most successful in milder cases, but may be tried in curves up to 60 degrees to maintain, but not correct, the deformity. Once patients enter the adolescent growth spurt, bracing is often ineffective.

In late-onset, adolescent, scoliosis, a higher risk of progression is seen the earlier in adolescence it presents. Although there is a slightly increased association with low back pain, overall patient function is not particularly affected. The primary concern is cosmetic in lower degree curves. Bracing for idiopathic scoliosis is controversial.[155] The general consensus is that curves less than 20 degrees are observed. Curves of 20 to 30 degrees may be observed, but if there is progression of more than 5 degrees in 6 months, then bracing should be instituted.

Curves between 30 and 40 degrees are braced if the patient is less skeletally mature than Risser stage 3. The Risser staging system estimates skeletal maturity from a pelvic radiograph. Normally, ossification of the iliac crest apophysis begins at the anterior superior iliac spine (ASIS). Mature ossification proceeds with age in a posteromedial direction along the crest. In the Risser staging system, the crest is divided into 4 quadrants. Risser stage 1 denotes ossification in the first quadrant only, while Risser stage 4 denotes complete ossification of the iliac crest apophysis. Risser stage 5 indicates that all quadrants of the apophysis are ossified and that they are completely fused to the iliac crest. Children generally progress over a two-year period from Risser stage 1 to 5.

Some spinal curves between 40 and 45 degrees can be treated successfully with bracing, but generally it will not work for curves greater than 45 degrees. With the apex at T8 or lower, a Wilmington or Boston back brace may be used. Higher thoracic curves may require a Milwaukee brace. Greater effectiveness is seen with braces the more hours each day they are worn. It must be noted that bracing reduces vital capacity significantly. Surgical treatment for the deformity can be quite effective. In general, progressive curves, and those above 30 degrees in the adolescent are considered for surgery.

Patients with scoliosis have no particular contraindications to swimming or other contact sports. In children who are treated with a brace, sports participation may be encouraged during the few hours they are out of the brace. Some sports such as cheerleading, horseback riding, and bicycling allow participation with a brace.

Lumbosacral Spine Pain

Presentation

Low back pain is said to affect 70% of people at some point in their lives.[131] Specific incidence data are available for individual sports. Low back pain affects 10% to 30% of professional golfers per year.[156] The incidence of low back pain among American football players and male dancers is about 30%.[157,158] Female gymnasts at high levels of competition are said to have a 45% to 65% incidence of spine abnormalities seen on MRI, compared to 15% seen in comparable elite swimmers[159]; 10% to 30% of female gymnasts have been shown to have pars interarticularis defects, a level four times as high as their nonathletic peers.[160] Finally, back pain has been shown to account for about 15% of the visits to a sports medicine clinic by tennis and squash players.[161]

Most athletes with low back pain present with mild to moderate pain. In some, the pain will be severe. Acute low back pain is usually of sudden onset, triggered by a trivial movement such as bending over to pick up an object. The pain may increase over a period of several hours. Patients with chronic (i.e., greater than 3 months' duration) back pain describe acute exacerbations that may become increasingly frequent, severe, and longer lasting over the course of months. The pain is usually in the lower lumbar area. It may be unilateral, central or bilateral. It may extend to the buttocks, posterolateral thigh, or lower leg.

Natural History

Nonspecific low back pain recovery is generally rapid, with one third of patients significantly improved within a week, and two thirds by 7 weeks. However, recurrences are common, affecting up to 40% of patients within 6 months. The overall picture can be a chronic problem with intermittent exacerbations.[110] Recovery from acute radicular pain due to a herniated disk is favorable, with sequential MRI studies showing regression of disk herniations and good resolution of symptoms in many cases by 6 months.[122,162]

Pathophysiology

It is convenient to think of back pain in terms of location, existing either as a central or axial (nonradiating) pain versus a radicular pain involving the lower extremities. Axial low back pain has several potential etiologies. These include injury to the intervertebral disks, in the form of annulus fibrosus tears and degenerative disk disease, apophyseal joints, and vertebral bodies. Excessive rotational stress may injure the annulus fibrosus and apophyseal joints. The outer half of the posterior annulus fibrosus is innervated.[163] A tear in the annulus may provoke an inflammatory response with chemical irritation of the nociceptors, and may predispose to a frank disk herniation. Pure axial compression of the disk will increase the radial and hoop strains in the disk and also provoke pain. Tears or fractures at the disk–vertebral endplate junction may also arise from excessive weight bearing. The apophyseal joints are common sites of pain, and may arise from injury due to subchondral fracture, capsular tears, synovial tissue irritation, or hemorrhage into the joint space.

Differentiation between injuries of disk and apophyseal joints may be appreciated by pain-provoking activities (flexion with disk injuries, and extension with apophyseal joints). Spondylolysis, or stress fracture of the pars interarticularis, is seen in sports with back extension and rotation, such as gymnastics and tennis. Spondylolisthesis or slippage of one vertebra upon the other may be seen in athletes with bilateral pars defects. Any of the pain-producing structures of the spine has been implicated in low back pain, including the vertebral venous plexus, dura mater, intervertebral ligaments, and muscles and their fascia. Such structures may cause pain simply due to functional instability of the spine arising from weakness and spasm of the core muscles. Radicular pain is sharp and lancinating along a dermatomal distribution. This suggests nerve root irritation. Radicular pain can be associated with numbness and tingling, as well as somatic pain, a deep ache, referred along the buttocks or posterior thigh. Abnormalities in sensation, motor strength, and deep tendon reflexes will be seen in patients presenting with nerve root irritation. Commonly, in athletes, such nerve root irritation is a result of disk protrusion or extrusion. With older patients, the irritation can also result from degenerate apophyseal joints and ligamentum flavum hypertrophy. Spinal canal stenosis, both degenerative and congenital, can cause symptoms about the hips. It is characterized by pain aggravated with walking and typically relieved by forward flexion and rest. Each of these components must be evaluated. Overall, the diagnosis is made by corroborating the clinical history, physical exam, and imaging findings.

Treatment

Many patients affected by nonspecific low back pain experience spontaneous recovery quickly. For most, the best recommendation in the acute phase is neither bed rest nor physical exercise, but a general emphasis on the avoidance of painful activities with a gradual return to normal activities. Heavy lifting and trunk rotation should be discouraged. Positions of comfort vary, and may involve lying prone, supine, or commonly side-lying with a degree of lumbar flexion. Bed rest for more than a day or two is inadvisable.[108,110]

Nonsteroidal antiinflammatory drugs, taken regularly, are effective for symptom relief. No one antiinflammatory has been shown to be superior to another. The prescription of so-called muscle relaxants is common, but it is not entirely clear which patients stand to benefit.[164] The class of medications is broad, and includes benzodiazepines (diazepam), barbiturate precursors (SOMA, carisoprodol), tricyclic antidepressants (cyclobenzaprine), and other centrally acting depressants such as the -aminobutyric-acid-b (GABA-b) agonist baclofen.[165] Side effects (drowsiness, dizziness, and nausea) are common, and there is abuse potential. Drug interactions, withdrawal symptoms, and serious medical complications are also pos-

sible.[110,165] These so-called muscle relaxants are undoubtedly helpful in individuals suffering with actual central nervous system pathology, where loss of central control leads to spastic, hyper-reflexic muscle. In patients without upper motor neuron damage, it is not clear whether the medications actually "relax" spasmodic peripheral skeletal muscle. Nevertheless, the nonbenzodiazepine sedatives seem to show some benefit in perceived low back pain. Such benefits are not seen as often in the treatment of neck pain (see below).

Because nonspecific low back pain generally resolves spontaneously, an automatic prescription for physical therapy is not always warranted. Indeed, in the treatment of acute and subacute back pain, the scientific literature addressing exercise versus no treatment is not particularly supportive.[166] However, in the long-term, a generalized conditioning program with aerobic fitness, combined with education and specific trunk and leg strengthening, has been shown to be helpful in reducing pain and improving overall function.[110]

It is helpful to think of the physical therapy treatment of mechanical low back pain as a series of six phases, and an individual decision must be made to determine the correct emphasis of therapies in a particular patient:

1. Control of pain and inflammation can be accomplished with modalities such as ice, transcutaneous electrical nerve stimulation (TENS), spinal manipulation/manual therapy, massage, trigger point therapies, acupuncture, traction, education, and relative rest. Many of these interventions may be individually perceived as helpful, but scientific efficacy is mostly anecdotal.[110,166] Massage can address the abnormalities of the muscles and fascia, which are often seen in patients with low back pain.[108] Unfortunately, massage therapy has not been rigorously studied.

   Spinal manipulation and mobilization techniques have moderate evidence to support their effectiveness for short-term pain relief.[166,167] The goals are to restore movement to hypomobile intervertebral segments and reduce pain. Mobilization techniques include PA central, PA unilateral, rotations, and transverse vertebral pressure. The details may be found in various manual medicine textbooks.[167] Traction maneuvers are not well substantiated for treating the lumbar spine; in the cervical spine there is somewhat better science supporting its use.[132] In many interdisciplinary centers, these manual medicine maneuvers are performed usually by osteopathic physicians, chiropractors, or medical physicians, and sometimes by physical therapists.

2. Restore full range of pain-free motion. In contrast to the passive modalities emphasized in phase 1, the patient should graduate to an active program of fitness. The program should involve stretching, range of motion, strengthening, and core stability. The exercises should be performed in a direction away from movement that aggravates symptoms. For example, extension exercises may reduce neural tension or disk protrusions in patients with degenerative disks for which flexion increases pain. Conversely, patients

with spinal stenosis or posterior spinal column pathology, who have pain with extension, should be treated with trunk flexion exercises. In general, strengthening should first involve isometrics, with progression to isotonic exercises with concentric strengthening. However, there has been no strong scientific evidence to support one specific exercise program over another.[166]

3. Identify and address possible contributors to pain, such as poor posture, abnormal biomechanics, sports technique, other joint injuries. The two principles are activity modification and correction of the biomechanical abnormalities that predispose the patient to injury. Activities should be modified to reduce stress to the lumbar spine, and involve new techniques of awareness and activation for posture, activities of daily living, and sports technique.

Biomechanical imbalances (muscle weakness, tight muscles, poor muscle control) must be addressed. These imbalances may increase the stresses experienced by the spine. Here, the exercise principles of Janda[168] are particularly enlightening. In athletes it is common to find relative weakness of gluteal and hamstring muscles. These muscles are important for pelvic control and tilt, and usually require some training to activate during lifting and bending activities. Muscle tightness is commonly found in the erector spinae, psoas, iliotibial band, hip external rotators, hamstrings, rectus femoris, and gastrocnemius-soleus complex.

Motor control rehabilitation focuses on the transversus abdominis and lumbar multifidi core muscles. In patients with back pain there are changes in the firing patterns of these muscles. The rehabilitation begins with formal motor skill training using core strengthening exercises and the concept of the neutral spine, incorporation of muscle activation patterns during daily activity, and progress toward the incorporation into sports-specific tasks.[108]

4. Enable the patient to achieve strength, endurance, coordination, and speed. Dynamic exercises are structured to maximize coordinated muscular activities, which emphasize postural control and spinal stability.

5. Improve the patient's general cardiovascular condition. Patients are encouraged to remain active and to socialize. These activities may increase native endorphin levels to promote a sense of well-being. Indeed, 20 to 30 minutes of aerobic exercise performed three to four times a week at an intensity level of 60% of cardiac maximum has been shown to increase endorphin levels up to 100 times.[169]

6. Maintenance. An individual training program is developed for the patient athlete to be continued after discharge from formal physical therapy.

Selected Lumbosacral Spine Syndromes

Spondylolysis

Spondylolysis is a defect of the pars interarticularis, which is the junction of the lamina with the pedicle. The L5 vertebra is most commonly involved. When the condition is bilateral,

the superior articular processes remain attached to the vertebral body, but there is a defect through the pars such that the spinous process and inferior articular processes are detached. If the defect only is present, the condition is referred to as "spondylolysis." If there is slip displacement of the vertebral body as a result of the defect, the condition is referred to more generally as "spondylolisthesis" (see following discussion). Spondylolysis may be hereditary or acquired, and is associated with spina bifida occulta. First-degree relatives are at increased risk, and higher prevalence has been seen in Eskimo population studies. Gender and race play a role, with an incidence of 6.5% in white men, 3% in black men, 2.5% in white women, and 1% in black women. For most, the condition is thought to be an acquired stress fracture, and is seen particularly with athletes involved in sports that entail episodic hyperextension and rotation, such as gymnastics, tennis, diving, rowing, dance, weight-lifting, wrestling, pole vaulting, high jump, javelin, discus, hammer throw, volleyball, American football linemen, and baseball pitching. The fracture usually is seen on the opposite side to the side performing the activity (i.e., left-sided fracture in a right-handed javelin thrower).[108] While noted in 5% of the general population, the incidence of spondylolysis in divers, weight-lifters, wrestlers, and gymnasts has been reported to be 10% to 60%.[153] Furthermore, only 10% of those individuals in the general population are symptomatic with a spondylolysis. But among athletes, 50% of those individuals with a spondylolysis report associated low back pain. Three phases of stress fracture are described: early, progressive, and terminal. The early stage is characterized by focal bony absorption or a hairline defect seen on imaging. The progressive stage has a wide defect with small fragments. The terminal stage demonstrates sclerotic bony changes.

Patients complain of a unilateral low back pain with possible involvement of the buttock and posterior thigh. The pain is typically provoked with prolonged standing or back extension-rotation maneuvers. There is poor tolerance of activities that load the spine such as running and jumping, while sitting is better tolerated. On exam the pain is provoked by the single-legged hyperextension test. This maneuver has the athlete standing on the leg of the affected side and then placed into lumbar extension with rotation. The hamstring muscles are often tight. There is unilateral tenderness to palpation over the fracture site.

Radiographs may not show the fracture acutely. However, in longer-standing cases, the pars interarticularis defect may be revealed on the oblique views (an absent neck in the "Scottie dog'; see above, also see Figs. 4.14, 4.15, and 4.32). Overall, the sensitivity of lateral and oblique radiographs in diagnosing spondylolysis is 75% to 77%.[153] When a pars defect is suspected clinically, a SPECT scan is important to direct management.[170] The SPECT scan uses small amounts of radionucleotide tracer, which is retained by osteoclasts involved in the acute and progressive bony phases of fracture remodeling. Because of this, SPECT scans should not be used with pregnant women. A positive SPECT can also be seen in chronic degenerative arthritic conditions, in the facet joint, for example, where bony resorption and remodeling are also occurring. Usually in the youthful athletic population this is not a concern. The SPECT can be followed by CT, if the SPECT was positive or "hot," to better image the fracture site. Other conditions picked up by the SPECT scan can be assessed with the CT scan, such as osteoid osteoma, osteoblastoma, facet joint osteoarthritis, or fracture in other elements of the posterior column (pedicle or facet joint itself). The patient may be monitored during healing with repeat CT scan of the fracture. If the SPECT was negative or "cold," an MRI is suggested to evaluate degenerative disk disease, the presence of nerve root compression, tumor, or infection. With high-quality images, proper technique and greater interpretive skill, an MRI examination may also visualize marrow edema at the site of an acute spondylotic defect.[171] Even in the best circumstances, however, bony anatomy is not as well defined in MRI as with CT scanning, nor is the pathology as well demonstrated to patients as with SPECT scanning.

The goals of treatment are pain relief, defect healing, healthy return to sports, and prevention of future injury. The first treatment step is restriction of the offending maneuver or activity. Second, a stretching program focused on the hamstrings and gluteal muscles is instituted. Hip range of motion and control is as important as trunk strengthening. Core trunk strength exercises are prescribed as soon as they can be performed in a pain-free fashion. As always, there is a progression starting with isometrics, and moving on toward closed and open chain exercises. Emphasis of core muscle group co-contractions should be made, and training must incorporate the use of these coordinated co-contractions into sports and daily activities. When aggravating maneuvers (lumbar extension and rotation) are pain-free and there is no local tenderness, the athlete may be progressed to 4 to 6 weeks of sports-specific drills with an emphasis on balance, speed, and endurance training using pain as a guide. Technique adjustments should be identified to limit lumbar extension. Specific strengthening and stretching routines should be incorporated into the warm-up and cool-down routine of the athlete. The use of rigid bracing is debatable.[108,139,170] Repeat imaging may not be required, although younger athletes (ages 9 to 13) with spina bifida occulta and spondylolisthesis may require surveillance every 6 months until age 16.

Most cases of early stage fracture proceed to radiographic healing. Unilateral defects are more likely to heal than bilateral defects. There is improved success with L4 defects compared to L5 defects, and with defects that are closer to the vertebral body. About half of the patients with progressive stage defects demonstrate bony healing, while almost none of the terminal-stage patients with sclerotic changes show healing. However, excellent and good clinical outcomes have been reported even in the absence of radiographic healing.[153] Surgical intervention is rarely indicated, but when performed, successful fusion rates of 80% to 90% are reported.[172] In patients with a healthy intervertebral disk, this can involve direct repair of the pars fracture using a lag screw and grafting across the defect. In cases with a coexistent degenerate disk, a one-level fusion utilizing a posterior approach may be preferred.

Spondylolisthesis

Spondylolisthesis is defined as the slippage of one vertebral body forward on the one below. Six categories of spondylolisthesis have been proposed: congenital, isthmic, degenerative, traumatic, pathologic, and postsurgical. Isthmic spondylolisthesis is the most common type seen in children and young adults. It is associated with bilateral pars defects that develop usually in early childhood. It is commonly seen in children between the ages of 9 and 14, and is often asymptomatic during this period. The vast majority of cases involve a slip of L5 on S1 (Fig. 4.32). The Meyerding classification relies upon radiographic imaging and denotes slippage in percent terms of the superior endplate of the underlying vertebral body (usually S1). Grade 1 slip denotes a vertebral body that has slipped 5% to 25% of the total distance of the underlying endplate. Grade 2 denotes 26% to 50% slip, grade 3 denotes 51% to 75%, and grade 4 denotes 76% to 100% slip. Complete dislocation is grade 5, which is termed spondyloptosis. Most (i.e., 60% to 75%) of slips are grade 1, with less than 2% grade 3, 4, or 5.[173] The likelihood of spondylolisthesis progression is low. When seen, progression occurs in children with skeletal immaturity.

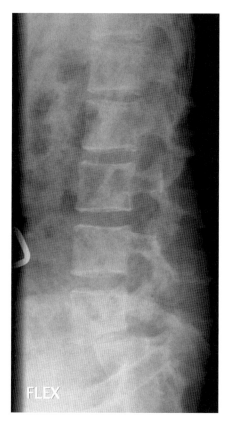

FIG. 4.32. Bilateral pars defects with resultant grade 2 anterolisthesis of L5 on S1 in a 31-year-old woman. There was no evidence of abnormal motion in the flexio and extension views.

Children and adolescents with high-grade slip are at risk for further progression. Females are at greater risk than males.[172]

Grade 1 slips are usually asymptomatic. Patients with grade 2 or higher slips may complain of low back pain, usually without radicular leg pain. The pain is exacerbated with lumbar extension activities. Pain may be mild to severe, and usually is more severe in those cases associated with an acute spondylosis. However, most cases are not associated with increased pain, disability, or abnormal radiographic motion.[173] On exam there may be a palpable "step-off" defect corresponding to a severe slip, and there may be abnormal soft tissue tone or point tenderness. Lumbar extension may be pain-limited. It is important to realize that the back pain may not be exclusively arising from an incidentally noted spondylolisthesis. Neurologic deficits are rare, but when present usually involve the L5 spinal nerve roots.

The treatment of athletes with symptomatic grade 1 or 2 spondylolisthesis involves relative rest, followed by stretching and trunk strengthening exercises. The program is similar to that described above for symptomatic spondylolysis. Anti-lordotic bracing may help control pain, but will not decrease slippage. Manual medicine techniques involve gentle joint mobilization to stiff joints above and below the slip. Manipulation should not be performed at the level of the slip. Return to sports is allowed after the athlete is pain free on lumbar extension, and is able to demonstrate good spinal stabilization. A recurrence of pain mandates cessation of the exacerbating activity. Athletes with grade 3 or 4 spondylolisthesis must avoid high speed and contact sports. Usually these patients are too symptomatic to participate in such sports anyway. Again, slip progression is rare. Injection therapies into the pars defect or facet joints have been reported anecdotally, without consistent benefit. Surgical fusion may be indicated for those athletes with evidence of slip progression or pain not relieved by nonoperative measures.[108,173] Fusions require about 6 to 12 months before solid fusion is obtained and an athlete can return to compete in contact sports.[139]

Acute Nerve Root Compression

Lumbar herniated disks are relatively uncommon in young competitive athletes. When they do occur, prolapse of the disk releases contents of the nucleus pulposus into the spinal canal and neuroforamen. There, irritation of the spinal nerve roots may occur. Three types of herniations are described: protrusions, in which the surrounding disk annulus remains intact; extrusions, in which the annulus is violated, but the posterior longitudinal ligament (PLL) is intact; and sequestered disk, in which both the annulus and PLL are violated and free disk fragments are seen in the spinal canal[153] (Fig. 4.33). Clinical and animal research studies suggest that radicular pain is the result of inflammation of the nerve root, and this may occur from chemical irritation by disk materials, compression and ischemia of the nerve root epineurial vasculature, or mechanical compression of the dorsal root ganglion. In older athletes, nerve roots may be affected anteriorly by the disk, but also posteriorly by facet joint osteoarthritic processes. A disk prolapse

may develop after a trivial event, which triggers a painful episode. Ninety-five percent of lumbosacral disk herniations occur at the L4-L5 or L5-S1 levels with involvement of the L5 or S1 nerve roots. They occur more commonly in males than females, and in patients between 20 and 50 years of age. A weak association between the activity of bowling and lumbar disk herniation has been reported. No association was noted with other sports (baseball, softball, golf, swimming, diving, weight lifting, or racket sports).[153] About 2% of the general

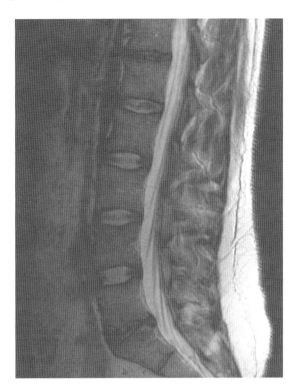

A

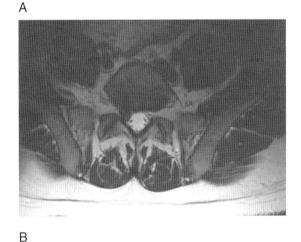

B

FIG. 4.33. Acute right paracentral disk extrusion, seen at the L5-S1 level on sagittal (A) and axial (B) T2-weighted MRIs, in a 33-year-old man with a 6-week history of right leg pain, numbness, and tingling. The disk mass impinges on the traversing right S1 nerve root. Two epidural steroid injections helped manage his pain and the patient improved over 5 months.

population is affected, but only 10% to 25% are symptomatic for more than 6 weeks.[145] Because less than 10% are affected more than 3 months, urgent surgical intervention is generally not required in most cases (unless there is a cauda equina syndrome). Similar resolution is seen over 6 to 12 weeks in cervical spine radiculopathies.[145,162]

Patients complain of lancinating pain down the limb in a characteristic dermatomal pattern. This is associated with paresthesias. A position of comfort is difficult to find. Upper or midlumbar radiculopathies generally refer pain to the anterior thigh, whereas lower lumbosacral radiculopathies refer pain along the lateral or posterior thigh to the side of the foot. Physical exam findings include positive nerve root tension signs, altered deep tendon reflexes, and sometimes myelopathic findings on motor exam. Palpatory exam usually reveals marked tenderness and paraspinal muscles that are tight in spasm. The diagnostic impression may be confirmed with MRI, which helps verify the level of compression and exclude other forms of spinal pathology. Electrodiagnostic studies may help rule-in a radiculopathy in difficult cases, but as mentioned previously they may not be used to exclude a radiculopathy.

Supportive care, as detailed above, is appropriate, which includes NSAIDs prescribed on a regularly scheduled basis, short prescriptions of sedative "muscle relaxant" medications, exercise, manual medicine techniques, and waiting for symptom resolution. Weak narcotic medications and bed rest have not been shown to be effective compared to alternative treatments for any patient outcomes such as pain relief, recovery rate, return to daily activities, or days lost from work.[166] Staying active, to the extent possible, has strong evidence for positive outcomes, as do back exercise programs. No one exercise program has been shown superior to another. Patients should be reassured that most disk problems resolve without residual impairments, but that episodic exacerbations are not unexpected. As the acute phase resolves, the focus of treatment is restoration of range of motion, active stabilization of the trunk through strengthening and motor firing control, postural advice, adjustment of sporting technique, and aerobic conditioning.[108]

Injections of epidural steroids can improve patient satisfaction, decrease pain, increase tolerance for walking and standing, and prevent surgery in many patients. Contraindications to an interventional procedure include anticoagulation, allergy to injectates (contrast dye, steroid, local anesthetic), and, depending on the treatment, pregnancy. Relative caution should be exercised with patients who are concurrently taking aspirin or other NSAIDs, or with other poorly controlled medical conditions. The three routes for delivery of epidural medications are caudal, interlaminar, and transforaminal. All of these routes should be performed with fluoroscopic guidance, because there is a 30% to 40% "miss" rate seen with even experienced interventionalists. Other risks include vasovagal reaction, dural violation, hematoma, and infection. Nerve root injury and meningitis have also been reported.[126]

An abundant literature exists regarding the efficacy of epidural steroid injection therapy, most of it uncontrolled, poorly designed, and retrospective. Such studies have been unable to demonstrate much of a positive treatment effect. On the other hand, there are several well-designed studies that show substantive long-term benefit.[122,123,126] The optimal timing, frequency, or medication dosing of injections is unknown. Typically, an athlete's response to an injection is evaluated about 2 weeks later, and a second injection may be recommended. A total of three to four injections may be scheduled over 6 to 8 weeks, depending on the clinical response. Urgent surgical consideration should be given to patients who experience cauda equina syndrome, which is progressive neurologic deficit with motor loss. Surgery is also a useful consideration for those with intractable pain, symptoms lasting longer than 6 weeks, or recurrent episodes that interfere with the patient's activities.

For those patients who have severe pain, or weakness, during 8 to 12 weeks of nonoperative management, surgery may be strongly considered. Microdiskectomy is the preferred procedure. In elite and professional athletes, a study showed that after surgery, 53 of 60 returned to their chosen sport in an average of 5 months.[139]

Degenerative Disk Disease

The intervertebral disk is a poorly vascularized, fibrous structure with pain sensing nerve fibers innervating the outer one-third layer. Microtrauma, annular tears, and disk degeneration may allow the release of inflammatory mediators, which are irritating to the surrounding structures. The risks for disk disruption are prolonged sitting, repetitive impact loading, and twisting. Athletes seem to be at risk compared to nonathletes. For example, 75% of male gymnasts have been reported to have signs of disk degeneration, compared to 30% of age-matched controls.[153] Patients complain of axial low back pain. The diagnosis is made with MRI, diskography or CT-diskography. Treatment is controversial. Some promote nonoperative therapy, others surgical intervention. Nonoperative techniques include basic spine rehabilitation protocols and experimental interventional techniques to treat axial low back pain, which include the use of epidural steroid injections, intradiskal steroid injections, and intradiskal electrothermal therapy.[174] The operative management of degenerative disk disease involves fusion by a variety of techniques, or experimental intervertebral disk replacement technologies.[175]

Zygapophyseal Pain

The zygapophyseal joint, also known as the facet joint, has been said to be a source of pain for 15% to 40% of patients with chronic low back pain. However, there are several spinal structures that may contribute to axial low back pain. A definitive diagnosis of lumbosacral facet joint syndrome is challenging to confirm. Facet joint arthropathy may arise from degenerative or traumatic etiologies. Many athletes, such as

American football players, experience repetitive forceful lumbar hyperextension, which might be injurious to the facet joints. The patient with facet joint syndrome typically presents with axial low back pain that can refer to the buttocks. Certain combined extension and rotation maneuvers can exacerbate the pain. Facet joints are not directly palpable, but the palpatory exam may have localized paravertebral pain unilaterally. Plain radiographs do not reliably diagnose early facet joint arthropathy (Fig. 4.34). Magnetic resonance imaging or CT examinations will show facet joint degenerative changes more exactly, but anatomic morphology does not correlate well with pain. Medial-branch blocks, or intraarticular injections of the facet joint with local anesthetic, using fluoroscopic guidance, are currently used to help make the diagnosis. Each joint is dually innervated. Medial branch blocks should address both branches. If there is a significant positive response, longer term relief may be obtained with radiofrequency ablation procedures. However, there is controversy regarding the effectiveness of such interventional procedures to treat facet joint arthropathy in the lumbosacral spine. While there is good science to support their use in the cervical spine facet joints,[125] their use in the lumbosacral spine remains largely anecdotal.[176] Therefore, they may be attempted in patients with persistent symptoms despite adequate nonoperative care. Otherwise the treatment plan involves relative rest, medications, and progressive exercise as symptoms dictate. For many athletes, such a basic treatment plan works well.

Conclusion

Magnetic resonance imaging has revolutionized our understanding of the spine. It is the modality of choice to evaluate soft tissue lesions, neurologic lesions, neoplasms, or infection. In most cases practically, MRI need not be the immediate diagnostic study of choice. This is important because there are many asymptomatic abnormalities seen with imaging. Patients should understand that typical degenerative changes will be spotted on their MRI examinations. However, when there is specific clinical concern and the possibility of treatment altering decisions, MRI can be very helpful to detect structural abnormalities of both the soft tissues (e.g., intervertebral disk) and hard tissues (bone).

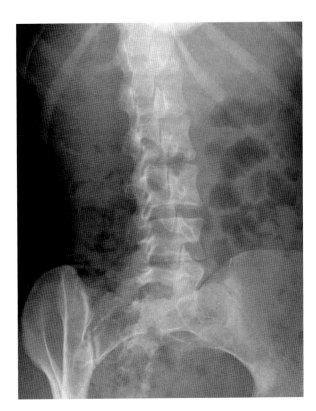

A

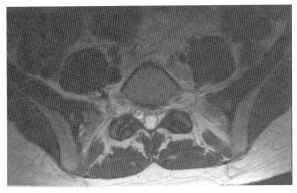

B

FIG. 4.34. A 23-year-old woman with a 1-year history of axial right-sided low back pain. Her pain was reproducible with the palpatory exam as well as the single-legged hyperextension test. (A) Oblique radiograph demonstrates sclerosis of the right L5-S1 facet joint. (B) Axial T2-weighted MRI of the L5-S1 level shows moderate facet joint arthropathy, right worse than left.

References

1. Pathria MN. Physical injury: spine. In: Resnick D, Niwayama G, eds. Diagnosis of Bone and Joint Disorders, 3rd ed. Philadelphia: WB Saunders, 1995:2825–98.
2. Pretorius ES, Fishman EK. Volume-rendered three-dimensional spiral CT: musculoskeletal applications. Radiographics 1999;19(5):1143–60.
3. Daffner RH. Helical CT of the cervical spine for trauma patients: a time study. AJR Am J Roentgenol 2001;177(3):677–9.
4. Berlin L. CT versus radiography for initial evaluation of cervical spine trauma: what is the standard of care? AJR Am J Roentgenol 2003;180(4):911–5.
5. Dublin AB, McGahan JP, Reid MH. The value of computed tomographic metrizamide myelography in the neuroradiological evaluation of the spine. Radiology 1983;146:79–86.
6. Rupani HD, Holder LE, Espinola DA, Engin SI. Three-phase radionuclide bone imaging in sports medicine. Radiology 1985;156(1):187 96.

7. Papanicolaou N, Wilkinson RH, Emans JB, Treves S, Micheli LJ. Bone scintigraphy and radiography in young athletes with low back pain. AJR Am J Roentgenol 1985;145(5):1039–44.

8. De Maeseneer M, Lenchik L, Everaert H, et al. Evaluation of lower back pain with bone scintigraphy and SPECT. Radiographics 1999;19(4):901–12.

9. Kanal E, Borgstede JP, Barkovich AJ, et al. American College of Radiology white paper on MR safety. AJR Am J Roentgenol 2002;178(6):1335–47.

10. Trainor TJ, Trainor MA. Etiology of low back pain in athletes. Curr Sports Med Rep 2004;3(1):41–6.

11. Olmarker K, Rydevik B, Nordborg C. Autologous nucleus pulposus induces neurophysiologic and histologic changes in porcine cauda equina nerve roots. Spine 1993;18(11):1425–32.

12. Franson RC, Saal JS, Saal JA. Human disc phospholipase A2 is inflammatory. Spine 1992;17(6 suppl):S129–32.

13. Spitzer WO, Leblanc FE, Dupuis M. Scientific approach to the assessment and management of activity-related spinal disorders. A monograph for clinicians. Report of the Quebec Task Force on Spinal Disorders. Spine 1987;12(suppl 7S):1–59.

14. Staal JB, Hlobil H, van Tulder MW, et al. Occupational health guidelines for the management of low back pain: an international comparison. Occup Environ Med 2003;60(9):618–26.

15. Modic MT, Obuchowski NA, Ross JS, et al. Acute low back pain and radiculopathy: MR imaging findings and their prognostic role and effect on outcome. Radiology 2005;237(2):597–604.

16. Fardon DF, Milette PC; Combined Task Forces of the North American Spine Society, American Society of Spine Radiology, and American Society of Neuroradiology. Nomenclature and classification of lumbar disc pathology. Recommendations of the Combined task Forces of the North American Spine Society, American Society of Spine Radiology, and American Society of Neuroradiology. Spine 2001;26(5):E93–E113

17. Jensen MC, Brant-Zawadzki MN, Obuchowski N, Modic MT, Malkasian D, Ross JS. Magnetic resonance imaging of the lumbar spine in people without back pain. N Engl J Med 1994;331(2):69–73.

18. Torgerson WR, Dotter WE. Comparative roentgenographic study of the asymptomatic and symptomatic lumbar spine. J Bone Joint Surg Am 1976;58(6):850–3.

19. Maroon JC, Bailes JE. Athletes with cervical spine injury. [Spine Update]. Spine 1996;21(19):2294–9.

20. Mintz DN. Magnetic resonance imaging of sports injuries to the cervical spine. Semin Musculoskelet Radiol 2004;8:99–110.

21. Sluckey AP, et al. Magnetic resonance imaging in spinal trauma: indications, techniques, and utility. J Am Acad Orthop Surg 1998;6:134–45.

22. Harris JH Jr. The cervicocranium: its radiographic assessment. Radiology 2001 218:337–51.

23. Lustrin ES, Karakas SP, Ortiz AO, et al. Pediatric cervical spine: normal anatomy, variants, and trauma. Radiographics 2003;23(3):539–60.

24. Hanson JA, Deliganis AV, Baxter AB, et al. Radiologic and clinical spectrum of occipital condyle fractures: retrospective review of 107 consecutive fractures in 95 patients. AJR Am J Roentgenol 2002;178(5):1261–8.

25. Deliganis AV, Baxter AB, Hanson JA, et al. Radiologic spectrum of craniocervical distraction injuries. Radiographics 2000;20(Spec. No.):S237–50.

26. Cremers MJ, Bol E, de Roos F, van Gijn J. Risk of sports activities in children with Down's syndrome and atlantoaxial instability. Lancet 1993;342(8870):511–4.

27. Singer SJ, Rubin IL, Strauss KJ. Atlantoaxial distance in patients with Down syndrome: standardization of measurement. Radiology 1987;164(3):871–2.

28. Braganza SF. Atlantoaxial dislocation. Pediatr Rev 2003;24(3):106–7.

29. Rogers LF. The spine. Radiology of Skeletal Trauma, 2nd ed. New York, Churchill Livingstone, 1992:439–592.

30. Kim KS, Chen HH, Russell EJ, et al. Flexion teardrop fracture of the cervical spine: radiographic characteristics. AJR 1989;152:319.

31. White AA, Southwick WO, Panjabi MM. Clinical instability in the lower cervical spine: a review of past and current concepts. Spine 1976;1:15.

32. Terk MR, Hume-Neal M, Fraipont M, et al. Injury of the posterior ligament complex in patients with acute spinal trauma: evaluation by MR imaging. AJR 1997;168:1481–6.

33. Emery S, Pathria MN, Wilber RG, Masaryk T, Bohlman HH. MRI of posttraumatic spinal ligament injury. J Spinal Disorders 1989;2:229–33.

34. Yetkin Z, Osborn AG, Giles DS, et al. Uncovertebral and facet joint dislocations in cervical articular pillar fractures: CT evaluation. AJNR 1985;6:633.

35. Marar BC. Hyperextension injuries of the cervical spine: the pathogenesis of damage to the spinal cord. J Bone Joint Surg [Am] 1974;56:1655.

36. Edeiken-Monroe B, Wagner LK, Harris JH Jr. Hyperextension dislocation of the cervical spine. AJR 1986;146:803.

37. Regenbogen VS, Rogers LF, Atlas SW, et al: Cervical spinal cord injuries in patients with cervical spondylosis. AJR 1986;146:277.

38. Taylor AR. The mechanism of injury to the spinal cord in the neck without damage to the vertebral column. J Bone Joint Surg [Br] 1951;33:543.

39. Schneider RC, Crosby EC, Russo RH, et al. Traumatic spinal cord syndromes and their management. Clin Neurosurg 1973;20:424.

40. Torg JS, Pavlov H, Genuario SE, et al. Neurapraxia of the cervical spinal cord with transient quadriplegia. J Bone Joint Surg [Am] 1986;68:1354.

41. Goldberg AL, Rothfus WE, Deeb ZL, et al. The impact of magnetic resonance on the diagnostic evaluation of acute cervicothoracic spinal trauma. Skel Radiol 1988;17:89.

42. Flanders AE, Schaefer DM, Doan HY, et al. Acute cervical spine trauma: Correlation of MR imaging findings with degree of neurologic deficit. Radiology 1990;177:25.

43. Maiman DJ, Pintar FA. Anatomy and clinical biomechanics of the thoracic spine. Clin Neurosurg 1992;38:296.

44. Rogers LF, Thayer C, Weinberg PE, et al. Acute injuries of the upper thoracic spine associated with paraplegia. AJR 1980;134:67.

45. Wintermark M, Mouhsine E, Theumann N, et al. Thoracolumbar spine fractures in patients who have sustained severe trauma: depiction with multi-detector row CT. Radiology 2003;227(3):681–9.

46. Lenchik L, Rogers LF, Delmas PD, Genant HK. Diagnosis of osteoporotic vertebral fractures: importance of recognition and description by radiologists. AJR Am J Roentgenol 2004;183(4):949–58.

47. Kaplan PA, Orton DF, Asleson RJ. Osteoporosis with vertebral compression fractures, retropulsed fragments, and neurologic compromise. Radiology 1987;165:533.

48. Yuh WT, Zachar CK, Barloon TJ, et al. Vertebral compression fractures: Distinction between benign and malignant causes with MR imaging. Radiology 1989;172:215.

49. Denis F. The three column spine and its significance in the classification of acute thoracolumbar spinal injuries. Spine 1983;8:817.

50. Finn GA, Stauffer ES: Burst fracture of the fifth lumbar vertebra. J Bone Joint Surg [Am] 1992;74:398.

51. Patten RM, Gunbarg SR, Brandenburger DK. Frequency and importance of transverse process fractures in the lumbar vertebrae at helical abdominal CT in patients with trauma. Radiology 2000;215:831–4.

52. Sturm JT, Perry JF. Injuries associated with fractures of the transverse processes of the thoracic and lumbar vertebrae. J Trauma 1984;24:597.

53. Wiltse LL, Newman PH, Macnab I. Classification of spondylolysis and spondylolisthesis. Clin Orthop 1976;117:23.

54. Afshani E, Kuhn JP. Common causes of low back pain in children. RadioGraphics 1991;11:269–91.

55. Cope R. Acute traumatic spondylolysis: report of a case and review of the literature. Clin Orthop 1988;230:162.

56. Hensinger RN. Current concepts review: spondylolysis and spondylolisthesis in children and adolescents. J Bone Joint Surg [Am] 1989;71:1098.

57. Amato M, Totty WG, Gilula LA. Spondylolysis of the lumbar spine: Demonstration of defects and laminal fragmentation. Radiology 1984;153:627.

58. Sherman FC, Wilkinson RH, Hall JE, et al. Reactive sclerosis of a pedicle and spondylolysis in the lumbar spine. J Bone Joint Surg [Am] 1977;59:49.

59. Teplick GJ, Laffey PA, Berman A, et al. Diagnosis and evaluation of spondylolisthesis and/or spondylolysis on axial CT. AJNR 1986;7:479.

60. Ulmer JL, Mathews VP, Elster AD, Mark LP, Daniels DL, Mueller W. MR imaging of lumbar spondylolysis: the importance of ancillary observations. AJR Am J Roentgenol 1997;169(1):233–9.

61. Jinkins JR, Matthes JC, Sener RN, et al. Spondylolysis, spondylolisthesis, and associated nerve root entrapment in the lumbosacral spine: MR evaluation. AJR 1992;159:799.

62. Pennell RG, Maurer AH, Bonakdarpour A. Stress injuries of the pars interarticularis: radiologic classification and indications for scintigraphy. AJR 1985;145:763.

63. Bellah RD, Summerville DA, Treves ST, et al. Low-back pain in adolescent athletes: detection of stress injury to the pars interarticularis with SPECT. Radiology 1991;180:509.

64. Connolly LP, Drubach LA, Connolly SA, Treves ST. Young athletes with low back pain: skeletal scintigraphy of conditions other than pars interarticularis stress. Clin Nucl Med 2004;29(11):689–93.

65. Sairyo K, Katoh S, Sasa T, et al. Athletes with unilateral spondylolysis are at risk of stress fracture at the contralateral pedicle and pars interarticularis: a clinical and biomechanical study. Am J Sports Med 2005;33(4):583–90.

66. Major NM, Helms CA. Sacral stress fractures in long-distance runners. AJR Am J Roentgenol 2000;174(3):727–9.

67. Bick EM, Copel JW. The ring apophysis of the human vertebra: Contribution to human osteogeny. II. J Bone Joint Surg [Am] 1951;33:783.

68. Epstein NE, Epstein JA, Mauri T. Treatment of fractures of the vertebral limbus and spinal stenosis in five adolescents and five adults. Neurosurgery 1989;24:595.

69. Takata K, Inoue S, Takahashi K, et al. Fracture of the posterior margin of a lumbar vertebral body. J Bone Joint Surg [Am] 1988;70:589.

70. Hollingworth P. Back pain in children. Br J Rheumatol 1996;35(10):1022–8.

71. Horne J, Cockshott WP, Shannon HS. Spinal column damage from water ski jumping. Skeletal Radiol 1987;16(8):612–6.

72. Rachbauer F, Sterzinger W, Eibl G. Radiographic abnormalities in the thoracolumbar spine of young elite skiers. Am J Sports Med 2001;29(4):446–9.

73. Ogon M, Riedl-Huter C, Sterzinger W, Krismer M, Spratt KF, Wimmer C. Radiologic abnormalities and low back pain in elite skiers. Clin Orthop Rel Res 2001;(390):151–62.

74. Swischuk LE, John SD, Allbery S. Disk degenerative disease in childhood: Scheuermann's disease, Schmorl's nodes, and the limbus vertebra: MRI findings in 12 patients. Pediatr Radiol 1998;28(5):334–8.

75. Gustavel M, Beals RK. Scheuermann's disease of the lumbar spine in identical twins. AJR Am J Roentgenol 2002;179(4):1078–9.

76. Pfirrmann CW, Resnick D.Schmorl nodes of the thoracic and lumbar spine: radiographic-pathologic study of prevalence, characterization, and correlation with degenerative changes of 1,650 spinal levels in 100 cadavers. Radiology 2001;219(2):368–74.

77. Stabler A, Bellan M, Weiss M, Gartner C, Brossmann J, Reiser MF. MR imaging of enhancing intraosseous disk herniation (Schmorl's nodes). AJR Am J Roentgenol 1997;168(4):933–8.

78. Hauger O, Cotten A, Chateil JF, Borg O, Moinard M, Diard F. Giant cystic Schmorl's nodes: imaging findings in six patients. AJR Am J Roentgenol 2001;176(4):969–72.

79. Tall RL, DeVault W. Spinal injury in sport: epidemiologic considerations. Clin Sports Med 1993;12(3):441–8.

80. Tomaszewski D, Avella D. Vertebral osteomyelitis in a high school hockey player: a case report. J Athl Train 1999;34(1):29–33.

81. Heck JF, Sparano JM. A classification system for the assessment of lumbar pain in athletes. J Athl Train 2000;35(2):204–11.

82. Algra PR, Heimans JJ, Valk J, Nauta JJ, Lachniet M, Van Kooten B. Do metastases in vertebrae begin in the body or the pedicles? Imaging study in 45 patients. Am J Roentgenol 1992;158:1275–9.

83. Van Lom KJ, Kellerhouse LE, Pathria MN, et al. Infection versus tumor in the spine: criteria for distinction with CT. Radiology 1988;166:851.

84. Vanel D, Bittoun J, Tardivon A. MRI of bone metastases. Eur Radiol 1998;8(8):1345–51.

85. Algra PR, Bloem JL, Tissing H, Falke THM, Arndt JW, Verboom LJ. Detection of vertebral metastases: comparison between MR imaging and bone scintigraphy. RadioGraphics 1991;11:219–32.

86. Munday TL, Johnson MH, Hayes CW, Thompson EO, Smoker WR. Musculoskeletal causes of spinal axis compromise: beyond the usual suspects. Radiographics 1994;14(6):1225–45.

87. Murphey MD, Andrens CL, Flemming DJ, et al. Primary tumors of the spine: radiologic-pathologic correlation. Radiographics 1996;16:1131–58.

88. Angtuaco EJ, Fassas AB, Walker R, Sethi R, Barlogie B. Multiple myeloma: clinical review and diagnostic imaging. Radiology 2004;231(1):11–23.

89. Laredo J, Assouline E, Gelbert F, et al. Vertebral heman-
    giomas: fat content as a sign of aggressiveness. Radiology
    1990;177:467–72.

90. Woods ER, Martel W, Mandell SH, Crabbe JP. Reactive soft-
    tissue mass associated with osteoid osteoma: correlation of
    MR imaging features with pathologic findings. Radiology
    1993;186(1):221–5.

91. Kothari NA, Pelchovitz DJ, Meyer JS. Imaging of musculosk-
    eletal infections. Radiol Clin North Am 2001;39(4):653–71.

92. Ledermann HP, Schweitzer ME, Morrison WB, Carrino JA.
    MR imaging findings in spinal infections: rules or myths?
    Radiology 2003;228(2):506–14.

93. Gillams AR, Chaddha B, Carter AP. MR appearances of the
    temporal evolution and resolution of infectious spondylitis.
    AJR Am J Roentgenol 1996;166(4):903–7.

94. Namaguchi Y, Rigamonti D, Rothman MI, et al. Spinal epidural
    abscess: Evaluation with gadolinium-enhanced MR imaging.
    RadioGrahics 1993;13:545–559.

95. Moorthy S, Prabhu NK. Spectrum of MR imaging findings in
    spinal tuberculosis. AJR Am J Roentgenol 2002;179(4):979–
    83.

96. de Roos A, Kressel H, Spritzer C, Dalinka M. MR imaging of
    marrow changes adjacent to end plates in degenerative lumbar
    disk disease. AJR Am J Roentgenol 1987;149(3):531–4.

97. Modic MT, Steinberg PM, Ross JS, Masaryk TJ, Carter JR.
    Degenerative disk disease: assessment of changes in vertebral
    body marrow with MR imaging. Radiology 1988;166(1 pt
    1):193–9.

98. Bouchaud-Chabot A, Liote F. Cervical spine involve-
    ment in rheumatoid arthritis. A review. Joint Bone Spine
    2002;69(2):141–54.

99. Bundschuh C, Modic MT, Kearney F et al. Rheumatoid
    arthritis of the cervical spine: surface-coil MR imaging. AJR
    1988;151:181–7.

100. Hermann KG, Althoff CE, Schneider U, et al. Spinal
    changes in patients with spondyloarthritis: comparison of
    MR imaging and radiographic appearances. Radiographics
    2005;25(3):559–69

101. Zunkeler B, Schelper R, Menezes AH. Periodontoid cal-
    cium pyrophosphate dihydrate deposition disease: "pseudog-
    out" mass lesions of the craniocervical junction. J Neurosurg
    1996;85(5):803–9.

102. Kakitsubata Y, Boutin RD, Theodorou DJ, et al. Calcium pyro-
    phosphate dihydrate crystal deposition in and around the atlan-
    toaxial joint: association with type 2 odontoid fractures in nine
    patients. Radiology 2000;216(1):213–9.

103. Ring D, Vaccaro AR, Scuderi G, Pathria MN, Garfin SR.
    Acute calcific retropharyngeal tendinitis. Clinical presenta-
    tion and pathological characterization. J Bone Joint Surg Am
    1994;76(11):1636–42.

104. Park YH, Taylor JA, Szollar SM, Resnick D. Imaging findings
    in spinal neuroarthropathy. Spine 1994;19(13):1499–504.

105. Wagner SC, et al. Can imaging findings help differentiate spi-
    nal neuropathic arthropathy from disk space infection? Initial
    experience. Radiology 2000;214(3):693–9.

106. Cobby MJ, Adler RS, Swartz R, Martel W. Dialysis-related
    amyloid arthropathy: MR findings in four patients. AJR Am J
    Roentgenol 1991;157(5):1023–7.

107. Flipo RM, Cotten A, Chastanet P, et al. Evaluation of destruc-
    tive spondyloarthropathies in hemodialysis by computerized

108. Brukner P, Khan K. Clinical Sports Medicine. San Francisco:
    McGraw-Hill, 2001.

109. Borenstein D, Wiesel S, Boden S, eds. Epidemiology of Back
    Pain. Philadelphia: WB Saunders, 1995.

110. Deyo R, Weinstein J. Low back pain. N Engl J Med
    2001;344:363–70.

111. Boden S. Current concepts review—the use of radiographic
    imaging studies in the evaluation of patients who have degen-
    erative disorders of the lumbar spine. J Bone Joint Surg [Am]
    1996;78(1):114–24.

112. Humphreys S, Eck J, Hodges S. Neuroimaging in low back
    pain. Am Fam Physician 2002;65(11):2299–306.

113. Slipman C, Patel R, Botwin K, et al. Epidemiology of spine
    tumors presenting to musculoskeletal physiatrists. Arch Phys
    Med Rehabil 2003;84(4):492–5.

114. Deyo R, Rainville J, Kent D. What can the history and
    physical examination tell us about low back pain? JAMA
    1992;68(6):760–5.

115. Hoppenfeld S. Physical Examination of the Spine and Extremi-
    ties. Norwalk, CT: Appleton and Lange, 1976.

116. Yoss R, Corbin K, Maccarty C, Love J. Significance of symp-
    toms and signs in localization of involved roots in cervical disk
    protrusion. Neurology 1957;7:673–83.

117. Wilbourn A, Aminoff M. AAEM minimonograph 32: the elec-
    trodiagnostic examination in patients with radiculopathies.
    Muscle Nerve 1998;21:1612–31.

118. Panjabi M, Chang D, Dvorak J. An analysis of errors in kine-
    matic parameters associated with in vivo functional radio-
    graphs. Spine 1992;17(2):200–5.

119. Dvorak J, Panjabi M, Novotny J, Chang D, Grob D. Clinical
    validation of functional flexion-extension roentgenograms of
    the lumbar spine. Spine 1991;16(8):943–50.

120. Dvorak J, Panjabi M, Chang D, Theiler R, Grob D. Functional
    radiographic diagnostics of the lumbar spine. Flexion-exten-
    sion and lateral bending. Spine 1991;16(5):562–71.

121. Carragee E, Hannibal M. Diagnostic evaluation of low back
    pain. Orthop Clin North Am 2004;35:7–16.

122. Bush K, Cowan N, Katz D, Gishen P. The natural history of sciatic
    associated with disc pathology. A prospective study with clinical
    and independent radiologic follow-up. Spine 1992;10:1205–12.

123. Riew D, Yin Y, Gilulu L, et al. The effect of nerve-root injec-
    tions on the need for operative treatment of lumbar radicular
    pain. J Bone Joint Surg 2000;82–A(11):1589–93.

124. Carette S, Leclaire R, Marcous S, et al. Epidural corticosteroid
    injections for sciatica due to herniated nucleus pulposus.
    N Engl J Med 1997;336(23):1634–40.

125. Lord S, Barnsley L, Wallis B, McDonald G, Bogduk N.
    Percutaneous radio-frequency neurotomy for chronic cervical
    zygapophyseal-joint pain. N Engl J Med 1996;335(23):1721–6.

126. Cannon D, Aprill C. Lumbosacral epidural steroid injections.
    Arch Phys Med Rehabil 2000;81(3 suppl 1):S87–100.

127. Dvorak J, Panjabi M, Grob D, Novotny J, Antinnes J. Clinical
    validation of functional flexion/extension radiographs of the
    cervical spine. Spine 1993;18(1):120–7.

128. Brockmeyer D. Down syndrome and craniovertebral instabil-
    ity. Pediatr Neurosurg 1999;31:71–7.

129. Boden S, McCowin P, Davis D, Dina T, Mark A, Wiesel S.
    Abnormal magnetic-resonance scans of the cervical spine in

asymptomatic subjects. A prospective investigation. J Bone Joint Surg [Am] 1990;72(8):1178–84.

130. Boden S, Davis D, Dina T, Patronas N, Wiesel S. Abnormal magnetic-resonance scans of the lumbar spine in asymptomatic subjects. A prospective investigation. J Bone Joint Surg [Am] 1990;72(3):403–8.

131. Nachemson A, Waddell G, Norlund A. Epidemiology of neck and low back pain. In: Nachemson A, Jonsson E, eds. Neck and Back Pain: The Scientific Evidence of Causes, Diagnosis, and Treatment. Philadelphia: Lippincott Williams and Wilkins, 2000:495.

132. Nachemson A, Jonsson E, eds. Neck and Back Pain: The Scientific Evidence of Causes, Diagnosis, and Treatment. Philadelphia: Lippincott Williams and Wilkins, 2000.

133. Date E, Gray L. Electrodiagnostic evidence for cervical radiculopathy and suprascapular neuropathy in shoulder pain. Electromyogr Clin Neurophysiol 1996;36(6):333–9.

134. van Tulder M, Goossens M, Hoving J. Nonsurgical treatment of chronic neck pain. In: Nachemson A, Jonsson E, eds. Neck and Back Pain: The Scientific Evidence of Causes, Diagnosis, and Treatment. Philadelphia: Lippincott Williams and Wilkins, 2000:495.

135. Harms-Ringdahl K, Nachemson A. Acute and subacute neck pain: nonsurgical treatment. In: Nachemson A, Jonsson E, eds. Neck and Back Pain: The Scientific Evidence of Causes, Diagnosis, and Treatment. Philadelphia: Lippincott Williams and Wilkins, 2000:495.

136. Schuldt. On neck muscle activity and load reduction in sitting postures. An electromyographic and biomechanical study with applications in ergonomics and rehabilitation. Scand J Rehabil Med Suppl 1988;19:1–49.

137. Hurwitz E, Aker P, Adams A, Meeker W, Shekelle P. Manipulation and mobilization of the cervical spine. A systemic review of the literature. Spine 1997;22(14):1746–59.

138. Pearson N, Walmsley R. Trial into the effects of repeated neck retractions in normal subjects. Spine 1995;20(11):1245–50.

139. Eddy D, Congeni J, Loud K. A review of spine injuries and return to play. Clin J Sports Med 2005(15):453–8.

140. McDonald G, Lord S, Bogduk N. Long-term follow-up of patients treated with cervical radiofrequency neurotomy for chronic neck pain. Neurosurgery 1999;45(1):61–7.

141. Bush K, Hillier S. Outcome of cervical radiculopathy treated with periradicular/epidural corticosteroid injections: a prospective study with independent clinical review. Eur Spine J 1996;5(5):319–25.

142. Clendenin R, Nichols J. Football injuries. In: Lennard T, Crabtree H, eds. Spine in Sports. Philadelphia: Elsevier Mosby, 2005:226.

143. Vaccaro A, Klein G, Ciccoti M, et al. Return to play criteria for the athlete with cervical spine injuries resulting in stinger and transient quadriplegia/paresis. Spine J 2002;2(5):351–6.

144. Chang DG, Tencer AF, Ching RP, Treece B, Senft D, Anderson PA. Geometric changes in the cervical spinal canal during impact. Spine 1994;19(8):973–80.

145. Snider R, Brodke D, Fischgrund J, et al. Spine. In: Greene W, ed. Essentials of Musculoskeletal Care. Rosemont: American Academy of Orthopedic Surgeons, 2001:756.

146. Panjabi M, Cholewicki J, Nibu K, Grauer J, Babat L, Dvorak J. Mechanism of whiplash injury. Clin Biomech 1998;13(4):239–49.

147. Winnell J, Burke S. Sports participation of children with Down syndrome. Orthop Clin North Am 2003;34:439–43.

148. Atlantoaxial instability in Down syndrome: subject review. (American Academy of Pediatrics Committee on Sports Medicine and Fitness). Pediatrics 1995;96(1):151–4.

149. Lin J, Boop F. Common spinal disorders in the young athlete. In: Lennard T, Crabtree H, eds. Spine in Sports. Philadelphia: Elsevier Mosby, 2005:226.

150. Morganti C. Recommendations for return to sports following cervical spine injuries. Sports Med 2003;33(8):563–73.

151. Pfeifer M, Begerow B, Minne H. Effects of a new spinal orthosis on posture, trunk strength, and quality of life in women with postmenopausal osteoporosis: a randomized trial. Am J Phys Med Rehabil 2004;83(3):177–86.

152. Wenger D, Frick S. Scheuermann kyphosis. Spine 1999;24(24):2630–9.

153. Lennard T, Crabtree H, eds. Spine in Sports. Philadelphia: Elsevier Mosby, 2005.

154. Asher M, Burton D. Adolescent idiopathic scoliosis: natural history and long term treatment effects. Scoliosis 2006;1(1):2–12.

155. Dickson R, Weinstein S. Bracing (and screening)-yes or no? J Bone Joint Surg [Br] 1999;81(2):193–8.

156. McCarroll J. The frequency of golf injuries. Clin Sports Med 1996;15(1):1–7.

157. Saal J. Common American football injuries. Sports Med 1991;12(2):132–47.

158. Drake D, Nadler S, Chou L, Toledo S, Akuthota V. Sports and performing arts medicine. 4. Traumatic injuries in sports. Arch Phys Med Rehabil 2004;85(3 suppl 1):S67–71.

159. Goldstein J, Berger P, Windler G, Jackson D. Spine injuries in gymnasts and swimmers. An epidemiologic investigation. Am J Sports Med 1991;19(5):463–8.

160. Jackson D, Wiltse L, Cirincoine R. Spondylolysis in the female gymnast. Clin Orthop Rel Res 1976(117):68–73.

161. Chard M, Lachmann S. Racquet sports—patterns of injury presenting to a sports injury clinic. Br J Sports Med 1987;21(4):150–3.

162. Bush K, Chaudhuri R, Hillier S, Penny J. The pathomorphologic changes that accompany the resolution of cervical radiculopathy. A prospective study with repeat magnetic resonance imaging. Spine 1997;22(2):183–6.

163. Bogduk N. Clinical Anatomy of the Lumbar Spine and Sacrum, 4th ed. Melbourne: Churchill Livingstone; 2005.

164. van Tulder M, Touray T, Furlan A, Solway S, Bouter L. Muscle relaxants for nonspecific low back pain: a systematic review within the framework of the Cochrane collaboration. Spine 2003;28(17):1978–92.

165. Meleger A. Muscle relaxants and antispasticity agents. Phys Med Rehabil Clin North Am 2006;17(2):401–13.

166. van Tulder M, Waddell G. Conservative treatment of acute and subacute low back pain. In: Nachemson A, Jonsson E, eds. Neck and Back Pain: The Scientific Evidence of Causes, Diagnosis, and Treatment. Philadelphia: Lippincott Williams and Wilkins, 2000.

167. Dvorak J, Haldeman S, Gilliar W. Manual therapy in patients with low back pain. In: Herkowitz H, Dvorak J, Bell G, Nordin M, Grob D, eds. The Lumbar Spine, 3rd ed. Philadelphia: Lippincott Williams and Wilkins, 2004:943.

168. Janda V. Muscle Function Testing. Boston: Butterworths, 1983.

169. Appenzeller O, Wood S. Peptides and exercise at high and low altitudes. Int J Sports Med 1992;13(suppl 1):S135–S40.

TABLE 5.1. Indications for shoulder magnetic resonance imaging in sports medicine.

Shoulder instability
Rotator cuff pathology
Bursitis
Sequelae of different forms of impingement
Rotator interval disorders
Adhesive capsulitis
Biceps tendon pathology
Acromioclavicular (AC) joint abnormalities
Osteochondral injury
Occult fractures
Intraarticular bodies
Denervation

positioning, imaging planes, and pulse sequences. The use of direct and indirect magnetic resonance arthrography (MRA) will also be addressed.

Magnetic Field Strength

In general, as the magnetic field strength increases, there is a linear increase in the signal-to-noise ratio (SNR) and contrast-to-noise ratio (CNR). The increased SNR results in shorter acquisition times and thinner slice thickness. This reduces the risk of patient motion and increases spatial resolution. The increased CNR determines the extent to which adjacent structures can be distinguished from one another, as well as determining the general conspicuity of lesions on MRI studies. Clinical MRI is done on units ranging between 0.2 and 3 tesla (T). Low-field imaging tends to be below 0.5 T. Between 0.5 and 1.0 T there is midfield imaging. High-field imaging is above 1.0 T.

High-field imaging is preferred for shoulder imaging. Although one cannot use the extremity magnets for shoulder MRI, low-field imaging is also an option. Unfortunately, with low-field imaging there are significant limits in pulse sequences, SNR, and CNR. Since imaging time has an inverse relationship to field strength, low-field units take a significantly longer time for imaging, increasing the chance for motion artifact. Open MRI units that have a field strength between 0.2 and 1.0 T are an alternate option to the more confining high-field-strength closed-bore units for claustrophobic patients in place of antianxiety medication. The low-field magnet is also attractive from an economic standpoint, costing less to purchase and maintain, reducing the cost per imaging study. It demonstrates large labral and rotator cuff tears as well as bursitis and marrow edema, but more subtle abnormalities including small full-thickness or partial rotator cuff tears as well as labral tears are difficult to detect. For this reason, MRA may be useful for low-field MRI of the shoulder.

A prospective study comparing low-field- and high-field-strength imaging of rotator cuff and labral pathology suggested that diagnostic accuracy for small lesions of the rotator cuff and labrum encountered with low-field-strength studies was less than that of high-field-strength studies and could be enhanced by the addition of intraarticular injection of a gadolinium-based contrast material in conjunction with MRI.[1] The disadvantages of noncontrast low field shoulder MRI have been confirmed in several studies. One study prospectively evaluated a patient population with rotator cuff and labral pathology.[2] The study design included imaging at low field strength (0.2 T) and at high field strength (1.5 T) with arthroscopy as the gold standard in the same patient population. Contrary to other studies, these authors found that high-field-strength units allow more accurate interpretation than their low-field-strength counterparts, affecting clinical treatment. Earlier, two retrospective studies comparing diagnostic accuracy and sensitivity of low-field- versus high-field-strength systems found no significant difference in sensitivity, specificity, and accuracy for rotator cuff and labral lesions. These two studies were retrospective in nature and were performed in less ideal circumstances, comparing two different sets of patients, one imaged on a low-field-strength system, the other on a high-field-strength system.[3–5]

Coil Selection

It is important to image the glenohumeral joint with a dedicated shoulder coil. The choice of coil depends on the manufacturer and field strength of the magnet. Coils are available either from the manufacturer or a subcontractor. Challenges that affect shoulder MRI include inherent off-center magnet placement of this joint with reduction in the SNR and less homogeneous fat suppression.

Patient Positioning

Standard high-field-strength magnets offer limited alternatives for patient positioning when imaging the shoulder. The small-bore size and circumferential gantry of most closed systems necessitate that the shoulder be imaged with the patient in the supine position, with the arm extended along the side. Hand position may be neutral (thumb pointing upward) or externally rotated during imaging of the shoulder.[6–8] Internal rotation of the shoulder is not advocated for routine imaging since there is overlap between the supraspinatus and infraspinatus tendon.[9]

Additional provocative positions can aid in further evaluation of shoulder structures in certain situations, such as the abduction and external rotation (ABER), adduction internal rotation (ADIR), and traction positions. These maneuvers can be done after the rest of the study, preferably with MRA. The ABER position is used primarily during MRA to bring out subtle tears of the anteroinferior labrum, such as Perthes lesions. This position also opens the articular surface of the supraspinatus and infraspinatus tendons.[10,11] Patients with instability and suspected internal impingement can benefit from this assessment. The ABER position has the potential to demonstrate scapulohumeral imbalance and decentering of the humeral head relative to the glenoid fossa. Decentering can occur in traumatic or atraumatic instability as well as glenohumeral osteoarthritis. Subtle shoulder subluxation not demonstrated with the arm at the patient's side may be revealed in this position. To attain the ABER position, the palm of the hand is placed behind the head and neck of the supine patient. A coil is placed anteriorly over the region (Fig. 5.1). Coronal scout images demonstrate the humerus and glenoid. Cursors are drawn parallel to the long axis of the humerus (Fig. 5.2) to obtain oblique axial images of the glenohumeral joint (Fig. 5.3). More superior images are identified by the presence of the biceps tendon (Fig. 5.4). Below these images one will see the posterior superior labrum and mid-anterior labrum. The supraspinatus is seen demonstrated on the higher images. Inferiorly, further away from the biceps, the anterior inferior labrum and infraspinatus are identified (Fig. 5.5).

The newly described ADIR positioning is more limited in scope but can be used to evaluate anterior labroligamentous periosteal sleeve avulsion (ALPSA) lesions of the anterior inferior labrum.[12] In this position, the hand of the affected arm is placed behind the back (Fig. 5.6).

The diagnosis of SLAP lesions is improved with arm traction.[13] The wrist is pulled with a 3-kg nonferromagnetic weight that separates the torn labrum from the glenoid (Fig. 5.7).

Kinematic imaging is possible on a clinical MR unit. Internal and external rotation of the shoulder is used to assess anterior and posterior labral tears, respectively, and for assessment of subcoracoid impingement.[14–16] An open magnet allows for dynamic abduction external rotation of

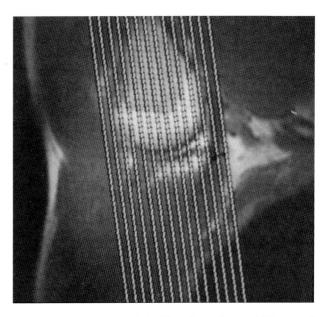

FIG. 5.2. An ABER scout. A localizer for oblique axial images for the ABER images represents a coronal scout of the area with cursors aligned along the long axis of the humerus. This results in oblique axial images of the glenohumeral joint.

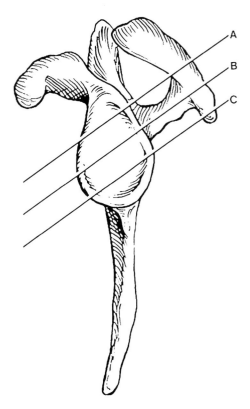

FIG. 5.3. ABER orientation. ABER positioning results in oblique axial images along the glenoid. A, the superior portion of the glenoid, near the biceps anchor and supraspinatus tendon. It also includes the posterosuperior labrum. B, the midportions of the anterior and posterior labrum and the junction between the supraspinatus and infraspinatus tendons. C, the anterior inferior portion of the glenoid and the infraspinatus and teres minor tendons. (From Steinbach et al.,[78] with permission.).

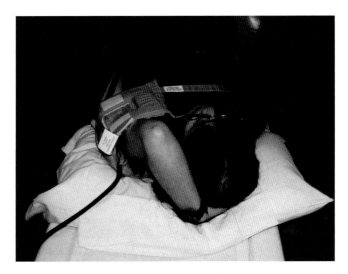

FIG. 5.1. Abduction and external rotation (ABER) positioning. The hand is placed behind the head of the supine patient. In this example, a flex coil is located anteriorly.

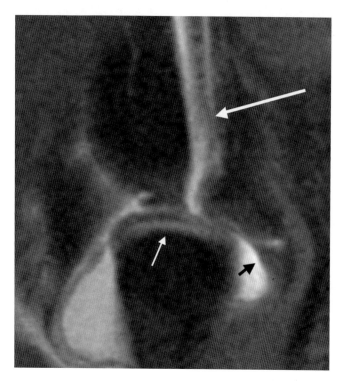

FIG. 5.4. Normal superior ABER MRI. ABER oblique axial image obtained in the superior portion of the glenoid labrum demonstrates the landmark biceps tendon (long white arrow), as well as the smooth undersurface of the supraspinatus tendon (black arrow) and superior glenoid cartilage and labrum (short white arrow).

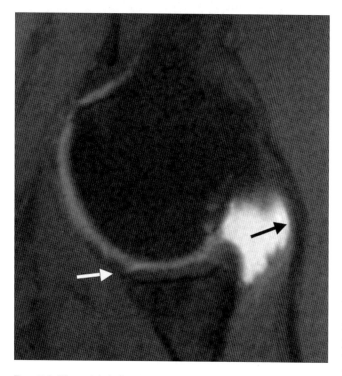

FIG. 5.5. Normal inferior ABER MRI. ABER oblique axial image obtained in the inferior portion of the glenoid labrum demonstrates that anterior inferior labrum being pulled by the inferior glenohumeral ligament (white arrow). The undersurface of the infraspinatus tendon is also visualized (black arrow).

the shoulder. The question remains as to the value of these additional sequences during clinical imaging time.[17,18]

Imaging Planes and Pulse Sequences

Many different MR pulse sequences have been used to evaluate the glenohumeral joint. Sequence protocols depend on the available MR equipment. Fat suppression, desirable for some musculoskeletal imaging to increase lesion conspicuity and to distinguish high signal intensity fluid or contrast from fat, is not always available on older and lower field equipment. Choice of pulse sequences include fast spin echo (FSE) (General Electric) sequences, with equivalent sequences on other scanners—fast low angle shot (FLASH) (Siemens), turbo spin echo (TSE) (Philips), with proton density (PD), and T2-weighted technique with or without fat suppression. The FSE images are typically obtained with a repetition time (TR) of 3000 to 5000 ms and an echo time (TE) of 30 to 50 ms. T1-weighted images, gradient echo sequences, and short-tau inversion recovery (STIR) imaging are classic spin echo sequences that were the original sequences used on MRI. They take more time and are mainly performed these days on lower field units that cannot handle the faster protocols. Spin echo sequences are generally obtained with a TR of 600 to 2000 ms and an TE of 25 to 80 ms. Each of these sequences has different strengths and weaknesses. Our routine noncontrast General Electric 1.5-T shoulder MR protocol is listed in Table 5.2.

Routine MRI of the shoulder is obtained in three orthogonal planes. The protocol begins in the axial plane with images extending from the top of the acromion through the inferior margin of the glenoid. Routinely, an axial FSE PD-weighted and fat-suppressed FSE T2-weighted sequence are both performed in this plane. It is important to include the acromion in patients over the age of 20 to assess for the presence of an os acromiale. The axial plane also allows for evaluation of the disk and cartilage of the acromioclavicular joint. The subscapularis, infraspinatus, and teres minor muscles and tendons are particularly well seen in this plane. The anterior and posterior labrum and glenohumeral ligaments can be seen on axial images, especially in the presence of an effusion or contrast. The hyaline cartilage along the glenoid and humeral head are also evaluated. If the patient has had previous surgery and it is not known which type, one might also include a gradient echo sequence to look for micrometallic foci that would lead to the surgical bed (700/15; flip angle, 40 degrees) (Fig. 5.8).

To prescribe the oblique coronal plane, cursors can be placed along the axis of the central supraspinatus tendon on the axial images. Alternatively, for the technologist who is not as informed about tendon anatomy, the scapular axis or a plane perpendicular to the glenoid surface can be used to define the oblique coronal plane. It is important to angle the coronal images along the oblique coronal axis, so that the rotator cuff muscles and tendons can be seen in continuity. Both T1- and T2-weighted FSE sequences in the oblique coronal plane are obtained from the region in front of the coracoid process through the posterior musculature. The oblique coronal plane

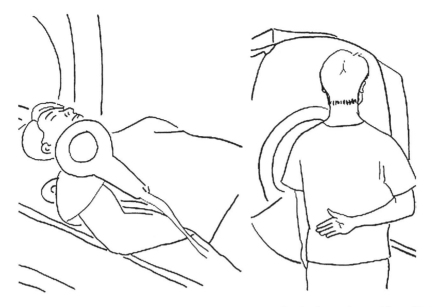

FIG. 5.6. Adduction internal rotation (ADIR) position is obtained by placing the patient in the supine position with the arm behind the back. A shoulder coil is placed in front of the region. (From Song et al.,[12] with permission.).

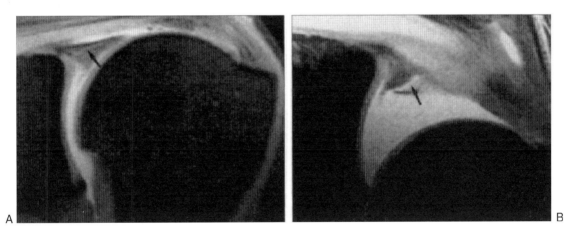

FIG. 5.7. Superior labrum anterior to posterior (SLAP) lesion with and without traction. Traction provides improved visualization of a SLAP lesion. (A) There is nonspecific intermediate signal intensity in the superior labrum (arrow) without traction. (B) An image obtained in the same labrum with traction demonstrates a definite tear with contrast entering the labrum (arrow). (From Chan et al.,[13] with permission.).

TABLE 5.2. Routine shoulder magnetic resonance protocol (General Electric 1.5 T).

Plane/sequence	TR	TE	ET	Flip
3-plane location				
1. Axial PD	2000	26	4	
2. Axial T2 FS	3000	50	8	
3. Cor T1 obl	600	20	4	
4. Cor T2 obl FS	3000	50	8	
5. Sag T2 obl FS	3000	50	8	
6. Sag PD obl	2000	26	4	
9. Axial MPGR (optional)	600	20		20

Cor, coronal; ET, _____; FS, fat suppression; MPGR, _____; obl, oblique; PD, proton density; Sag, sagittal; TE, echo time; TR, repetition time.
Field of view (FOV) = 12–16 cm
Slice thickness = 3–4 mm; no skip
NEX = 3
Matrix = 224 × 256 up to 512 × 512 for high resolution

is helpful for evaluation of the supraspinatus, infraspinatus, and teres minor muscles and tendons as well as the superior labrum, acromioclavicular joint, deltoid muscle, and SA-SD bursa. The bone marrow can be assessed using a combination of T1-weighting and fluid-sensitive sequences.

An oblique sagittal plane is then selected perpendicular to the oblique coronal images and parallel to the glenoid rim. The field of view should include the acromion, the entire humeral head, and the scapula. It is important to obtain this sequence with a fluid-sensitive sequence to further evaluate the rotator cuff muscles and tendons in cross section. I use both a proton density and fat-suppressed T2-weighted FSE sequence for this purpose. The muscles are well seen around the scapula more medially. Further out into the periphery, the cuff tendons predominate, forming a dark crescent over the humeral head.

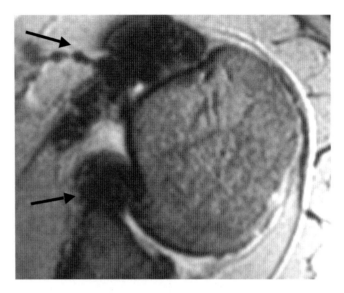

Fig. 5.8. Micrometallic foci from surgery appear as large low signal intensity dots in front of the biceps tendon and anterior labrum (arrows) on this axial gradient echo image.

An increase in signal intensity representing degeneration, inflammation, or a tear is appreciated on images obtained with this orientation. Rotator interval tears are also well seen in this plane. Oblique sagittal images also provide excellent visualization of the intraarticular biceps tendon, acromion, and SA-SD bursa.

When compared to spin echo imaging, FSE PD and T2-weighted images have the advantage of increased spatial resolution, improved SNR, and decreased imaging time.[19,20] The FSE sequences may be blurred, especially the PD sequences. This can be minimized by adjusting the echo train length of each FSE sequence to a particular MR unit.

Frequency-selective fat suppression differentiates fat from fluid when using the FSE fluid-sensitive sequences; however, the fat may not be completely saturated. This occurs because of the bulk susceptibility artifact/magnetic field inhomogeneity related to the curved external surface of the shoulder. When this happens, it is helpful to compare this sequence with the T1-weighted sequence, in which fat is routinely high signal intensity and fluid is low signal intensity. True fluid-like pathology presenting as high signal intensity on fat-suppressed FSE T2-weighted sequences would be low signal intensity on T1-weighted images. Alternatively, a fast or regular inversion recovery (STIR on General Electric units) sequence can be added that shows fluid signal intensity without relying on frequency selective fat saturation. A disadvantage of STIR is that it does not have as much signal to noise as FSE or spin echo sequences. It also does not cover as large an area as the other sequences.

Magnetic Resonance Arthrography

Although high-resolution nonenhanced MRI has been shown to have high accuracy rates for the demonstration of labral

tears,[21] direct MRA with intraarticular injection of a dilute gadolinium solution has gained popularity during the last decade because of its ability to distend the joint and outline labral and capsular structures as well as the undersurface of the rotator cuff.[22–26] Because it costs more than routine MRI and involves joint intervention and labor, we utilize MRA in certain situations where it will give us more information than the routine MRI. Indications are listed in Table 5.3.

For direct MRA, blind injection techniques without image guidance have been shown to frequently result in extraarticular injections.[27] Ultrasound-guided techniques can be used.[28] Most radiologists prefer to inject the glenohumeral joint with fluoroscopic guidance. Under sterile conditions, a 20- to 23-gauge 6-to 7-cm-long (spinal) needle is advanced into the middle to lower third of the glenohumeral joint along the medial humeral head (Fig. 5.9). Care is taken to avoid the joint space and glenoid to reduce the small risk of damaging the cartilage and labrum. A standard anterior approach is often utilized, although some institutions prefer to use the posterior approach

TABLE 5.3. Indications for magnetic resonance arthrography.

Under the age of 35 years
Shoulder instability
SLAP lesions
Joint bodies
Rotator interval pathology
Adhesive capsulitis
Postoperative shoulder
Solving question of partial- vs. full-thickness rotator cuff tear

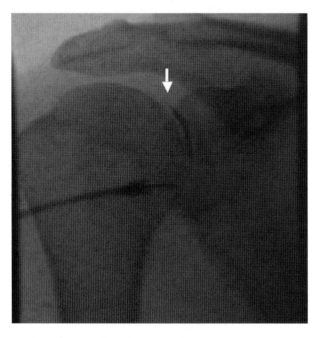

Fig. 5.9. Arthrogram injection under fluoroscopy. During an arthrogram, the needle is positioned at the junction of the middle and inferior third of the humeral head. Note iodinated contrast within the joint (arrow).

when evaluating the anterior labrocapsular structures.[29,30] This approach avoids injection into the subscapularis tendon, which can mimic a tear. Another fluoroscopic approach that has been recently described is through the rotator interval[31] (Fig. 5.10). This can be helpful in the obese patient since the distance to the humeral head is less than to the lower glenohumeral joint.

In most practices, injectate is composed of dilute gadolinium rather than pure saline. Dilute gadolinium has high signal intensity on T1-weighting, distinguishing it from low signal intensity joint fluid and other fluid-containing structures such as the SA-SD bursa and paralabral cysts. This allows for evaluation of communication between the glenohumeral joint and these other compartments and extracapsular tissues. Use of dilute gadolinium also shortens protocols by using T1-weighted fat-suppressed sequences, which have high signal-to-noise and contrast. Shoulder movement is less of a problem when the sequence is shorter. Up to 12 cc of a dilute gadolinium mixture is usually injected into the joint. I prefer to inject a small amount (2 cc) of iodinated contrast first to ensure intraarticular location of the needle tip before injecting a dilute gadolinium mixture with a ratio of 1:200 to 1:250 gadolinium to saline (approximately 2 mmol/L). Iodinated contrast can be substituted for some of the saline in this mixture if the user wants to see the contrast in the joint by fluoroscopy. Occasionally this can be helpful if the patient becomes claustrophobic in the MR scanner and the study is aborted. Additionally, being able to monitor the flow of contrast into the joint with iodinated contrast added to the mixture prevents extravasation of fluid from the joint during injection. The small amount of gadolinium used for the direct MRA injection is drawn from a larger commercially available

vial of gadolinium. This adds some cost to the procedure. One could potentially use the same bottle of gadolinium for up to 3 days if sterile techniques are used.[32] Epinephrine (1/1000) is added to this mixture in the amount of 0.3 cc/20 cc dilute contrast to avoid loss of injected contrast if there is a delay of over 1 1/2 hours.

Protocols for MR arthrography vary widely. A sample protocol is shown in Table 5.4. The rationale for this protocol is as follows: We obtain fat-suppressed T1-weighted axial, oblique-coronal and oblique sagittal sequences to evaluate the labral and capsular structures. Fat-suppressed FSE proton density or T2-weighted oblique-coronal and sagittal sequences are helpful for detecting rotator cuff tears that do not contact the articular surface, paralabral cysts, bursitis, cartilage, and marrow and muscle processes with long T2 relaxation times such as contusions and strains. A non–fat-suppressed T1-weighted oblique coronal sequence is also added so that fatty infiltration of muscles and marrow content can be assessed. Muscle quality is important for determining prognosis and treatment. Many centers also add an abduction external rotation oblique axial fat-suppressed T1-weighted sequence at the end of the study if the patient is able tolerate this position. As mentioned previously, this provocative maneuver pulls on the anterior-inferior glenohumeral ligament and labrum, enabling detection of anterior-inferior labral avulsions and tears as well as subtle undersurface tears of the rotator cuff.[10] Also noted previously in this chapter is the newly described provocative position of the glenohumeral joint in internal rotation, the ADIR position. This has been advocated as a way to best evaluate anterior labroligamentous periosteal sleeve avulsion (ALPSA) lesions of the anterior inferior labrum.[12]

Complications of direct MR arthrography are rare. They include infection, bleeding, allergy, and postprocedural pain. Gadolinium is an uncommon allergen, although mild to severe reactions have been reported. A known allergy to iodinated contrast or anesthetic requires premedication or removal of the substance from the injection. Vasovagal reactions and

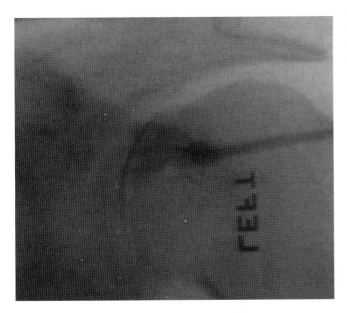

FIG. 5.10. Rotator interval injection under fluoroscopy. For an arthrogram injected through the rotator interval, the needle is placed along the superomedial aspect of the humeral head.

TABLE 5.4. Shoulder magnetic resonance arthrography Protocol (General Electric 1.5 T).

Plane/sequence	TR	TE	ET
3-plane location			
1. Axial T1	600	20	4
2. Cor T1 Obl	600	20	4
3. Cor T2 Obl	3000	50	8
4. Sag T2 Obl	3000	50	8
5. Axial T2	3000	50	8
6. Cor obl T1	600	20	4
7. ABER T1	600	20	3

ABER, abduction and external rotation.
FOV = 12–14
Slice thickness = 3–4 mm; no skip
NEX = 3
Matrix = 224 × 256 up to 512

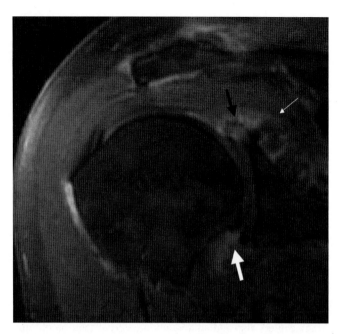

FIG. 5.11. Indirect MR arthrogram. On this fat-suppressed T1–weighted indirect MR arthrographic image, high signal intensity intravenous gadolinium extends into the glenohumeral joint (thick white arrow) and into a SLAP lesion (black arrow) with extension around a multiloculated paralabral cyst (thin white arrow).

nausea are sometimes present during intraarticular injections, while infection and bleeding are unusual.[33] Joint pain is often encountered a few hours after the procedure and may last for up to 72 hours, It is most likely related to injected contrast and joint distention.[34]

Some centers are using intravenous (indirect) MRA to evaluate the shoulder for instability.[25,35,36] A standard intravenous injection of gadolinium is injected approximately 10 to 20 minutes prior to the MR examination followed by imaging with a protocol identical to that of the direct MRA (Fig. 5.11). This technique does not require fluoroscopy or intraarticular injection, thus increasing patient acceptance. The gadolinium outlines the labrum and undersurface of the tendons. A major disadvantage of this technique is a lack of joint distention if there is no preexisting effusion. It is also more difficult to be certain about the significance of sites of contrast enhancement since intravenous contrast flows to vascularized tissues, including the subacromial subdeltoid bursa, labral base, and degenerated or vascularized portions of the tendons of the rotator cuff.

Shoulder Instability

The most unstable joint in the body, the glenohumeral joint is subject to subluxation and dislocations. During the last decade, MRI has enabled direct visualization of many of the lesions related to instability, aiding in diagnosis as well as therapeutic planning and follow-up.

Shoulder Anatomy Related to Instability

Currently the entire capsular mechanism is believed to be important in the development of instability. The most important of these structures are the glenoid labrum, the fibrous capsule, the glenohumeral ligaments, the rotator cuff tendons, and the coracoacromial arch. The anterior complex includes the supraspinatus muscle and tendon, subscapularis muscle and tendon, rotator interval between the supraspinatus and subscapularis, anterior capsule, glenohumeral ligaments, synovial membrane, and the anterior labrum and osseous glenoid. The posterior complex includes the infraspinatus muscle and tendon, teres minor muscle and tendon, posterior capsule, synovial membrane, posterior labrum, and osseous glenoid.

Normal Labrum and Anatomic Variants

The fibrous connective tissue labrum is an important structure that stabilizes the shoulder joint. It deepens the shallow glenoid fossa, increasing the contact area for the humeral head. The intact labrum also acts as a pressure seal, allowing negative pressure to occur within the shoulder joint during motion, aiding in the dynamic stabilization of the joint. In addition, the labrum serves as an anchor for some of the glenohumeral ligaments as well as the long head of the biceps tendon.

The usually low signal intensity labrum lies on hyaline articular cartilage that is of intermediate signal intensity on T1- and T2-weighted MRI (Fig. 5.12). The cartilage demonstrates intermediate signal intensity on FSE images and increased signal on gradient echo images obtained with a flip angle of 30 degrees or less. The hyaline cartilage can be

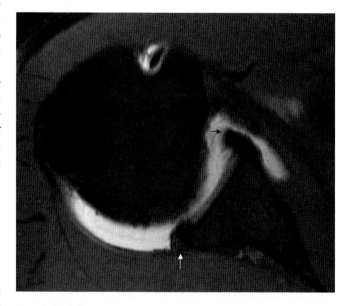

FIG. 5.12. Normal anterior and posterior labra. The normal anterior (black arrow) and posterior labra (white arrow) are low signal triangular structures attached to the intermediate signal intensity hyaline cartilage on this fat-suppressed T1-weighted magnetic resonance arthrogram (MRA).

deficient either at or near the center of the ovoid glenoid fossa, a region referred to as the bare area.[37] The labrum can be triangular or round, as well as anteriorly cleaved, notched, or even absent in asymptomatic individuals.[38,39]

Absence of the anterosuperior labrum may be congenital, and this has been termed the Buford complex. This variant of normal seen in 1% to 2% of shoulder arthroscopies and is associated with a "cord-like" middle glenohumeral ligament[40–42] (Fig. 5.13). Another labral variant seen in 11% to 15% of shoulders in the anterosuperior region of the glenoid labrum is the sublabral foramen.[40] This foramen or hole is seen at the base of the anterosuperior labrum and is associated with a "cord-like" middle glenohumeral ligament in 75% of cases[40] (Fig. 5.14). One should not mistake the cord-like middle glenohumeral ligament for a labral detachment. Although not common, both the Buford complex and the sublabral foramen can extend into the anterior inferior portion of the labrum.[43] In addition, it is interesting to note that a sublabral foramen is usually accompanied by a sublabral recess in the superior labrum.

The sublabral recess is a normal recess that can exist between the superior labrum and the glenoid articular cartilage.[44–46] This anatomic variant is smooth, 1 to 2 mm in width, and does not extend to the top of the labrum (Fig. 5.15). It is not associated with a paralabral cyst, as are some superior labral tears. Although many have written that this recess does not extend posterior to the long head of the biceps attachment to the superior labrum,[47] it has been our experience and that of others that this recess can do so in the absence of a tear.[48]

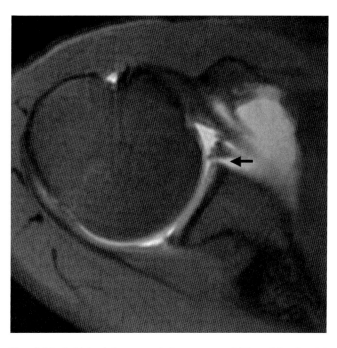

FIG. 5.14. Sublabral foramen. A fat-suppressed T1-weighted axial image from an MR arthrogram shows that the anterior superior labrum is separated from the glenoid by a normal variant termed a sublabral foramen (arrow).

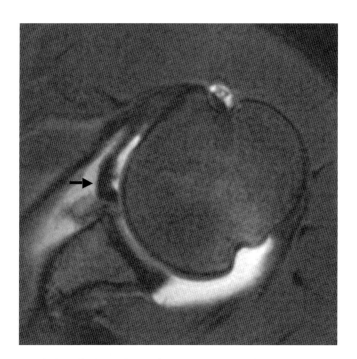

FIG. 5.13. Buford complex. A fat-suppressed T1-weighted axial image from an MRA shows that the anterior-superior labrum is absent, consistent with a normal variant termed the Buford complex. This is associated with a cord-like middle glenohumeral ligament (arrow).

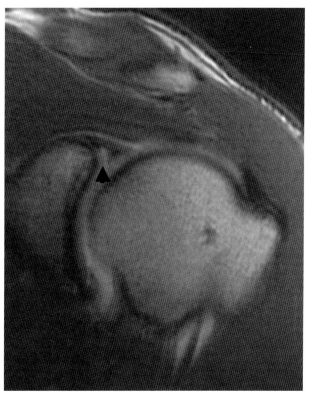

FIG. 5.15. Sublabral recess. A T1-weighted coronal image from an MRA shows a recess at the base of the superior labrum consistent with a normal variant (arrowhead).

Glenohumeral Ligaments

The superior, middle, and inferior glenohumeral ligaments are infoldings of the capsule that provide shoulder stability. The superior glenohumeral ligament (SGHL) originates at the superior glenoid tubercle anterior to the insertion of the long head of the biceps tendon and inserts into the fovea capitis line just superior to the lesser tuberosity of the humerus. It is best seen on axial images obtained directly beneath or adjacent to the origin of the long head of the biceps tendon. The SGHL lies just medial and parallel to the coracoid and is located in the rotator interval, just underneath the extraarticular coracohumeral ligament (CHL) (Fig. 5.16). The SGHL and CHL together form a sling around the intraarticular portion of the biceps tendon in the rotator interval.

The middle glenohumeral ligament (MGHL) has a variable origin from the glenoid, scapula, anterior labrum, biceps tendon, inferior glenohumeral ligament, or superior glenohumeral ligament.[49] It attaches to the anterior aspect of the proximal humerus just below the attachment of the SGHL. It can be absent in up to 27% of individuals.[49,50] Absence of this ligament is not associated with increased incidence of instability, but the subscapularis recess may be enlarged and the inferior glenohumeral ligament usually originates more superiorly than when the MGHL is absent. The MGHL merges with the subscapularis tendon as it inserts on the lesser tuberosity of the humerus. This ligament is usually seen en face on axial images as it takes an oblique course from the glenoid to the subscapularis tendon (Fig. 5.17). It lies in a linear fashion in front of the glenoid on oblique sagittal images (Fig. 5.18). Occasionally this ligament can be duplicated, simulating a longitudinal tear and cleavage.

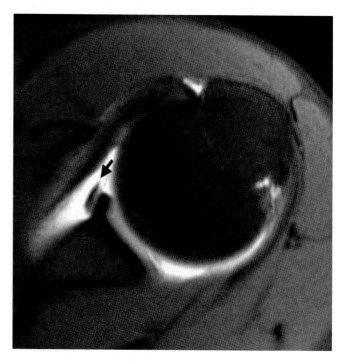

FIG. 5.17. Normal middle glenohumeral ligament axial view. The middle glenohumeral ligament (MGHL) is seen in front of the anterior labrum (arrow) on this axial fat-suppressed T1-weighted image from an MRA.

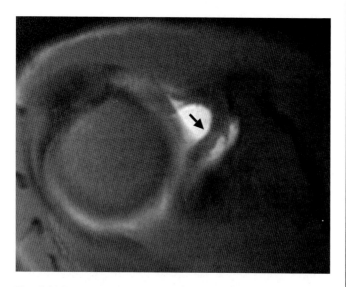

FIG. 5.16. Normal superior glenohumeral ligament. A fat-suppressed T1-weighted axial image from an MRA demonstrates a normal superior glenohumeral ligament (SGHL) parallel and mesial to the coracoid process (arrow).

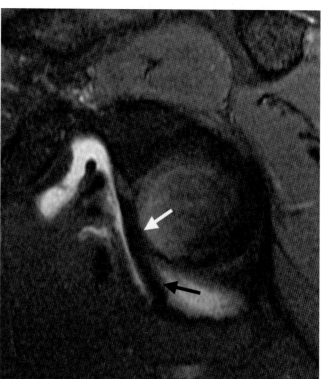

FIG. 5.18. Normal MGHL sagittal view. A fat-suppressed T1-weighted sagittal image from an MRA shows a normal linear MGHL anterior to the glenoid (arrows).

The inferior glenohumeral ligament (IGHL), considered the most important stabilizer of the glenohumeral joint, is a complex that originates at the middle to inferior portion of the anterior glenoid labrum. It drapes for a variable distance from anterior to posterior and inserts on the anatomic neck of the humerus (see Fig. 5.19, below). This ligament is inseparable from the labrum, forming a labroligamentous complex. It is composed of strong collagenous thickenings at its anterior and posterior margins—the anterior and posterior bands, joined by a fibrous thickening of the capsule called the axillary pouch or recess (Fig. 5.19). The IGHL functions as a sling to support the humeral head and prevents abnormal anterior and posterior instability. It reinforces the anterior capsule between the subscapularis muscle and the inferior aspect of the glenoid at or near the origin of the long head of the triceps.

The glenohumeral ligaments are best assessed in the presence of capsular distention, which is produced if there is a large amount of joint fluid or contrast in the shoulder joint.[46,49,51,52] The addition of ABER or ADIR postioning optimizes visualization of portions of the labroligamentous complex including the anterior labrum and inferior glenohumeral ligament.[8,10,12]

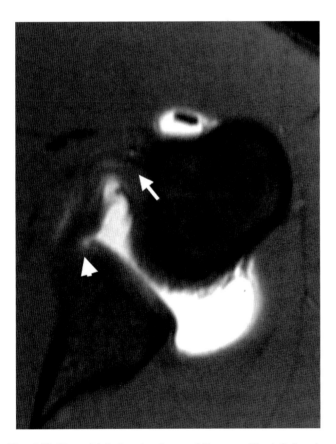

FIG. 5.19. Normal inferior glenohumeral ligament. The inferior glenohumeral ligament (IGHL) spans from the anterior inferior labrum (arrowhead) to the anatomic neck of the humerus (arrow) on this image from a fat-suppressed axial T1-weighted MRA.

Labral Tears Associated with Anterior Glenohumeral Instability

Tears of the labrum are common in athletes with instability, especially in sports that require forceful and repetitive abduction and overhead rotation of the humerus. Arthro–computed tomography (Artho-CT) and MRI have been utilized to evaluate the capsular and labral structures.[53–56] Due to limited soft tissue contrast, arthro-CT is too weak for evaluation of internal characteristics of tissues including tendon degeneration; intrasubstance tears of the tendons, ligaments, and fibrocartilage; and bone marrow pathology. These days, arthro-CT is usually reserved for patients who cannot undergo MRI due to contraindications such as the presence of a cardiac pacemaker. Some countries that do not have much access to MRI also still rely on arthro-CT for this assessment.

Studies using conventional (unenhanced) MRI in the evaluation of glenohumeral instability have produced mixed results in the detection of labral tears, with sensitivities and specificities ranging from 44% to 100% and 66% to 95%, respectively.[21,57–61] Magnetic resonance arthrography has generally produced sensitivies of 86% to 91% and specificities of 86% to 98%.[24,56,62] Although controversial and related to circumstance, many believe that labral tears are best evaluated when there is a joint effusion or with MRA.[22,52,63] High-resolution MRI can also be of value for evaluating the labrum when MRA is not available.[60]

It is best to use morphologic criteria such as absence, fraying, detachment, displacement, or deformity to identify labral tears. Fluid or contrast within the labral substance (if not one of the described normal variants) is also a good indication of a labral tear. Labral tears occasionally present on MRI as a focal or diffuse increase in signal intensity extending to the surface on all imaging sequences, but this is less reliable. Variations have been seen in signal intensity in the labra using multiplanar gradient echo sequences. We have found that some of this may be attributable to the magic angle phenomenon, which occurs on spin echo and gradient echo images when the labrum lies approximately 55 degrees to the main magnetic field on images obtained with a short TE. The transitional zone between the labrum and the articular cartilage may have areas of intermediate signal intensity beneath the labrum.[64] Fibrovascular tissue, eosinophilic or mucoid degeneration, synovialization, calcification, ossification, or combinations of these tissue types can lead to alterations in signal intensity of the labrum.[64]

Labrocapsular Lesions Associated with Anterior Glenohumeral Instability

The anterior inferior labrum is the most frequently affected site of labral pathology related to instability. Injury to the anterior inferior labrum may demonstrate findings mentioned above for routine tears of the labrum but often reach predictable patterns in the form of a Bankart, ALPSA, or Perthes lesion. Sometimes one may see that these lesions change with time. For example, a Perthes lesion may turn into a Bankart or ALPSA lesion.

The most common lesion resulting from an anterior dislocation is the Bankart lesion. This represents an avulsion of the labrum from the glenoid rim. The avulsed labrum is not attached to the scapular periosteum (Fig. 5.20). The labrum may be hemorrhagic, fragmented, or pulled away from the glenoid.

Neviaser[65] described a variant of the Bankart lesion known as the ALPSA lesion. It represents an avulsion of the inferior glenohumeral ligament complex from the anteroinferior glenoid with an intact periosteum. The avulsed anteroinferior labrum displaces medially and rotates inferiorly along the denuded anterior scapular neck (Fig. 5.21). These lesions eventually heal in this medially displaced position, leading to recurrent anterior instability because of persistent incompetence of the inferior glenohumeral ligament labral complex.

The third variant in this location is termed the Perthes lesion, named after a German physician who described it in the early 1900s.[66] This lesion is an avulsion of the anterior-inferior labrum with an intact scapular periosteum. The Perthes lesion is well visualized with abduction and external rotation of the shoulder (Figs. 5.22 and 5.23).

Avulsion of the inferior glenohumeral ligament complex from the humerus has also been described, and is termed a humeral avulsion of the glenohumeral ligament (HAGL) lesion.[67,68] This latter injury is occasionally associated with a tear of the subscapularis tendon and recurrent anterior instability.[69] The HAGL lesion typically results from a first-time

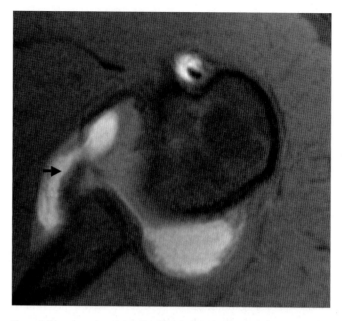

FIG. 5.21. Anterior labroligamentous periosteal sleeve avulsion (ALPSA) lesion. The anterior inferior labrum is medially displaced with respect to the glenoid (arrow) and attached to the scapular periosteum on this axial fat-suppressed T1-weighted image from an MRA.

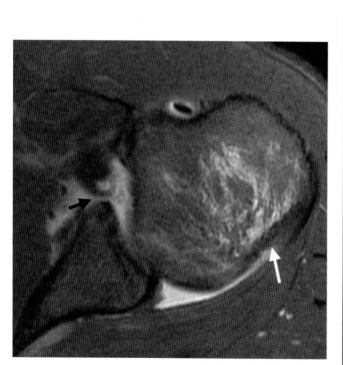

FIG. 5.20. Bankart lesion. An axial T2-weighted MRI demonstrates a Bankart lesion with the labrum separated from the glenoid (black arrow) as well as a Hill-Sachs lesion along the posterior humeral head (white arrow).

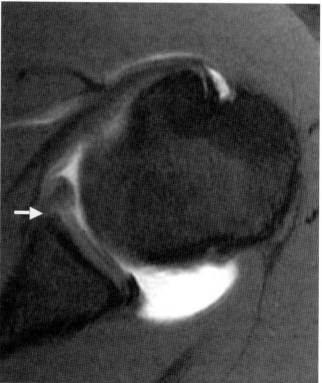

FIG. 5.22. Perthes lesion hidden on MRA. The anterior-inferior labrum appears intact on this axial fat-suppressed T1-weighted image from an MRA (arrow).

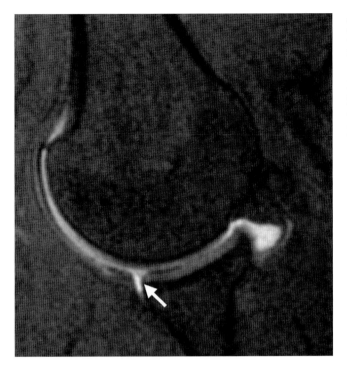

FIG. 5.23. Perthes lesion (from Fig. 5.22) visualized with ABER positioning. Upon abduction and external rotation of the shoulder, the labrum in Figure 5.22 demonstrates a defect at the base on a fat-suppressed T1-weighted image (arrow). There is still labral attachment to scapular periosteum. These findings are consistent with a Perthes lesion.

dislocation in persons older than 35 years of age.[68] The HAGL lesion is seen on axial images as a disruption at the humeral neck attachment. On coronal MRI, the normal U-shape of the anterior band of the IGHL looks like a J-shape when the ligament is disrupted (Fig. 5.24). Sometimes a patient can avulse a bony fragment along with the inferior glenohumeral ligament from the humeral attachment. This bony HAGL injury is termed a BHAGL lesion.[70] When the inferior glenohumeral ligament is avulsed at the humeral and labral attachments, it is called a floating anterior-inferior glenohumeral ligament (AIGHL).[71] Occasionally the inferior glenohumeral ligament can tear in midportion and not at either attachment. It has been noted that one can have an avulsion of the inferior glenohumeral ligament at the glenoid attachment without tearing the anterior-inferior labrum. This is known as the anterior ligamentous inferior periosteal sleeve avulsion (ALIPSA) lesion.

Although not related to instability, a glenolabral articular disruption (GLAD) is a superficial tear of the anteroinferior labrum that is accompanied by fibrillation and erosion of the adjacent articular cartilage[72,73] (Fig. 5.25). It results from a forced adduction injury to the shoulder with the arm in abduction and external rotation. The GLAD lesion can progress to rapid degenerative joint disease and loose bodies.

Posterior Glenohumeral Instability

Posterior labral and capsular tears are less common than anterior ones and are usually seen in association with posterior or multidirectional instability. Similar to the anterior labral tears, posterior tears present with absence, morphologic distortion, or contrast or fluid extending into the substance of the labrum.

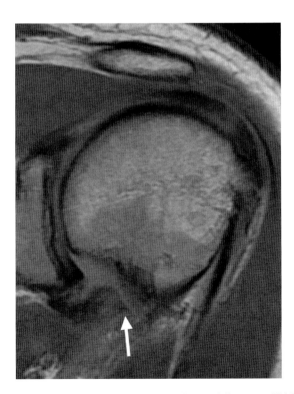

FIG. 5.24. Humeral avulsion of the glenohumeral ligament (HAGL) lesion. A coronal T1-weighted MR image from an arthrogram reveals avulsion of the inferior glenohumeral ligament (IGHL) from the humeral attachment (arrow).

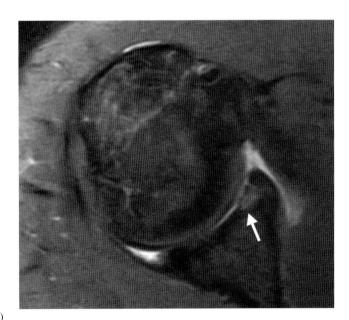

FIG. 5.25. Glenolabral articular disruption (GLAD) lesion. A cartilage defect is seen at the base of the torn anterior labrum on this fat-suppressed axial T2-weighted MRI (arrow).

A particular type of posterior labral tear is the posterior labro-capsular periosteal sleeve avulsion (POLPSA) injury.[74,75] This lesion is an avulsion of the attachment of the posterior capsule and the periosteum, resulting in a patulous recess posteriorly (Fig. 5.26). It may represent an acute Bennett lesion. The Bennett lesion is an extraarticular posterior capsule avulsive injury caused by traction of the inferior glenohumeral ligament during the deceleration phase of pitching.[76,77] It usually occurs in patients with overhead-overuse activity. This lesion is associated with posterior labral injury and posterior under-surface type 1 and 2 tears of the rotator cuff. The patient may develop crescentic mineralization adjacent to the posterior-inferior osseous glenoid and sclerosis of the posterior glenoid (Fig. 5.27). The mineralization may occasionally be identified on MRI but is better seen on axillary radiographs and CT.

A posterior HAGL lesion can also be seen following posterior dislocation.[78,79] This is often caused by a posteriorly directed force on an abducted shoulder. It may also be related to microinstability. Bony avulsion of the inferior glenohumeral ligament is termed the posterior BHAGL lesion. Fluid may be seen between the infraspinatus muscle and the scapula, suggesting a capsular tear.

Additional Abnormalities Associated with Instability

The rotator cuff tendons may also be affected by instability through a secondary extrinsic impingement mechanism, so it is important to evaluate them carefully in these patients. The anteriorly unstable humeral head produces narrowing of the coracoacromial outlet, leading to rotator cuff pathology. This mimics primary impingement and should be evaluated, particularly in the younger patient (adolescent and young adult) who is more likely to have instability rather than impingement.

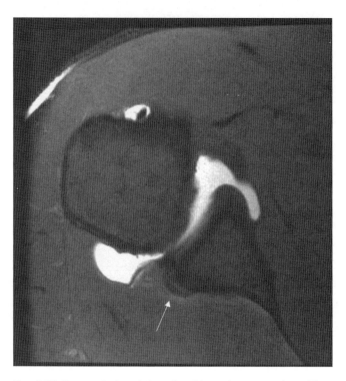

FIG. 5.27. Bennett lesion. A low signal intensity crescentic ossification lies posterior to the glenoid on this fat-suppressed T1-weighted image from an MRA (arrow).

Tears of the subscapularis tendons are often associated with anterior or posterior dislocation. Tears of the teres minor and infraspinatus tendons can be seen more frequently with posterior dislocation.[80]

Other abnormalities that can be seen with instability include subluxation or dislocation of the humeral head and compression fractures of the humeral head. Subluxation or dislocation are well demonstrated on axial MRI. Provocative maneuvers such as the abduction external rotation postioning of the shoulder have the potential to bring out subtle subluxation. Osseous lesions including the Hill-Sachs lesion of the humeral head and the Bankart lesion of the anterior-inferior glenoid rim may be better seen on MRI than on conventional radiographs.[81] The Hill-Sachs lesion manifests as a depression along the postero-lateral aspect of the humeral head superiorly in the top 2 cm usually above the level of the coracoid (Fig. 5.28). It is seen in approximately 75% of patients with anterior instability. On MRI, there often is abnormal signal intensity within the marrow indicative of acute trauma (contusion) that will not be detected by CT. In Workman et al.'s[81] series, MRI was 97% sensitive, 91% specific, and 94% accurate for detecting Hill-Sachs lesions. It was also found to be superior to arthroscopy in detecting Hill-Sachs lesions. One must be careful not to overcall a Hill-Sachs lesion when there are cysts or erosions in the same area. Symptomatic cystic change in this area has been seen at the infraspinatus attachment in pitchers. Many other patients have asymptomatic cysts or vessels in this location.[82] Also there is a normal anatomic groove located

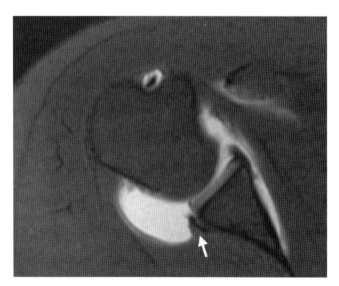

FIG. 5.26. Posterior labrocapsular periosteal sleeve avulsion (POLPSA) lesion. There is a periosteal sleeve avulsion of the posterior labrum on this fat-suppressed axial T1-weighted MRA (arrow).

posterolaterally on the humeral head that should not be confused with a Hill-Sachs lesion.[83] This groove can be distinguished from the Hill-Sachs lesion by its location along the long axis of the humerus. It usually lies at least 20mm distal to the top of the humeral head, while the Hill-Sachs lesion is usually located in the first 18mm of the proximal humeral head. The lesion related to posterior superior glenoid impingement (PSGI) may be difficult to distinguish from a Hill-Sachs lesion. This syndrome is often described in truck drivers and throwing athletes as well as others who repeatedly place the shoulder in abduction and external rotation.[84–87] This position causes anterior subluxation of the humerus with impingement of the humeral head against the posterosuperior labrum, resulting in posterosuperior labral damage as well as a defect in the humeral head that may be similar to a Hill-Sachs lesion. There is often associated disruption of the inferior aspect of the supraspinatus and infraspinatus tendons. The history of an absence of prior dislocation and associated abnormalities discussed in the last section can aid in distinction between the Hill-Sachs lesion and the PSGI lesion on the humeral head.

An osseous Bankart lesion is well seen on CT as a small fragment of bone associated with irregularity of the adjacent glenoid rim. On MRI, low signal cortical fragments or glenoid deficiency are seen in all planes, but particularly on axial images (Fig. 5.28). Very small osseous Bankart lesions may be missed on MRI.

The osseous lesions associated with posterior instability carry the familiar eponyms associated with anterior instability except that the word *reverse* is added to them. A reverse Bankart lesion refers to an impaction fracture of the posterior glenoid resulting from a posteriorly dislocated humerus (Fig. 5.29). A reverse Hill-Sachs lesion results from an impaction fracture of the anterosuperior humerus (Fig. 5.30). A deficiency of the posterior glenoid rim has also been linked with posterior instability.[88] Avulsion of the lesser tuberosity may also occur with posterior instability.

A unique subset of shoulder ganglion cysts has been described that rise from glenoid labral tears.[89] The mechanism for formation of these paralabral cysts is similar to a meniscal cyst with extrusion of joint fluid through labrocapsular tears into adjacent tissue planes. The most common locations for the labral cyst/tear complex are posterior (associated with a posterosuperior labral tear) (Fig. 5.31) and superior (associated with a SLAP lesion). Extraarticular extension of the labral cyst into the spinoglenoid notch or suprascapular notch is common. Intraosseous extension can also occur in the bony glenoid. When located adjacent to SLAP or posterior labral lesions, these cysts can produce suprascapular nerve entrapment, which is a cause of shoulder pain that can be evaluated with MRI.[90] In addition, cysts associated with inferior labral tears can produce axillary nerve compression in the quadrilateral space.[91] Anterior dislocation of the glenohumeral joint may also damage the axillary nerve or its branches. In one

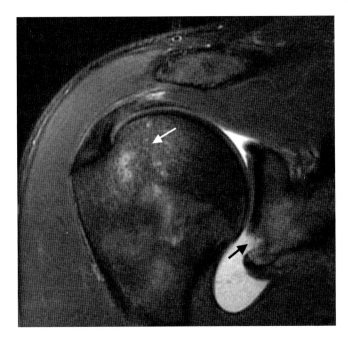

FIG. 5.28. Osseous Hill-Sachs and Bankart lesions following anterior shoulder dislocation. Edema is present in the posterior-superior humeral head consistent with a Hill-Sachs lesion (white arrow). A glenoid fracture is present anteroinferiorly (black arrow) on this fat-suppressed coronal T2-weighted image from an MRA.

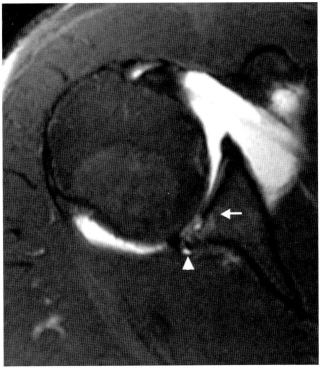

FIG. 5.29. Reverse Bankart lesion. A fat-suppressed T2-weighted axial MRI displays high signal intensity within the glenoid and overlying cartilage consistent with a compression fracture (arrow) in a patient with multidirectional instability. A small paralabral cyst extends from a posterior labral tear (arrowhead). The humeral head is also posteriorly subluxed.

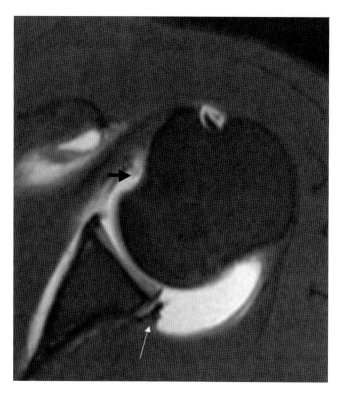

Fig. 5.30. Reverse Hill-Sachs lesion. The concavity in the anterior humeral head represents a compression fracture (black arrow) on this fat-suppressed axial T1-weighted image from an MR arthrogram. Notice the POLPSA lesion posteriorly (white arrow).

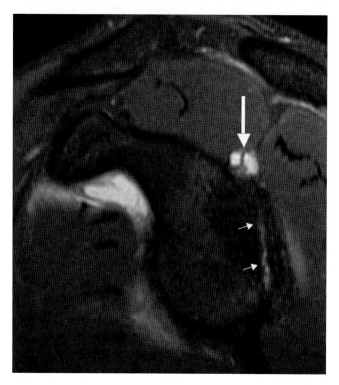

Fig. 5.31. Paralabral cyst. A multiloculated cyst (large arrow) lies just above an extensive posterior labral tear (small arrows) on this fat-suppressed sagittal T2-weighted MRI.

series, 43% of patients with anterior shoulder dislocation developed axillary nerve damage.[92]

Lesions of the rotator interval have also been implicated in posterior and inferior instability of the glenohumeral joint. Stretching or interruption of the capsule of the rotator interval produces increased anterior translation of the humeral head at 60 degrees of flexion. Damage to this region is most commonly associated with enlargement or tearing from a shoulder dislocation; however, some individuals with abnormalities in the rotator interval do not have glenohumeral instability.[93]

Superior Labrum and Biceps Tendon

The long head of the biceps tendon originates through and is continuous with the superior labrum. A superior labral tear with anterior and posterior components of the tear relative to the origin of the long head of the biceps is called a superior labrum from anterior to posterior (SLAP) lesion.[94,95] Identification and classification of SLAP lesions by CT and MRI can be challenging. These lesions can be seen by CT arthrography,[96] but they are best seen on MRI and especially MRA, due to improved soft tissue contrast (see Fig. 5.7, above). Magnetic resonance imaging has demonstrated sensitivity of 41% to 98%, specificity of 86% to 100%, and accuracy of 63% to 95% in detection of SLAP lesions. This compares with MRA, which has been shown to achieve 89% to 100% sensitivity, 69% to 91% specificity, and 74% to 92% accuracy.[56,63,97]

One can evaluate the superior labrum and biceps tendon in all three planes, with the tear most easily characterized in the oblique-coronal and axial planes (Fig. 5.32). The SLAP lesions are best demonstrated on MRI with the shoulder in external rotation, which provides traction on the long head of the biceps, enhancing the detection of imbibition of contrast, posterior and superior extent of the tear, and separation at the site of the tear. The diagnosis of SLAP lesions is also improved with arm traction.[13] The wrist is pulled with a 3-kg nonferromagnetic weight.

It is difficult sometimes to completely characterize the lesions according to the various subtypes using MRI. The main function of the MRI is to identify the lesions of the superior labrum and biceps tendon. One should also look for SLAP lesions when imaging in the abduction external rotation (ABER) position. This provocative position may enhance evaluation of the SLAP lesion by causing fluid to be further pushed into the superior labrum.

The SLAP lesions can also be associated with paralabral cysts. At times, these cysts may be the red flag that alerts the radiologist to the underlying labral tear. They often lie medial to the tear in the suprascapular notch and can produce entrapment of the suprascapular nerve, which courses through this region. Associated denervation changes may be identified in the supraspinatus or infraspinatus muscles.

Fifteen percent to 25% of SLAP lesions are associated with a full- or partial-thickness tear of the rotator cuff,

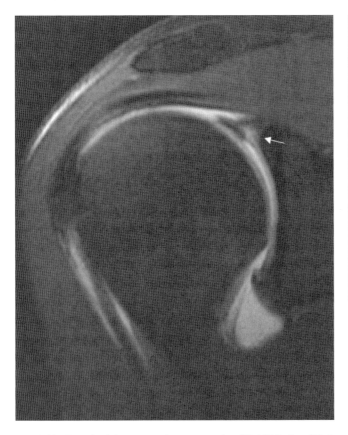

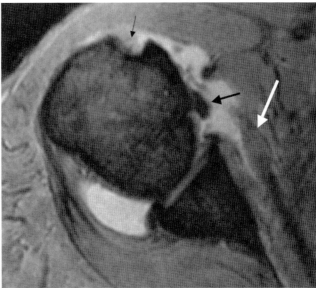

FIG. 5.33. Biceps dislocation with subscapularis tendon tear. There is medial dislocation of the biceps tendon (large black arrow) associated with a complete tear of the subscapularis tendon (white arrow) on this axial gradient echo MRI. Note the empty bicipital groove (small black arrow).

FIG. 5.32. Superior labrum anterior to posterior (SLAP) lesion. High signal intensity gadolinium extends into the superior labrum (arrow) consistent with a tear on this coronal fat-suppressed T1-weighted image from an MRA.

anterosuperior impingement, anterior instability, humeral head fracture, chondromalacia of the humeral head, and acromioclavicular (AC) joint arthritis.[98] It is especially important to remember to carefully scrutinize the superior labrum and biceps tendon in these situations.

Labral fraying and irregularity can be seen in asymptomatic shoulders, often in patients of older age.[45] This appearance can simulate a type I or II SLAP lesion. It is crucial to keep this in mind and to correlate symptoms with the appearance on MRI.

It can be difficult to distinguish a SLAP lesion from the sublabral recess, the normal variant involving the superior labrum that was described previously in this chapter. A type II SLAP lesion may simulate a sublabral recess, which is located anterior and inferior to the biceps tendon insertion of the superior glenoid tubercle and has been seen in 19 of 26 (73%) cadaver shoulders in one study.[45] Contrast material or fluid accumulates in this area. This normal variant is smoothly marginated, usually symmetric, and lacks imbibition of contrast into the superior labrum. It usually does not extend posterior to the long head of the biceps, but this is not a hard-and-fast rule. The sublabral recess is distinguishable from a type III SLAP lesion where fluid signal intensity extends into the substance of the superior labrum, resembling a bucket-handle tear of the knee.

The sublabral recess and the Buford complex are frequently associated with a cord-like middle glenohumeral ligament, which should further distinguish them from a SLAP lesion.

The long head of the biceps tendon extends from the supraglenoid tubercle through the glenohumeral joint and into the bicipital groove. As with all tendons, this tendon can undergo tendinosis, and partial- and full-thickness tears anywhere along its course. As described above, tears at the origin are common with SLAP lesions. Biceps long head subluxation or dislocation in the region of the rotator interval and biceps groove occurs with injury to the soft tissue restraints including the supraspinatus tendon, rotator interval, and the superior subscapularis tendon (Fig. 5.33). Normal variants of the biceps tendon include congenital absence, duplication, and mesenteric attachment. The intraarticular biceps tendon is viewed in all three planes. Sagittal images show the tendon in cross section and is best for showing tendinosis and partial tears. Axial images are helpful for evaluating the origin of the long head of the biceps and its relationship to a sublabral recess or SLAP lesion. Axial images also demonstrate biceps tendon subluxation and dislocation as well as tears in the region of the bicipital groove.

Rotator Cuff

The rotator cuff complex is composed of the supraspinatus, infraspinatus, teres minor, and subscapularis tendons and muscles, along with the capsular covering between the supraspinatus and subscapularis known as the rotator interval.

Rotator cuff tears are more common in association with aging and impingement. Microtrauma and instability can also be associated with rotator cuff tear. Although less common, occult greater tuberosity fractures and complete subscapularis tendon tears are seen on MRI following traumatic injury.

Rotator cuff disease may include tendinosis and partial- and full-thickness tears. Magnetic resonance imaging characterizes the degree of tendon pathology and displays tendon retraction and associated muscle atrophy or fatty infiltration. It demonstrates abnormal distention of the SA-SD bursa or subcoracoid bursa. Magnetic resonance imaging can also show damage to the rotator interval, located in the region devoid of tendons between the supraspinatus and subscapularis tendons. There may be synovitis, tears of the superior glenohumeral and coracohumeral ligaments and tendinosis, subluxation, or tears of the biceps tendon in this region.

Impingement

Sports injuries result from various forms of shoulder impingement. These include primary extrinsic, internal, subcoracoid, and anterosuperior impingement. Supraspinatus muscle hypertrophy, greater tuberosity fractures that are displaced or surrounded by abundant callus, and scapulothoracic instability also contribute to impingement. Each type of impingement is associated with different clinical symptoms, pathology, and treatment. This has been described in the clinical chapter. The imaging of these disorders will be discussed individually in this section.

Primary Extrinsic Impingement

Magnetic resonance imaging demonstrates abnormalities associated with the primary extrinsic impingement syndrome. This common form of impingement in young and middle-aged athletes results in progressively painful compression of the supraspinatus tendon, SA-SD bursa, and long head of the biceps tendon between the humeral head and the coracoacromial arch.[99]

Although controversial, many believe that variations in the architecture of the coracoacromial arch, including one or more of the following, are related to this form of impingement; osseous changes that can lead to primary extrinsic impingement include subacromial enthesophytes, and osteophytes and capsular hypertrophy along the inferior aspect of the AC joint.[99,100] Anteriorly hooked, anteroinferiorly and inferolaterally downsloping, and low-lying acromia are believed by some researchers to predispose to impingement of the supraspinatus tendon by narrowing the acromiohumeral distance.[101-105] Many of these anatomic features may be present in asymptomatic shoulders, and clinical correlation is imperative.[154,106-109] Additionally, the diagnosis of impingement is based on clinical criteria, and therefore should not be made from static MRI studies.

An os acromiale can also predispose to impingement.[110] Careful preoperative imaging evaluation is necessary to exclude the presence of an os acromiale. This ossification center may be difficult to find on conventional radiographs.[111-114] It is best seen on an axillary view that displays the long axis of the acromion. It can also be seen on an axial CT or on an MR study, in which it is important to include high axial sections that demonstrate the entire acromion (Fig. 5.34). The os acromiale is easiest to identify in the axial plane, although it can usually be noticed in all three planes, especially if it is larger. The clinician should be careful not to miss the synchondrosis, which can have an appearance similar to the neighboring AC joint. This is especially easy to do on the oblique sagittal images. Magnetic resonance imaging has an advantage over conventional radiographs and CT in that it can reveal underlying, frequently associated rotator cuff tendon abnormalities.

Secondary injury that affects the supraspinatus tendon, biceps tendon, and subacromial bursa from abnormalities of the coracoacromial arch are best evaluated with MRI. Analysis of signal intensity changes in the supraspinatus and biceps tendons should be correlated with clinical findings. Focal regions of intermediate or high signal intensity may be seen in asymptomatic individuals because of degeneration rather than inflammation or partial thickness tear.[115-117]

The biceps tendon often becomes impinged by the coracoacromial arch right before it enters the bicipital groove. Neer[99] has shown that a shallow or laterally placed bicipital groove also exposes the long head of the biceps tendon to impingement by the anterior third of the acromion, resulting in inflammation or rupture of the intraarticular portion of the tendon. Fluid in the biceps tendon sheath is often seen in asymptomatic individuals because this structure communicates with the glenohumeral joint. It can be difficult to diagnose tenosynovitis of the biceps from an MRI since fluid naturally surrounds this

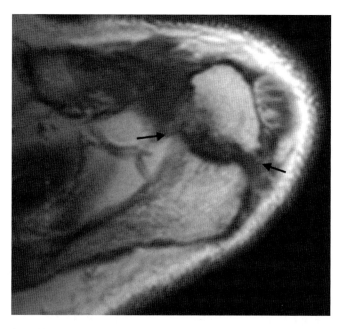

FIG. 5.34. An os acromiale is identified in the anterior aspect of the acromion separated by the synchondrosis (arrows) on this axial T1-weighted MRI.

tendon. Multiple low signal intensity bands in the tendon sheath are associated with tenosynovitis. With tendinosis, the tendon may be increased in size and may concomitantly or alternatively demonstrate internal high signal intensity on T2 weighting. This is common in the long head of the biceps right before it enters the intertubercular groove. Sagittal images of the biceps are best for assessment of this location. Partial-thickness tears may be difficult to distinguish from tendinosis if the tendon is not thinned, split, or irregular. The full-thickness biceps tendon rupture is seen with discontinuity of the tendon and several axial MRIs showing an empty intertubercular groove.

A thickened or ossified coracoacromial ligament has been associated with the extrinsic impingement syndrome.[63] Some believe that it is a cause of impingement,[118] whereas others postulate that it is thickened as a result of alteration of the soft tissue structures from the impingement process.[119] The criteria for thickening of the ligament on MRI are somewhat subjective. In one study, the coracoacromial ligament was considered to be thickened when the major part of the ligament was smoothly or irregularly enlarged or thicker than 2.0mm.[108] This definition was arbitrarily chosen by the study's authors based on clinical experience. There was a statistically significant association between a thickened coracoacromial ligament and rotator cuff tear in that study. An anatomic study of the coracoacromial ligament demonstrated that the subacromial thickness can vary from 2 to 5.6mm, with an average measurement of 3.9mm.[120] Posttraumatic calcification or ossification of the coracoacromial ligament is another rare cause of impingement.[121]

Internal Impingement

Internal impingement (also referred to as posterosuperior glenoid impingement) of the glenoid rim can produce shoulder pain and can lead to partial-thickness tears of the undersurface of the rotator cuff. This form of internal impingement was first described by Walch et al.[85] and then Liu and Boynton[86] in overhead-throwing athletes; it has also been recognized in nonathletes who frequently rotate the shoulder into the extremes of abduction and external rotation.[84] The mechanism that leads to this form of impingement involves superior or posterosuperior angulation of the humerus with respect to the glenoid. In this syndrome, the articular side of the rotator cuff tendons and the greater tuberosity are compressed against the posterosuperior glenoid labrum, resulting in partial-thickness tendon tears, especially of the posteroinferior supraspinatus and the infraspinatus, a degenerative tear of the posterior surface of the posterior superior labrum or underlying glenoid, and an osteochondral compression fracture in the region of the greater tuberosity of the humeral head (which can simulate a Hill-Sachs lesion) (Fig. 5.35). The inferior glenohumeral ligament and adjacent labrum can also be injured. The tears can be well seen on MRAs obtained in the ABER position.[87] Treatment has mixed results and is aimed at controlling extremes of shoulder elevation and abduction external rotation by exercise or surgery and at repair of the injured structures.[122]

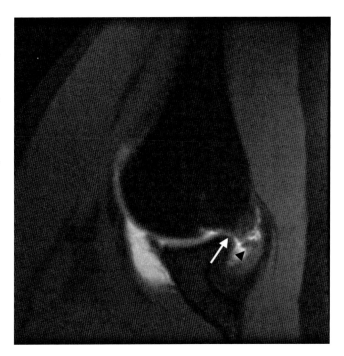

FIG. 5.35. Posterosuperior glenoid impingement. There is an articular-sided tear of the supraspinatus tendon (black arrowhead) as well as a tear of the posterior superior labrum (white arrow) on this fat-suppressed T1-weighted image from an MRA obtained with the glenohumeral joint in abduction and external rotation.

More recently there has been some question as to the association of partial undersurface tears of the rotator cuff and superior labral lesions with internal impingement. One study found that these "kissing" lesions were not associated with major sports activity.[123] Therefore, it should not always be assumed that an undersurface rotator cuff and posterosuperior labral tear that are seen in the same patient are caused by abduction and external rotation.

Coracoid Impingement

Subcoracoid impingement is an uncommon form of impingement that occurs when the coracoid–lesser tuberosity distance narrows, encroaching upon the subscapularis tendon in the vicinity of its attachment to the lesser tuberosity.[124,125] Subscapularis tendon tears result from this type of impingement. Symptoms are produced with the humeral head in forward flexion and medial rotation, which reduces the distance between the coracoid and humerus. Narrowing of this distance can be caused by congenital hypertrophy or elongation of the coracoid or acquired conditions including coracoid or lesser tuberosity fractures, glenoid osteotomy, and coracoid process transfer during surgery.

Because the coracohumeral distance is narrowed in internal rotation, it has been suggested that imaging of the glenohumeral joint be obtained in internal rotation when specifically evaluating this form of impingement.[126] Although a distance of 10.5 to 11.5mm between the coracoid and humeral head is statistically significant, it is not a good predictor of subcoracoid impingement. It is recommended that imaging play a supporting role in this evaluation, with the confirmation of this disorder remaining a clinical diagnosis.

Anterosuperior Impingement

Anterosuperior impingement (ASI) is a newly described form of internal shoulder impingement caused by trauma or degeneration. It is responsible for some anterior shoulder pain in middle-aged patients.[127–129] It is the result of an impingement of the long head of the biceps and the subscapularis tendon with the anterosuperior glenoid rim. It occurs in the region of the biceps pulley, where the SGHL and the CHL merge together around the biceps tendon and subscapularis tendon, resulting from horizontal adduction and internal rotation of the arm.[128]

There are four patterns of anterosuperior impingement[127]: (1) isolated lesion of the SGHL, (2) SGHL lesion and a partial articular-sided supraspinatus tendon tear, (3) SGHL lesion and deep surface tear of the subscapularis tendon, and (4) SGHL lesion and a partial articular-sided supraspinatus and subscapularis tendon tears. The long head of the biceps tendon is often involved, demonstrating synovitis, subluxation, dislocation, and partial or complete tearing.

Lesions of the long head of the biceps tendon, SGHL, and undersurface of the supraspinatus and subscapularis tendons are well seen with MRI.[130,131] Magnetic resonance arthrography is particularly useful for their demonstration[132] (Fig. 5.36).

Rotator Cuff Tendon Evaluation by Magnetic Resonance

Rotator Cuff Tendinosis and Tendinopathy

When a tendon has a signal intensity abnormality without focal disruption or associated findings to suggest a partial-thickness tear, the terms *tendinosis* and *tendinopathy* have been used to signify an underlying tendon degeneration or inflammation.[115] These terms suggest that there is a chronic, often preexisting, degenerative process. In general, the signal intensity of the lesion is not as marked as that of a tear on T2-weighting (Fig. 5.37). There is usually some thickening of the tendon (the normal thickness of the supraspinatus tendon is between 2 and 4 mm, with a mean of 3.2 mm) which distinguishes the signal change from magic angle phenomenon.[133]

Partial-Thickness Rotator Cuff Tears

Partial thickness tears of the rotator cuff are defined as tears that do not extend all the way from the articular to the bursal side of the tendon. They can be seen inferiorly at the articular surface, superiorly at the bursal surface, or intrasubstance,

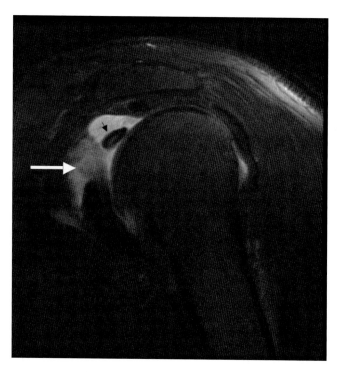

FIG. 5.36. Anterosuperior impingement. The coracohumeral and superior glenohumeral ligament bicipital sling is disrupted around the biceps tendon (white arrow) on this fat-suppressed sagittal MR image from a shoulder arthrogram. There is also an intrasubstance partial tear of the biceps tendon (black arrow) and enlargement of the rotator interval around the biceps. These are all consistent with a clinical history of anterior superior impingement.

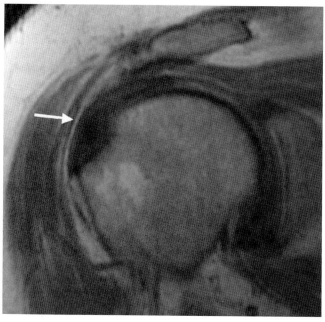

FIG. 5.37. Supraspinatus tendinosis. The supraspinatus tendon is thickened with intermediate signal intensity on this oblique coronal T1-weighted MRI of the shoulder (arrow).

within the tendon. One should describe partial tears according to location (articular, bursal, interstitial), area (in square millimeters), and depth of the tear.[134] Normal tendon thickness is 10 to 12mm. A grade 1 tear is up to 3mm in depth. Grade 2 tears extend 3 to 6mm into the cuff but do not exceed half the thickness of the tendon. Grade 3 lesions involve more than 6mm of the tendon depth without extending all the way across from the articular to the bursal surface.

Tears at the articular surface are the most common type of partial-thickness tears.[135] These are frequently seen at the footprint attachment of the supraspinatus tendon to the greater tuberosity.[136] Originally described by Codman, supraspinatus and infraspinatus partial tears at the footprint are termed rim rent tears. These tears are often overlooked and can be difficult to see on oblique-coronal images alone. It is a good practice to search for them on axial and sagittal images. When more than 7mm of exposed bone is identified at the footprint lateral to the articular cartilage edge of the greater tuberosity, the partial tear is considered significant and should be repaired.[136] A partial articular supraspinatus tendon avulsion is known as the PASTA lesion.[137] The identification of extension of an articular sided partial tear into the substance of the tendon is important for diagnosis and treatment. These tears have been termed Partial Articular tears with Intratendinous extension (PAINT) by Conway.[138]

Focal increased signal intensity extending through a portion of the tendon is suggestive of a partial-thickness tear on MRI. Partial-thickness rotator cuff tears occasionally present with irregularity or thinning without abnormal signal intensity. Partial- and full-thickness tears can propagate within the tendon extending in the longitudinal plane of the tendon fibers. This is known as delamination. There may be varying degrees of retraction of the various layers.

When describing a partial-thickness tear, it is important to mention the morphologic features of the tear, the location of the tear, its size and extent from the articular to the bursal surface, and whether more than one tendon is involved. Thinning, irregularity, delamination, and the presence of an undersurface flap of tissue are also important to mention. This information is helpful for prognosis and preoperative planning.

It is more difficult to detect a partial-thickness tear than a full-thickness tear.[19] Partial-thickness tears may occasionally be tough to distinguish from tendinosis or nondisplaced full-thickness tears if they are elevated in signal intensity on all imaging sequences. The use of higher resolution techniques improves the sensitivity of MRI for detecting partial-thickness tears. Fluid accumulation in the SA-SD bursa, which is common with full-thickness rotator cuff tears, may also be seen in patients with all types of partial-thickness tears. Increased intraarticular fluid may also be found in the setting of a partial- or full-thickness rotator cuff tear.

Magnetic resonance arthrography has been shown to be more accurate than conventional MRI for evaluation of partial tears located on the articular surface of the rotator cuff.[51,139,140] Additional detection and characterization of

articular-sided partial-thickness tears can be obtained if the arm is in the ABER position during the MR examination.[11,87] Abduction of the arm allows the undersurface to be depicted free from the superior surface of the humerus and also promotes spreading of the frayed and torn edges of the inferior surface[85,87] (Fig. 5.38).

Full-Thickness Rotator Cuff Tears

Full-thickness rotator cuff tears often begin anteriorly at the footprint or in the critical zone of the supraspinatus tendon and propagate posteriorly. Because of this pattern, larger tears show a greater amount of tendon retraction anteriorly than posteriorly. Approximately 40% of supraspinatus tendon tears extend into the infraspinatus tendon. Tears of the supraspinatus tendon also have a tendency to extend anteriorly into the rotator interval and subscapularis tendon.

A full-thickness rotator cuff tear involves a complete disruption of the tendon from the articular to the bursal surface. Magnetic resonance findings in full-thickness rotator cuff tears include one or more of the following signs: disruption of the low signal intensity tendon by an area of high signal intensity on T1- and T2- or T2*-weighted images, tendon retraction, muscle atrophy and fatty replacement, absence of the tendon, acromiohumeral articulation, and fluid in the SA-SD bursa (Fig. 5.39).

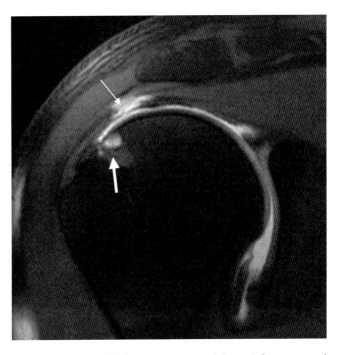

FIG. 5.38. Articular-sided supraspinatus partial tear. A fat-suppressed T1-weighted oblique coronal image from an MRA reveals a greater than 50% partial articular-sided tear of the supraspinatus (small arrow). Cysts lie in the humeral head across from the tear as a result of posterosuperior glenoid impingement (large arrow).

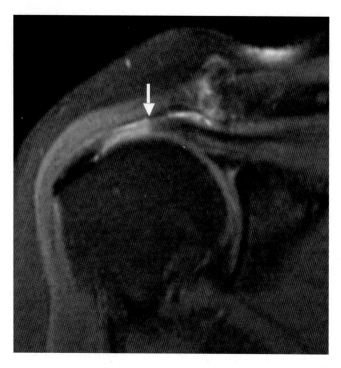

Fig. 5.39. Full-thickness tear supraspinatus. There is a 2-cm gap in the critical zone of the supraspinatus tendon associated with retraction (arrow) on this fat-suppressed oblique coronal T2-weighted MRI.

It has been shown in 10% of cases with partial- and full-thickness tears that fibrous and granulation tissue can fill in the tear, producing low signal intensity on T2 weighting.[116] In such cases, the clinician can look for abnormal tendon morphology such as attenuation or irregularity of the rotator cuff.[116]

Full-thickness tears of the rotator cuff tendons can be accurately identified using conventional nonarthrographic MRI with high sensitivity and specificity.[108,117,141–143] Increased signal intensity extending from the inferior to the superior surface of the tendon on all imaging sequences is an accurate sign of a full-thickness rotator cuff tear.[115] Use of the fat-saturation technique with FSE imaging can improve detection of both full-thickness and partial-thickness tears compared to standard spin-echo imaging techniques.[19] In one study, the fat-saturation technique increased sensitivity for detection of full-thickness tears from 80% to 100%.[19]

Tendon retraction is a specific sign of full-thickness rotator cuff tear.[108] The musculotendinous junction should lie no further medial than 15 degrees from a line drawn through the 12 o'clock position of the humeral head.[108] Retraction can also be defined when the musculotendinous junction lies medial to the glenoid rim. Severe muscle atrophy and fatty replacement are common in patients with large rotator cuff tears.[54,135,144]

Absence of the tendon and acromiohumeral articulation are signs of a chronic rotator cuff tear. The conventional radiograph is useful for identifying acromiohumeral articulation. When the distance between the acromion and the humeral

head is less than 7 mm, a rotator cuff tear is likely. There is no need to perform other studies to exclude a tear in this situation. However, additional studies such as MRI would be indicated if the referring clinician desires information about which tendons are torn as well as other structures in and around the glenohumeral joint. In addition to internal glenohumeral joint derangement, deltoid dehiscence is seen following massive rotator cuff tears.

Fluid in the SA-SD bursa is a sensitive but relatively non-specific finding in patients with rotator cuff tears.[108] The fluid escapes from the glenohumeral joint through the articular surface tear into the bursa that lies above the superior surface of the tear. Small amounts of fluid in the bursa can be seen as an isolated finding in asymptomatic patients.[107,109,133,142,145,146] Cases of isolated SA-SD bursitis without rotator cuff tear are identified following trauma and in association with inflammatory disorders such as rheumatoid arthritis or infection. Subacromial-subdeltoid bursitis is also common with impingement syndrome. Previous injection of a local anesthetic or steroid preparation may cause difficulty in interpretation of the rotator cuff tendons and bursa.[106,147–149] The area of injection is high signal intensity on MRI and can mimic a bursitis, tendinopathy, or tear. Injected fluid can remain in the subacromial subdeltoid bursa for up to 3 days following injection.[147] It is important for the referring physician to know of this phenomenon and request an MR study prior to injection or to delay the MR examination for a few months if such treatment has been performed. The patient should be questioned and counseled about recent injections at the time of the MR appointment. The interpreting radiologist needs to be aware of such injections and their date of administration when evaluating the MR study.

If there is any question concerning the distinction of a full- and partial-thickness tear, MRA is recommended, particularly if the abnormal signal intensity extends from the undersurface of the tendon.[140] When gadolinium is injected into the glenohumeral joint, it fills a defect in the rotator cuff that extends to the articular surface, including partial-thickness undersurface tears. It does not demonstrate a partial tear in the substance or at the superior surface of the rotator cuff tendons. The gadolinium spreads into regions of tendinosis that are not torn. The contrast also fills in frayed and friable tendon margins. Tendons that imbibe contrast have increased signal intensity on fat-suppressed T1-weighted images. These tendons are often friable and swollen, related to degeneration and inflammation. Damaged tendon edges that imbibe contrast are debrided prior to repair of the cuff. If the tear is full thickness, the contrast enters the SA-SD bursa. The SA-SD bursa must be carefully evaluated for the presence of contrast in patients with equivocal full-thickness tears. It is important to use fat-suppression to decrease the signal from fat without affecting the high signal intensity of the gadolinium on T1-weighted images.[140]

An intramuscular "sentinel" cyst may form in the sheath or substance of the rotator cuff muscles when fluid from the joint propagates along a partial- or full-thickness tear into

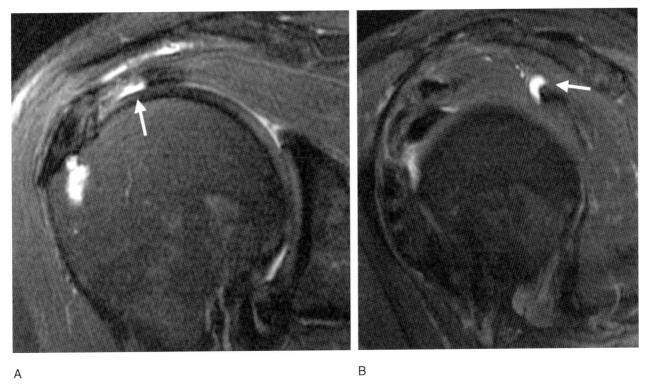

A   B

FIG. 5.40. Intramuscular cyst associated with tendon tear. (A) A partial articular-sided supraspinatus tendon tear is noted on this fat-suppressed T2-weighted oblique coronal MRI (arrow). (B) Fluid from the tear extended posteromedially into the infraspinatus muscle in the form of a cyst (arrow).

the musculotendinous junction.[150,151] These cysts are strongly associated with rotator cuff tears and present as a high signal intensity mass on T2-weighting and STIR images with rim enhancement following intravenous gadolinium injection. When seen on MRI, intramuscular rotator cuff cysts suggest that there is a high likelihood of an underlying rotator cuff tendon tear (Fig. 5.40). The cysts are more commonly seen in association with laminar partial-thickness tears, comprising half of the tears in one study.[151] It is interesting that in some cases the cyst can propagate from a torn tendon into an adjacent rotator cuff muscle with an intact tendon related to interdigitation of tendons as they insert on the humerus. Magnetic resonance arthrography and ABER positioning aid in depiction of partial undersurface tears related to an intramuscular cyst, demonstrating intrasubstance propagation of the tear through delaminated layers of the torn tendon.

Infraspinatus, Teres Minor, and Subscapularis Tendon Tears

Although commonly torn in association with supraspinatus tendon tears, isolated tears of the infraspinatus tendon are rare.[152] An increasing role is being placed on this tendon as a source of symptoms.[153] Tears of the infraspinatus are more frequent in younger athletes who use an overhead-throwing motion. This tendon may also be affected by the previously described internal impingement syndrome. Tears of this tendon

are best identified with the aid of all three imaging planes (Fig. 5.41).

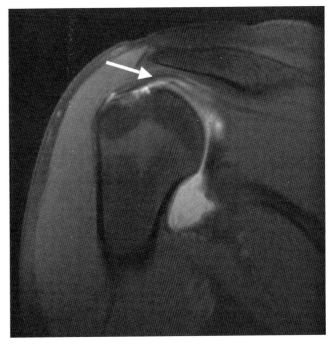

FIG. 5.41. Infraspinatus tendon tear. Partial disruption in the form of a laminar tear is seen in the infraspinatus tendon on this fat-suppressed T1-weighted oblique coronal MR image from an arthrogram (arrow).

Subscapularis tendon tears are seen in patients with antero-superior and subcoracoid impingement as well as in middle-aged and older patients with recurrent shoulder dislocation or in association with massive tears of the other rotator cuff tendons.[68,69,124,125,154,155] A recent article confirms the relationship between subscapularis tendon abnormality and chronicity of supraspinatus tendon tears.[156] Tears may also be seen following direct trauma to the anterior aspect of the shoulder joint and with hyperextension or external rotation of the adducted arm.[157] In the latter case, the patient experiences pain and weakness when the arm is used below shoulder level. On MRI, subscapularis tendon tears are often identified on axial and oblique sagittal images. Partial tears can be subtle and are commonly seen along the articular surface. Full-thickness tears are frequently seen at the attachment to the lesser tuberosity and are associated with retraction (Fig. 5.33). In the presence of a subscapularis tendon tear, the biceps tendon may sublux or dislocate out of the intertubercular groove (Figs. 5.33 and 5.42). Occasionally, it may dislocate into a partial subscapularis tendon tear (Fig. 5.42). The biceps tendon occasionally lies in front of the glenohumeral joint. This is because a disruption of an extension of the subscapularis tendon over the intertubercular groove, formerly known as the transverse humeral ligament, allows the tendon to escape the bicipital groove.[158,159] Cysts or edema are common in the lesser tuberosity in the presence of partial- and full-thickness subscapularis tendon tears as well as supraspinatus tears.

Teres minor tendon tears are rare. Posterior dislocation is a common predisposing mechanism. It is important for the clinician to check the posterior labrocapsular structures for abnormalities when such a tear is present. Teres minor muscle strains may also be an important clue to underlying posterior glenohumeral instability.

Rotator Interval Pathology

Lesions of the rotator interval produce anterior shoulder pain. The long head of the biceps brachii tendon and the rotator interval are intimately related structures that can be linked to specific abnormalities termed "pulley lesions" that were also described in the anterosuperior impingement section.[132] Tears of the rotator cuff interval cause enlargement of the capsule and may allow fluid to escape from the joint and frequently into the SA-SD and subcoracoid bursae.[160] Magnetic resonance arthrography and fluid-sensitive sequences with fat suppression in the axial and sagittal planes are particularly useful for demonstrating these tears as a region of high signal intensity often in association with biceps tendon and coraco-humeral ligament abnormalities (Fig. 5.43).

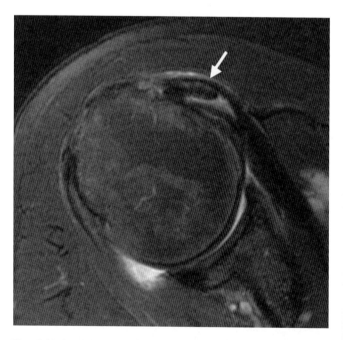

FIG. 5.42. Partial subscapularis tendon tear with biceps tendon dislocation. The biceps extends medial to the groove inside the partial subscapularis tendon tear (arrow) on this fat-suppressed axial T2-weighted MRI.

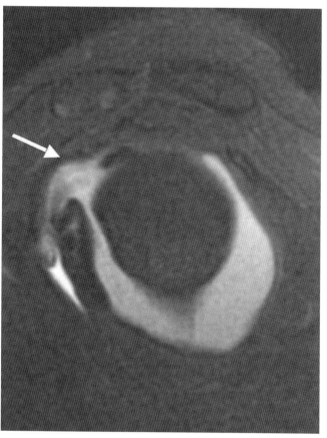

FIG. 5.43. Rotator interval tear. The rotator interval is disrupted (arrow) on this fat-suppressed sagittal T1-weighted image from an MRA.

B. Orthopedic Perspective: The Shoulder in Sports Medicine

Benjamin Shaffer and Patrick J. Murray

The shoulder is a common site of athletic injury. As such, these injuries encompass the full spectrum of shoulder pathology, from acute to chronic, and from minimally symptomatic to athletically disabling. The discipline of sports medicine requires accurate and prompt diagnoses, in part consequent to the unique and potentially season-threatening or career-ending impact on players and teams alike. Imaging tools that facilitate diagnostic accuracy are a crucial part of the orthopedist's armamentarium.

Magnetic resonance imaging has become an important diagnostic adjunct in the evaluation of shoulder conditions, providing an unprecedented level of soft tissue detail. Recent developments have furthered the utility of MR technology, including direct MRA, diagnosis-specific sequencing such as fat suppression and spin-echo techniques, and special positioning such as ABER views. In conjunction with an experienced musculoskeletal radiologist, these newer applications have added an important dimension to our diagnostic accuracy. For example, the detection of labral pathology is considerably improved with the use of MRA. In overhead-throwing athletes in which undersurface cuff pathology is common, ABER sequencing is critical to visualize the cuff footprint. Because of the variable sequencing available, these studies are best requested based on the suspected diagnosis. Certainly, good communication between the clinician and the radiologist will likely improve the diagnostic yield.

Although it is an important tool, it must be remembered that MRI is no substitute for a thorough history, physical exam, and radiographic exam. The fact that many referred patients have already been imaged does not justify the general overutilization of this imaging technique. Magnetic resonance imaging is best indicated in confirming suspected pathology, assisting in clinical decision making, and helping to exclude conditions that may confound or otherwise influence the treatment plan.

Instability

Shoulder instability is most commonly classified by direction, including anterior, posterior, and multidirectional. Anterior instability is further divided into two main groups known for their acronyms TUBS and AMBRII. Patients with TUBS typically have a *t*raumatic onset of *u*nidirectional instability, in which a *B*ankart lesion is typically present, usually requiring *s*urgery. Conversely, AMBRII patients have symptoms whose onset is *a*traumatic, *m*ultidirectional, often *b*ilateral, often responds to *r*ehabilitation, and when unresponsive to nonoperative measures requires an *i*nferior capsular shift and rotator interval closure.[161] Differentiating between these types of instability is critical for successful treatment. Athletes may suffer from either type.

Traumatic Anterior Instability

Anterior shoulder dislocations and subluxations (partial dislocations) account for approximately 90% of traumatic shoulder instability. They are associated with contact and collision sports, and most commonly occur when the athletes' vulnerable abducted and externally rotated shoulder is subjected to a sudden external rotation or extension force.[162]

The glenohumeral joint is stabilized by both static and dynamic mechanisms. The interaction between these two types of restraints allows stability of the glenohumeral joint throughout a wide range of motion. Static restraints include the glenohumeral articular geometry, surrounding glenoid-deepening labrum, and the glenohumeral ligaments and capsule. Of these various ligaments, the most important restraint to anterior instability is the anterior band of the inferior glenohumeral ligament.[163] In addition to deepening the glenoid fossa, the labrum also serves as the attachment site of the glenohumeral ligaments and joint capsule.

Dynamic restraints of the glenohumeral joint include the muscles of the rotator cuff (supraspinatus, infraspinatus, subscapularis, and teres minor), biceps long head tendon, and the scapular stabilizers (serratus anterior, latissimus dorsi, trapezius, rhomboids).

Pathoanatomy and Pathophysiology

The most common pathoanatomy in patients with traumatic anterior glenohumeral instability is a Bankart lesion, which is a detachment of the anteroinferior labrum and glenohumeral ligament from the glenoid rim.[164] Although initially perceived as the "essential lesion" responsible for anterior glenohumeral instability, we now appreciate that a number of associated pathologic lesions can occur with or instead of the Bankart lesion. The most common associated such pathology is capsular patholaxity, with a stretch or plastic deformation of the capsuleligamentous structures from the dislocation event.[165] The Perthes lesion is a nondisplaced labral tear whose attachment to the glenoid rim appears intact but whose medial attachment along the glenoid neck is in fact stripped.[166] An ALPSA lesion represents a Bankart equivalent in which the avulsed anteroinferior capsulolabrum is healed in a nonanatomic position along the medial neck of the glenoid.[167] A HAGL lesion, occurring in up to 9% of some reported series,[168] occurs when failure of the glenohumeral ligament occurs on the humeral side.[169]

Injury often occurs to the bony structures as well, with a high incidence of Hill-Sachs lesions, in which the posterolateral humeral head demonstrates articular or osteochondral impression fracture. Occasionally, the anterior-inferior glenohumeral ligament/labrum complex avulses a portion of the anterior glenoid at the site of attachment, known as a "bony Bankart" lesion. Recognition of the presence and dimensions of such bony lesions has important implications in treatment, as these shoulders may pose a higher risk of failure with arthroscopic stabilization procedures.[170] Other less common associated problems include fractures of the proximal humerus (most commonly the greater tuberosity) and tears of the rotator cuff (usually in patients over age 40).[171]

Diagnosis and Treatment

Diagnosis of anterior instability is established through a careful history and physical, complemented by x-rays. Acutely, patients with a dislocated shoulder hold their arm in slight abduction and external rotation at their side. Normal deltoid contour is lost. Neurologic exam may demonstrate injury to the axillary nerve. Recurrent instability events can generally be diagnosed by history and physical exam.[161] The apprehension sign is the most common physical finding, generated when positioning the patients' shoulder in abduction and external rotation, and applying an anterior-directed force. The test is considered positive if the patient demonstrates apprehension during this maneuver (Fig. 5.44). The relocation sign is positive when this apprehension is relieved by a posterior-directed force. Laxity tests include the load and shift test and the sulcus sign (Fig. 5.45). In the load and shift test, the humeral head is "loaded" through an

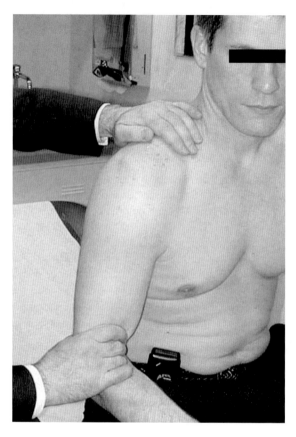

FIG. 5.45. Sulcus sign. Downward traction of the arm will create a gap between the acromion and the humeral head. (From Flatow E. Mini-incision Bankart repair for shoulder instability. In: Scuderi G, Tria A, Berger R, eds. MIS Techniques in Orthopedics. New York: Springer, 2006, with permission.).

axial force into the glenoid, followed by attempted translation posteriorly, comparing the amount and the quality of the end point to the opposite side. Shoulder laxity tests may be difficult to interpret, however, demonstrating poor inter- and intraobserver reliability.[172] Because some patients may have instability in directions other than anteriorly, all patients, particularly those with recurrent instability, must be assessed for generalized ligamentous laxity, which may indicate multidirectional instability.

Treatment of an acute anterior instability episode involves transient immobilization followed by a rehabilitation program. Recent evidence has suggested the possible value of immobilization in external rotation compared to traditional sling immobilization, with improved coaptation of the anterior capsulolabral complex to the glenoid.[173–175]

Unfortunately, nonoperative treatment has led to a fairly predictable recurrence incidence, varying with patient age. Generally, the younger the patient, the higher the risk, with patients under age 20 thought to have a nearly 90% incidence.[176] This high recurrence risk has led some clinicians to consider surgical treatment of the first-time dislocator, especially among athletes in whom recurrence risks subsequent seasons. Treatment of recurrent instability is primarily surgical, with traditional open techniques, or, more commonly, arthroscopic approaches.

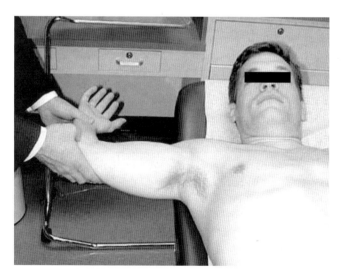

FIG. 5.44. Apprehension test. Abduction and external rotation will produce a sense of impending subluxation/dislocation with anterior glenohumeral instability. (From Flatow E. Mini-incision Bankart repair for shoulder instability. In: Scuderi G, Tria A, Berger R, eds. MIS Techniques in Orthopedics. New York: Springer, 2006, with permission.).

Imaging

Plain radiographs are indicated in cases of an acute dislocation. Prior to or following reduction, a true anteroposterior (AP) view and either a scapular Y lateral or axillary view help confirm the direction of the dislocation and the adequacy of reduction, and delineate any associated fractures, particularly of the posterolateral humeral head (Hill-Sachs lesion) or anterior glenoid (bony Bankart lesion). Special views may facilitate detection of either the Hill-Sachs lesion (Stryker notch view)[177] or the bony Bankart lesion (West Point view).[178] Bony defects may require further more sophisticated imaging such as CT or CT arthrogram, which may help quantify the dimensions of the lesions. Such assessment is critical in that it may influence the surgical approach.

Magnetic resonance imaging is rarely necessary, but often obtained in the patient with acute instability. However, it is of particular value in the patient over age 40, in whom there is an increasingly statistical likelihood of associated rotator cuff tear.[171] In patients with recurrent instability, in which the direction of humeral head displacement is unclear, MRI may be valuable. Signs suggestive of anterior instability include abnormalities of the anterior glenohumeral ligament or labrum, or the presence of a Hill-Sachs lesion. Historically, MRI has not consistently allowed for a high accuracy in assessing pathology of the glenoid labrum. This is due in part to variations in labral anatomy and significant inter- and intraobserver variability in image interpretation. Multiple studies have examined the efficacy of MRI in the identification of labral tears associated with anterior shoulder instability. They have shown sensitivity of 44% to 100% and specificity of 66% to 100%.[179–183]

Intraarticular injection of contrast media prior to MRI (direct MRA) has enhanced diagnostic accuracy.[184–188] For example, in a direct comparison of MRI and MRA compared with surgical findings, Chandnani et al.[184] found the two techniques to be roughly equivalent in ability to detect labral tears, at 96% and 93%, respectively. However, MRA was significantly more accurate in detecting detached labral fragments (96% vs. 46%) and correctly identifying labral degeneration (56% vs. 11%). Waldt et al.[188] evaluated the accuracy of MRA in detection of labroligamentous pathology associated with shoulder instability, compared with surgical findings, and found the overall accuracy to be 89% in detection and 84% in classification of pathology. Overall, 80% of Bankart lesions, 77% of ALPSA lesions, and 50% of Perthes lesions were correctly identified. In studies by Palmer et al.[185] and Palmer and Caslowitz,[186] MRA demonstrated sensitivity of 91% and 92%, and specificity of 93% and 92%, respectively, in detection of labral pathology associated with anterior shoulder instability. Overall, MRI and MRA are valuable tools in evaluating patients with instability, but neither is 100% accurate in labral interpretation.

Recent developments have permitted improvements in detection of associated pathology by shoulder positioning during the MR. Specifically, ABER sequences, in which the shoulder is positioned in abduction and external rotation following intraarticular injection, improves accuracy of labral interpretation, as well as recognition of undersurface cuff tears. For example, Cvitanic et al.,[189] in a study comparing MR and operative findings in 92 patients, demonstrated 89% sensitivity and 95% specificity in the diagnosis of anterior labral injuries with MRA in the ABER position, compared with 48% sensitivity and 91% specificity with MRA in the conventional position. Using both in conjunction increased sensitivity to 96% and specificity to 97%. In a cadaver study, Kwak et al.[190] found that MRA in the ABER position achieved the best visualization of the inferior glenohumeral ligament. Clinicians should consider obtaining MR arthrograms in the ABER position for patients who are suspected of having a lesion of the anterior capsulolabral complex.

Magnetic resonance imaging and MRA can also assist in evaluating patients with recurrent instability following previous surgical stabilization. Conventional MRI in this population, particularly in the presence of metal anchors, may make interpretation difficult. For example, Wagner et al.[191] reported 80% sensitivity, 79% specificity and 79% accuracy in the detection of recurrent labral tears in 24 patients at an average of 10 months postoperatively. This study, however, was limited by a small number of patients, and variable radiographic technique (MRI, direct and indirect MRA).

Traumatic Posterior Instability

Acute posterior shoulder dislocations are markedly less common in comparison to anterior instability patterns, accounting for only 2% to 4% of all glenohumeral dislocations. The mechanism of injury is typically an axial load with the arm in an adducted and internally rotated position. Posterior shoulder dislocations may also occur as a result of seizure or electric shock. Commonly, posterior instability is more subtle and recurrent, often seen in football linemen or in association with inferior laxity (multidirectional instability).[192] Acute traumatic posterior dislocation is typically accompanied by a reverse Bankart lesion, in which the ligament/labrum complex is avulsed from the posterior glenoid rim. In patients with recurrent instability, attenuation of the capsule may be the pathologic finding rather than labral disruption. Other pathology may include posterior capsular laxity, posterior HAGL lesions, and posterior labrocapsular periosteal sleeve avulsions (POLPSA lesions). Posterior instability may be associated with a hypoplastic glenoid or excessively retroverted humerus or glenoid.[193] Osseous injury may include anterior humeral head impaction fractures, also called "reverse" Hill-Sachs lesions or rim fractures of the posterior glenoid rim.

The diagnosis of acute posterior shoulder dislocation is frequently missed.[194] Clinically, patients present with pain and hold their arm in adduction and internal rotation, unable to externally rotate. Differences from the shoulders' normal contour may be subtle. An AP and axillary radiographs are mandatory whenever dislocation is suspected. The AP view may be unremarkable, but the axillary view confirms the diagnosis.

Clinical examination should include the load and shift test, and the jerk test (also called the clunk test).[161] The jerk test attempts to elicit actual transient instability of the joint, and may be voluntarily demonstrated by the patient. In this test, the arm is first flexed to 90 degrees and an axial load applied, translating the humeral head posteriorly. The patients' arm is then extended in the plane of abduction, with a resultant "clunk" indicating reduction of the subluxed or dislocated humeral head. Physical exam findings however, are often subtle and may be underwhelming. For this reason, MRI is especially valuable in this population.

Acute treatment of posterior shoulder dislocation is rarely necessary as it most commonly reduces spontaneously. Early treatment involves postreduction sling immobilization and rehabilitation. Surgery may be appropriate in athletes after a first-time dislocation, although most surgical cases are indicated with recurrent instability. Definitive treatment involves anatomic repair of the typically detached posterior labrum/inferior glenohumeral ligament from the glenoid.[195]

Anteroposterior and axillary radiographs are required in cases of suspected posterior shoulder dislocation. Further studies are not typically necessary, but may include CT to evaluate bony pathology or MRI to evaluate the labrum. These advanced diagnostic imaging tests may be of value in clinical decision making.[196]

Multidirectional Instability

Multidirectional instability (MDI) of the shoulder represents an atraumatic condition in which patients develop functional symptoms due to an inherently lax capsule. Often associated with generalized ligamentous laxity, it may also reflect underlying soft tissue connective disorders such as Ehlers-Danlos syndrome. Patients typically present with chronic symptoms related to repetitive activities, such as swimming or overhead throwing. Pain is the most common symptom, but they may complain of a sense of instability or the arm "going dead." Infrequently patients may be able to voluntarily demonstrate their instability, particularly by subluxing the shoulder inferiorly.

In addition to an appropriate history, the diagnosis of MDI is established by physical exam. Laxity tests may reveal increased translation in anterior, posterior, or inferior directions, which may or may not be symptomatic. The hallmark of MDI, however, is the presence of a sulcus test. When positive, a "sulcus" develops between the acromion and the proximal humerus upon inferior passive translation of the humeral head. This sulcus is readily appreciated, though it may be normal in some patients with generalized laxity. The sulcus sign can be graded based on the measured amount of inferior translation, with 3 cm the likely threshold for significant translation. Recent modifications of the sulcus test include repeating it with the patients' arm externally rotated, which if positive suggests deficiency of the tissue within the rotator interval. When the arm is positioned in combined abduction/external rotation, persistent translation suggests capsular patholaxity in the axillary pouch.

Radiographic studies are unhelpful. Plain films are normal, and MRI does not show any pathologic findings, although there may be a relatively capacious pouch. The primary treatment of MDI is nonoperative for most patients, with cuff and scapular stabilizer strengthening sufficient to resolve most symptoms. Failure to respond may warrant operative intervention with an inferior capsular shift or arthroscopic plication.[197] Most patients do not have actual labral pathology or bony Bankart lesion.

Superior Labrum and Biceps Tendon

Injury to the superior glenoid labrum is a common and increasingly recognized cause of shoulder pain, particular in the athletic population. The superior labrum serves as the attachment site for the tendon of the long head of the biceps muscle. Structurally, the superior labrum, like the anterior and posterior labrum, is a rim of fibrocartilage that is triangular in cross section, and is continuous with the glenoid articular cartilage. The superior labrum has a number of normal variants.[198] In the central detachment type, or sublabral recess, the central portion of the meniscus-like labrum is free and not attached to the articular margin, though peripherally attached.[199] The sublabral hole, located anterior to the biceps anchor, consists of a band-like middle glenohumeral ligament (MGHL) associated with a bare space between the labrum and anterosuperior glenoid. This variant is found in 11% to 15% of patients.[200,201] A Buford complex is another normal variant, similar to the sublabral hole with a cord-like MGHL, but the anterosuperior labrum is absent. The cord-like MGHL is continuous with the superior labrum. This normal variant occurs in approximately 1.5% of patients.[202] The significance of all these variations is in the difficulty in differentiating a true SLAP tear from a normal variant by MRI.

The tendon of the long head of the biceps is a fairly constant intraarticular structure that exits the joint at the bicipital groove. However, its relationship to the glenohumeral ligaments is somewhat variable, and congenital anomalies, such as the presence of a double tendon, an aberrant mesentery-like attachment, and complete absence of the tendon, have been described.[161,203]

Pathoanatomy and Pathophysiology

Injuries to the superior labrum have been dubbed SLAP lesions, which have been classified into as many as 10 different types,[201] but the most common classification as initially proposed by Snyder et al.[204] involves four types. Type I represents degenerative fraying and is the most common. Type II is a detachment of the superior labrum from the underlying glenoid. Type III and IV are relatively uncommon; type III is a bucket-handle equivalent tear in which the superior labrum is split and subluxed inferiorly into the joint, and Type IV is a detachment of the superior labrum like a type II, but with tear extension into the root of the biceps.

The SLAP lesions are common in athletes and often coexist with other pathology. There are multiple described mechanisms of injury with variable symptomatology. One of the most common presentations is an acute injury, such as sliding into base with arm extended overhead, or a fall onto an outstretched arm with the shoulder in abduction and forward flexion, generating a traction force that pulls on the biceps anchor. Such an event is typically accompanied by sudden onset of pain, and subsequent mechanical clicking or catching. Another mechanism in the overhead-throwing athlete is the "peel-back" phenomenon,[205] in which repetitive stresses in the throwing position leads to progressive peeling back of the superior labrum/biceps anchor complex medially off the glenoid neck, seen in overhead-throwing athletes with an abduction and external rotation force during the throwing motion.

Injuries to the biceps tendon include degenerative fraying, partial or complete tears, as well as subluxation or dislocation. Injury mechanism includes both acute trauma and repetitive stress. Tears may be associated with SLAP lesions. Biceps long head subluxation or dislocation occurs with injury to the soft tissue restraints. Medially this includes tearing of the upper portion of the subscapularis tendon.[206] Laterally this can occur with a rotator cuff tear of the supraspinatus extending into the rotator interval. Axial MRI cuts in which the biceps can be seen to be displaced from its normal position within the intertubercular groove demonstrate the diagnosis.

Diagnosis and Treatment

In addition to a careful history including mechanism of injury, the physical exam can assist in diagnosis of SLAP lesions. Clinical tests described to help detect SLAP lesions include the O'Brien active-compression test and the biceps load test. The O'Brien active-compression test[207] is performed with the patient's arm held in 90 degrees of forward flexion and 10 degrees of adduction. With the thumb pointing toward the floor, the patient is asked to resist a downward force. Pain with this maneuver that is located in the shoulder (not the acromioclavicular joint) and relieved when the thumb is pointed upward is indicative of a SLAP lesion. No physical exam finding has been shown to be sensitive or specific for SLAP lesions, however. To further complicate matters, SLAP lesions, particularly in the throwing population, often accompany other shoulder pathology, and are rarely isolated findings. For these reasons, SLAP lesions present a diagnostic challenge.

Biceps tendon pathology may be diagnosed by a careful history and physical exam. Patients with acute complete ruptures usually present with a sudden event in which they feel a pop and notice a "Popeye" muscle, with distal displacement of the biceps muscle belly and ecchymosis over the next few days. Often there is a preceding history of pain. Biceps tendon instability accompanies other shoulder pathology and itself is not readily diagnosed by physical exam. Multiple physical exam tests have been described aimed at diagnosing biceps pathology, although none has been shown to be specific. Speed's test is performed with the patient's palm facing up with the elbow in full extension. A positive test consists of the presence of pain located in the bicipital groove with resisted forward flexion. While this test has been shown to be 90% sensitive in detecting anterior shoulder pathology, its specificity for biceps pathology is only 13%.[208]

Symptomatic SLAP lesions may respond to nonoperative treatment. However, in the athletic population, particularly overhead-throwing athletes, repetitive stresses may make nonoperative treatment unrealistic. The surgical approach depends on arthroscopic findings, and includes debridement for types I and III SLAP lesions and repair for types II and IV.[209]

Biceps tendon pathology may also be successfully managed nonoperatively, typically with corticosteroid injections into the bicipital sheath. Persistent symptoms may warrant arthroscopic evaluation with definitive treatment based on the extent of the pathology. Generally, less than 50% tendon diameter involvement leads to debridement, with greater than 50% requiring either tenodesis (reattaching the biceps tendon to the proximal humerus) or tenolysis (releasing or cutting the biceps tendon). In cases of biceps instability, tenodesis is usually performed, along with adjunctive treatment of associated cuff pathology.[210]

Imaging

Diagnosis of SLAP lesions requires a careful history and physical exam, because imaging studies are not reliably accurate. Plain radiography is of no value except to exclude other diagnoses. Because SLAP lesions are often only part of a spectrum of pathology, and because of known anatomic variability, MRI is an important adjunct in diagnostic evaluation.

An MRI or MRA is indicated when superior labral pathology is suspected. In evaluation of the superior labrum, paracoronal (in the plane of the scapula) T2 images are of greatest value.[211] As in meniscus pathology, the interpretation of true SLAP tears (from an intralabral signal) requires extension of the increased signal to the articular margin of the labrum. Intraarticular gadolinium may help differentiate between intralabral signal and nondisplaced tears. Distinguishing true labral pathology from variants such as a sublabral hole requires MR expertise. In general, the sublabral recess tends to be more medial than SLAP tears, and located between the biceps tendon and the glenoid articular cartilage. Conversely, SLAP tears often extend posterior to the biceps tendon and more laterally than the sublabral recess.[212]

In terms of biceps evaluation, axial imaging permits visualization of the biceps attachment on the superior labrum, as well as the course of the tendon within the intertubercular groove. Intrasubstance signal in the biceps tendon may be indicative of a partial tear. Absence of the long head indicates a complete tear. Subluxation or dislocation is easily seen on axial and sometimes coronal images,[213] usually in association with other pathology (supraspinatus or subscapularis tendon tears).

Several authors have reported on the efficacy of MRI and MRA to detect and identify superior labral pathology.

Magnetic resonance imaging has demonstrated sensitivity from 41% to 98%, specificity of 86% to 100%, and accuracy of 63% to 95% in detection of SLAP lesions.[181,183,214,215] This compares with MRA, which has been shown to achieve 89% to 100% sensitivity, 69% to 91% specificity and 74% to 92% accuracy.[216–218] Despite the purported value of the addition of intraarticular contrast to conventional MRI, few studies have borne out the increased sensitivity or accuracy of this approach in the diagnosis of SLAP lesions.[219] Nevertheless, such imaging, in particular for evaluation of the throwing athlete and in suspected cases of labral pathology, has become fairly standard.

For visualization of the biceps tendon, MRI and MRA are useful. In one study, MRI was shown to have 67% sensitivity and 90% specificity in the detection of biceps tendon instability.[213] The authors found that visualization of the tendon perched on the lesser tuberosity in the presence of an obtusely angled intertubercular groove was a good indicator of biceps tendon instability. Zanetti et al.[220] were able to demonstrate 86% sensitivity and 87% to 94% specificity in the diagnosis of biceps tendon rupture using MRA. They stressed the importance of visualization of the tendon in both the axial and sagittal oblique images. They also observed that biceps tendinopathy was most closely associated with observed caliber changes and intrasubstance signal as seen by MRA. Some authors advocate MRA over MRI alone when there is clinical suspicion of biceps tendon pathology due to the superior visualization of the tendon in the presence of contrast agents.

Rotator Cuff and Impingement

The rotator cuff consists of the musculotendinous units of four muscles: supraspinatus, infraspinatus, teres minor, and subscapularis. Each of these muscles has its origin on the scapula and insertion on the proximal humerus. The tendons come together to form a cuff of tissue that represents the largest single tendinous structure in the human body. Anatomically, from superior to posterior, the supraspinatus, infraspinatus, and teres minor insert on the greater tuberosity. Anteriorly, the subscapularis inserts on the lesser tuberosity, and is separated from the rest of the rotator cuff by the rotator interval (Fig. 5.46).

In the normal shoulder, the rotator cuff serves an important function that has been described as the "compressor" cuff.[221] In the midrange of glenohumeral motion during which the static shoulder stabilizers are relatively lax, the rotator cuff acts to stabilize the glenohumeral joint by compressing the humeral head into the glenoid, thereby maintaining a constant center of rotation. The rotator cuff also acts as a humeral head depressor with the arm at higher degrees of elevation. While the cuff is biomechanically critical in ensuring head centering, the deltoid and other parascapular muscle groups account for the majority of force generation about the shoulder.

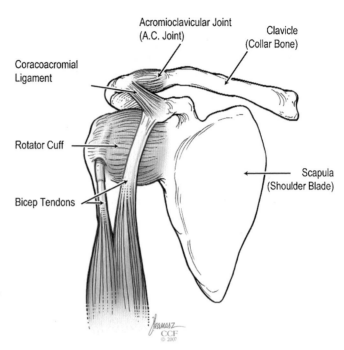

FIG. 5.46. The attachments of the shoulder ligaments, rotator cuff, and biceps tendon to the bones are shown. (Courtesy of the Cleveland Clinic Center for Medical Art and Photography. © 2007. All rights reserved.).

Rotator cuff pathology may occur in isolation in the aging population, in which progressive degenerative changes are well established. Yet the cuff is also involved to a great degree in younger athletic patients, particularly in throwing athletes, in which underside cuff tearing due to tension overload failure and internal impingement conspire to compromise normal function. Cuff pathology in this group often coexists with other structural damage. In these cases, MRI has proven invaluable to better understand and help direct treatment.

Pathoanatomy and Pathophysiology

The spectrum of cuff pathology ranges from mild tendonitis to full-thickness retracted tears. There are many different theories to explain rotator cuff pathology, but none is universal. The most common theory is that of subacromial impingement, in which mechanical pressure on the bursal side of the cuff leads to progressive cuff changes and eventual tearing. In this model, anterior acromial spurring and coracoacromial (CA) ligament thickening account for the observed cuff changes.[222,223] Pathologic lesions associated with external impingement include rotator cuff tendinopathy, partial- or full-thickness tears, and labral tears.

Many observations subsequent to this theory, however, have led to the current realization that in fact, most problems of the rotator cuff are not actually caused by this outlet impingement, though some may occur secondarily. The most likely primary cause of cuff problems is inherent degenerative pathology in the cuff that has been shown to be age related.[224] Another described cause of cuff problems, particularly in the overhead-throwing athlete, has been termed "internal impingement," which is created by the direct contact of the posterior cuff against the posterior superior glenoid as the arm is positioned in abduction and external rotation (i.e., the throwing position).[225] The pathologic lesions typically seen with internal impingement include posterosuperior labral degeneration or tear, partial-thickness tears of the supraspinatus or anterior edge of infraspinatus tendons, and cystic changes in the posterolateral humeral head.[226] Extrinsic, or "external," impingement in athletes occurs secondary to microinstability patterns, allowing the humeral head to translate superiorly.[227]

Another type of impingement is anterosuperior impingement, a relatively uncommon cause of cuff pathology. In this phenomenon, the anterior cuff (supraspinatus and upper subscapularis tendons), along with the biceps sling (coracohumeral ligament and superior glenohumeral ligament) become mechanically compressed within the confines of the rotator interval. A "roller Wringer" effect has been described in which the coracoid can actually lead to undersurface fiber failure of the subcapularis, particularly in cases in which the coracoid process is elongated, or the space between the coracoid and lesser tuberosity are narrowed.[228]

Rotator cuff tears occur when there is mechanical failure, usually at the tendinous attachment. Tearing can occur as an acute event, insidiously, or as an acute-on-chronic phenomenon. The supraspinatus is the most commonly involved cuff tendon, with extension into the infraspinatus a close second. Subscapularis pathology is an increasingly recognized entity, with partial tearing, detachment, and/or "cabling" of the upper fibers. Usually this subscapularis involvement is in conjunction with other cuff findings. Teres minor tendon involvement is decidedly uncommon. Tears of the cuff may be nonretracted or demonstrate considerable retraction, often associated with atrophy and fatty infiltration of the affected muscle(s).[229]

Partial-thickness tears, on both the bursal and the articular side, are relatively common, perhaps more common in fact than full-thickness detachments. Their diagnosis is difficult clinically, and may present with chronic symptoms of impingement or acute pain suggestive of a full-thickness cuff tear. Definitive diagnosis may require arthroscopic evaluation, as MRI cannot easily distinguish signal changes due to partial tearing from tendinosis and degenerative changes.

Diagnosis and Treatment

Diagnosis of shoulder impingement and rotator cuff tears is clinical. The most common complaints are pain and weakness. Many shoulder conditions, however, present in a similar manner, and the differential diagnosis includes AC joint arthritis/osteolysis, calcific tendonitis, and an early adhesive capsulitis (frozen shoulder).

The classic tests for subacromial impingement are those described by Neer and modified by Hawkins.[161] These classic impingement signs rely on re-creating symptoms through a mechanical maneuver in which the cuff is "impinged" between the humeral head and the coracoacromial arch (anterior acromial undersurface and CA ligament). A positive Neer's sign occurs when pain is elicited as the arm is passively flexed while fixing the scapula. The Hawkins maneuver adds a component of internal rotation and adduction. Neither has been shown to have a high accuracy rate, and certainly many other conditions can lead to a positive impingement sign. Selective injection of local anesthetic into the subacromial space may offer acute relief of symptoms and decreased provocation of symptoms with repeat impingement testing. This is another sign of subacromial impingement. Unfortunately, scrutiny of this injection technique's accuracy has shown a high rate of infiltration into other surrounding structures, thereby limiting the value of this adjunctive clinical tool.[230]

Range-of-motion testing usually reveals no restriction in passive motion assessment, although pain may limit active motion. Restriction may suggest the presence of concomitant or masquerading adhesive capsulitis. Clinical evaluation of the individual cuff muscles has been described.[231] Integrity of the supraspinatus involves testing the arm against resistance when positioned in the plane of the scapula at 90 degrees of forward elevation. Testing with the thumb pointed down and up have both been described. The infraspinatus is best examined by evaluating the strength of the shoulder in external rotation, with the arm positioned at the side. Since the infraspinatus accounts for the majority of strength in this position, weakness or pain implicates this muscle. The infraspinatus and teres minor can be examined together with strength testing of external rotation with the arm at 90 degrees of abduction. Subscapularis tendon involvement can be assessed by performing the lift-off test or the belly-press test. In the lift-off test, the arm is placed behind the patient's back, and the patient is asked to lift it away. The inability to do so suggests a tear of the subscapularis. The belly-press test may be more reliable, however, because it does not rely on patients' ability to place the arm behind their back, a painful maneuver for many patients regardless of pathology. In the belly-press test, patients are asked to place their hand on their belly and bring their "wing" forward while keeping the wrist straight. Inability to do so suggests a subscapularis tendon tear.[161]

Diagnostic tests for internal impingement are fraught with even greater difficulty. A number of physical exam tests have been described, but independent evaluation has failed to confirm the accuracy as typically observed by the doctor describing them. The diagnosis of subcoracoid impingement relies on local tenderness about the coracoid, and pain elicited upon adducting the flexed shoulder across the body, reproducing the patients' symptoms.[232]

With the exception of acute traumatic cuff ruptures, initial treatment for cuff pathology is usually nonoperative. Physical therapy programs usually focus on the restoration of normal motion, limiting provocative activities to the cuff, and emphasizing strengthening of the scapular rotators (and eventual cuff).[233] There is also a considerable role for analgesics (nonsteroidal antiinflammatory medications) and judicious use of corticosteroid injections. Surgery is appropriate when symptoms are refractory to nonoperative management, patient impairment, or both. Surgically correctable lesions may include partial or complete rotator cuff tears, labral injuries, and biceps pathology.

Imaging

Plain radiographs are of great value in the patient with cuff symptoms. A "true" AP view in the plane of the scapula rules out the presence of glenohumeral arthritis or calcific deposits, as well as permitting assessment of the subacromial space. When narrowed beyond 6 mm, there is probably caudal migration of the humeral head, indicative of a large and possibly irreparable tear of the rotator cuff.[234] An axillary view helps evaluate the glenohumeral joint to exclude glenohumeral arthritis and demonstrates an os acromiale if it exists. An outlet view is important to help determine acromial morphology, with those patients demonstrating a considerable "hook" or spur (type III acromion) potentially more likely to have cuff pathology (and potentially require surgical "decompression" of the spur).[235] A "Zanca" view, in which an AP of the shoulder is directed at the AC joint, tilting it 10 degrees cephalad, demonstrates any arthritis of the AC joint, which occasionally causes or contributes to cuff problems.[236]

Ultrasound has been recently applied to evaluation of the rotator cuff, with some studies suggesting a high accuracy rate.[237] Unfortunately, despite the fact that it has proven an effective and relatively inexpensive cuff and biceps evaluation technique, it is extremely operator-dependent. Furthermore, accuracy in capsulolabral imaging has not been demonstrated. These current shortcomings limit the utility of ultrasound for shoulder evaluation.

Magnetic resonance imaging, however, has proven to be of considerable value. It remains the diagnostic test of choice for most authors, and is commonly included in the diagnostic workup of suspected cuff pathology. It is appropriate in patients who have failed nonoperative treatment, present with acute trauma, pain and weakness, or in cases in which there is some diagnostic uncertainty. In younger throwing athletes for whom return to play may be a factor, earlier MRI is likely to be considered.

Magnetic resonance imaging evaluation of the rotator cuff is best performed using T1 and T2 images in the oblique coronal and oblique sagittal planes. T1 fat-suppressed, T1 spin-echo, T2 FSE fat-saturated, and proton-density sequences are necessary to fully assess the cuff.[238–241] The addition of intraarticular gadolinium may assist in the diagnosis of partial articular-sided tears, more accurately determine cuff tear size, and help identify any associated labral pathology.[242–244]

Rotator cuff tendinopathy is indicated by increased signal within the substance of the cuff on the T1 and T2 images. Partial cuff tears are indicated by increased signal extending to the articular side or bursal side of the cuff, and in the case of intraarticular gadolinium, the presence of contrast material extending into the cuff undersurface. Full-thickness rotator cuff tears show lack of integrity of the tendon, typically near the insertion site. Fluid present on both the glenohumeral and subacromial side usually suggests communication and indirectly, a likely cuff tear. Axial MRIs are important to assess the subscapularis and to demonstrate the presence of long head biceps rupture or subluxation. Sagittal views help assess acromial morphology similar to those seen with plain x-rays. Computed tomography and MRI have both been evaluated for muscle atrophy and fatty infiltration, which may help guide clinical decision making in terms of cuff reparability.[229,245]

In the overhead-throwing athlete, MRIs must be interpreted in conjunction with a thorough clinical evaluation. Up to 93% of these patients demonstrate some abnormality by MRI, but most of them are asymptomatic.[246,247] Magnetic resonance imaging findings consistent with internal impingement are common, and include increased signal within the supraspinatus and infraspinatus tendons, partial-thickness cuff tears, cystic changes in the superolateral humeral head, and posterosuperior labral degeneration.[248] It is important to distinguish potentially incidental observations by comparing them with actual clinically relevant findings. For this reason, many authors have advocated MRA and utilizing the ABER position during imaging in this patient population.

Magnetic resonance imaging may have value in assessment of coracoid impingement. Several recent studies have examined the interval between the coracoid and lesser tuberosity.[232,249,250] This likely requires positioning of the shoulder in internal rotation, the position in which this condition occurs. Thus, if ordering an MR for the purpose of evaluating for coracoid impingement, the study ought to be ordered with the shoulder so positioned.

In evaluating the rotator cuff, multiple studies of conventional MRI have demonstrated a sensitivity and specificity of around 90%.[251,252] Magnetic resonance imaging more accurately detects full-thickness tears than partial-thickness tears. Magnetic resonance arthrography has been compared favorably with MRI in diagnosis of partial-thickness cuff tears, specifically articular-sided tears, as well as full-thickness tears. Toyoda et al.,[244] in a direct comparison between MRI and MRA, found a sensitivity of 90.2% for MRI and 100% for MRA in detection of full-thickness tears. Furthermore, they found that MRA more accurately estimated the size and morphology of the tear when compared to intraoperative findings. Meister et al.[243] demonstrated 84% sensitivity and 96% specificity in diagnosis of articular-sided partial-thickness tears with MRA. Subscapularis tears are also well visualized with MRA, with a sensitivity of 91% and specificity of 79% to 86% in a study by Pfirrmann et al.[253]

Magnetic resonance arthrography with the arm in the ABER position may increase the accuracy in detecting and characterizing partial-thickness tears. Tirman et al.[254] found an increased rate of detection of articular-sided partial infraspinatus tears with imaging in the ABER position in overhead-throwing athletes. Lee and Lee[255] found that ABER MRA views detected the horizontal component of partial-thickness articular-sided tears 100% of the time, whereas oblique coronal MRA views detected such tears 21% of the time.

When rotator cuff pathology is discovered, biceps tendon pathology should also be suspected. Chen et al.[256] reported a 76% incidence of biceps tendon pathology in surgically confirmed case of complete rotator cuff tears. Magnetic resonance imaging and MRA can help detect biceps pathology prior to surgery. Beall et al.[257] reported 52% sensitivity and 86% specificity of unenhanced MRI in detection of biceps pathology in the presence of rotator cuff pathology. Identifiable biceps tendon pathology was strongly associated with subscapularis tendon tears. The use of MRA significantly increases the sensitivity for detection of biceps pathology.

Overall, many studies have shown that MRI has demonstrated a high sensitivity and specificity in the detection of rotator cuff pathology. Magnetic resonance arthrography may be used to improve the diagnostic accuracy, especially in the detection of partial-thickness articular-sided tears, and evaluation of concomitant capsulolabral injury. Utilizing the ABER position for MRA may further increase the ability to detect and characterize partial-thickness tears of the infraspinatus.

Muscle and Tendon Injuries

Pectoralis Major Injury

Injury to the pectoralis major musculotendinous unit occurs infrequently, usually when the muscle is at maximal tension and subjected to additional stress. This occurs in weight-lifters during the bench press or may occur with direct blows, such as in a football tackle. Patients describe the appropriate mechanism, and often feel a "pop" followed by intense pain. Tears may be partial or complete and can typically be detected by history and physical exam. Ecchymosis, swelling, and, in cases of complete rupture, deformity may be present with abnormal contour of the retracted muscle. The anterior axillary fold may be webbed with the arm at 90 degrees of abduction. Active contraction of the shoulder in adduction, internal rotation, and forward flexion is painful or weak.[258]

Ruptures of the pectoralis major may occur in the substance of the muscle, at the musculotendinous junction, or at the tendinous insertion lateral to the biceps tendon on the proximal humerus. The tendinous insertion consists of the clavicular head, which inserts more distally, and the sternal head. Complete ruptures are rare, and typically occur at the bone–tendon junction. Partial tears may be characterized as high grade (over 50%) or low grade (under 50%). Optimal treatment of these injuries depends on the type of tear that is present. Low-grade partial tears and tears of the muscle belly tend to do well with nonoperative management, whereas high-grade partial and complete tears have been shown to have better functional and cosmetic outcomes with surgery. Operative treatment in athletes allows for quicker return to sports, and surgery performed within 8 weeks of injury yields better results than delayed surgical repair.[259]

Determining the type and location of injury is important in clinical decision making. In cases of complete rupture, physical exam is usually sufficient. Plain radiographs are indicated to rule out (uncommon) bony avulsion injury. Ultrasound has been used with some success in accurately determining the location of the injury.[258] However, MRI is the imaging modality of choice because it offers excellent detail of the soft tissues, permits assessment of the location and degree of the tear, and is readily available. Axial images are useful in examining the normal insertion, which is consistently identifiable between the quadrilateral space and the deltoid tuberosity.[260] The tendinous insertion and musculotendinous junction are best visualized on axial images, but coronal images may be useful to determine the grade of partial tears. Acute injury is best seen as increased signal on T2 sequences because hematoma may be isointense with muscle on T1.[261] T1 images are useful in evaluation of chronic tears.

Multiple authors have examined the diagnostic utility of MRI in diagnosis of pectoralis major injuries. Connell et al.[261] performed MRI in 15 patients with clinically suspected pectoralis major injuries. Primary repair was performed in nine patients with apparent injuries of the tendinous insertion, and the injury as seen on MRI was confirmed at surgery in every case. Zvijac et al.[262] compared clinical diagnosis with MRI results in 27 patients with pectoralis major injuries. The MRI findings more accurately diagnosed the pathology, and showed that clinical exam often overestimated the severity of the injury. The MRI findings changed the treatment plan in three patients from operative to nonoperative when less significant injury was shown.

Neurologic Injuries

In evaluating athletes and active patients with complaints of shoulder pain, clinicians must consider neurologic etiologies in the differential diagnosis. Though rare, injuries to the brachial plexus and axillary nerve may simulate other pathology. Other neurologic entities include brachial neuritis and supra-scapular nerve compression (secondary to cyst formation in the spinoglenoid notch). An MRI is a useful tool in diagnosis or exclusion of these conditions.

Brachial Plexus

Brachial plexus injuries most often occur in contact and collision athletes. The mechanism of injury is usually a direct compression or stretch. This injury, referred to as a "burner" or "stinger," causes acute unilateral weakness, pain, and sensory changes in the affected extremity. This is typically a transient neuropraxia, and usually resolves within several minutes. However, weakness of the deltoid or rotator cuff muscles may occur days later, and other symptoms may also persist. In the event that symptoms do not resolve, diagnostic testing is indicated to evaluate for injury to the brachial plexus.[263] Nerve conduction studies and MRI assist in determining the level and severity of the lesion. An MRI is particularly useful in identifying nerve root avulsion injuries.[264]

Brachial neuritis, also known as Parsonage-Turner syndrome, may be clinically confused with rotator cuff or labral pathology. Brachial neuritis is idiopathic, and usually presents with sudden onset of neuritic pain accompanied by weakness. Physical exam demonstrates atrophy with hollowing out of the supraspinatus or infraspinatus fossa, although other muscle groups may be involved. The syndrome is usually self-limited, with resolution of pain within a few weeks, but recovery of muscle mass and strength can take a long time and may be incomplete. Specific MRI findings make this the diagnostic study of choice, with marked edema of muscles innervated by the involved nerves on T2 images.[265] Electrodiagnostic tests have also been found useful both diagnostically and prognostically.

Axillary Nerve

Axillary nerve injury is the most common neurologic sequela of anterior shoulder dislocations, occurring in 5% to 54%, depending on the method of assessment (physical exam vs. EMG).[266] The axillary nerve courses from anterior to posterior through the quadrilateral space, which is defined superiorly by the teres minor, inferiorly by the teres major, medially by the long head of the triceps, and laterally by the shaft of the humerus. It innervates the teres minor and deltoid muscles. It courses along with the posterior humeral circumflex vessels. In this anatomic position, the nerve may be subject to compression by fibrous bands or paralabral cysts, leading to a clinical syndrome known as quadrilateral space syndrome.[267] Patients with this syndrome present with complaints of poorly localized shoulder pain and paresthesias, and may have tenderness over the quadrilateral space. The vague nature of the signs and symptoms and the rarity of the condition combine to make this a difficult diagnosis, easily confused with rotator cuff pathology or impingement.

Some authors have found arteriography useful in demonstrating constriction of the posterior circumflex humeral artery with the arm in the ABER position.[268] Electromyographic studies may show denervation of the deltoid, and nerve conduction studies may reveal slowed conduction through the axillary nerve.[267] However, the presence of specific MRI findings and the noninvasive nature of the test have made MRI the diagnostic tool of choice for this syndrome. Magnetic resonance imaging shows selective atrophy of the teres minor, which is seen as reduced volume or fatty infiltration of the muscle on oblique sagittal spin-echo T1 images. Diffuse increased signal on oblique sagittal T2 fat-suppressed images is also seen, which is indicative of neurogenic edema.[269] The deltoid muscle may also be involved. These findings contrast with MRI findings of brachial neuritis, which involve muscles innervated by other nerves. In addition to the findings in the teres minor and deltoid, any space-occupying lesion that could be causing the syndrome, such as a paralabral cyst, can be easily visualized by MRI.

In the absence of identifiable compression from an extrinsic mass (paralabral cyst), treatment for quadrilateral space syndrome is nonoperative, with expectant spontaneous resolution in most cases. In those refractory to nonoperative management, or in which there is compression due to mass effect from a paralabral cyst, surgical intervention can be successful. Treatment involves arthroscopic debridement and possible repair of the inciting labral pathology, and cyst decompression. In the absence of identifiable mass, fibrous bands in the quadrilateral space are debrided.

Suprascapular Nerve

The suprascapular nerve, a branch of the superior trunk of the brachial plexus, innervates the supraspinatus and infraspinatus muscles, in addition to providing sensory fibers to the acromioclavicular and glenohumeral joints. It travels through the suprascapular notch underneath the transverse scapular ligament, through the supraspinatus fossa, spinoglenoid notch, and deep to the infraspinatus in its fossa. The nerve may be injured or compressed along its course, most commonly beneath the transverse scapular ligament or at the spinoglenoid notch in association with labral pathology and a spinoglenoid cyst. This nerve can also be injured from fractures, shoulder dislocation, or iatrogenic injury during surgery. Suprascapular nerve entrapment is often not appreciated until visible atrophy of the supraspinatus or infraspinatus has developed. Symptoms include vague shoulder pain and weakness, with physical exam findings of atrophy and/or weakness. Although electrodiagnostic tests (EMG and nerve conduction velocity) can aid in the diagnosis, MRI is the study of choice due to its ability to identify a compressive mass (typically a ganglion cyst).[270] Additionally, MRI permits evaluation of associated labral pathology and occasionally tears of the rotator cuff.

Ganglion cysts are easily visualized by increased signal on coronal, sagittal, and axial T2 images. Uncommon other causes of suprascapular nerve entrapment include synovial sarcoma, Ewing's sarcoma, chondrosarcoma, metastatic carcinoma, and posttraumatic hematoma. Ganglion cysts may spontaneously resolve, although surgical intervention to arthroscopically decompress the cyst and address any labral pathology is probably the most common approach.

Miscellaneous

Glenolabral Articular Disruption Lesions

The glenolabral articular disruption (GLAD) lesion was first described by Thomas Neviaser[271] in 1993 as a superficial tear in the anteroinferior labrum associated with articular cartilage injury. Patients typically present with a history of trauma and nonspecific shoulder pain. Instability is an uncommon component of the presentation. The MRI appearance of the GLAD lesion may be similar to that of a Bankart lesion. The inferior glenohumeral ligament, however, is intact. Magnetic resonance arthrography in the ABER position may increase study sensitivity.[272] Often these lesions are appreciated arthroscopically for persistent symptoms that are refractory to nonoperative treatment.

Adhesive Capsulitis

Originally described by Julius Neviaser[273] in 1945, adhesive capsulitis, also known colloquially as frozen shoulder, is an idiopathic process of shoulder pain and stiffness. The process has been divided into clinical stages, beginning with an initial inflammatory painful phase (stage 1), in which there is no identifiable motion restriction. In stage 2, ongoing inflammation is accompanied by progressive restriction in motion in all planes. During stage 3, inflammation and pain typically resolve, with stiffness the hallmark of presentation. Finally, in stage 4 the shoulder thaws, with near-complete resolution of symptoms and restoration of motion. Each of these stages varies in duration, and may take up to year or more to resolve.[274]

Physical exam findings vary depending on the stage. Diagnosis of this condition is clinical based on presentation and physical findings. Diagnostic imaging is useful only in excluding other possible conditions. Because of acute pain in the initial presentation, diagnosis of calcific tendonitis, shoulder sepsis, and brachial neuritis must be considered. Plain x-rays are otherwise unhelpful. Likewise, MRI has no real value in establishing or confirming the diagnosis, with the exception in the early inflammatory phase of effusion in the glenohumeral joint. Magnetic resonance imaging and MRA findings include increased capsular thickness in the axillary recess, increased thickness of the rotator interval including the coracohumeral ligament, obliteration of the fat triangle between the coracohumeral ligament and coracoid process, and decreased volume of the axillary recess.[275,276]

Because the disorder is considered self-limiting in most patients, treatment is nonoperative in the form of activity modification, analgesic management (including intraarticular corticosteroid injection in the initial painful phases), and gentle physical therapy to restore mobility in the latter stiff and thawing phases. Rarely, persistent stiffness requires operative intervention, including manipulation and usually adjunctive arthroscopic capsular release.

Acromioclavicular Pathology

The acromioclavicular (AC) joint is commonly injured in athletes, especially in contact or collision sports. An AC instability can result from disruption of the capsule, extracapsular ligaments (the conoid and trapezoid), and the surrounding clavipectoral fascia. Acromioclavicular degeneration can develop as age-related or posttraumatic pathology, and may represent part of the spectrum of subacromial impingement and rotator cuff pathology. Distal clavicular osteolysis can occur as an atraumatic process that represents a stress failure syndrome of the distal clavicle, or in response to a single traumatic event.

Diagnosis of AC pathology relies on clinical evaluation and plain radiographic studies. Magnetic resonance imaging does not contribute to diagnosis or affect treatment of these injuries. It can demonstrate degenerative changes in the AC joint, and can identify arthritis in this joint earlier than can plain radiographs.[277] However, degenerative changes can also be seen by MRI in a large proportion of young, asymptomatic patients,[278] and so clinical correlation is critical. Acromioclavicular joint cysts associated with degenerative changes may present as a mass, raising concern of malignancy. Magnetic resonance imaging can demonstrate the degenerative nature of these cysts.[279]

Distal clavicular osteolysis develops in about 6% of patients after AC joint injury.[280] Plain radiographs may show osteopenia in the distal clavicle, joint space widening, and articular erosions, but may also be equivocal. When this diagnosis is suspected in patients with chronic AC pain with normal radiographs, MRI can be helpful. Magnetic resonance imaging findings include soft tissue swelling, bone marrow edema in the distal clavicle, cortical irregularity associated with periarticular cyst-like erosions, joint space widening, clavicular periostitis, and marrow edema in the acromion.[281]

Treatment of AC instability is nonoperative for mild injuries. More significant injures can be treated with a variety of surgical reconstruction procedures. The painful AC joint may require resection of the distal clavicle if conservative measures are ineffective.

Conclusion

General indications for MRI or MRA include patients in whom symptoms persist despite appropriate nonoperative treatment, situations in which clinical decision making may be influenced, and cases of diagnostic uncertainty or concern of malignancy. With these exceptions, MRI can be inappropriately utilized as an extension of the clinical workup. Because MRI findings are often incidental, their interpretation must be considered in the context of the clinical presentation. In athletes with suspected labral or cuff pathology, the addition of intraarticular gadolinium contrast will likely improve imaging sensitivity and accuracy. The ABER sequences are invaluable in examining internal impingement and cuff pathology in the overhead-throwing athlete.

References

1. Merl T, Scholz M, Gerhardt P, et al. Results of a prospective multicenter study for evaluation of the diagnostic quality of an open whole-body low-field MRI unit. A comparison with high-field MRI measured by the applicable gold standard. Eur J Radiol 1999;30:43–53.

2. Magee T, Shapiro M, Williams D. Comparison of high-field-strength versus low-field-strength MRI of the shoulder. AJR Am J Roentgenol 2003;181:1211–15.

3. Tung GA, Entzian D, Green A, Brody JM. High-field and low-field MR imaging of superior glenoid labral tears and associated tendon injuries. AJR Am J Roentgenol 2000;174:1107–14.

4. Allmann KH, Walter O, Laubenberger J, et al. Magnetic resonance diagnosis of the anterior labrum and capsule. Effect of field strength on efficacy. Invest Radiol 1998;33:415–20.

5. Shellock FG, Bert JM, Fritts HM, Gundry CR, Easton R, Crues JV, 3rd. Evaluation of the rotator cuff and glenoid labrum using a 0.2-tesla extremity magnetic resonance (MR) system: MR results compared to surgical findings. J Magn Reson Imaging 2001;14:763–70.

6. Tuite MJ, DeSmet AA, Norris MA, Orwin JF. MR diagnosis of labral tears of the shoulder: value of T2*-weighted gradient-recalled echo images made in external rotation. AJR 1995;164:941–4.

7. Tuite MJ, Asinger D, Orwin JF. Angled oblique sagittal MR imaging of rotator cuff tears: comparison with standard oblique sagittal images. Skeletal Radiol 2001;30:262–9.

8. Kwak SM, Brown RR, Trudell D, Resnick D. Glenohumeral joint: comparison of shoulder positions at MR arthrography. Radiology 1998;208:375–80.

9. Davis SJ, Teresi LM, Bradley WG, Ressler JA, Eto RT. Effect of arm rotation on MR imaging of the rotator cuff. Radiology 1991;181:265–8.

10. Tirman PFJ, Bost FW, Steinbach LS, et al. MR arthrographic depiction of tears of the rotator cuff: benefit of abduction and external rotation of the arm. Radiology 1994;192:851–6.

11. Lee SY, Lee JK. Horizontal component of partial-thickness tears of rotator cuff: imaging characteristics and comparison of ABER view with oblique coronal view at MR arthrography initial results. Radiology 2002;224:470–6.

12. Song HT, Huh YM, Kim S, et al. Anterior-inferior labral lesions of recurrent shoulder dislocation evaluated by MR arthrography in an adduction internal rotation (ADIR) position. J Magn Reson Imaging 2006;23:29–35.

13. Chan KK, Muldoon KA, Yeh L, et al. Superior labral anteroposterior lesions: MR arthrography with arm traction. AJR Am J Roentgenol 1999;173:1117–22.

14. Friedman RJ, Bonutti PM, Genez B. Cine magnetic resonance imaging of the subcoracoid region. Orthopedics 1998;21:545–8.

15. Sans N, Richardi G, Railhac JJ, et al. Kinematic MR imaging of the shoulder: normal patterns. AJR Am J Roentgenol 1996;167:1517–22.

16. Cardinal E, Buckwalter KA, Braunstein EM. Kinematic magnetic resonance imaging of the normal shoulder: assessment of the labrum and capsule. Can Assoc Radiol J 1996;47:44–50.

17. Beaulieu CF, Hodge DK, Bergman AG, et al. Glenohumeral relationships during physiologic shoulder motion and stress testing: initial experience with open MR imaging and active imaging-plane registration. Radiology 1999;212:699–705.

18. Allmann KH, Uhl M, Gufler H, et al. Cine-MR imaging of the shoulder. Acta Radiol 1997;38:1043–6.

19. Reinus WR, Shady KL, Mirowitz SA, Totty WG. MR diagnosis of rotator cuff tears of the shoulder: value of using T2–weighted fat-saturated images. AJR 1995;164:1451–5.

20. Sonin AH, Peduto AJ, Fitzgerald SW, Callahan CM, Bresler ME. MR imaging of the rotator cuff mechanism: comparison of spin-echo and turbo spin-echo sequences. AJR 1996;167:333–8.

21. Gusmer PB, Potter HG, Schatz JA, et al. Labral injuries: accuracy of detection with unenhanced MR imaging of the shoulder. Radiology 1996;200:519–24.

22. Chandnani VP, Yeager TD, DeBerardino T, et al. Glenoid labral tears: prospective evaluation with MR imaging, MR arthrography, and CT arthrography. AJR 1993;161:1229–35.

23. Shankman S, Bencardino J, Beltran J. Glenohumeral instability: evaluation using MR arthrography of the shoulder. Skeletal Radiol 1999;28:365–82.

24. Palmer WE, Brown JH, Rosenthal DI. Labral-ligamentous complex of the shoulder: evaluation with MR arthrography. Radiology 1994;1994:645–51.

25. Steinbach LS, Palmer WE, Schweitzer ME. Special focus session. MR arthrography. RadioGraphics 2002;5:1223–46.

26. Beltran J, Rosenberg ZS, Chandnani VP, Cuomo F, Beltran S, Rokito A. Glenohumeral instability: evaluation with MR arthrography. RadioGraphics 1997;17:657–73.

27. Sethi PM, Kingston S, Elattrache N. Accuracy of anterior intra-articular injection of the glenohumeral joint. Arthroscopy 2005;21:77–80.

28. Zwar RB, Read JW, Noakes JB. Sonographically guided glenohumeral joint injection. AJR Am J Roentgenol 2004;183:48–50.

29. Chung CB, Dwek JR, Feng S, Resnick D. MR arthrography of the glenohumeral joint: a tailored approach. AJR 2001;177:217–9.

30. Farmer KD, Hughes PM. MR arthrography of the shoulder: fluoroscopically guided technique using a posterior approach. AJR Am J Roentgenol 2002;178:433–4.

31. Depelteau H, Bureau NJ, Cardinal E, Aubin B, Brassard P. Arthrography of the shoulder: a simple fluoroscopically guided approach for targeting the rotator cuff interval. AJR Am J Roentgenol 2004;182:329–32.

32. Kamishima T, Schweitzer ME, Awaya H, Abraham D. Utilization of "used" vials: cost-effective technique for MR arthrography. J Magn Reson Imaging 2000;12:953–5.

33. Newberg AH, Munn CS, Robbins AH. Complications of arthrography. Radiology 1985;155:605–6.

34. Hall FM, Rosenthal DI, Goldberg RP, Wyshak G. Morbidity from shoulder arthrography: etiology, incidence, and prevention. AJR Am J Roentgenol 1981;136:59–62.

35. Sommer T, Vahlensieck M, Wallny T, et al. Indirect MR arthrography in the diagnosis of lesions of the labrum glenoidale. Rofo Fortschr Geb Rontgenstr Neuen Bildgeb Verfahr 1997;1:46–51.

36. Maurer J, Rudolph J, Lorenz M, Hidajat N, Schroder R, Sudkamp NP. A prospective study on the detection of lesion of the labrum glenoidale by indirect MR arthrography of the shoulder. Rofo Fortschr Geb Rontgenstr Neuen Bildgeb Verfahr 1999;14:307–12.

37. Rockwood CA, Matsen FAI. The Shoulder. Philadelphia: WB Saunders, 1990.

38. Neumann CH, Petersen SA, Jahnke AH. MR imaging of the labral-capsular complex: normal variations. AJR 1991;157:1015–21.

39. Park YH, Lee JY, Moon SH, et al. MR arthrography of the labral capsular ligamentous complex in the shoulder: imaging variations and pitfalls. AJR 2000;175:667–72.

40. Williams MM, Snyder SJ, Buford D. The Buford complex- the cord-like middle glenohumeral ligament and absent anterosuperior labrum complex: a normal anatomic capsulolabral variant. Arthroscopy 1994;10:241–7.

41. Tirman PFJ, Feller JF, Palmer WE, Carroll KW, Steinbach LS, Cox I. The Buford Complex—a variation of normal shoulder anatomy. MR arthrographic imaging features. AJR 1996;166:869–73.

42. Tuite MJ, Orwin JF. Anterosuperior labral variants of the shoulder: appearance on gradient-recalled-echo and fast spin-echo MR images. Radiology 1996;199:537–40.

43. Tuite M, Blankenbaker DG, Siefert M, Aiegert AJ, Orwin JF. Sublabral foramen and Buford complex: inferior extent of the unattached or absent labrum in 50 patients. Radiology 2002;223:137–42.

44. Detrisac DA, Johnson LL. Arthroscopic Shoulder Anatomy: Pathologic and Surgical Implications. Thorofare, NJ: Slack, 1987.

45. Smith DK, Chopp TM, Aufdemorte TB, et al. Sublabral recess of the superior glenoid labrum: study of cadavers with conventional nonenhanced MR imaging, MR arthrography, anatomic dissection, and limited histologic examination. Radiology 1996;201:251–6.

46. Yeh L, Kwak S, Kim YS, et al. Anterior labroligamentous structures of the glenohumeral joint: correlation and anatomic dissection in cadavers. AJR 1998;171:1229–36.

47. Beltran J, Bencardino J, Mellado J, Rosenberg ZS, Irish RD. MR arthrography of the shoulder: variations and pitfalls. RadioGraphics 1997;17:1403–12.

48. Tuite MJ, Rutkowski A, Enright T, Kaplan L, Fine JP, Orwin J. Width of high signal and extension posterior to biceps tendon as signs of superior labrum anterior to posterior tears on MRI and MR arthrography. AJR Am J Roentgenol 2005;185:1422–8.

49. Beltran J, Bencardino J, Padron M, Shankman S, Beltran L, Ozkarahan G. The middle glenohumeral ligament: normal anatomy, variants and pathology. Skeletal Radiol 2002;31:253–62.

50. Moseley HF, Overgaard B. The anterior capsular mechanism in recurrent anterior dislocation of the shoulder. J Bone Joint Surg 1962;44:913–27.

51. Flannigan B, Kursunoglu-Brahme S, Snyder S, et al. MR arthrography of the shoulder: comparison with conventional MR imaging. AJR 1990;155:829–32.

52. Roger B, Skaf A, Hooper AW, Lektrakul N, Yeh L, Resnick D. Imaging findings in the dominant shoulder of throwing athletes: comparison of radiography, arthrography, CT arthrography, and MR arthrography with arthroscopic correlation. AJR 1999;172:1371–80.

53. Kieft GJ, Bloem JL, Rozing PM, Obermann WR. MR imaging of recurrent anterior dislocation of the shoulder: comparison with CT arthrography. AJR 1988;150:1083–87.

54. Seeger LL, Gold RH, Bassett LW, Ellman H. Shoulder impingement syndrome: MR findings in 53 shoulders. AJR 1988;150:343–7.

55. Wilson AJ, Totty WG, Murphy W, et al. Shoulder joint: arthrographic CT and long-term follow-up, with surgical correlation. Radiology 1989;173:329–33.

56. Applegate GR, Hewitt M, Snyder SJ, Watson E, Kwak S, Resnick D. Chronic labral tears: value of magnetic resonance arthrography in evaluating the glenoid labrum and labral-bicipital complex. Arthroscopy 2004;20:959–63.

57. Pappas AM, Goss TP, Kleinman PK. Symptomatic shoulder instability due to lesions of the glenoid labrum. Am J Sports Med 1983;11:279–88.

58. Coumas JM, Waite RJ, Goss TP, Ferrari DA, Kanzaria PK, Pappas AM. CT and MR evaluation of the labral capsular ligamentous complex of the shoulder. AJR 1992;158:591–7.

59. Garneau RA, Renfrew DL, Moore TE, El-Khoury GY, Nepola JV, Lemke JH. Glenoid labrum: evaluation with MR imaging. Radiology 1991;179:519–22.

60. Legan JM, Burkhard TK, Goff WB II, et al. Tears of the glenoid labrum: MR imaging of 88 arthroscopically confirmed cases. Radiology 1991;179:241–6.

61. McCauley TR, Pope CF, Jokl P. Normal and abnormal glenoid labrum: assessment with multiplanar gradient-echo MR imaging. Radiology 1992;183:35–7.

62. Tirman PFJ, Stauffer AE, Crues JV, et al. Saline magnetic resonance arthrography in the evaluation of glenohumeral instability. Arthroscopy 1993;9:550–9.

63. Magee T, Williams D, Mani N. Shoulder MR arthrography: which patient group benefits most? AJR Am J Roentgenol 2004;183:969–74.

64. Loredo R, Longo C, Salonen D, et al. Glenoid labrum: MR imaging with histologic correlation. Radiology 1995;196:33–41.

65. Neviaser TJ. The anterior labroligamentous periosteal sleeve avulsion lesion: a cause of anterior instability of the shoulder. Arthroscopy 1993;9:17–21.

66. Perthes G. Uber operationen bei habitueller schulterluxation. Deutsch Ztshr Chir 1906;85:199–227.

67. Tirman PFJ, Steinbach LS, Feller JF, AE S. Humeral avulsion of the anterior shoulder stabilizing structures after anterior shoulder dislocation: demonstration by MR and MR arthrography. Skeletal Radiol 1996;25:743–8.

68. Neviaser RJ, Neviaser TH, Neviaser JS. Anterior dislocation of the shoulder and rotator cuff rupture. Clin Orth Rel Res 1993:103–6.

69. Neviaser RJ, Neviaser TJ, Neviaser JS. Concurrent rupture of the rotator cuff and anterior dislocation of the shoulder in the older patient. J Bone Joint Surg 1988;70–A:1308–11.

70. Oberlander MA, Morgan BE, Visotsky JL. The BHAGL lesion: a new variant of anterior instability. Arthroscopy 1996;12:627.

71. Warner JJP, Beim GM. Combined Bankart and HAGL lesion associated with anterior shoulder instability. Arthroscopy 1997;13:749.

72. Sanders TG, Tirman PFJ, Linares R, Feller JF, Richardson R. The glenolabral articular disruption lesion: MR arthrography with arthroscopic correlation. AJR 1999;172:171–5.

73. Neviaser TJ. The GLAD lesion: another cause of anterior shoulder pain. Arthroscopy 1993;9:22–3.

74. Simons P, Joekes E, Melissen RGHH, Bloem JL. Posterior labrocapsular periosteal sleeve avulsion complicating locked posterior shoulder dislocation. Skeletal Radiol 1998;27:588–90.

75. Yu JS, Ashman CJ, Jones G. The POLPSA lesion: MR imaging findings with arthroscopic correlation in patients with posterior instability. Skeletal Radiol 2002;31:396–9.

76. Bennett GE. Shoulder and elbow lesions of the professional baseball pitcher. JAMA 1941;117:510–4.

77. De Maeseneer M, Jaovisidha S, Jacobson JA, et al. The Bennett lesion of the shoulder. J CAT 1998;22:31–4.

78. Steinbach LS, Tirman PFJ, Peterfy CA, Feller JF. Shoulder Magnetic Resonance Imaging. Philadelphia: Lippincott-Raven, 1998.

79. Chung CB, Sorenson S, Dwek JR, Resnick D. Humeral avulsion of the posterior band of the inferior glenohumeral ligament: MR arthrography and clinical correlation in 17 patients. AJR Am J Roentgenol 2004;183:355–9.

80. Hottya GA, Tirman PFJ, Bost FW, Montgomery WH, Wolf EM, Genant HK. Tear of the posterior shoulder stabilizers after posterior dislocation: MR imaging and MR arthrographic findings with arthroscopic correlation. AJR 1998;171:763–8.

81. Workman TK, Burkhard TK, Resnick D, et al. Hill-Sachs lesion: comparison of detection with MR imaging, radiography, and arthroscopy. Radiology 1992;185:847–52.

82. Jin W, Ryu KN, Park YK, Lee WK, Ko SH, Yang DM. Cystic lesions in the posterosuperior portion of the humeral head on MR arthrography: correlations with gross and histologic findings in cadavers. AJR Am J Roentgenol 2005;184:1211–15.

83. Richards RD, Sartoris DJ, Pathria MN, Resnick D. Hill-Sachs lesion and normal humeral groove: MR imaging features allowing their differentiation. Radiology 1994;190:665–8.

84. Jobe CM. Posterior superior glenoid impingement: expanded spectrum. Arthroscopy 1995;11:530–6.

85. Walch G, Boileau P, Noel E, Donell ST. Impingement of the deep surface of the supraspinatus tendon on the posterosuperior glenoid rim: an arthroscopic study. Shoulder Elbow Surg 1992;1:238–45.

86. Liu SH, Boynton E. Posterior superior impingement of the rotator cuff on the glenoid rim as a cause of shoulder pain in the overhead athlete. Arthroscopy 1993;9:697–9.

87. Tirman PFJ, Bost F, Garvin GJ, et al. Posterosuperior glenoid impingement of the shoulder: findings at MR imaging and MR arthrography with arthroscopic correlation. Radiology 1994;193:431–6.

88. Weishaupt D, Zanetti M, Nyffeler RW, et al. Posterior glenoid rim deficiency in recurrent (atraumatic) posterior shoulder instability. Skeletal Radiol 2000;29:204.

89. Tirman PFJ, Feller JF, Janzen DL, Peterfy CG, Bergman AG. Association of glenoid labral cysts with labral tears and glenohumeral instability: radiologic findings and clinical significance. Radiology 1994;190:653–8.

90. Fritz R, Helms CA, Steinbach LS, et al. MR imaging of suprascapular nerve entrapment. Radiology 1992;182:437–44.

91. Sanders TG, Tirman PFJ. Paralabral cyst: an unusual cause of quadrilateral space syndrome. Arthroscopy 1999;15:632–7.

92. Visser CP, Coene LN, Brand R, Tavy DL. The incidence of nerve injury in anterior dislocation of the shoulder and its influence on functional recovery. A prospective clinical and EMG study. J Bone Joint Surg Br 1999;81:679–85.

93. Nobuhara K, Hitoshi I. Rotator interval lesion. Clin Orthp Rel Res 1987;223:44.

94. Snyder SJ, Karzel RP, Del Pizzo W, Ferkel RD, Friedman MJ. SLAP lesions of the shoulder. Arthroscopy 1990;6:274–9.

95. Andrews JR, Carson WG, McLeod WD. Glenoid labrum tears related to the long head of the biceps. Am J Sports Med 1985;13:337–41.

96. Hunter JC, Blatz DJ, Escobedo EM. SLAP lesions of the glenoid labrum: CT arthrographic and arthroscopic correlation. Radiology 1992;184:513–8.

97. Waldt S, Burkart A, Lange P, Imhoff AB, Rummeny EJ, Woertler K. Diagnostic performance of MR arthrography in the assessment of superior labral anteroposterior lesions of the shoulder. AJR Am J Roentgenol 2004;182:1271–8.

98. Rames RD, Karzel RP. Injuries to the glenoid labrum, including SLAP lesions. Orthop Clin North Am 1993;24:45–53.

99. Neer CS. Anterior acromioplasty for the chronic impingement syndrome in the shoulder. J Bone Joint Surg 1972;54–A:41–50.

100. Watson M. Rotator cuff function in the impingement syndrome. J Bone Joint Surg 1989;71–B:361–6.

101. Morrison DS, Bigliani LU. The clinical significance of variations in acromial morphology. Orthop Trans 1986;11:234.

102. Edelson JG, Taitz C. Anatomy of the coraco-acromial arch. Relation to degeneration of the acromion. J Bone Joint Surg 1992;74B:589.

103. Gill TJ, McIrvin E, Kocher MS, Homa K, Mair SD, Hawkins RJ. The relative importance of acromial morphology and age with respect to rotator cuff pathology. J Shoulder Elbow Surg 2002;11:327–30.

104. Hirano M, Ide J, Takagi K. Acromial shapes and extension of rotator cuff tears: magnetic resonance imaging evaluation. J Shoulder Elbow Surg 2002;11:576–8.

105. Aoki M, Ishii S, Usui M. The slope of the acromion and rotator cuff impingement. Proc Am Shoulder Elbow Surg 1986.

106. Kieft GJ, Bloem JL, Rozing PM, Obermann WR. Rotator cuff impingement syndrome: MR imaging. Radiology 1988;166:211–4.

107. Chandnani V, Ho C, Gerharter J, et al. MR findings in asymptomatic shoulders: a blind analysis using symptomatic shoulders as controls. Clin Imaging 1992;16:25–30.

108. Farley TE, Neumann CH, Steinbach LS, Jahnke AJ, Petersen SS. Full-thickness tears of the rotator cuff of the shoulder: diagnosis with MR imaging. AJR 1992;158:347–51.

109. Liou JTS, Wilson AJ, Totty WG, Brown JJ. The normal shoulder: common variations that simulate pathologic conditions at MR imaging. Radiology 1993;186:435–41.

110. Mudge MK, Wood VE, Frykman GK. Rotator cuff tears associated with os acromiale. J Bone Joint Surg 1984;66–A:427–429.

111. Liberson F. Os acromiale: a contested anomaly. J Bone Joint Surg 1937;19:683–9.

112. Edelson JG, Zuckerman J, Hershkovitz I. Os acromiale: anatomy and surgical implications. J Bone Joint Surg 1993;74–B:551–555.

113. Andrews JR, Byrd TJW, Kupfferman SP, Angelo RL. The profile view of the acromion. Clin Orthop 1991;263.

114. McClure JG, Raney RB. Anomalies of the scapula. Clin Orthop 1975;110:22–31.

115. Kjellin I, Ho CP, Cervilla V, et al. Alterations in the supraspinatus tendon at MR imaging: correlation with histopathologic findings in cadavers. Radiology 1991;181:837–41.

116. Rafii M, Firooznia H, Sherman O. Rotator cuff lesions: signal patterns at MR imaging. Radiology 1990;177:817–23.

117. Robertson PL, Schweitzer ME, Mitchell DG, et. al. Rotator cuff disorders: interobserver and intraobserver variation in diagnosis with MR imaging. Radiology 1995;1995:831–5.

118. Burns WC, Whipple TL. Anatomic relationships in the shoulder impingement syndrome. Clin Orthop Rel Res 1993:96–102.

119. Sarkar K, Taine W, Uhthoff HK. The ultrastructure of the coracoacromial ligament in patients with chronic impingement syndrome. Clin Orthop Rel Res 1990:49–54.

120. Gallino M, Battiston B, Annartone G, Terragnoli F. Coracoacromial ligament: a comparative arthroscopic and anatomic study. Arthroscopy 1995;11:564–7.

121. Morimoto K, Mori E, Nakagawa Y. Calcification of the coracoacromial ligament. A case report of the shoulder impingement syndrome. Am J Sports Med 1988;16:80.

122. Sonnery-Cottet B, Edwards TB, Noel E, Walch G. Results of arthroscopic treatment of posterosuperior glenoid impingement in tennis players. Am J Sports Med 2002;30:227–32.

123. Budoff JE, Nirschl RP, Ilahi OA, Rodin DM. Internal impingement in the etiology of rotator cuff tendinosis revisited. Arthroscopy 2003;19:810–4.

124. Gerber C, Terrier F, Ganz R. The role of the coracoid process in the chronic impingement syndrome. J Bone Joint Surg 1985;67B:703.

125. Dines DM, Warren RF, Inglis AE, Pavlov H. The coracoid impingement syndrome. J Bone Joint Surg 1990;72–B:314–6.

126. Giaroli EL, Major NM, Lemley DE, Lee J. Coracohumeral interval imaging in subcoracoid impingement syndrome on MRI. AJR Am J Roentgenol 2006;186:242–6.

127. Habermeyer P, Magosch P, Pritsch M, Scheibel MT, Lichtenberg S. Anterosuperior impingement of the shoulder as a result of pulley lesions: a prospective arthroscopic study. J Shoulder Elbow Surg 2004;13:5–12.

128. Gerber C, Sebesta A. Impingement of the deep surface of the subscapularis tendon and the reflection pulley on the anterosuperior glenoid rim: a preliminary report. J Shoulder Elbow Surg 2000;9:483–90.

129. Le Huec JC, Schaeverbeke T, Moinard M, et al. Traumatic tear of the rotator interval. J Shoulder Elbow Surg 1996;5:41–6.

130. Krief OP. MRI of the rotator interval capsule. AJR Am J Roentgenol 2005;184:1490–4.

131. Beall DP, Williamson EE, Ly JQ, et al. Association of biceps tendon tears with rotator cuff abnormalities: degree of correlation with tears of the anterior and superior portions of the rotator cuff. AJR Am J Roentgenol 2003;180:633–9.

132. Morag Y, Jacobson JA, Shields G, et al. MR arthrography of rotator interval, long head of the biceps brachii, and biceps pulley of the shoulder. Radiology 2005;235:21–30.

133. Mirowitz SA. Normal rotator cuff: MR imaging with conventional and fat-suppression techniques. Radiology 1991;180:735–40.

134. Ellman H. Diagnosis and treatment of incomplete rotator cuff tears. Clin Orthop Rel Res 1990;254:64–74.

135. Tamai K, Ogawa K. Intratendinous tears of the supraspinatus tendon exhibiting winging of the scapula. Clin Orthop Rel Res 1985;194:159.

136. Ruotolo C, Fow JE, Nottage WM. The supraspinatus footprint: an anatomic study of the supraspinatus insertion. Arthroscopy 2004;20:246–9.

137. Millstein ES, Snyder SJ. Arthroscopic management of partial, full-thickness, and complex rotator cuff tears: indications, techniques, and complications. Arthroscopy 2003;19(suppl 1):189–99.

138. Conway JE. Arthroscopic repair of partial-thickness rotator cuff tears and SLAP lesions in professional baseball players. Orthop Clin North Am 2001;32:443–56.

139. Hodler J, Kursunoglu-Brahme S, Snyder SJ, et al. Rotator cuff disease: assessment with MR arthrography versus standard MR imaging in 36 patients with arthroscopic confirmation. Radiology 1992;182:431–6.

140. Palmer WE, Brown JH, Rosenthal DI. Rotator cuff: evaluation with fat-suppressed MR arthrography. Radiology 1993;1993:683–7.

141. Burk DL Jr, Karasick D, Mitchell DG, et al. Rotator cuff tears: prospective comparison of MR imaging with arthrography, sonography, and surgery. AJR 1989;152:87–92.

142. Kaplan PA, Bryans KC, Davick JP, Otte M, Stinson WW, Dussault RG. MR imaging of the normal shoulder: variants and pitfalls. Radiology 1992;184:519–24.

143. Tsai JC, Zlatkin MB. Magnetic resonance imaging of the shoulder. Radiol Clin North Am 1990;28:279–91.

144. Ianotti JP, Zlatkin MB, Esterhai JL, et al. Magnetic resonance imaging of the shoulder. J Bone Joint Surg 1991;73–A:17–29.

145. Neumann CH, Holt RG, Steinbach LS, Jahnke AH, Petersen SA. MR imaging of the shoulder: appearance of the supraspinatus tendon in asymptomatic volunteers. AJR 1992;158:1281–7.

146. Mitchell MJ, Causey G, Berthoty DP, et al. Peribursal fat plane of the shoulder: anatomic study and clinical experience. Radiology 1988;168:699–704.

147. Major NM. MR imaging after therapeutic injection of the subacromial bursa. Skeletal Radiol 1999;28:628–31.

148. Bergman AG, Fredericson M. Shoulder MRI after impingement test injection. Skeletal Radiol 1998;27:365–8.

149. Wright RW, Fritts HM, Tierney GS, Buss DD. MR imaging of the shoulder after an impingement test: how long to wait. AJR Am J Roentgenol 1998;171:769–73.

150. Sanders TG, Tirman PF, Feller JF, Genant HK. Association of intramuscular cysts of the rotator cuff with tears of the rotator cuff: magnetic resonance imaging findings and clinical significance. Arthroscopy 2000;16:230–5.

151. Kassarjian A, Torriani M, Ouellette H, Palmer WE. Intramuscular rotator cuff cysts: association with tendon tears on MRI and arthroscopy. AJR Am J Roentgenol 2005;185:160–5.

152. Bryan W, Wild J. Isolated infraspinatus atrophy. Am J Sports Med 1989;17:130–3.

153. Ferrari JD, Ferrari DA, Coumas J, Pappas AM. Posterior ossification of the shoulder: the Bennett lesion. Am J Sports Med 1994;22:171–6.

154. Symeonides PP. The significance of the subscapularis muscle in the pathogenesis of recurrent anterior dislocation of the shoulder. J Bone Joint Surg Br 1972;54:476–83.

155. Sakurai G, Ozaki J, Tomita Y, Kondo T, Tamai S. Incomplete tears of the subscapularis tendon associated with tears of the supraspinatus tendon: cadaveric and clinical studies. J Shoulder Elbow Surg 1998;7:510–5.

156. Bergin D, Parker L, Zoga A, Morrison W. Abnormalities on MRI of the subscapularis tendon in the presence of a full-thickness supraspinatus tendon tear. AJR Am J Roentgenol 2006;186:454–9.

157. Gerber C, Krushell RJ. Isolated rupture of the tendon of the subscapularis muscle. J Bone Joint Srug 1991;73–B:389–94.

158. Chan TW, Dalinka MK, Kneeland BJ, Chevrot A. Biceps tendon dislocation: evaluation with MR imaging. Radiology 1991;179:649–52.

159. Cervilla V, Schweitzer ME, Ho C, Mott A, Kerr R, Resnick D. Medial dislocation of the biceps brachii tendon: appearance at MR imaging. Radiology 1991;180:523–6.

160. Seeger LL, Lubowitz J, Thomas BJ. Case report 815. Skeletal Radiol 1993;22:615–7.

161. Rockwood CA, Matsen FA, Wirth MA, et al. The Shoulder, 3rd ed. Philadelphia: Elsevier, 2004.

162. Lintner SA, Speer KP. Traumatic anterior glenohumeral instability: the role of arthroscopy. J Am Acad Orthop Surg 1997;5:233–9.

163. Burkart AC, Debski RE. Anatomy and function of the glenohumeral ligaments in anterior shoulder instability. CORR 2002;400:32–9.

164. Bankart ASB. Recurrent or habitual dislocation of the shoulder joint. Br Med J 1923;2:1132–3.

165. Pollack RG, Wang VM, Bucchieri JS, et al. Effects of repetitive subfailure strains on the mechanical behavior of the inferior glenohumeral ligament. J Shoulder Elbow Surg 2000;9:427–35.

166. Wischer TK, Bredella MA, Genant HK, et al. Perthes lesion (a variant of the Bankart lesion): MR imaging and MR arthrographic findings with surgical correlation. AJR 2002;178:233–7.

167. Neviaser TJ. The anterior labroligamentous periosteal sleeve avulsion lesion: a cause of anterior instability of the shoulder. Arthroscopy 1993;9:17–21.

168. Bokor DJ, Conboy VB, Olson C. Anterior instability of the glenohumeral joint with humeral avulsion of the glenohumeral ligament: review of 41 cases. J Bone Joint Surg Br 1999;81:93–6.

169. Wolf EM, Cheng JC, Dickson K. Humeral avulsion of glenohumeral ligaments as a cause of anterior shoulder instability. Arthroscopy 1995;11:600–7.

170. Burkhart SS, DeBeer JF. Traumatic glenohumeral bone defects and their relationship to failure of arthroscopic Bankart repairs: significance of the inverted-pear glenoid and the humeral engaging Hill-Sachs lesion. Arthroscopy 2000;16:677–94.

171. Neviaser RJ, Neviaser TJ, Neviaser JS. Concurrent rupture of the rotator cuff and anterior dislocation of the shoulder in the older patient. J Bone Joint Surg 1988;70:1308–11.

172. Ellenbecker TS, Bailie DS, Mattalino AJ, et al. Intrarater and interrater reliability of a manual technique to assess anterior humeral head translation of the glenohumeral joint. J Shoulder Elbow Surg 2002;11(5):470–5.

173. Itoi E, Sashi R, Minagawa H, et al. Position of immobilization after dislocation of the glenohumeral joint. J Bone Joint Surg 2001;83A:661–7.

174. Miller BS, Sonnabend DH, Hatrick C, et al. Should acute anterior dislocations of the shoulder be immobilized in external rotation? A cadaveric study. J Shoulder Elbow Surg 2004;13:589–92.

175. Hart WJ, Kelly CP. Arthroscopic observation of capsulolabral reduction after shoulder dislocation. J Shoulder Elbow Surg 2005;14:134–7.

176. Douoguih WA. Treatment of traumatic anterior shoulder instability in the contact and collision athlete. Curr Opin Orthop 2005;16:82–8.

177. Hall RH, Isaac F, Booth CR. Dislocations of the shoulder with special reference to accompanying small fractures. J Bone Joint Surg 1959;41:489–94.

178. Roukos JR, Feagin JA, Abbott HG. Modified axillary roentgenogram: a useful adjunct in the diagnosis of recurrent instability of the shoulder. CORR 1972;82:84–6.

179. Garneau RA, Renfrew DL, Moore TE, et al. Glenoid labrum: evaluation with MR imaging. Radiology 1991;179:519–22.

180. Iannotti JP, Zlatkin MB, Esterhai JL, et al. Magnetic resonance imaging of the shoulder: sensitivity, specificity and predictive value. J Bone Joint Surg 1991;73:17–29.

181. Legan JM, Burkhard TK, Goff WB, et al. Tears of the glenoid labrum: MR imaging of 88 arthroscopically confirmed cases. Radiology 1991;179:241–6.

182. Green MR and Christensen KP. Magnetic resonance imaging of the glenoid labrum in anterior shoulder instability. Am J Sports Med 1994;22:493–8.

183. Gusmer PB, Potter HG, Schatz JA, et al. Labral injuries: accuracy of detection with unenhanced MR imaging of the shoulder. Radiology 1996;200:519–24.

184. Chandnani VP, Yeager TD, DeBerardino T, et al. Glenoid labral tears: prospective evaluation with MR imaging, MR arthrography, and CT arthrography. AJR 1993;161:1229–35.

185. Palmer WE, Brown JH, Rosenthal DI. Labral-ligamentous complex of the shoulder: evaluation with MR arthrography. Radiology 1994;190:645–51.

186. Palmer WE, Caslowitz PL. Anterior shoulder instability: diagnostic criteria determined from prospective analysis of 121 MR arthrograms. Radiology 1995;197:819–25.

187. Willemsen UF, Wiedemann E, Brunner U, et al. Prospective evaluation of MR arthrography performed with high-volume intraarticular saline enhancement in patients with recurrent anterior dislocations of the shoulder. AJR 1997;170:79–84.

188. Waldt S, Burkart A, Imhoff AB, et al. Anterior shoulder instability: accuracy of MR arthrography in the classification of anteroinferior labroligamentous injuries. Radiology 2005;237:578–83.

189. Cvitanic O, Tirman PF, Feller JF, et al. Using abduction and external rotation of the shoulder to increase the sensitivity of MR arthrography in revealing tears of the anterior glenoid labrum. AJR 1997;169:837–44.

190. Kwak SM, Brown RR, Trudell D, et al. Glenohumeral joint: comparison of shoulder positions at MR arthrography. Radiology 1998;208:375–80.

191. Wagner SC, Schweitzer ME, Morrison WB, et al. Shoulder instability: accuracy of MR imaging performed after surgery in depicting recurrent injury—initial findings. Radiology 2002;222:196–203.

192. Tung GA, Entzian D, Green A, et al. High-field and low-field MR imaging of superior glenoid labral tears and associated tendon injuries. AJR 2000;174:1107–14.

193. Pollock R, Bigliani L. Recurrent posterior shoulder instability. CORR 1993;291:85–96.

194. Rowe CR, Zarins B. Chronic unreduced dislocations of the shoulder. J Bone Joint Surg 1982;64A:494–505.

195. Bottoni CR, Franks BR, Moore JH, et al. Operative stabilization of posterior shoulder instability. Am J Sports Med 2005;33:996–1002.

196. Hottya GA, Tirman PF, Bost FW, et al. Tear of the posterior shoulder stabilizers after posterior dislocation: MR imaging and MR arthrographic findings with arthroscopic correlation. AJR 1998;171:763–8.

197. Yamaguchi K, Flatow EL. Management of multidirectional instability. Clin Sports Med 1995;14:885–902.

198. Palmer WE, Caslowitz PL, Chew FS. MR arthrography of the shoulder: normal intraarticular structures and common abnormalities. AJR 1995;164:141–6.

199. Smith DK, Chopp TM, Aufdemorte TB, et al. Sublabral recess of the superior glenoid labrum: study of cadavers with conventional nonenhanced MR imaging, MR arthrography, anatomic dissection, and limited histologic examination. Radiology 1996;201:251–6.

200. Park YH, Lee JY, Moon SH, et al. MR arthrography of the labral capsular ligamentous complex in the shoulder: imaging variations and pitfalls. AJR 2000;175:667–72.

201. Mohana-Borges AVR, Chung CB, Resnick D. Superior labral anteroposterior tear: classification and diagnosis on MRI and MR arthrography. AJR 2003;181:1449–62.

202. Williams MM, Snyder SJ, Buford D Jr. The Buford complex—the "cord-like" middle glenohumeral ligament and absent

anterosuperior labrum complex: a normal anatomic capsulolabral variant. Arthroscopy 1994;10:241–7.

203. Keefe DT, Lowe WR. Symptomatic superior labral anterior posterior lesion with absence of the long head of the biceps tendon. Am J Sports Med 2005;33:1746–50.

204. Snyder SJ, Karzel RP, DelPizzo W, et al. SLAP lesions of the shoulder. Arthroscopy 1990;6:274–9.

205. Burkhart SS, Morgan CD. The peel-back mechanism: its role in producing and extending posterior type II SLAP lesions and its effect on SLAP repair rehabilitation. Arthroscopy 1998;14:637–40.

206. Morag Y, Jacobson JA, Shields G, et al. MR arthrography of rotator interval, long head of the biceps brachii, and biceps pulley of the shoulder. Radiology 2005;235:21–30.

207. O'Brien SJ, Pagnani MJ, Fealy S, et al. The active compression test: a new and effective test for diagnosing labral tears and acromioclavicular joint abnormality. Am J Sports Med 1998;26:610–3.

208. Bennett WF. Specificity of the Speed's test: arthroscopic technique for evaluating the biceps tendon at the level of the bicipital groove. Arthroscopy 1998;14:789–96.

209. Nam EK, Snyder SJ. The diagnosis and treatment of superior labrum, anterior and posterior (SLAP) lesions. Am J Sports Med 2003;31:798–810.

210. Eakin CL, Faber KJ, Hawkins RJ, et al. Biceps tendon disorders in athletes. J Am Acad Orthop Surg 1999;7:300–10.

211. Sanders TG, Miller MD. A systematic approach to magnetic resonance imaging interpretation of sports medicine injuries of the shoulder. Am J Sports Med 2005;33:1088–105.

212. Tuite MJ, Cirillo RL, DeSmet AA, et al. Superior labral anterior-posterior (SLAP) tears: evaluation of three MR signs on T2–weighted images. Radiology 2000;215:841–5.

213. Spritzer CE, Collins AJ, Copperman A, et al. Assessment of instability of the long head of the biceps tendon by MRI. Skeletal Radiol 2001;30:199–207.

214. Yoneda M, Izawa K, Atsushi H, et al. Indicators of superior glenoid labral detachment on magnetic resonance imaging and computed tomography arthrography. J Shoulder Elbow Surg 1998;7(1):2–12.

215. Connell DA, Potter HG, Wickiewicz TL, et al. Noncontrast magnetic resonance imaging of superior labral lesions: 102 cases confirmed at arthroscopic surgery. Am J Sports Med 1999;27:208–13.

216. Bencardino JT, Beltran J, Rosenberg ZS, et al. Superior labrum anterior-posterior lesions: diagnosis with MR arthrography of the shoulder. Radiology 2000;214:267–71.

217. Jee W-H, McCauley TR, Katz LD, et al. Superior labral anterior posterior (SLAP) lesions of the glenoid labrum: reliability and accuracy of MR arthrography for diagnosis. Radiology 2001;218:127–32.

218. Applegate GR, Hewitt M, Snyder SJ, et al. Chronic labral tears: value of magnetic resonance arthrography in evaluating the glenoid labrum and labral-bicipital complex. Arthroscopy 2004;20:959–63.

219. Magee T, Williams D, Mani N. Shoulder MR arthrography: which patient group benefits most? AJR 2004;183:969–74.

220. Zanetti M, Weishaupt D, Gerber C, et al. Tendinopathy and rupture of the tendon of the long head of the biceps brachii muscle: evaluation with MR arthrography. AJR 1998;170:1557–61.

221. Lee SB, Kim KJ, O'Driscoll SW, et al. Dynamic glenohumeral stability provided by the rotator cuff muscles in the mid-range and end-range of motion: a study in cadavera. J Bone Joint Surg 2000;82–A:849–57.

222. Neer CS. Anterior acromioplasty for the chromic impingement syndrome in the shoulder. J Bone Joint Surg 1972;54A:41–50.

223. Watson M. Rotator cuff function in the impingement syndrome. J Bone Joint Surg Br 1989;71:361–6.

224. Uhthoff HK, and Sano H. Pathology of failure of the rotator cuff tendon. Orthop Clin North Am 1997;28:31–41.

225. Walch G, Boileau J, Noel E, et al. Impingement of the deep surface of the supraspinatus tendon on the posterior superior glenoid rim: an arthroscopic study. J Shoulder Elbow Surg 1992;1:238–43.

226. Paley KJ, Jobe FW, Pink MM, et al. Arthroscopic findings in the overhand throwing athlete: evidence for posterior internal impingement of the rotator cuff. Arthroscopy 2000;16:35–40.

227. Jobe CM. Posterior superior glenoid impingement: expanded spectrum. Arthroscopy 1995;11:530–6.

228. Lo IKY, Burkhart SS. The etiology and assessment of subscapularis tendon tears: a case for subcoracoid impingement, the roller-wringer effect, and TUFF lesions of the subscapularis. Arthroscopy 2003;19:1142–50.

229. Goutallier D, Postel JM, Bernageau J, et al. Fatty muscle degeneration in cuff ruptures: pre- and post-operative evaluation by CT scan. CORR 1994;304:78–83.

230. Mathews PV, Glousman RE. Accuracy of subacromial injection: anterolateral versus posterior approach. J Shoulder Elbow Surg 2005;14:145–8.

231. Itoi E, Minagawa H, Yamamoto N, et al. Are pain location and physical examinations useful in locating a tear site of the rotator cuff? Am J Sports Med 2006;34:256–64.

232. Giaroli EL, Major NM, Lemley DE, et al. Coracohumeral interval imaging in subcoracoid impingement syndrome on MRI. AJR 2006;186:242–6.

233. Kibler WB, McMullen J. Scapular dyskinesis and its relation to shoulder pain. J Am Acad Orthop Surg 2003;11:142–51.

234. Weiner DS. Superior migration of the humeral head: a radiologic aid in the diagnosis of tears of the rotator cuff. J Bone Joint Surg Br 1970;52B:524–7.

235. Bigliani LU, Morrison D, April EW. The morphology of the acromion and its relationship to rotator cuff tears. Orthop Trans 1986;10:228.

236. Zanca P. Shoulder pain: involvement of the acromioclavicular joint: analysis of 1000 cases. AJR 1971;112:493–506.

237. Teefey SA, Rubin DA, Middleton WD, et al. Detection and quantification of rotator cuff tears: comparison of ultrasonographic, magnetic resonance imaging, and arthroscopic findings in seventy-one consecutive cases. J Bone Joint Surg 2004;86A:708–16.

238. Palmer WE, Brown JH, Rosenthal DI. Rotator cuff: evaluation with fat-suppressed MR arthrography. Radiology 1993;188:683–7.

239. Singson RD, Hoang T, Dan S, et al. MR evaluation of rotator cuff pathology using T2–weighted fast spin-echo technique with and without fat-suppression. AJR 1996;166:1061–5.

240. Parsa M, Tuite M, Norris M, et al. MR imaging of rotator cuff tendon tears: comparison of T2–weighted gradient-echo and conventional dual-echo sequences. AJR 1997;168:1519–24.

241. Seibold CJ, Mallisee TA, Erickson SJ, et al. Rotator cuff: evaluation with US and MR imaging. Radiographics 1999;19:685–705.

242. Tirman PFJ, Bost FW, Garvin GJ, et al. Posterosuperior glenoid impingement of the shoulder: findings at MR imaging and MR arthrography with arthroscopic correlation. Radiology 1994;193:431–36.

243. Meister K, Thesing J, Montgomery WJ, et al. MR arthrography of partial thickness tears of the undersurface of the rotator cuff: an arthroscopic correlation. Skeletal Radiol 2004;33:136–41.

244. Toyoda H, Ito Y, Tomo H, et al. Evaluation of rotator cuff tears with magnetic resonance arthrography. CORR 439:109–15.

245. Schaefer O, Winterer J, Lohrmann C, et al. Magnetic resonance imaging for supraspinatus muscle atrophy after cuff repair. CORR 2002;403:93–9.

246. Miniaci A, Mascia AT, Salonen DC, et al. Magnetic resonance imaging of the shoulder in asymptomatic professional baseball pitchers. Am J Sports Med 2002;30:66–73.

247. Jost B, Zumstein M, Pfirrmann CWA, et al. MRI findings in throwing shoulders. CORR 2005;434:130–7.

248. Kaplan LD, McMahon PJ, Towers J, et al. Internal impingement: findings on magnetic resonance imaging and arthroscopic evaluation. Arthroscopy 2004;20:701–4.

249. Giaroli EL, Major NM, Higgins LD. MRI of internal impingement of the shoulder. AJR 2005;185:925–9.

250. Richards DP, Burkhart SS, Campbell SE. Relation between narrowed coracohumeral distance and subscapularis tears. Arthroscopy 2005;21:1223–8.

251. Zlatkin MB, Iannotti JP, Roberts MC, et al. Rotator cuff tears: diagnostic performance of MR imaging. Radiology 1989;172:223–9.

252. Davidson JFJ, Burkhart SS, Richards DP, et al. Use of preoperative magnetic resonance imaging to predict rotator cuff tear pattern and method of repair. Arthroscopy 2005;21:1428e1–e10.

253. Pfirrmann CW, Zanetti M, Weishaupt D, et al. Subscapularis tendon tears: detection and grading at MR arthrography. Radiology 1999;213:709–14.

254. Tirman PFJ, Bost FW, Steinbach LS, et al. MR arthrographic depiction of tears of the rotator cuff: benefit of abduction and external rotation of the arm. Radiology 1994;192:851–6.

255. Lee SY, Lee JK. Horizontal component of partial-thickness tears of the rotator cuff: imaging characteristics and comparison of ABER view with oblique coronal view at MR arthrography—initial results. Radiology 2002;224:470–6.

256. Chen C-H, Hsu K-Y, Chen W-J, et al. Incidence and severity of biceps long-head tendon lesion in patients with complete rotator cuff tears. J Trauma 2005;58:1189–93.

257. Beall DP, Williamson EE, Ly JQ, et al. Association of biceps tendon tears with rotator cuff abnormalities: degree of correlation with tears of the anterior and superior portions of the rotator cuff. AJR 2003;180:633–9.

258. Petilon J, Carr DR, Sekiya JK, et al. Pectoralis major muscle injuries: evaluation and management. J Am Acad Orthop Surg 2005;13:59–68.

259. Schepsis AA, Grafe MW, Jones HP, et al. Rupture of the pectoralis major muscle: outcome after repair of acute and chronic injuries. Am J Sports Med 2000;28:9–15.

260. Lee J, Brookenthal KR, Ramsey ML, et al. MR imaging assessment of the pectoralis major myotendinous unit: an MR imaging-anatomic correlative study with surgical correlation. AJR 2000;174:1371–5.

261. Connell DA, Potter HG, Sherman MF, et al. Injuries of the pectoralis major muscle: evaluation with MR imaging. Radiology 1999;210:785–91.

262. Zvijac JE, Schurhoff MR, Hechtman KS, et al. Pectoralis major tears: correlation of magnetic resonance imaging and treatment strategies. Am J Sports Med 2006;34(2):289–94.

263. Thomas BE, McMullen GM, Yuan HA. Cervical spine injuries in football players. J Am Acad Orthop Surg 1999;7:338–47.

264. Koffler KM, Kelly JD. Neurovascular trauma in athletes. Orthop Clin North Am 2002;33:523–34.

265. Helms CA, Martinez S, Speer KP. Acute brachial neuritis (Parsonage-Turner syndrome): MR imaging appearance—report of three cases. Radiology 1998;207:255–9.

266. Perlmutter GS. Axillary nerve injury. CORR 1999;368:28–36.

267. Cothran RL, Helms CA. Quadrilateral space syndrome: incidence of imaging findings in a population referred for MRI of the shoulder. AJR 2005;184:989–92.

268. Cahill B, Palmer R. Quadrilateral space syndrome. J Hand Surg 1983;8:65–9.

269. Linker CS, Helms CA, Fritz RC. Quadrilateral space syndrome: findings at MR imaging. Radiology 1993;188:675–6.

270. Fritz RC, Helms CA, Steinbach LS, et al. Suprascapular nerve entrapment: evaluation with MR imaging. Radiology 1992;182:437–44.

271. Neviaser TJ. The GLAD lesion: another cause of anterior shoulder pain. Arthroscopy 1993;9:22–3.

272. Sanders TG, Tirman PFJ, Linares R, et al. The glenolabral articular disruption lesion: MR arthrography with arthroscopic correlation. AJR 1999;172:171–5.

273. Neviaser JS. Adhesive capsulitis of the shoulder: a study of the pathological findings in periarthritis of the shoulder. J Bone Joint Surg 1945;27:211–22.

274. Neviaser TJ. Adhesive Capsulitis. In: McGinty JB, Caspari RB, Jackson RW, Poehling GG, eds. Operative Arthroscopy. Philadelphia: Lippincott-Raven, 1996:785–91.

275. Mengiardi B, Pfirrmann CW, Gerber C, et al. Frozen shoulder: MR arthrographic findings. Radiology 2004;233:486–92.

276. Lefevre-Colau MM, Drape JL, Fayad F, et al. Magnetic resonance imaging of shoulders with idiopathic adhesive capsulitis: reliability of measures. Eur Radiol 2005;15:2415–22.

277. De Abreu MR, Chung CB, Wessely M, et al. Acromioclavicular joint osteoarthritis: comparison of findings derived from MR imaging and conventional radiography. Clin Imaging 2005;29:273–7.

278. Stein BE, Wiater JM, Pfaff HC, et al. Detection of acromioclavicular joint pathology in asymptomatic shoulders with magnetic resonance imaging. J Shoulder Elbow Surg 2001;10:204–8.

279. Tshering Vogel DW, Steinbach LS, Hertel R, et al. Acromioclavicular joint cyst: nine cases of a pseudotumor of the shoulder. Skeletal Radiol 2005;34:260–5.

280. Yu YS, Dardani M, Fischer RA. MR observations of posttraumatic osteolysis of the distal clavicle after traumatic separation of the acromioclavicular joint. J Comput Assist Tomogr 2000;24:159–64.

281. De la Puente R, Boutin RD, Theodorou DJ, et al. Post-traumatic and stress-induced osteolysis of the distal clavicle: MR imaging findings in 17 patients. Skeletal Radiol 1999;28:202–8.

6
Elbow

A. Radiologic Perspective: Magnetic Resonance Imaging Evaluation of Sports-Related Injury to the Elbow

Romulo Baltazar, Benjamin May, and Javier Beltran

Injury to the myotendinous, ligamentous, osseus, and nervous structures of the elbow can result from acute macrotrauma or recurrent microtrauma. Acute macrotrauma primarily results from direct impact of the elbow with the ground, collision of an outstretched hand with the ground, or high intensity movement involving the elbow joint in an unconditioned individual. Recurrent or chronic repetitive microtrauma to the elbow is usually the result of either eccentric overuse of the extensors of the forearm or repetitive valgus stress overload, as occurs with overhead throwing or work-related tasks. In these settings, the ability of MRI to achieve superb soft tissue contrast is of particular utility. It can evaluate for and distinguish between myotendinous, ligamentous, osseus, cartilaginous, and nervous etiologies in the athlete who presents with non-specific symptoms.

Myotendinous Pathology

While some overlap exists, it is useful to group myotendinous injury of the elbow according to anatomic and, consequently, functional divisions. This approach promotes a structured understanding of pathology about the elbow joint and emphasizes the parallelism that exists between form and function. The lateral compartment of the elbow includes the supinator, the brachioradialis, and the common tendon of the extensor muscles of the hand and wrist, which arise from the lateral epicondyle. The medial compartment of the elbow includes the pronator teres and the common tendon of the flexor-pronator muscles of the hand and wrist. The most commonly seen pathology involving the tendons of the lateral and medial compartments of the elbow is tendinosis. This typically occurs in the setting of chronic repetitive microtrauma, as seen in work-related and sports-related overuse stress. Acute disruption is also seen but less frequently and more so in the case of the medial compartment than of the lateral compartment. The anterior compartment of the elbow includes the biceps and the brachialis muscles. The posterior compartment includes the triceps and the anconeus muscles. In contrast to pathology within the lateral and medial compartments, the most commonly seen pathology involving the tendons in the anterior and posterior compartments of the elbow is rupture due to acute macrotrauma. This usually occurs in the setting of pre-existing changes that weaken the tendon attachments, though the individuals may have been totally asymptomatic prior to rupture.

Magnetic resonance imaging (MRI) offers excellent soft tissue contrast detection and is extremely useful in diagnosing and directing treatment of myotendinous injury. Myotendinous injury has been characterized in terms of clinical stage and clinical grade with the MRI appearance paralleling the pathomorphologic changes. There are three stages of myotendinous injury. In acute injury, there is disruption of the muscle fibers and bleeding at the myotendinous juncture or avulsion of the tendon from the bony insertion. In recurrent injury, there are microtears at the myotendinous juncture or within the tendon. Without an adequate period of recovery and repair, these microtears will scar and the tendon will demonstrate decreased flexibility and increased predisposition to reinjury. In chronic injury, the myotendinous structures experience progressive myotendinous mucoid degeneration and angiofibrotic hyperplasia.[1-5] This process is referred to as tendinosis (or tendinopathy).

On MRI, tendons normally appear as smooth linear extensions of uniformly very low signal on T1- and T2-weighted images. They are prominent against a background of subcutaneous fat. In tendinosis, the tendon demonstrates a bulbous morphology and increased signal on T1-weighted images and decreased signal on T2-weighted images. A partially torn tendon demonstrates a focus of increased signal on T2-weighted images. A completely torn tendon demonstrates focal discontinuity with or without retraction and tendon redundancy. The void left by the disrupted tendon is filled by high signal on T2-weighted images. In all three cases, the tendinous finding may be accompanied by adjacent traumatic effusion, the degree of which reflects the acuteness of the injury. Traumatic effusion manifests on magnetic resonance (MR) as high signal surrounding the injured tendon or interdigitating between intact myotendinous fibers on T2-weighted images.

Normal Anatomy of the Lateral Compartment

The lateral compartment structures include the supinator, the brachioradialis, and the common tendon of the extensor muscles of the hand and wrist, which arise from the lateral epicondyle. These muscles are best seen on coronal and axial MRI. The wrist extensor tendons assist in the stabilization of the elbow against varus stress. Upon repetitive varus stress, the musculotendinous complex may be subjected to eccentric loading and potential overuse.

Lateral Epicondylitis ("Tennis Elbow")

Lateral epicondylitis is chronic overuse tendinopathy of the extensor muscles of the hand and wrist related to eccentric overuse of the extensors of the forearm[6] and less commonly varus stress overload. It is the most commonly encountered

sports-related injury to the elbow. While originally described in a tennis player[7] (hence the term *tennis elbow*)l, it is much more commonly seen in the general population as the result of repetitive work-related activity.[6,8] As many as 50% of athletes involved in overhead-throwing sports go on to develop lateral epicondylitis.[9] Patients present with lateral elbow pain that is insidious in onset and progressive in course. They complain of pain gripping, especially heavy objects, though the pain can progressively become constant. On pathology, there is degeneration and tearing of the common extensor tendon. The extensor carpi radialis brevis tendon is the most frequently injured structure and may be partially avulsed from the lateral epicondyle leading to scar formation.[1] Lateral epicondylitis may be associated with injury to the lateral collateral ligament complex (discussed in greater detail below). This relationship should not surprise; the common extensor tendon works closely with the lateral collateral ligament complex both spatially and functionally.

Magnetic resonance imaging is useful in making the initial diagnosis and in grading the severity of a myotendinous injury.[10] This includes the degree of tendon damage and the presence of associated ligamentous or osseous abnormality. Thus, its role may help direct medical or surgical management.

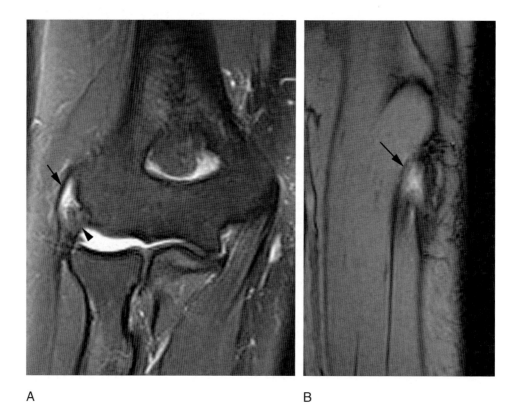

A   B

FIG. 6.1. Lateral epicondylitis. Coronal T2 (A) and sagittal gradient echo (GRE) (B) images demonstrate focal area of increase signal intensity in the region of the common extensor tendons (arrows). There is some thickening and irregularity of the radial collateral ligament (arrowhead in A) representing degeneration.

The common extensor tendon must be scrutinized on coronal MRI in terms of morphology and signal intensity. Tendinopathy manifests as thickening or thinning of the tendon and high signal on T2-weighted images at the attachment onto the lateral epicondyle. This high signal may extend into the common extensor muscle mass. Partial tears are evident when hyperintensity is seen on T2-weighted images (Fig. 6.1). Complete tears are identified as a focal segment of discontinuity with a fluid-filled gap in the expected site of tendon attachment. Finally, the lateral collateral ligament complex,[9] the anconeus muscle,[11] and the radial nerve[7] must be evaluated since concomitant injury may exist. These entities are discussed in greater detail in the next section. Treatment is discussed in the orthopedic section of the chapter.

Normal Anatomy of the Medial Compartment

The medial compartment structures include the pronator teres and common tendon of the flexor-pronator muscles of the hand and wrist, which arise from the medial epicondyle.[12] These muscles are best seen on coronal and axial MRI. The wrist flexor-pronator tendons assist in stabilizing the elbow against valgus stress. Upon repetitive valgus stress, the musculotendinous complex may be subjected to overuse.

Medial Epicondylitis ("Golfer's Elbow")

Medial epicondylitis is chronic overuse tendinopathy of the flexor-pronator muscles of the hand and wrist. It is seen much less commonly than lateral epicondylitis[13]; however, it occurs more commonly in professional tennis players than does lateral epicondylitis (tennis elbow). It is thought to result from repetitive valgus stress, such as that seen in sports and work-related tasks involving grasping and carrying, causing overload of the pronator-flexor muscle group. Not surprisingly, it is alternatively referred to in the literature as "golfer's elbow" and "medial tennis elbow" and is known also to occur in bowlers, javelin throwers, racquetball players, and swimmers.[12] Patients present with medial elbow pain that is insidious in onset and progressive in course. It may result in pain with gripping, and may also result in concomitant ulnar nerve symptoms, such as numbness in the ulnar digits and hand. Pathology involving the common flexor tendon parallels that of the common extensor tendon and ranges from tendinosis to partial and complete tears. However, unlike the common extensor tendon, the common flexor tendon is more susceptible to acute disruption.[7] In either case, the close spatial and functional relationship of the common flexor tendon to the ulnar collateral ligament complex renders the two susceptible to concomitant injury.[14,15] Injury to the ulnar nerve is also commonly seen in this context.[14,16] These entities are discussed in greater detail below.

Magnetic resonance imaging is useful in identifying the injury, grading its severity, and assessing the integrity of the underlying ulnar collateral ligament complex. Preoperative MRI delineates the anatomy and facilitates surgical planning, obviating the need for extensive surgical exploration. As in lateral epicondylitis, medial epicondylitis manifests on coronal MRI as tendinopathy, partial tear, and tendon disruption. As above, tendinopathy manifests as thickening or thinning of the tendon with high signal on T1-weighted images within the tendon. A partial tear appears as a focus of high signal on T2-weighted images (Fig. 6.2). Complete tears are identified when a fluid-filled gap is present in the expected site of tendon attachment.

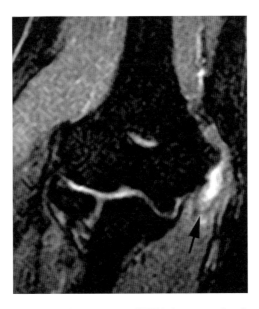

FIG. 6.2. Medial epicondylitis. Coronal short-tau inversion recovery (STIR) demonstrating focal area of increased signal intensity in the region of the common flexor tendons (arrow).

Normal Anatomy of the Anterior Compartment

The structures that comprise the anterior compartment of the elbow include the biceps and brachialis muscles. The biceps is the most powerful supinator of the forearm, while also assisting in elbow flexion. It lies superficially within the anterior compartment and inserts distally at the radial tuberosity. The distal tendon is notable for the absence of any surrounding muscle. In addition to its superficial location, the tendon has an area of relative hypovascularity just proximal to its insertion onto the radial tuberosity.[17] These characteristics render it susceptible to injury and makes it the most commonly torn tendon in the elbow. The bicipital aponeurosis, also referred to as the lacertus fibrosis, originates from the biceps tendon, extends across the flexor-pronator group of muscles superficially, and inserts on the antebrachial fascia. The brachialis is the primary flexor of the forearm. It lies deep to the biceps, abuts the joint capsule anteriorly, and inserts on the ulnar tuberosity. The distal brachialis tendon is surrounded by muscle. Subsequently, injury to the brachialis muscle is less common than to the biceps. The two muscles are best seen on sagittal and axial MRI.

Distal Rupture of the Biceps Tendon

As in any tendon, the entire spectrum of injury to the biceps tendon is possible and has been reported in the literature, ranging from tendinosis to partial and complete tears.[1,5] In the case of the biceps tendon, however, the vast majority of cases are the result of acute injury and involve complete rupture, as the injury is a few millimeters proximal to the bony insertion. Distal rupture of the biceps tendon is at least ten times less common than proximal rupture.[18–20] It occurs as a result of a sudden, forceful overload with the elbow in mid-flexion. This is seen most commonly in male weight-lifters and rugby players.[19] One study has also identified smokers as a population at risk.[19] Anoxia is thought to weaken the tendon and cause fiber degeneration, weakening, and susceptibility to rupture (Figs. 6.3 and 6.4). Treatment is discussed in the orthopedic section of the chapter.

On MRI, the biceps tendon must be evaluated for abnormal morphology or signal intensity and, in the event of rupture, the lacertus fibrosis must be evaluated to assess the need for early operation. The appearance of biceps tendon pathology mimics those already discussed. The partially torn distal bicipital tendon demonstrates high signal on T2-weighted images in and adjacent to the tendon. The completely torn biceps tendon is retracted, forming a pseudotumor with a fluid-filled gap present in the expected site of tendon attachment (Fig. 6.3).

Strain of the Brachialis Tendon ("Climber's Elbow")

Strain of the brachialis tendon can result from (1) repetitive movement including climbing, pull-ups, and supination; or (2) traumatic blow to the tendon. It has been referred to as "climber's elbow."[7] Pathology of the brachialis is best seen on axial MRI with findings that parallel those of the tendinopathies, discussed above.

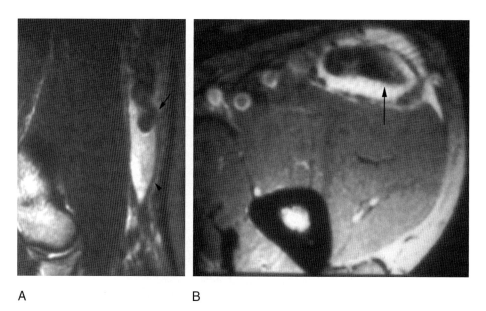

A   B

FIG. 6.3. (A–B) Complete rupture of the distal biceps tendon. Sagittal T2 (A) and axial T2 (B) images demonstrating the ruptured distal biceps tendon retracted proximally (arrows). Note the hematoma distally, contained within the peritenon (arrowhead in B).

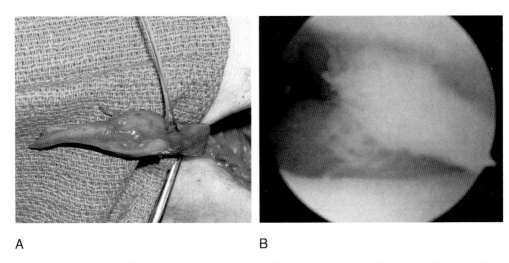

A   B

FIG. 6.4. (A) Surgical picture of a patient with a symptomatic partial distal biceps tendon rupture. Notice the bulbous end of the tendon indicating the degeneration that preceded the partial rupture. (B) View via tenoscopy of a partial distal biceps avulsion from the radial tuberosity.

Normal Anatomy of the Posterior Compartment

The structures that comprise the posterior compartment of the elbow include the triceps and the anconeus muscles. The triceps functions as the primary extensor of the forearm and inserts on the proximal olecranon. The anconeus, a small and functionally insignificant muscle, resists abduction of the ulna during pronation of the forearm. It lies within the lateral aspect of the posterior elbow, originating from the posterior aspect of the lateral epicondyle and inserting on the distal olecranon. The two muscles are best seen on sagittal and axial MRI. Of special note, the insertion of the triceps at the proximal olecranon is characterized by the presence of fibrofatty slips, which interdigitate between tendon fibers. These may be misidentified as partial tears by the novice MRI interpreter.

Rupture of the Triceps Tendon

Rupture of the triceps tendon is an uncommon cause of acute posterior elbow pain.[18,21] Seen most commonly in weight-lifters and football players, it may result from (1) decelerating counterforce during active extension or (2) a direct blow to the tendon. Disruption occurs at the site of insertion onto the proximal olecranon. It may be associated with steroid use, cortisone injections to the triceps tendon, total elbow arthroplasty, olecranon bursitis, subluxation of the ulnar nerve, or fracture of the radial head.[7]

Magnetic resonance imaging distinguishes between tendinosis, which also occurs only rarely, and tears.[6] It thus aids in making the diagnosis and doing preoperative planning. On MRI, evaluation of the triceps is sensitive to the degree of flexion, appearing taut on flexion and redundant in full extension. As above, the partially torn triceps tendon appears thickened or thinned with high signal on T2-weighted MRI. The completely torn triceps tendon is retracted to form a pseudotumor, and a fluid-filled gap is present in the expected site of tendon attachment (Fig. 6.5). Olecranon bursitis is evident on T2-weighted images when a well-defined high signal fluid collection is present posterior to the triceps tendon within the olecranon bursa.

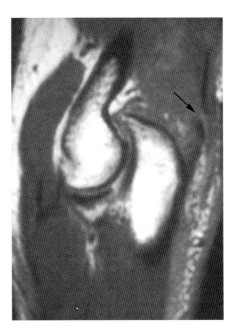

FIG. 6.5. Ruptured triceps tendon. Sagittal T1 image demonstrating a complete rupture of the triceps tendon with minimal tendon retraction (arrow).

Snapping Triceps Syndrome

First described in 1970, snapping triceps syndrome is the transient subluxation of the medial head of the triceps over the medial epicondyle during elbow flexion beyond 100 degrees.[22] The etiology is variable and may include congenital, developmental, and posttraumatic causes. It has also been described in weight-lifters in relation to hypertrophy of the triceps muscle.[23] Clinically, a painful snapping sensation is encountered as the tendon relocates during elbow extension from the flexed position.[24] Symptoms related to ulnar nerve neuropathy may also be present due to chronic nerve irritation given the close proximity of the cubital tunnel. This entity often coexists with ulnar nerve dislocation in which a double snap may be experienced. The diagnosis in this setting is key for preoperative planning since the patient's complaints may be rooted in both abnormalities. Correction of one without the other would result in persistent symptomatology. Individuals with symptomatic persistent snapping elbow are usually treated surgically by rerouting the medial head of the triceps.

While the argument has been made that ultrasound is the superior imaging tool in diagnosing snapping triceps syndrome,[25–27] the advantage of MRI in mapping the relevant elbow anatomy is indisputable. Additionally, MRI is superior in its ability to concomitantly identify tendinous, ligamentous, osseus, or nervous pathology in the workup of medial elbow pain. Magnetic resonance imaging of the snapping triceps syndrome was first described in 1996.[28] Standard MRI of the elbow fails to identify subluxation since it is performed in the extended position and the medial head of the triceps will have relocated. Thus, a modified protocol with the elbow flexed beyond 100 degrees must be employed in addition to the standard. In this position, the finding of the medial head of the triceps subluxed over the cubital tunnel is easily made.

Ligamentous Pathology

The ligaments of the elbow provide structural support in both flexion-extension and rotation of the forearm. They are subdivided into the ulnar (medial) collateral ligament complex (UCLC) and the lateral (radial) collateral ligament complex (LCLC), based on their anatomy and their function. The UCLC, particularly the anterior band of the anterior oblique ligament (AOL), is the primary ligamentous stabilizer against valgus stress to the elbow, and the radial lateral collateral ligament complex (RCLC) is the primary ligamentous stabilizer against varus stress. Not surprisingly, injuries to the ligaments of the elbow result from pathologic valgus stress or varus stress. Injury is the result of either chronic repetitive microtrauma or acute macrotrauma. Chronic repetitive microtrauma results in scar tissue formation, which in turn diminishes the functional capability of the ligament and renders it susceptible

to additional injury. The progressive damage erodes performance and causes clinical symptoms. Conversely, acute macrotrauma to the supportive ligaments can occur as the result of a high-intensity movement, for example, an erratic golf swing in a poorly conditioned individual. As the term *acute macrotrauma* implies, clinically significant injury is immediate.

Magnetic resonance imaging is invaluable in discriminating among myotendinous, ligamentous, and osseus etiologies in the patient who presents with medial elbow pain. The MR manifestations of ligament sprain parallel the pathomorphologic changes. Normal ligaments are composed primarily of type I collagen and appear homogeneously low in signal.[29] A grade I sprain, characterized clinically by intact function, demonstrates increased signal on T1-weighted images.[30] This reflects hemorrhage and edema within the substance of the ligament.[31] A grade II sprain, characterized clinically by partial loss of function, may be related to a partial tear of the ligament. On MR, the ligament demonstrates focal partial discontinuity or confined intracapsular extravasation of joint fluid.[30,32] A grade III sprain, characterized clinically by absence of function, may be related to a complete tear.[30,32] On MR, the ligament demonstrates disruption gap, fiber redundancy, and extracapsular extravasation of joint fluid. In each case, the ligamentous finding may be accompanied by adjacent traumatic effusion, the degree of which reflects the acuteness of the injury. Traumatic effusion manifests on MR as high signal on T2-weighted images surrounding the injured ligament.

Normal Anatomy of the Ulnar Collateral Ligament Complex

The ulnar collateral ligament complex is the primary soft tissue stabilizer against valgus stress on the elbow[33] (Fig. 6.6). It is composed of the anterior oblique, posterior oblique, and transverse (Cooper's) ligaments. The anterior oblique ligament is the most functionally important of the elbow ligaments. It is the primary ligamentous supporter against valgus stress on the

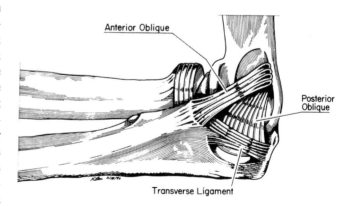

FIG. 6.6. Drawing of the three bundles of the ulnar collateral ligament. (From Safran,[6] with permission.).

elbow.[34,35] It is a cord-like structure that extends from the distal aspect of the medial epicondyle along the medial capsule and attaches onto the sublime tubercle of the medial coronoid process. It is easily identified on coronal MRI as focal thickening of the medial capsule. Its broad attachment at the medial epicondyle may be intermediate in signal on T1-weighted images and may be mistaken for sprain.[32] The remainder is homogeneously low in signal on all MR images. The posterior oblique ligament is more important in resisting valgus stress in greater degrees of elbow flexion, while the transverse ligament is structurally and functionally less important.

Injury to the Ulnar Collateral Ligament Complex

Injury to the ulnar collateral ligament complex occurs in overhead throwing athletes as a result of chronic repetitive valgus stress or, less frequently, acute trauma.[36] The former may be an isolated finding or seen as a component of the so-called valgus extension overload syndrome, discussed below. The latter can result from falling on an outstretched arm or may be a sequela of posterior dislocation of the elbow. When injured as a result of repetitive microtrauma, such as seen in the overhead-throwing athlete, the anterior oblique ligament is usually injured in its mid-substance. In the setting of acute macrotrauma, rupture occurs most commonly in the proximal aspect of the anterior oblique ligament of the ulnar collateral ligament complex.[37] Avulsion of the sublime tubercle, also described below, fills out the spectrum of possible injury involving the ulnar collateral ligament complex.

Chronic repetitive valgus stress results in a collection of microtraumatic injuries that occur when the elbow is repeatedly subjected to the considerable valgus stress intrinsic to overhead throwing.[38–40] In particular, the late-cocking (phase 3) and early-acceleration (phase 4) phases of overhead throwing cause medial distraction (tensile forces) and lateral impaction (compressive forces) with the elbow flexed and the forearm supinated.[38,41] Athletes involved in baseball, tennis football, volleyball, ice hockey, and water polo can be affected. Medially, the distraction forces, if excessive, outmatch the tensile strength of the ulnar collateral ligament complex. In the absence of the required period of recovery following this insult, the functional integrity of the ulnar collateral ligament complex is compromised. The end result can include (1) sprain of the ulnar collateral ligament complex, (2) medial epicondylitis, (3) ulnar nerve traction injury, and (4) avulsion injury to the medial epicondyle in the skeletally immature. Laterally, the compressive forces can result in chondral or osteochondral injury within the radiocapitellar joint with possible loose body formation.[32,42] In this setting, valgus subluxation may also occur due to laxity of the ulnar collateral ligament complex.

On MRI, injury to the anterior bundle of the ulnar collateral ligament complex is best seen on coronal images.[32] The anterior bundle appears bulbous and ill-defined with increased signal on T1-weighted sequences.[32,43,44] Periligamentous edema

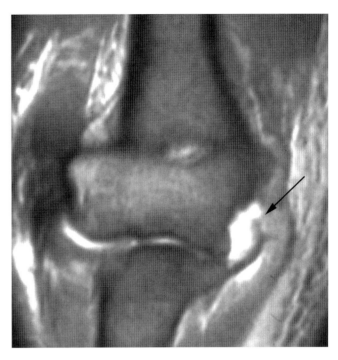

FIG. 6.7. Tear of the ulnar collateral ligament. Coronal T2 image demonstrating a complete disruption of the ulnar attachment of the anterior oblique band of the ulnar collateral ligament (arrow), surrounded by extensive soft tissue edema.

may be seen in acute injury (Fig. 6.7). Scarring may be seen in chronic injury. Partial tears of the anterior bundle appear as focal partial discontinuity or confined intracapsular extravasation of joint fluid. In the skeletally immature, this occurs more commonly at the medial epicondyle attachment. (Again, the high signal normally seen at the attachment onto the medial epicondyle should not be confused with abnormality.) In adults, partial tears occur more commonly at the insertion onto the sublime tubercle. This is typified by the T-sign on MRI,[45,46] in which the articular joint fluid meets the extravasated joint fluid along the medial margin of the coronoid process (Fig. 6.8). This finding signifies a partial-thickness tear of the undersurface of the anterior bundle. Grade III sprains demonstrate disruption gap, fiber redundancy, and extracapsular extravasation of joint fluid.

It should be noted here that partial tears may be undergraded because (1) ligament laxity may be overlooked without stress views, and (2) chronic partial tears may be missed in the absence of joint fluid. Intraarticular injection of gadolinium may be of particular help in making this diagnosis,[45] although this is controversial.[2]

Avulsion of the Sublime Tubercle

Avulsion of the sublime tubercle is an underreported cause of chronic medial elbow pain that has received growing attention in recent years.[47–50] Due to similarities in clinical presentation

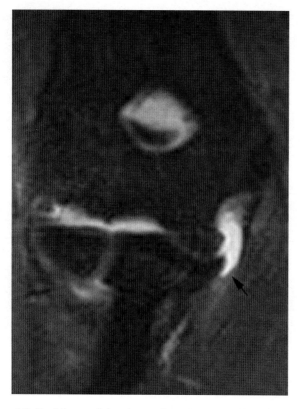

FIG. 6.8. Partial tear of the ulnar collateral ligament. Coronal STIR image demonstrating a partial detachment of the ulnar insertion of the ulnar collateral ligament (T sign) (arrow).

and pathophysiology, it is best conceptualized as an extension of the known spectrum of injury to the ulnar collateral ligament due to chronic repetitive valgus stress. First described in 1972,[51] the finding has been reported primarily in the dominant arm of young male baseball pitchers who present with chronic medial elbow pain.[47,48,50] One published case was believed to result from a single clear episode of trauma.[48]

Magnetic resonance imaging distinguishes among ligamentous, tendinous, osseus, and nervous causes of an overhead-throwing athlete's medial elbow pain. When avulsion is identified as the cause, it can aid the surgeon in determining the necessary type of fixation.[50] The avulsed bone fragment is best seen on coronal gradient echo images as a hypointense fragment that demonstrates continuity with the ulnar collateral ligament.[47] This finding may be difficult to appreciate on T1-weighted images[47] (Fig. 6.9).

Normal Anatomy of the Lateral Collateral Ligament Complex

The lateral collateral ligament complex is the primary soft tissue stabilizer against varus stress on the elbow.[33,34] It accounts for 15% of the varus stability of the elbow joint. It is composed of the lateral ulnar (posterolateral) collateral ligament (LUCL), radial (lateral) collateral ligament (RCL) proper, the annular ligament, and the accessory collateral ligament. While

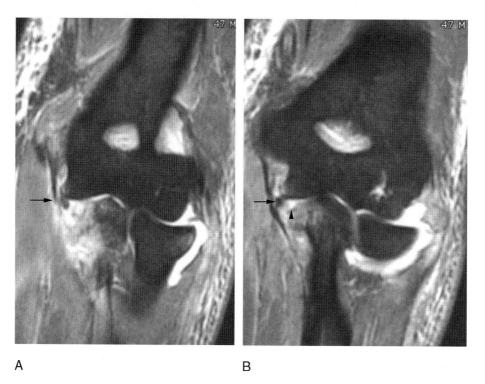

A   B

FIG. 6.9. (A–B) Avulsion fracture of the ulnar collateral ligament. Coronal STIR images demonstrating a bony fragment corresponding to the sublime tubercle (arrows in A,B) avulsed from the ulna (arrowhead in B). There is a joint effusion, bone marrow edema of the proximal ulna, and extensive soft tissue edema.

controversy remains, the LUCL is thought to be the most functionally significant of the above ligaments and the primary posterolateral stabilizer of the elbow. It extends as a sling from the lateral epicondyle, projects posteriorly and distally at the level of the radial head, and sweeps obliquely to its attachment onto the supinator crest of the ulna. The RCL extends from the anterior margin of the lateral epicondyle proximal to the origin of the LUCL and attaches onto the annular ligament and fascia of the supinator muscle. Both the LUCL and the RCL are best seen on coronal MRI. The annular ligament is the primary stabilizer of the proximal radioulnar joint. Its chondrified inner ring articulates circumferentially with the hyaline cartilage of the radial head. It appears best on axial MRI as a linear structure of uniformly low signal intensity.

Injury to the Lateral Ulnar Collateral Ligament

Injury to the lateral ulnar collateral ligament results (1) from chronic varus stress overload due to work, sports-related activity, or cubitus varus; (2) from an acute elbow injury such as posterior dislocation, hyperextension, or acute varus stress; or (3) as a complication of aggressive surgical treatment for lateral epicondylitis or radial head excision. Patients with insufficiency of the LUCL experience laxity of the ulnotrochlear joint and secondary subluxation/dislocation of the radiocapitellar joint, while the proximal radioulnar joint retains its normal relationship. As discussed above, lateral collateral ligament injury may accompany lateral epicondylitis.

Magnetic resonance imaging evaluation of the lateral ulnar collateral ligament is similar to evaluation of injury to the ulnar collateral ligament complex. Partial tears of the lateral ulnar collateral ligament are typically more conspicuous, and intraarticular injection of contrast is not necessary. Tears occur most commonly at the lateral epicondyle.[37] As in the ulnar collateral ligament complex, related structures of the elbow must be thoroughly evaluated to check for associated findings (Fig. 6.10). These can include lateral epicondylitis, medial ulnotrochlear chondromalacia, and joint bodies.[44,52]

Osseus Pathology

The range of osseus pathology to the elbow includes fracture, osteochondral injury including Panner's disease and osteochondritis dissecans, loose body formation, and osteophytes of the posteromedial ulna as seen with valgus extension overload.

Fractures Involving the Elbow

Acute macrotrauma to the osseus structures of the elbow primarily results from direct impact of the elbow with the ground or collision of an outstretched hand with the ground.

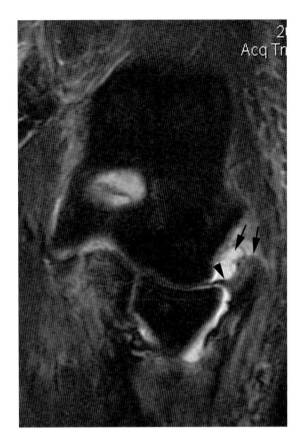

FIG. 6.10. Complete tear of the radial collateral ligament and lateral ulnar collateral ligament. Coronal STIR image demonstrating a retracted tear of the radial collateral ligament and the humeral origin of the lateral ulnar collateral ligament (arrows). Note the soft tissue edema and the joint effusion. There is a prominent synovial fold (arrowhead).

The former most frequently manifests as fracture of the olecranon. The latter results in varying pathology that is dependent on the degree of elbow flexion. If the elbow is flexed upon impact, posterolateral dislocation may occur. If the elbow is extended upon impact, force is transmitted proximally along the radius, and a fracture of the radius or capitellum may result. In the skeletally immature, valgus or varus sheer forces at the time of impact may result in fracture of the condylar and supracondylar structures.

Fractures about the elbow are adequately characterized on plain film in most cases. Additional MRI is most helpful in the diagnosis of occult or stress fractures, for instance in the setting of joint effusion without radiographic evidence of fracture.[53] It may also be useful to further characterize a known fracture in terms of the presence of intraarticular extension. The most common sports-related fractures of the elbow involve the radial head, olecranon, and capitellum (Fig. 6.11).

Stress fractures appear as linear or irregular decreased signal intensity on T1-weighted images. In the acute or subacute stages, marrow edema may be present as evidenced by increased signal intensity on fat-suppressed T2-weighted images or short-tau inversion recovery (STIR) images.

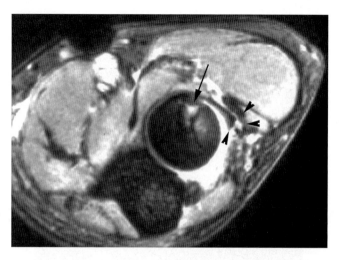

FIG. 6.11. Annular ligament tear and fracture of the head of the radius, following a posterior dislocation of the elbow and reduction. Axial GRE image demonstrates the fracture of the head of the radius (arrow). Note the detached end of the annular ligament (arrowheads).

Panner's Disease

Panner's disease is osteochondrosis of the capitellum or the radial head. It is a self-limited entity that usually affects the entire capitellum of predominantly male patients, most typically between the ages of 4 and 10 years of age. Patients present with pain and stiffness of the elbow and respond well to conservative treatment with no long-term sequelae. Treatment is usually restriction of activity while regaining full active elbow motion.

Plain films demonstrate increased density of the capitellum, which may be decreased in size, collapsed, or fragmented. Subsequent imaging reveals regeneration and reconstitution of the capitellum; in most cases, there is no residua of disease. On MRI, the entire capitellum may be abnormal in signal. The morphology of the capitellum may be irregular and flattened (Fig. 6.12).

Osteochondritis Dissecans of the Capitellum

Panner's disease must be distinguished from osteochondritis dissecans (OCD), a transchondral fracture that is not benign and may result in permanent disability.[54,55] As in Panner's disease, males are almost exclusively affected. Unlike in Panner's disease, the majority of patients with OCD are boys between the ages of 9 and 15 years who participate in gymnastics or throwing sports. They present with insidious and progressive pain in the lateral aspect of the elbow of the dominant arm, or, less likely, both arms. The etiology is unclear; it may be related to repetitive valgus stress and impaction at the radiocapitellar joint. On plain radiograph, an OCD lesion manifests as osteopenia at the capitellar epiphysis, which over time can

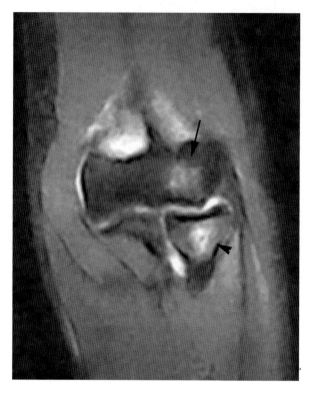

FIG. 6.12. Panner's disease. Coronal STIR image demonstrating intramedullary signal increase in the capitellum, with preservation of the articular surface (arrow). Note the reactive edema of the head of the radius (arrowhead).

progress to flattening of the capitellum sometimes associated with sclerosis. Unlike Panner's disease, loose body formation may occur and may be identified. These can be large and cause mechanical symptoms, including movement restriction or synovitis, joint effusion, and joint stiffness.

Magnetic resonance imaging allows earlier detection of osteochondral injury than is possible on plain radiography (Fig. 6.13). Furthermore, MRI can characterize the stability of osteochondral injury in terms of the integrity of the overlying articular cartilage, the viability of the separated fragment, and the presence of associated intraarticular bodies. Lesions are characterized as intact, separated and attached, or loose. The integrity of the articular surface overlying an OCD lesion dictates whether conservative or surgical treatment is warranted.

Each of the four stages of osteochondritis dissecans originally described by Berndt and Harty[56] in 1959 in surgical specimens may be demonstrated with characteristic findings on MRI. In stage I lesions, there is subchondral trabecular compression with intact overlying cartilage (Fig. 6.14). The intact cartilaginous covering designates this lesion as stable. On MRI, this manifests as focal hypointensity on T1-weighted images and proton-density–weighted images and variable signal intensity on T2-weighted images. In stage II lesions, there is compromise of the overlying cartilage with the resultant osteochondral fragment unseparated or incompletely separated. This is evident

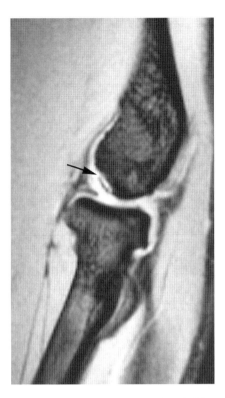

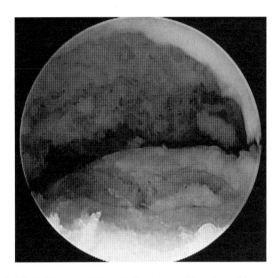

FIG. 6.15. A 13-year-old baseball pitcher with pain and intermittent catching of his elbow. The arthroscopic view reveals a completely detached but nondisplaced fragment.

FIG. 6.13. Osteochondritis dissecans (osteochondral fracture) of the capitellum. Sagittal GRE showing a partially detached osteochondral fragment of the capitellum (arrow), with fluid dissecting between the fragment and the underlying bone.

this manifests as a confluent rim of high signal on T2-weighted images (Fig. 6.15). In stage IV lesions, the fragment is displaced, constituting a loose body.

Loose Body Formation

Loose bodies can cause locking, clicking, or restricted movement in individuals, including athletes. They are seen in the context of OCD as well as in other clinical entities, such as chronic repetitive valgus stress and valgus extension overload syndrome (described above). Magnetic resonance imaging is useful in identifying and localizing loose bodies, particularly when there is joint fluid.[57,58] They usually settle within joint recesses, posteriorly at the olecranon recess (posteromedial or posterolateral elbow) or anteriorly at the radial and coronoid recesses, particularly the anterior radioulnar joint. They will manifest as well-circumscribed filling defects within joint fluid on both T1- and T2-weighted images (Fig. 6.16). Signal intensity varies with heterogeneity depending on the presence or absence of bone marrow, which appears bright on T1-weighted images. Intraarticular injection of gadolinium aids in the diagnosis of joint body when joint fluid is not present. This is best seen on fat-suppressed T1-weighted MRI. This technique also assists in the detection of a potential space between the osteochondral fragment and parent bone, which, as detailed above, would signify an unstable lesion.

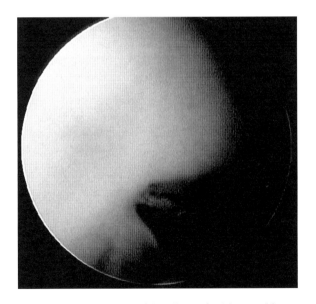

FIG. 6.14. Arthroscopic view of the elbow of a 14-year-old gymnast showing the capitellum and probe revealing soft, but intact, articular cartilage overlying the lesion.

from the presence of joint fluid or granulation tissue encircling an osteochondral fragment. Such a lesion is considered unstable. In stage III lesions, there is a completely separated but nondisplaced or minimally displaced fragment. On MRI,

Valgus Extension Overload Syndrome

Valgus extension overload syndrome[44,59,60] describes a collection of repetitive microtraumatic injuries that occur when the elbow is chronically subjected to the valgus stress of

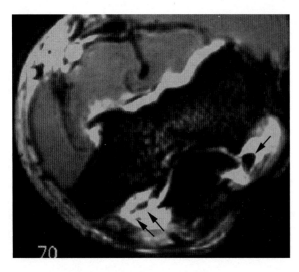

FIG. 6.16. Intraarticular loose bodies. Axial GRE image demonstrating multiple intraarticular loose bodies located medially and laterally in the posterior recesses of the joint (arrows).

throwing with elbow extension. Posteromedially, osseous or osteochondral injury can occur within the ulnotrochlear joint. Osteophytes can emerge from the medial olecranon due to the repeated abutment of the posteromedial olecranon upon the olecranon fossa, and may even detach within the joint compartment to form a loose body (Fig. 6.17). Fat interposed between the radiocapitellar and ulnotrochlear joints can become impinged. The resulting fibrosis and synovitis can obstruct normal joint articulation. An extreme of this condition may result in stress fractures of the olecranon.

As delineated above, there are a multitude of findings associated with valgus stress overload syndrome. A complete MRI evaluation of the osseus, chondral, ligamentous, and myotendinous structures of the elbow is warranted.

Nerve Pathology

In general, the nerves of the elbow demonstrate low to intermediate signal on all pulse sequences. Signal intensity is similar to muscle on T1 and slightly higher than that of muscle on T2. The nerves are hypointense to fat on T1 and T2, and detection is directly related to the amount of perineural fat (surrounding the nerve). Increased signal on fat suppression (FS), proton density (PD), and fast spin echo (FSE) can be a sign of neuropathy. Fusiform thickening or evidence of fibrosis around an area of interest are other signs of potential nerve damage.

Normal Anatomy of the Ulnar Nerve

As it approaches the elbow, the ulnar nerve passes with the ulnar collateral vessels dorsal to the medial humeral epicondyle and through the cubital tunnel. The cubital tunnel is delin-

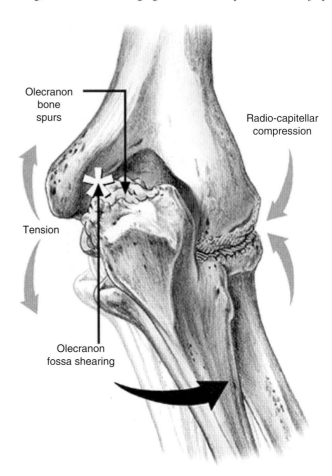

FIG. 6.17. Drawing illustrating the mechanism of forces leading to the formation of osteophytes and potential formation of loose bodies. (From Safran M. Injury to the ulnar collateral ligament: diagnosis and treatment. Sports Med Arthrosc Rev 2003;11:15–24, with permission.).

eated laterally by the medial surface of the trochlea and ulnar collateral ligament, anteriorly by the posterior aspect of the medial humeral epicondyle, and medially by the arcuate ligament. As it exits the cubital tunnel—and the elbow joint—the nerve courses anteriorly between the humeral and ulnar heads of the flexor carpi ulnaris muscle.

The ulnar nerve is the most consistently identified nerve on MRI elbow studies, and MRI is the best imaging tool for evaluation of neuropathy. It is best seen within the cubital tunnel in the axial plane with the forearm extended. The nerve is also well demonstrated in the sagittal plane medial to the olecranon and posterior to the medial humeral epicondyle.

Cubital Tunnel Syndrome

Due to its superficial location, the ulnar nerve is the most commonly injured nerve in the elbow.[61] The site of neuropathy is most often the cubital tunnel, where it is called the cubital tunnel syndrome. Common symptoms span from temporary paresthesias in the ring and small fingers to severe muscle atrophy that results in clawing of these fingers. Athletes may complain of loss of ball control or radicular symptoms with throwing. The natural physiology of the elbow joint can lead to this ulnar neuropathy. The internal volume of the cubital tunnel naturally decreases with flexion of the forearm secondary to tightening of the arcuate ligament and medial pressure from the ulnar collateral ligament and (bulging of) the medial head of the triceps. Furthermore, the ulnar nerve is stretched several millimeters against the medial epicondyle during flexion, further straining the nerve. The pressure within the nerve has been found to be six times greater than normal when the arm is in the throwers position of shoulder abduction-external rotation, elbow flexion, and wrist extension.[62,63]

A second cause of cubital tunnel syndrome is the so-called external compression syndrome. It can be an acute event resulting from a single direct force applied to the tunnel or a subacute process occurring from prolonged pressure to the region. The latter is commonly seen in the setting of extended hospitalization or following surgery,[64] where positioning and lack of movement cause prolonged compression of the ulnar aspect of the elbow.

A third form of ulnar neuropathy, referred to as chronic cubital tunnel syndrome, occurs secondary to (1) pressure from space-occupying lesions such as a tumors, hematoma, inflammatory pannus, osteophytes, ectopic calcification, ossification, scarring of the ulnar collateral ligament or capsule, and loose bodies[61,64–67]; or (2) from lateral shift of the ulna. The latter is commonly seen in athletes and is associated with chronic laxity of the ulnar collateral ligament and the increased valgus alignment seen in professional athletes who perform overhead maneuvers, such as throwing. In addition, posttraumatic changes in the region of the cubital tunnel can cause chronic cubital syndrome. Examples include scar tissue from a distal humeral or supracondylar fracture, avulsed medial epiphysis, previous surgery, and elbow dislocation.

In any of the three forms of ulnar neuropathy described above, the injured nerve may appear edematous on MRI (Fig. 6.18). The ulnar nerve, best seen within the cubital tunnel in the axial and sagittal planes with the forearm extended, demonstrates increased signal on FS, PD, and FSE sequences.[67]

Snapping triceps syndrome is a cause of ulnar neuropathy and is often seen in conjunction with ulnar nerve subluxation/dislocation. It is discussed in detail above.

Athletes may also have symptomatic ulnar nerve subluxation, where pain and radicular symptoms may result from the ulnar nerve snapping across the medial epicondyle with flexion.

Normal Anatomy of the Median Nerve

The median nerve is located superficially in the anterior aspect of the elbow, coursing beneath the lacertus fibrosis anteriorly and superficial to the brachialis muscle posteriorly.

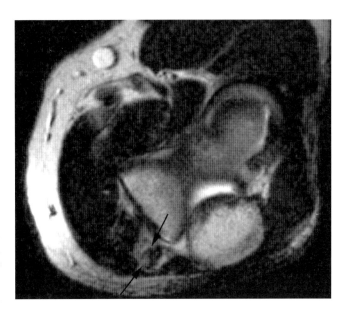

FIG. 6.18. Cubital tunnel syndrome. Axial T2 image demonstrating an enlarged and hyperintense ulnar nerve (arrows) within the cubital tunnel in the posterior medial aspect of the elbow.

It is bounded by the pronator teres medially and the brachialis muscle laterally. With the exception of the flexor carpi ulnaris muscle, the median nerve supplies the superficial muscles of the forearm.

Pronator Syndrome

Compressive injury to the median nerve at the elbow is called pronator syndrome (PS), and can occur anywhere between the distal humerus proximally and the flexor digitorum superficialis arch distally.[67] In order of decreasing frequency, the sites of median nerve compression in PS are (1) the fibrous bands at the ulnar and humeral heads of the pronator teres muscle approximately 3 cm distal to the medial epicondyle, (2) at the fibrous arch of the flexor digitorum superficialis muscle, (3) beneath an unusually thick lacertus fibrosus, and (4) between the supracondylar process (seen in approximately 3% of people[67]) and the ligament of Struthers.[61] Another uncommon cause of pronator syndrome includes masses of the forearm. Symptoms of pronator syndrome include an insidious onset of pain and discomfort in the proximal volar forearm without weakness or sensory loss.

Anterior Interosseus Nerve Syndrome

A lesser common neuropathy of the median nerve is the anterior interosseus nerve syndrome (AINS), which affects the motor branch as it diverges from the median nerve approximately 2 to 8 cm distal to the medial epicondyle. Compression of this branch may be the result of trauma (supracondylar fracture and posttraumatic thrombosis of the ulnar collateral vessels), vascular anomalies, fibrous bands, anomalous musculature, tendinosis of the ulnar head of the pronator teres, or an enlarged bicipital bursa.[61] Patients with AINS present with weakness or paralysis of the flexor pollicis longus, the flexor profundus tendon to the second and third digits, and the pronator quadratus. It can be distinguished from the pronator syndrome or carpal tunnel syndrome by the lack of sensory deficits on presentation.

As with the ulnar nerve, the median nerve is best visualized on axial MRI. However, given the minimal amount of fat around the median nerve at the level of the elbow, it is often difficult to identify.[67] Occasionally it can be seen in the coronal and sagittal projections. In median nerve neuropathy, T2-weighted images will demonstrate increased signal in the denervated musculature, during the early stages and atrophy and fatty infiltration during the late stages.

Normal Anatomy of the Radial Nerve

The radial nerve runs anterior to the lateral humeral epicondyle between the brachialis and brachioradialis muscles. At the level of the capitellum, the nerve divides into superficial (sensory) and deep (motor) branches. The superficial branch courses anterolaterally between the brachioradialis and the supinator muscles. The deep branch, also known as the posterior interosseous nerve, courses around the radial head, dives through the supinator muscle, continues between the superficial and deep portions of the supinator muscle at the so-called arcade of Frohse, and into the posterior aspect of the forearm deep to the extensor muscles. The radial nerve supplies the extensor muscles of the arm and forearm and provides sensory innervation of the skin of the thumb, index, and middle fingers.

Injury to the Radial Nerve

Direct trauma to the elbow or the presence of a mass lesion (lipoma or ganglion) can cause injury to the radial nerve, as well as pressure following cast application. The superficial branch of the radial nerve is typically injured from trauma to the lateral elbow or iatrogenically such as with elbow arthroscopy. Injury to the radial nerve may mimic deQuervain's tenosynovitis or pathology at the trapeziometacarpal joint.[67]

Radial Tunnel Syndrome

Compression to the nerve within the radial tunnel, which begins at the level of the capitellum and ends at the arcade of Frohse, is called Radial tunnel syndrome (RTS). Patients

with RTS typically present with tenderness and swelling over the anterolateral proximal forearm in the region of the radial neck. The most common site of compression injury to the deep branch of the radial nerve is at the level of the arcade of Frohse. Neuropathy occurring here is called the posterior interosseus nerve syndrome (PINS) or the supinator syndrome.

Posterior interosseus nerve syndrome can result from repeated pronation and extension of the forearm and flexion of the wrist. Patients generally include violinists, orchestra conductors, and swimmers. Mechanical compression from a mass lesion can also cause neuropathy and similar symptoms. Symptoms of PINS include an inability to extend the metacarpophalangeal (MCP) joints of the thumb and fingers with deviation of the wrist radially with extension. Patients may present with symptoms of tennis elbow that is refractory to treatment. However, on detailed examination, the pain is more distal than the typical location of tennis elbow. Since this is a purely motor nerve, there are no sensory deficits associated with this syndrome.

Findings on T1-weighted images include fibrosis at the arcade of Frohse. T2-weighted images demonstrates increased signal on FS, PD, and FSE in the muscles supplied by the posterior interosseous nerve during the early stages and atrophy with fatty infiltration during the late stages (Fig. 6.19). As with the other nerves of the elbow, the radial nerve is best seen on axial MRI, but can also been visualized in coronal and sagittal planes.

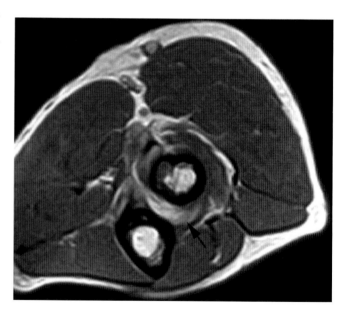

Fig. 6.19. Posterior interosseous nerve syndrome. Axial T1 image demonstrating atrophy of the supinator muscle (arrow), due to chronic denervation.

B. Orthopedic Perspective: Elbow Injuries

Marc R. Safran

Normal Elbow Anatomy and Physiology

The elbow is a compound synovial joint composed of three bones—the humerus, radius, and ulna—with three articulations—the ulnotrochlear, proximal radioulnar, and radiocapitellar—that result in complex movement with two planes of motion freedom—flexion-extension and forearm rotation. The extent of flexion-extension, normally between 0 and 150 degrees,[68] is defined by the articulation of the olecranon with the trochlea of the humerus. The range of motion that results is that of a nearly true hinge joint. The extent of forearm rotation, normally between 75 degrees of pronation and 85 degrees of supination,[68] is defined by the radial head's articulation with the radial notch of the ulna. The articulation of the radius with the rounded and smooth capitellum of the humerus forms a trochoid joint that allows axial rotation or pivoting. Elbow motion is guided by the capsuloligamentous structures about the elbow, specifically the ulnar collateral ligament complex and the lateral collateral ligament complex. The ulnar collateral ligament complex is composed of three ligaments: the anterior oblique ligament (AOL); the posterior oblique ligament (POL); and the transverse ligament, also known as Cooper's ligament. The AOL is functionally subdivided into an anterior band and posterior band. The anterior band of the AOL is the most important ligament in athletes involved in overhead sports, as this portion of the AOL resists the majority of valgus forces associated with throwing. The lateral collateral ligament complex is composed of the lateral ulnar collateral ligament, functionally similar to the AOL, the lateral (radial) collateral ligament, the annular ligament, and the accessory lateral collateral ligament. The anterior and posterior capsule also provide stability to the elbow, as do the muscles that cross the elbow joint.[69]

Treatment Options for Elbow Injuries

Orthopedic surgery and musculoskeletal medicine, like radiology, require an understanding of the anatomy of the joint and surrounding structures. To treat most of these injuries, an understanding of the anatomy is critical, as well as understanding the pathophysiology and degree of injury. The MRI is particularly helpful in assessing the severity of the injury and elucidating all the structures involved. This helps guide the orthopedist and musculoskeletal medicine practitioner in the management of these injuries. The anatomic descriptions and MRI examples are particularly helpful in reviewing the anatomy and providing examples of injuries about the elbow. This section of the chapter briefly reviews the treatment of these injuries.

Myotendonous Pathology

Lateral Musculotendinous Injuries: Lateral Epicondylitis ("Tennis Elbow") and Extensor Muscle Avulsion

When lateral epicondylitis is diagnosed, most patients are treated conservatively with a program of stretching and strengthening of the lateral musculature and modalities, such as ice. This is performed as a home exercise program or with physical therapy. Nonsteroidal antiinflammatory medications or cortisone injections may also be given to make the pain tolerable enough to perform the exercises. Iontophoresis has been shown effective to reduce pain in the short term, and may also be used as part of the conservative treatment regimen.[70] Other conservative measures such as extracorporeal shock wave therapy, prolotherapy, acupuncture, laser, and soft laser have not been shown to be effective in randomized controlled trials.[71] Current research in the use of topical nitric oxide has suggested that it may be beneficial.[72] Those individuals failing an adequate trial of conservative treatment, including stretching and strengthening of the wrist extensor/supinator muscles, may require surgical intervention. The pathology most often involves the extensor carpi radialis brevis, though it may also extend into other adjacent muscles-tendons. Many different surgical procedures have been advocated.[73] Arthroscopic debridement and release has been shown to be as effective as open surgical debridement or open surgical release, and adds the benefit of identifying and treating concomitant intraarticular pathology, such as a plica, synovitis, or radiocapitellar arthrosis.[73] It has been noted that up to two thirds of patients with lateral epicondylitis have a capsular injury underlying the area of damaged tendon[74] (Fig. 6.20). The significance of this capsular injury is unclear, as it does not appear to affect the results of treatment, though it does make one wonder if we truly understand the pathophysiology of tennis elbow. Percutaneous release has also been advocated and has very good results as well.[73] All procedures entail the risk of complications, including injury to the lateral collateral ligament complex.

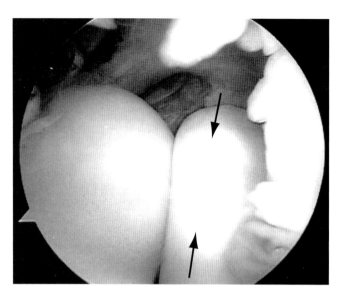

FIG. 6.20. Arthroscopic view of the elbow from the proximal medial portal. The open arrow points to the capitellum, while the lightening bolt points to the radial head (arrows). The closed thin arrow points to a rent or hole in the lateral capsule—a type III lesion seen in lateral epicondylitis.

Complete rupture of the common extensor origin of the wrist and hand is uncommon, but may occur acutely as part of an elbow dislocation. Individuals with extensor muscle origin avulsion should be treated with surgical repair, as persistent weakness would otherwise result.

Medial Musculotendinous Injury: Medial Epicondylitis ("Golfer's Elbow") and Flexor-Pronator Muscle-Tendon Avulsion

Medial epicondylitis is similar to lateral epicondylitis, and most patients are treated conservatively with a program of stretching and strengthening of the flexor-pronator musculature. Modalities such as ice may be used, taking care not to cause a thermal injury to the subcutaneous ulnar nerve. Treatment algorithms are based on knowledge from the more common lateral epicondylitis. Again, this may be performed as a home exercise program or with physical therapy. Nonsteroidal antiinflammatory medications, cortisone injections, or iontophoresis may also be used to make the pain tolerable to perform the exercises. Other measures such as extracorporeal shock wave therapy, prolotherapy, acupuncture, laser, and soft laser have not been shown to be effective. Individuals who fail an adequate trial of conservative treatment, including stretching and strengthening of the wrist flexor/pronator muscles, may require surgical intervention. The pathology usually involves the pronator teres, though the flexor muscle-tendon units may also be involved to varying degrees. Several different surgical procedures have been advocated, though not as many as for lateral epicondylitis. The common theme with surgical intervention for golfer's elbow is open surgical debridement of the degenerative tissue with or without detaching or reattaching the tendinous origin.[75] As with the lateral side, some surgeons may abrade or drill the medial epicondyle to increase blood flow to the area. If there is concomitant ulnar nerve symptomatology, consideration is given to transposition of the ulnar nerve. The results of surgery depend on the presence of ulnar nerve involvement, which reduces the likelihood of an asymptomatic outcome.[76] Surgery for medial epicondylitis has several potential risks, including injury to the ulnar collateral ligament complex.

Complete rupture of the common flexor origin of the wrist and hand also is uncommon, but may occur more frequently than a lateral rupture. It may be as a result of an elbow dislocation or repeated cortisone injections. Patients with flexor–pronator musculotendinous origin avulsion should be treated with surgical repair, as patients do not do well treated conservatively.

Rupture of the Distal Biceps Tendon

A meta-analysis has confirmed that the results of nonsurgical treatment are not very good for individuals with distal biceps tendon avulsions, and should likely be reserved for older, sedentary individuals whose distal biceps tendon avulsion involves their nondominant arm.[77] A nonanatomic repair to the brachialis tendon helps with flexion, but the loss of supination strength also results in less than satisfactory results. Thus, an anatomic surgical repair of the distal biceps tendon to the radius has been shown to provide the best results and is recommended to be performed in a timely manner to reduce the risk of impaired elbow flexion and supination.[78] In patients who present late after the injury, the bicipital aponeurosis is of particular importance in the ability to perform late repair of distal biceps tendon ruptures. If intact, the degree of retraction of the biceps tendon will be limited, the tendon end easily identifiable, muscle shortening minimal, and primary repair may be possible. If the aponeurosis is torn, the lacertus fibrosis may not anchor the ruptured biceps tendon, and the tendon will retract into the arm, resulting in scarring and muscle shortening, making delayed repair (more than 6 to 12 weeks) difficult, if not impossible.

Strain of the Brachialis Tendon ("Climber's Elbow")

Climber's elbow is usually treated conservatively, taking care to reduce the risk of elbow flexion contracture by stretching the elbow into extension and judicious use of antiinflammatory medications and modalities.

Rupture of the Triceps Tendon

Due to the uniformly poor results of nonoperative treatment, avulsion of the triceps tendon resulting in an inability to actively extend the elbow against gravity should be treated with urgent primary repair of the tendon to the olecranon.[79]

Ligmentous Pathology

Injury to the Ulnar Collateral Ligament Complex

Rarely does the ruptured ulnar collateral ligament require surgery. While it has been shown that chronic valgus laxity following a simple elbow dislocation is associated with an increased rate of degenerative change within the joint, recurrent instability is particularly uncommon.[80] Throwing athletes who wish to continue to participate in their sport are treated with a conservative treatment regimen, beginning with reduction of swelling, increase in elbow range of motion, and strengthening of the flexor–pronator muscles. The ability to return to the same level of sports with this regimen has been reported to be 42%.[81] Patients who fail two courses of an adequate rehabilitation program, or high-level throwers with an acute ulnar collateral ligament (UCL) rupture, are treated with UCL reconstruction. While there are several techniques for the UCL reconstruction, most use a free graft (palmaris longus or semitendinosus) through one or more tunnels in the ulna and humerus replicating the anterior oblique ligament anatomy and function.[82] Rehabilitation after this reconstruction may take 6 to 18 months to return to sports.

Avulsion of the Sublime Tubercle

While there are no series large enough to allow for an evidence-based analysis for the best treatment of avulsion of the sublime tubercle, the general consensus is that a displaced fragment of greater than 2 mm in a throwing athlete should be reattached surgically to the proximal ulna.[83]

Injury to the Lateral Ulnar Collateral Ligament

Individuals with injury to the LUCL may clinically have posterolateral rotatory instability (PLRI) of the elbow. These individuals present with symptoms of pain, locking, snapping, clicking, or recurrent instability, occasionally with driving/turning the steering wheel, or using their hands to push up on the arm rests from a seated position. Conservative treatment, including bracing, is usually unsuccessful. Reconstruction of the LUCL using a free graft, such as the palmaris longus or gracilis tendons, is used to replicate the anatomy of the LUCL by fixation to the lateral epicondyle proximally and the sublime tubercle of the ulna distally using one or more drill holes.[84]

Osteochondritis Dissecans of the Capitellum

The treatment of OCD is dependent on its stage.[85] If the overlying cartilage is intact and bone scan shows increased activity, these lesions have a high propensity to heal, particularly in the skeletally immature individual. If the cartilage is intact and the bone scan is not increased, drilling may be indicated to stimulate bone growth and healing. If the overlying articular cartilage is not completely intact, treatment is usually sur-

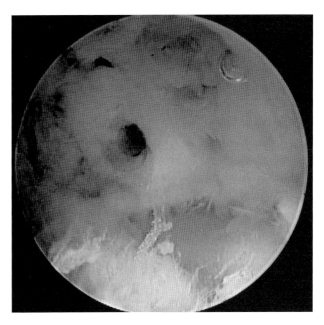

FIG. 6.21. The lesion of the case in FIG. 6.16 has been fixed in place with bioabsorbable pins. The arrow points to one of the pins in the fragment.

gical. If the MRI suggests the lesion is a stage II or III lesion, the elbow is usually treated with arthroscopy, debridement of the underlying bony bed, and fixation of the OCD fragment with pins, screws, or plugs (Fig. 6.21). However, the patient should be cautioned that even if these lesions heal, the ability to return to sports is highly variable, as is a persistence of elbow flexion contracture. In some cases the treatment is only debridement and microfracture (Fig. 6.22). Treatment of advanced stages of OCD with debridement alone usually results in degenerative arthritis at long-term follow-up; however, overgrown or fragmented lesions may not be amenable to internal fixation. Some surgeons have attempted filling of large lesions where fixation is not possible with autograft and allograft osteochondral plugs, as well as autologous chondrocyte implantation with bone grafting.

Loose Body Formation

Treatment of loose bodies entails removing the fragment(s) to prevent articular cartilage damage, reducing or eliminating mechanical symptoms, and maintaining normal elbow function. While this can be done with an open arthrotomy, elbow arthroscopy has become the standard of care for removal of loose bodies within the elbow (Figs. 6.23 and 6.24) due to its low morbidity, relatively quicker recovery, and ability to completely evaluate the joint.

Valgus Extension Overload Syndrome

Treatment of valgus extension overload syndrome (VEOS) is generally conservative, provided there are no loose bodies in

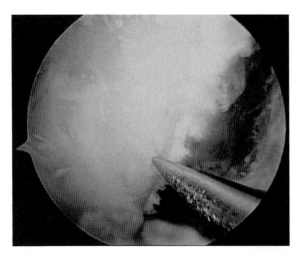

FIG. 6.22. Arthroscopic view of the capitellum of a 19-year-old collegiate water polo player with osteochondritis dissecans (OCD). The fragment was displaced and not reparable. Seen in this view is the capitellum with microfracture awl in place to start perforation to allow marrow elements to adhere to the site to undergo metaplasia and become fibrocartilage.

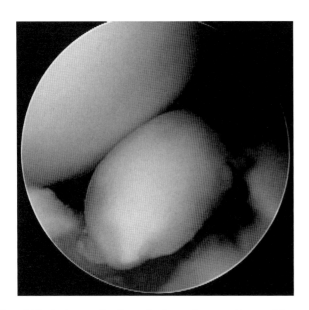

FIG. 6.23. Arthroscopic view of a loose fragment in an adolescent athlete with OCD of the elbow.

the elbow. When osteophytes are present on the olecranon, most surgeons have found conservative management not to be very successful at eliminating the symptoms. Thus, for those with loose bodies in the elbow, osteophytic spurring of the olecranon, or individuals who fail conservative management, osteophyte excision is usually recommended and quite successful. However, Andrews and Timmerman[86] noted that those undergoing aggressive osteophyte excision often have a high rate of subsequent surgery, including a significant rate of UCL reconstruction. It is unclear whether removing the osteophyte

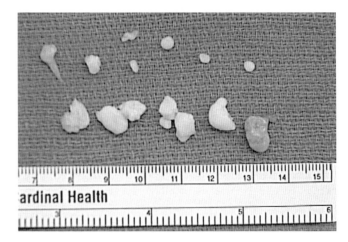

FIG. 6.24. Loose bodies removed from the elbow of a 58-year-old competitive tennis player.

uncovers preexisting valgus laxity or places more stress on the UCL, making it more susceptible to injury. Regardless, it is currently recommended that only the osteophyte be removed, and if concomitant UCL injury is identified, it is also treated with reconstruction.

Nervous Pathology

Cubital Tunnel Syndrome

Treatment of ulnar neuropathy depends on the cause.[87–89] Most patients undergo a regimen of conservative management, including modalities, and stretching and strengthening of the muscles that cross the elbow, provided no muscular atrophy is present. Those individuals with muscular atrophy, or those who fail conservative management are treated surgically. Surgical options include ulnar nerve in situ decompression, medial epicondylectomy, and ulnar nerve transposition, either submuscular or subcutaneous. Most athletes with ulnar neuropathy who undergo surgery usually have the nerve transposed.

Pronator Syndrome

Patients with this syndrome usually respond to conservative management, including stretching of the forearm musculature. Rarely, exploration of the nerve and surgical release are indicated.

Anterior Interosseus Nerve Syndrome

An uncommon syndrome, anterior interosseus nerve syndrome (AINS) is also usually responsive to nonoperative management. Surgery is reserved for those cases refractory to a couple of months of conservative management unless there is evidence of advanced changes of muscular denervation.

Injury to the Radial Nerve

Injury from penetrating trauma resulting in injury to the radial nerve, particularly the motor branch, may require nerve repair, bridge grafting, or tendon transfers, as loss of muscle function due to radial nerve injury is quite disabling. Otherwise, conservative management is often successful in treating nonpenetrating injury of the radial nerve.

Radial Tunnel Syndrome

Initial treatment of radial tunnel syndrome is conservative and typically includes relative rest and physical therapy with stretching of the supinator muscles. Surgical treatment involving exploration and release of constricting bands may be recommended in cases refractory to conservative treatment.

References

1. Field LD, Savoie FH. Common elbow injuries in sport. Sports Med 1998;26(3):193–205.
2. Regan W, Wold LE, Coonrad R, et al. Microscopic histopathology of chronic refractory lateral epicondylitis. Am J Sports Med 1992;20:746–9.
3. Nirschl RP, Pettrone FA. Tennis elbow. The surgical treatment of lateral epicondylitis. J Bone Joint Surg Am 1979;61(6A):832–9.
4. Potter HG, Hannafin JA, Morwessel RM, et al. Lateral epicondylitis: correlation of MR imaging, surgical, and histopathologic findings. Radiology 1995;196(1):43–6.
5. Regan W, Wold LE, Coonrad R, Morrey BF. Microscopic histopathology of chronic refractory lateral epicondylitis. Am J Sports Med 1992;20(6):746–9.
6. Safran MR. Elbow injuries in athletes. A review. Clin Orthop 1995;310:257–77.
7. Chung CB, Chew FS, Steinbach L. MR imaging of tendon abnormalities of the elbow. Magn Reson Imaging Clin North Am 2004;12(2):233–45.
8. Pasternack I, Tuovinen EM, Lohman M, et al. MR findings in humeral epicondylitis. A systematic review. Acta Radiol 2001;42(5):434–40.
9. Nirschl RP. Elbow tendinosis/tennis elbow. Clin Sports Med 1992;11:851–70.
10. Martin CE, Schweitzer M. MR imaging of epicondylitis. Skeletal Radiol 1998;27:133–8.
11. Coel M, Yamada CY, Ko J. MR imaging of patients with lateral epicondylitis of the elbow (tennis elbow): importance of increased signal of the anconeus muscle. AJR Am J Roentgenol 1993;161:1019–21.
12. Plancher K, Halbrecht J, Lourie GM. Medial and lateral epicondylitis in the athlete. Clin Sports Med 1996;15(2):283–305.
13. Ciccotti MC, Schwartz MA, Ciccotti MG. Diagnosis and treatment of medial epicondylitis of the elbow. Clin Sports Med 2004;23(4):693–705.
14. Gaary EA, Potter HG, Altchek DW. Medial elbow pain in the throwing athlete: MR imaging evaluation. AJR Am J Roentgenol 1997;168:795–800.
15. Conway JE, Jobe FW, Glousman RE, et al. Medial instability of the elbow in throwing athletes: treatment by repair or reconstruction of the ulnar collateral ligament. J Bone Joint Surg [Am] 1992;74:67–83.
16. Nirschl RP. Medial tennis elbow, surgical treatment. Orthop Trans Am Acad Orthop Surg 1980;7:298–302.
17. Seiler J, Parker L, Chamberland P, et al. The distal biceps tendon: Two potential mechanisms involved in its rupture: Arterial supply and mechanical impingement. J Shoulder Elbow Surg 1995;4:149–56.
18. Vidal AF, Drakos MC, Allen AA. Biceps tendon and triceps tendon injuries. Clin Sports Med 2004;23(4):707–22.
19. Safran MR, Graham SM. Distal biceps tendon ruptures. Clin Orthop 2002;404:275–83.
20. Rettig AC. Traumatic elbow injuries in the athlete. Orthop Clin North Am 2002;33:509–22.
21. Viegas SF. Avulsion of the triceps tendon. Orthop Rev 1990;19:533–6.
22. Rolfsen L. Snapping triceps tendon with ulnar neuritis. Report on a case. Acta Orthop Scand 1970;41(1):74–6.
23. Spinner RJ, An KN, Kim KJ, et al. Medial or lateral dislocation (snapping) of a portion of the distal triceps: a biomechanical, anatomic explanation. J Shoulder Elbow Surg 2001;10(6):561–7.
24. Spinner RJ, Goldner RD. Snapping of the medial head of the triceps and recurrent dislocation of the ulnar nerve. Anatomical and dynamic factors. J Bone Joint Surg [Am] 1998;80(2):239–47.
25. Jacobson JA, Jebson PJ, Jeffers AW, et al. Ulnar nerve dislocation and snapping triceps syndrome: diagnosis with dynamic sonography—report of three cases. Radiology 2001;220(3):601–5.
26. Spinner RJ, Goldner RD, Lee RA. Diagnosis of Snapping Triceps with US. Radiology 2002;224(3):933–4; author reply 934.
27. Yiannakopoulos CK. Imaging diagnosis of the snapping triceps syndrome. Radiology 2002;225(2):607–8; author reply 608.
28. Spinner RJ, Hayden FR Jr, Hipps CT, et al. Imaging the snapping triceps. AJR Am J Roentgenol 1996;167(6):1550–1.
29. Kaplan LJ, Potter HG. MR imaging of ligament injuries to the elbow. Magn Reson Imaging Clin North Am 2004;12(2):221–32.
30. Waite RJ, Cummings TM, Busconi B, et al. Elbow. In: Stark DD, Bradley WG, eds. Magnetic Resonance Imaging. St. Louis, Mosby, 1999:751–7.
31. Mirowitz SA, London SL. Ulnar collateral ligament injury in baseball pitchers: MR imaging evaluation. Radiology 1992;185(2):573–6.
32. Gaary EA, Potter HG, Altchek DW. Medial elbow pain in the throwing athlete: MR imaging evaluation. Am J Roentgenol 1997;168(3):795–800.
33. Regan WD, Korinek SL, Morrey BF, et al. Biomechanical study of ligaments around the elbow joint. Clin Orthop 1991;271:170–9.
34. Morrey BF, An K. Articular and ligamentous contributions to the stability of the elbow joint. Am J Sports Med 1983;11(5):315–9.
35. Hotchkiss RN, Weiland AJ. Valgus stability of the elbow. J Orthop Res 1987;5(3):372–7.
36. Safran MR. Ulnar collateral ligament injury in the overhead athlete: diagnosis and treatment. Clin Sports Med 2004;23(4):643–63.
37. Potter HG, Weiland AJ, Schatz JA, et al. Posterolateral rotatory instability of the elbow: usefulness of MR imaging in diagnosis. Radiology 1997;204(1):185–9.
38. Miller CD, Savoie FH. Valgus extension injuries of the elbow in the throwing athlete. J Am Acad Orthop Surg 1994;2(5):261–9.
39. Pappas AM, Zawacki RM, Sullivan TJ. Biomechanics of baseball pitching. A preliminary report. Am J Sports Med 1985;13(4):216–22.

40. Wilson FD, Andrews JR, Blackburn TA, et al. Valgus extension overload in the pitching elbow. Am J Sports Med 1983;11(2):83–8.

41. Conway JE, Jobe FW, Glousman RE, Pink M. Medial instability of the elbow in throwing athletes. Treatment by repair or reconstruction of the ulnar collateral ligament. J Bone Joint Surg Am 1992;74(1):67–83.

42. Wilson FD, Andrews JR, Blackburn TA, et al. Valgus extension overload in the pitching elbow. Am J Sports Med 1983;11(2):83–7.

43. Potter HG, Sofka CM. Imaging. In: Altchek DW, Andrews JR, eds. The Athlete's Elbow. New York: Lippincott Williams & Wilkins, 2001:59–80.

44. Potter HG. Imaging of posttraumatic and soft tissue dysfunction of the elbow. Clin Orthop 2000;370:9–18.

45. Schwartz ML, Al-Zahrani S, Morwessel RM, et al. Ulnar collateral ligament injury in the throwing athlete: evaluation with saline-enhanced MR arthrography. Radiology 1995;197(1):297–9.

46. Timmerman LA, Schwartz ML, Andrews JR. Preoperative evaluation of the ulnar collateral ligament by magnetic resonance imaging and computed tomography arthrography: evaluation in 25 baseball players with surgical confirmation. Am J Sports Med 1994;22(1):26–31.

47. Glajchen N, Schwartz ML, Andrews JR, et al. Avulsion fracture of the sublime tubercle of the ulna: a newly recognized injury in the throwing athlete. AJR Am J Roentgenol 1998;170(3):627–8.

48. Akagi M. Avulsion fracture of the sublime (coronoid) tubercle of the ulna in throwing athletes. AJR Am J Roentgenol 1999;173(3):849–50.

49. Akagi M, Ito T, Ikeda N, et al. Total avulsion fracture of the coronoid tubercle caused by baseball pitching. A case report. Am J Sports Med 2000;28(4):580–2.

50. Salvo JP, Rizio L, Zvijac JE, et al. Avulsion fracture of the ulnar sublime tubercle in overhead throwing athletes. Am J Sports Med 2002;30(3):426–31.

51. Tullos HS, Erwin WD, Woods GW, et al. Unusual lesions of the pitching arm. Clin Orthop Rel Res 1972;88:169–82.

52. Bredella MA, Tirman PF, Fritz RC, et al. MR imaging findings of lateral ulnar collateral ligament abnormalities inpatients with lateral epicondylitis. Am J Roentgenol 1999;173(5):1379–82.

53. Yao L, Lee JK. Occult intraosseous fracture: detection with MR imaging. Radiology 1988;167(3):749–51.

54. Bradley JP, Petrie RS. Osteochondritis dissecans of the humeral capitellum. Diagnosis and treatment. Clin Sports Med 2001;20(3):565–90.

55. Patel N, Weiner SD. Osteochondritis dissecans involving the trochlea: report of two patients (three elbows) and review of the literature. J Pediatr Orthop 2002;22(1):48–51.

56. Berndt AL, Harty M. Transchondral fractures (osteochondritis dissecans) of the talus. J Bone Joint Surg [Am] 1959;41–A:988–1020.

57. Quinn SF, Haberman JJ, Fitzgerald SW, et al. Evaluation of loose bodies in the elbow with MR imaging. J Magn Reson Imaging 1994;4(2):169–72.

58. Ho CP. Sports and occupational injuries of the elbow: MR imaging findings. AJR Am J Roentgenol 1995;164(6):1465–71.

59. Sugimoto H, Ohsawa T. Ulnar collateral ligament in the growing elbow: MR imaging of normal development and throwing injuries. Radiology 1994;192(2):417–22.

60. Ahmad CS, ElAttrache NS. Valgus extension overload syndrome and stress injury of the olecranon. Clin Sports Med 2004;23:665–76.

61. Rosenberg ZS, Bencardino J, Beltran J. MR features of nerve disorders at the elbow. Magn Reson Imaging Clin North Am 1997;5(3):545–65.

62. MacNichol MF. Extraneural pressure affecting the ulnar nerve at the elbow. Hand 1982;14:5–11.

63. Pechan J, Julis I. The pressure measurement in the ulnar nerve. A contribution to the pathophysiology of the cubital tunnel syndrome. J Biomechanics 1975;8:75.

64. Wadsworth TG, Fowley SB: Neurologic disorders. In: Wadsworth TG, Fowler SB, eds. The Elbow. New York: Churchill Livingstone, 1982:258–82.

65. Spinner M, Linchied RL. Nerve intrapment syndromes. In: Morbey BF, ed. The Elbow and Its Disorders. Philadelphia: Saunders, 1985:691–712.

66. Percina MM, Krymptoic-Nemanic J, Markowitz AD. Tunnel syndromes in the upper extremities. In: Pecina MM, Krympotic-Nemanic J, Markowitz AD, eds. Tunnel Syndromes. New York: CRC, 1991:29–53.

67. Rosenberg ZS, Beltran J, Cheung YY, et al. The elbow: MR features of nerve disorders. Radiology 1993;188(1):235–40.

68. Hutchinson MR, Wynn S. Biomechanics and development of the elbow in the young throwing athlete. Clin Sports Med 2004;23:531–44.

69. Safran MR, Baillargeon D. Soft tissue stabilizers of the elbow. J Shoulder Elbow Surg 2004;14(1 suppl):179S–185S.

70. Nirschl RP, Rodin DM, Ochiai DH et al. DEX-AHE-01–99 Study Group: iontophoretic administration of dexamethasone sodium phosphate for acute epicondylitis. A randomized, double-blinded, placebo controlled study. Am J Sports Med 2003;31:189–95.

71. Santini AJ, Frostick SP. How should you treat tennis elbow? In: MacAuley D, Best TM, eds. Evidence-Based Sports Medicine. London: BMJ Books, 2002:351–65.

72. Paoloni JA, Appleyard RC, Nelson J, Murrell GA. Topical glyceryl trinitrate application in the treatment of chronic extensor tendinosis at the elbow: A randomized, double-blinded, placebo controlled clinical trial. Am J Sports Med 2003;31:915–20.

73. Lo M, Safran MR. Surgical management of lateral epicondylitis—a systematic review. Clin Orthop Rel Res 2006; in press.

74. Baker CL Jr, Murphy KP, Gottlob CA, Curd DT. Arthroscopic classification and treatment of lateral epicondylitis: two year clinical results. J Shoulder Elbow Surg 2000;9:475–82.

75. Ollivierre CO, Nirschl RP, Pettrone FA. Reseaction and repair for medial tennis elbow. A prospective analysis. Am J Sports Med 1995;23:214–21.

76. Gabel GT, Morrey BF. Operative treatment of medial epicondylitis. Influence of concomitant ulnar neuropathy at the elbow. J Bone Joint Surg 1995;77(A):1374–79.

77. Rantanen J, Orava S. Rupture of the distal biceps tendon. A report of 19 patients treated with anatomic reinsertion, and a meta-analysis of 147 cases found in the literature. Am J Sports Med 1999;27:128–32.

78. Rettig AC. Traumatic elbow injuries in the athlete. Orthop Clin North Am 2002;33:509–22.

79. Viegas SF. Avulsion of the triceps tendon. Orthop Rev 1990;19:533–6.

80. Eygendaal D, Verdegaal SH, Obermann WR, et al. Posterolateral dislocation of the elbow joint. Relationship to medial instability. J Bone Joint Surg 2000;82(A):555–60.

81. Rettig AC, Sherrill C, Snead DS, et al. Non-operative treatment of ulnar collateral ligament injuries throwing athletes. Am J Sports Med 2001;29:15–17.

82. Safran MR, Ahmad C, ElAttrache N. Ulnar collateral ligament injuries of the elbow. Current concepts. J Arthrosc Rel Surg 2005;21(11):1381–95.

83. Glajchen N, Schwartz ML, Andrews JR, et al. Avulsion fracture of the sublime tubercle of the ulna: a newly recognized injury in the throwing athlete. AJR Am J Roentgenol 1998;170(3):627–8.

84. Sanchez-Sotelo J, Morrey BF, O'Driscoll SW. Ligamentous repair and reconstruction for posterolateral rotatory instability of the elbow. J Bone Joint Surg 2005;87(B):54–61.

85. Rudzki JR, Paletta GA. Juvenile and adolescent elbow injuries in sports. Clin Sports Med 2004;23:581–608.

86. Andrews JR, Timmerman LA. Outcome of elbow surgery in professional baseball players. Am J Sports Med 1995;23: 407–13.

87. Wadsworth TG, Fowley SB. Neurologic disorders. In: Wadsworth TG, Fowler SB, eds. The Elbow. New York: Churchill Livingstone, 1982:258–82.

88. Spinner M, Linchied RL. Nerve intrapment syndromes. In: Morbey BF, ed. The Elbow and Its Disorders. Philadelphia: Saunders, 1985:691–712.

89. Percina MM, Krympotic-Nemanic J, Markowitz AD. Tunnel Syndromes in the upper extremities. In: Pecina MM, Krympotic-Nemanic J, Markowitz AD, eds. Tunnel Syndromes. New York: CRC, 1991:29–53.

7
Wrist

A. Radiologic Perspective: Magnetic Resonance Imaging of the Wrist

Weiling Chang and Donald Resnick

Magnetic resonance imaging (MRI) is a noninvasive imaging method that offers remarkable information in assessing both the osseous and the soft tissue structures of the wrist. The ligaments, tendons, nerves, muscles, and cartilage can be resolved due to the high spatial and contrast resolution of this method. It is an excellent technique for evaluating patients with wrist pain to help establish or confirm underlying wrist abnormalities.

Normal Anatomy

The wrist connects the distal forearm to the hand. The distal portions of the radius and ulna articulate with the proximal carpal row, composed of the scaphoid, lunate, triquetrum, and pisiform bones. Unlike the remainder of the carpal bones, the pisiform is a sesamoid bone, being embedded within the fibers of the flexor carpi ulnaris tendon.

The distal radius has a normal radial and ulnar incline. It has a smooth C shaped concavity with two fossae that serve to accommodate the scaphoid and lunate bones.[1] The distal carpal row articulates with both the proximal carpal row and the metacarpal bases. It is composed of the trapezium, trapezoid, capitate, and hamate bones. On its volar surface, the carpus forms a osseous concavity that is sealed by the flexor retinaculum, creating the carpal tunnel[2] (Fig. 7.1).

Eight superficial and deep flexor tendons, the flexor pollicis longus tendon, the median artery and nerve, and the radial and ulnar bursae all pass through the carpal tunnel. The median nerve is identified by its intimate relationship with the flexor digitorum superficialis tendons of the second and third digits.[3] The ulnar bursa is the larger of the two bursae within the carpal tunnel. It forms a series of three invaginations which interdigitate superficial to, between, and deep to the flexor digitorum superficialis and profundus tendons.[4] Communication between these two bursae exists normally in many persons.

The distal radioulnar, radiocarpal, midcarpal, and carpometacarpal joints form some of the articulations of the wrist. The radiocarpal joint is separated from the distal radioulnar joint by the triangular fibrocartilage complex (TFCC) of the wrist. The scapholunate (SL) and lunotriquetral (LT) interosseous ligaments are horseshoe-shaped ligaments that separate the radiocarpal and midcarpal joints. There is no normal route of communication between the radiocarpal and midcarpal or the radiocarpal and distal radioulnar joints. If such a communication exists, a traumatic injury or degenerative process is the likely cause.

The TFCC is an anatomically complex structure composed of the following: (1) triangular fibrocartilage (TFC) articular disk, (2) meniscus homologue, (3) dorsal and volar radioulnar ligaments, (4) ulnar collateral ligament, and (5) the extensor carpi ulnaris tendon sheath.[5] Although the TFCC is composed of five separate structures, they imperceptibly blend with one another, and only the TFC itself can generally be identified as a discrete structure.

The normal magnetic resonance (MR) appearance of the TFC is a triangular region of homogeneous low signal intensity, best seen in coronal images (Fig. 7.2). At the ulnar styloid attachment site where the TFC normally thickens, it may have more intermediate signal intensity, although this signal is not as bright as the joint fluid. Thus, the finding can be distinguished from that of a TFC tear. In sagittal images the normal TFC appears as a biconcave disk that is thinner centrally than peripherally. Axial images are not as helpful in evaluating the TFC as are the coronal and sagittal images because the TFC is seen as a vague triangular region of low signal on one to two images only.

The TFCC attaches to the ulnar aspect of the distal radius via a short segment of hyaline cartilage, which appears relatively bright on T2-weighted images. The fibers of the TFCC insert upon the fovea at the base of the ulnar styloid via proximal and distal attachments, or laminae. The TFCC incorporates fibers of the ulnar collateral ligament which itself attaches to the lunate, triquetrum, hamate, and base of the fifth metacarpal bone.[5] The meniscal homologue is considered part of the TFCC. It is a region of relative thickening of the ulnar joint capsule, and it is bordered proximally by the prestyloid recess.

The TFCC acts as a stabilizer of the distal radioulnar joint. It has a cushioning effect in preventing disorders such as

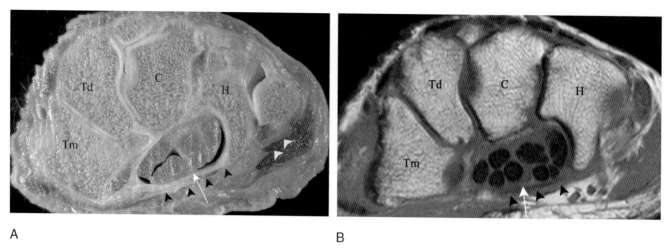

A   B

FIG. 7.1. (A,B) Carpal tunnel: normal anatomy. Axial anatomic section and MR image at the corresponding level reveals the flexor tendons within the carpal tunnel bounded along its volar surface by the flexor retinaculum (black arrowheads). The median nerve (white arrow) is intimate with the flexor superficialis tendons of the second and third digits and appears relatively bright compared to the remainder of the tendons. Tm, trapezium; Td, trapezoid; C, capitate, H, hamate.

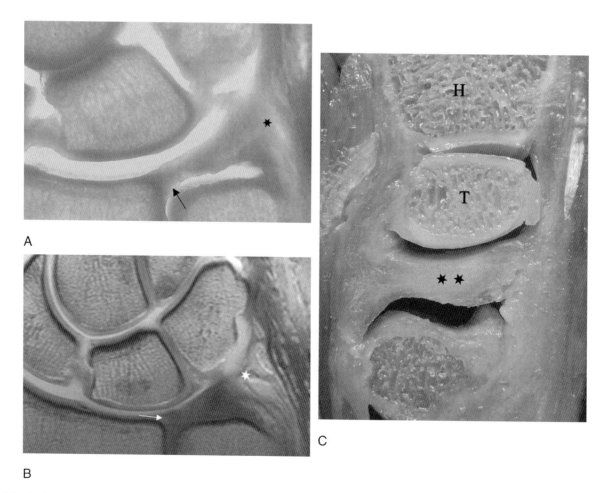

FIG. 7.2. (A–C) Triangular fibrocartilage complex: normal appearance. Coronal T1-weighted MRI through the triangular fibrocartilage complex (TFCC) and the corresponding anatomic section. (A,B) Articular cartilage is located at the radial limit of the triangular fibrocartilage complex (arrows), demonstrating intermediate signal intensity. Fibrofatty tissue is located in the region of the meniscal homologue (asterisk), also demonstrating intermediate signal intensity. The triangular fibrocartilage articular disk appears of low signal intensity on MRI. (C) Sagittal anatomic section of the wrist demonstrates the biconcave shape to the triangular fibrocartilage (asterisks) that is thicker toward its periphery. T, triquetrum; H, hamate.

ulnocarpal abutment. It transmits axial loads from the wrist to the forearm. The amount of force transmitted is related to the ulnar variance. Ulnar neutral variance is present when the ulna and radius are equal in length. In this situation, approximately 20% of an axial load is transmitted through the ulna.[5] In ulnar positive variance, the ulna is longer than the radius, and greater force is transmitted through the ulna. The converse occurs with ulnar minus variance.

The SL and LT ligaments are two examples of interosseous ligaments, linking the carpal bones of the proximal row (Fig. 7.3). They are both C-shaped, hammock-like structures demonstrating a thinner central membranous portion and relatively thicker palmar and dorsal portions. The palmar and dorsal portions are histologically composed of collagen fibers, typical of a true ligament, whereas the central membranous portion is formed from fibrocartilage.[6] The SL and LT ligaments appear as triangular-shaped low signal structures in the standard coronal plane. They can also be visualized exquisitely when using the axial or axial oblique imaging plane, providing an excellent second plane to confirm and to further characterize pathologic conditions.[7]

The scaphocapitate (SC) and triquetrohamocapitate (THC) ligaments are lesser known interosseous ligaments that function as an important link between the proximal and distal carpal rows. The SC ligament originates from the scaphoid tuberosity and then courses obliquely in a distal direction to attach to the body of the capitate. The THC ligament originates from the triquetrum and courses obliquely, also attaching to the body of the capitate. Together these two ligaments are known

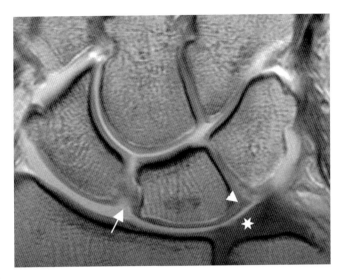

FIG. 7.3. Intercarpal ligaments: normal anatomy. Coronal MRI image demonstrates the normal appearance of the scapholunate (SL) ligament (white arrow) as a linear region of low signal. The MRI appearance of the lunotriquetral (LT) ligament (white arrowhead) is more difficult than the SL ligament to assess on MR imaging. Asterisk, TFC.

as the arcuate ligament of the wrist and are hypothesized to play a crucial role in maintaining midcarpal stability. They form an "inverted V" separated by an area devoid of ligamentous fibers that is located between the capitate and lunate, an area that is known as the space of Poirer (Fig. 7.4).

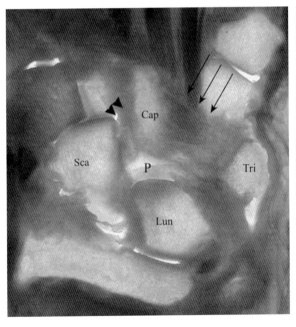

A

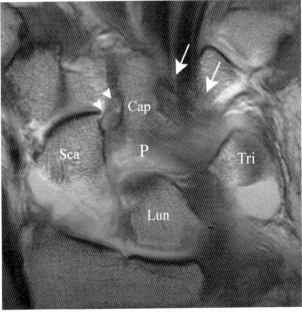

B

FIG. 7.4. (A,B) Intercarpal ligaments: normal anatomy. Coronal oblique MR arthrographic images of the volar aspect of the wrist show the THC ligament (straight arrows) extending from the triquetum to the capitate (Cap) over the volar aspect of the hamate. The SC ligament (arrowheads) arises from the scaphoid (Sca) and extends to the neck of the capitate. Together the two ligaments form an "inverted V". The potential space devoid of ligaments in the central portion of the "inverted V" is the space of Poirer (P). Lun, lunate.

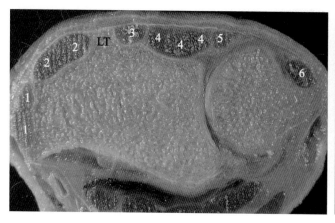

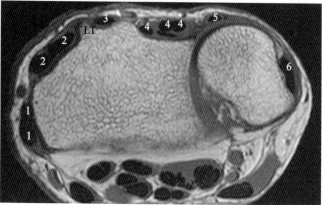

A   B

FIG. 7.5. (A,B) Dorsal extensor tendons: normal anatomy. Axial anatomic section and corresponding MRI through the level of the distal radio-ulnar joint demonstrates the dorsal tendons within six compartments: 1, abductor pollicis longus and extensor pollicis brevis; 2, extensor carpi radialis longus and brevis; 3, extensor pollicis longus; 4, extensor digitorum and indicis; 5, extensor digiti minimi; 6, extensor carpi ulnaris. The second and third dorsal extensor compartments are separated by an osseous landmark, Lister's tubercle (LT).

The dorsal extensor tendons are organized into six compartments separated by fascial investments and stabilized by the extensor retinaculum. These compartments are best identified at the level of the distal radioulnar joint (Fig. 7.5).

All but one of the flexor tendons extend through or very near the carpal tunnel. The exception is the flexor carpi ulnaris tendon, which lies just superficial to the flexor retinaculum. Both flexor and extensor tendons can be seen in all three imaging planes but are visualized to best advantage on axial images in which they normally appear as dark, ovoid structures.

Imaging Techniques

The preferred MRI technique for the wrist involves placing the patient in the supine position with the hand by the side or alternatively in the prone position with the arm extended above the head. The wrist is placed in a neutral position within a wrist coil. A comfortable position is essential to minimize motion artifact. In persons with palpable abnormalities or point tenderness, a vitamin E capsule is utilized as a marker to identify the area of interest.

Optimal images can be obtained in a high field magnet with a small field of view (8 to 12 cm) and thin slices. The standard coronal, axial, and sagittal imaging planes are obtained, although the study may be modified with oblique imaging planes to study a specific anatomic structure of interest.

An intravenous gadolinium solution is administered when there is concern for an underlying neoplastic or inflammatory process. An intraarticular gadolinium solution may be injected into the radiocarpal compartment of the wrist when there is concern regarding the integrity of the TFCC or the SL or LT ligament. Abnormalities in these structures are identi-

fied when there is abnormal passage of the injected intraarticular contrast material from the radiocarpal compartment to either the midcarpal or inferior radioulnar compartment.

Scaphoid Fractures and Their Complications

The scaphoid is the carpal bone most frequently fractured, an injury that usually results from a fall on an outstretched hand. Because radiographs may be negative initially, MRI is a method that can provide a definitive diagnosis when a fracture is suspected.[8] As with acute fractures elsewhere in the body, MRI exhibits exuberant edema with high signal on T2-weighted images accompanied by a dark linear fracture line best identified on T1-weighted images.

Scaphoid fractures are at risk for delayed union, nonunion, or osteonecrosis resulting from its vulnerable blood supply. There is an unusual distal to proximal orientation of the vascular supply to the scaphoid. The interosseous arterial feeders enter distally and then proceed to the proximal pole. When the scaphoid is fractured, its proximal pole is vulnerable to ischemia and osteonecrosis because its blood supply is disrupted. The risk of osteonecrosis correlates with the position of the fracture, with distal fractures carrying a better prognosis than proximal fractures.[2] Most frequently the scaphoid fractures occur through the waist of the bone. At this position, there is an associated 30% incidence of osteonecrosis.[9] Fracture healing time may also be increased, leading to potential delayed union or nonunion.[10]

Interfragmentary motion at the site of scaphoid fracture can occur secondary to normal carpal kinematics, resulting in a "humpback" deformity," which is characterized by a prominent

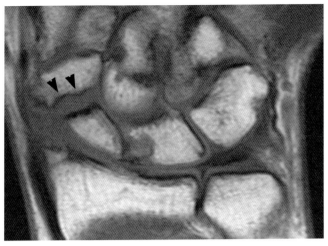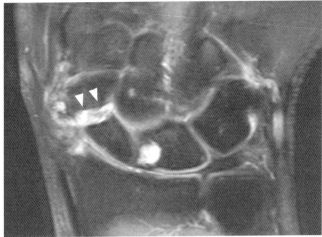

A   B

FIG. 7.6. (A,B) Scaphoid nonunion. Coronal T1 and fat-suppressed T2-weighted MRI of the wrist. There is fluid signal in the scaphoid waist fracture line (arrowheads). There is no marrow edema indicating that this is a chronic injury. A subchondral cyst is located at the radial aspect of the lunate.

dorsal protuberance.[10,11] It is the natural tendency for the distal fracture fragment to flex and the proximal fracture fragment to extend. This abnormal motion complicates normal fracture healing, and may result in a permanent dorsal intercalated segmental instability (DISI) pattern of malalignment.

Scaphoid nonunion is another potential complication when a fracture fails to heal within 9 months from the time of injury.[12] A pseudarthrosis or fibrous union may be present with no osseous bridging at the fracture site. By MRI, a definitive sign of scaphoid fracture union is a continuity of marrow across the fracture.[13] A persistent cleft of fluid signal at the fracture site suggests nonunion (Fig. 7.6). However, there is variability in the MR appearance of subacute and chronic fractures, and the stages of fracture healing are not well studied.

Osteonecrosis is suspected radiographically when there is increased sclerosis within the proximal pole of the scaphoid. However, radiographs have a relatively low sensitivity in identifying the early stages of osteonecrosis. Mild sclerosis may not correlate with osteonecrosis. The proximal fragment has a relatively diminished vascularity following fracture so there is less resorption of bone and preserved bone mineral density relative to the osteopenic bones in the remainder of the wrist. These changes do not necessarily progress to osteonecrosis.

Magnetic resonance imaging features of osteonecrosis include altered marrow signal with decreased signal in both T1- and T2-weighted images. However, signal alterations may be present with uncomplicated fractures related to the formation of granulation tissue, and a definitive diagnosis of avascular necrosis can be difficult. Studies have advocated the use of intravenous gadolinium administration to clarify the issue. Gadolinium enhancement correlates well with the presence of

viable tissue; nonenhancement suggests ischemia and osteonecrosis.[14]

Because of its multiplanar capabilities, MRI is also helpful in the evaluation of fractures that are difficult to identify with standard radiography. Fractures of the trapezial ridge occur from an avulsion at the attachment of the flexor retinaculum[7] (transverse carpal ligament) (Fig. 7.7). A second potential radiographically occult fracture involves the hook of the hamate (Fig. 7.8. Such fractures may result from a direct blow or an injury related to the flexor retinaculum (transverse carpal ligament). They are frequently associated with racquet sports or golf.[15] Hook of hamate fractures occasionally progress to nonunion and sometimes Guyon's canal syndrome.

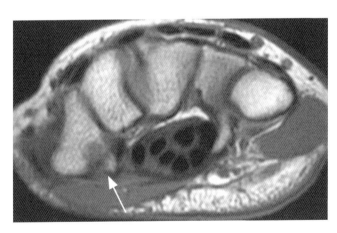

FIG. 7.7. Trapezial ridge fracture. Axial T1-weighted image of the wrist. A low signal intensity fracture line (white arrow) extends through the trapezial ridge. This occurs at the attachment site of the flexor retinaculum, and it is considered an avulsion fracture.

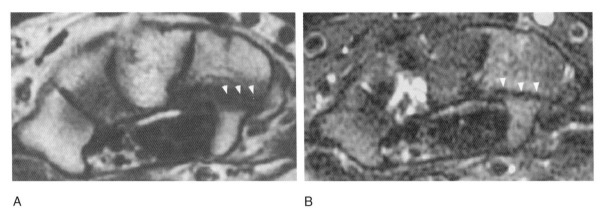

A   B

FIG. 7.8. (A,B) Hook of hamate fracture. Axial T1- and fat-suppressed T2-weighted images of the wrist. A low signal intensity fracture line is located at the base of the hook of hamate (arrowheads). The paucity of marrow edema suggests a chronic injury.

Interosseous Ligaments

Tears of the SL or LT ligament are established causes of chronic wrist pain. Both ligaments are biomechanically essential to the normal motion of the carpus. When untreated, these injuries can progress to wrist instability manifested by volar intercalated carpal instability (VISI) or dorsal intercalated carpal instability (DISI).

The SL ligament holds the scaphoid and lunate bones together with its thick dorsal and volar slips. An abnormality of the SL ligament is suspected when conventional radiographs reveal a scapholunate interosseous interval that is greater than 2 mm. Scapholunate ligament tears are almost definite when the interval is widened beyond 4 mm.

The SL ligament is larger in caliber than the LT ligament. However, the two ligaments are morphologically and structurally similar. Both are triangular in shape on coronal MRI. They are both low in signal intensity with all MR pulse sequences. Gradient echo images allow the acquisition of thin sections, and such images are advantageous in identifying focal abnormalities. Abnormalities are suspected when the SL and LT ligaments appear elongated, discontinuous, or absent[2] (Fig. 7.9). Secondary findings include increased signal within the adjacent bones, particularly at their ligamentous attachments.[16] The SL and LT ligaments can also have partial tears involving either their volar or dorsal slips, best diagnosed on axial images (Fig. 7.10). Volar slip failure is the more common injury.[16]

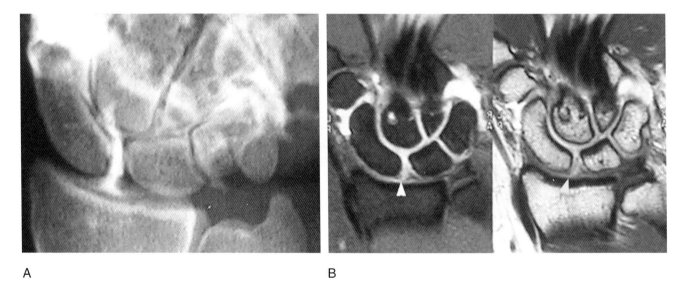

A   B

FIG. 7.9. Scapholunate ligament tear. (A) Fluoroscopic image of the wrist obtained immediately after midcarpal arthrography. There is abnormal communication of the contrast material between the midcarpal and radiocarpal compartments via a torn SL ligament. (B) Coronal T1- fat-suppressed and T1-weighted images following midcarpal arthrography of the wrist. High signal extends through a discontinuous scapholunate ligament (arrowhead). The ligament is disrupted at its scaphoid attachment. There is minimal widening of the scapholunate interval. A small cyst is also present in the capitate.

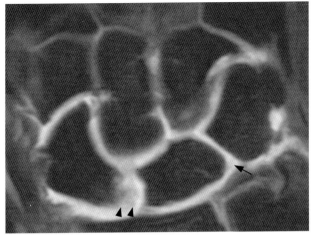
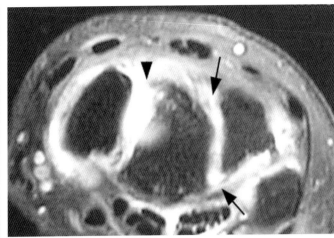

A

B

FIG. 7.10. Scapholunate and lunotriquetral ligament tears. Coronal T1- and axial T1-weighted fat-suppressed images following radiocarpal arthrography of the wrist. (A) There is discontinuity of the SL ligament (arrowheads) with intraarticular contrast material leaking into the midcarpal compartment. The LT ligament is absent (arrow). (B) Axial image shows the tear of the dorsal slip of the SL ligament (arrowhead). There is a widened gap between the dorsal scaphoid and lunate. Both volar and dorsal slips of the LT ligament are discontinuous (arrows).

The central membranous portion of the SL and LT ligaments is subjected to attritional changes with advancing age. This is manifested by intermediate signal within the central substance not reaching the same signal intensity as that of surrounding joint fluid. T2-weighted images are useful in distinguishing mucoid degeneration from tears. If the results of standard MRI are equivocal, MR arthrography can provide diagnostic confirmation.

Conventional MRI of the wrist allows the detection of SL ligament tears with a sensitivity of 50% to 93%, and LT ligament tears with a sensitivity of 40% to 56%.[17] When tears of the interosseous ligaments are suspected, MR arthrography can improve the diagnostic specificity.[17] When a dilute intraarticular gadolinium solution is injected into the midcarpal compartment and subsequently enters the radiocarpal compartment, a tear of the SL or LT ligament is inferred. Indirect MR arthrography has also been used in assessing internal derangements of the wrist, although it does not provide ideal distention of the joint space. Early research has documented equivocal results with this method with improved sensitivity in the evaluation of SL ligament injuries but no significant improvement over standard MRI in the evaluation of LT ligament injuries.[18]

A chronic tear of the SL ligament can lead to scapholunate advanced collapse (SLAC). When an SL ligament perforation is identified or suspected by MRI or conventional radiography, the study should be carefully scrutinized for features of a SLAC wrist (Fig. 7.11). Scapholunate advanced collapse is an end-stage osteoarthrosis of the wrist with findings occurring in a specific chronological order: (1) the SL ligament is disrupted; (2) rotatory subluxation of the scaphoid occurs, leading to an abnormal radioscaphoid articulation, resulting

in progressive radioscaphoid osteoarthrosis; (3) axial load is shifted toward the capitolunate articulation resulting in progressive capitolunate osteoarthrosis; and (4) proximal migration of the capitate occurs.[19]

Carpal Instability

Carpal instability can be classified into two broad patterns: carpal instability dissociative (CID) and carpal instability nondissociative (CIND). In the CID pattern, the abnormal kinematics results from dyssynchronous movement within the same carpal row. Examples include scapholunate dissociation resulting in DISI (Fig. 7.12) and lunotriquetral dissociation resulting in VISI. Although sometimes difficult to assess by MRI, abnormal lunate tilt is the hallmark of the CID pattern. This should be investigated carefully when a SL or LT ligament disruption is identified. In DISI, there is an exaggerated flexion of the scaphoid and extension of the lunate leading to a scapholunate angle that is greater than 60 degrees. In VISI, the scaphoid and lunate both reveal volar flexion, thereby diminishing the scapholunate angle to less than 30 degrees, diagnostic of the VISI pattern of malalignment.[20]

In the CIND category, the abnormal kinematics results from dyssynchronous motion between either the proximal and distal carpal rows or the distal radius and proximal carpal row.[21] Palmar midcarpal instability is a subtype of the CIND pattern of abnormality, and is associated with abnormal laxity of the SC and THC ligaments, which together form the arcuate ligament of the wrist. Clinically this entity is characterized by a painful and sudden clunking of the wrist with axial loading

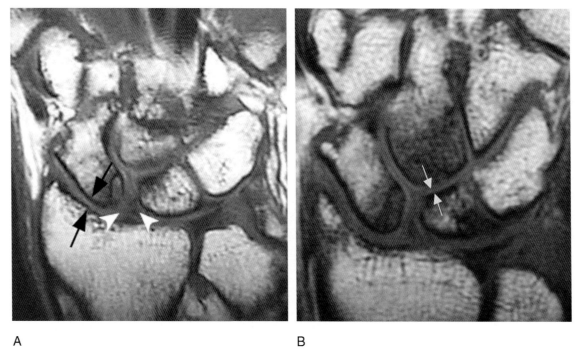

FIG. 7.11. (A,B) Scapholunate advanced collapse (SLAC) wrist. Coronal T1-weighted MRI of the wrist. The SL ligament is disorganized and discontinuous (white arrowheads). There is osteoarthrosis of the radioscaphoid joint with a decreased joint space and osteophyte formation (black arrows). Capitolunate osteoarthrosis is manifested by joint space loss and changes in marrow signal at the articular surfaces (white arrows).

and ulnar deviation. The arcuate ligament of the wrist can be visualized on standard MRI, although it is best seen in coronal oblique images. Magnetic resonance imaging abnormalities may result in abnormal high signal within the fibers of the ligament or a thickened appearance.

Triangular Fibrocartilage

Although not well understood, perforations and tears of the triangular fibrocartilage can be symptomatic and result in ulnar-sided pain. Traumatic injuries occur with a fall on an

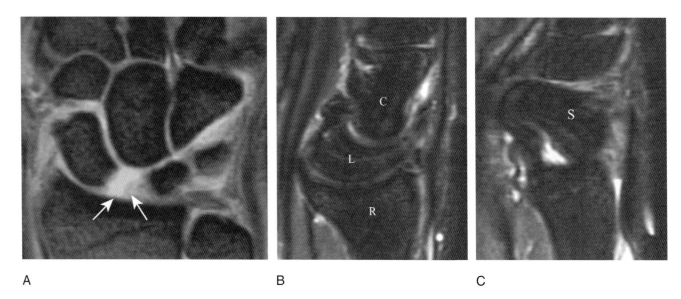

FIG. 7.12. Dorsal intercalated segmental instability. Coronal and sagittal T2-weighted fat-suppressed images of the wrist. (A) There is a SL ligament disruption with the ligament detached from its scaphoid attachment (white arrows). There is an increased scapholunate interval. (B,C) There is an exaggerated dorsal tilt of the lunate (L) relative to both the radius (R) and capitate (C). The scaphoid (S) has an abnormally flexed posture and demonstrates minimal dorsal subluxation.

outstretched hand with associated forearm rotation. Degenerative changes also occur within the TFC, and are considered a part of the normal aging process. An anatomic study found no degenerative lesions or perforations of the triangular fibrocartilage in persons in the first two decades of life. After the fifth decade of life, 100% of wrists had degenerative lesions of the triangular fibrocartilage, with 40% revealing perforations.[22] The incidence of these degenerative changes increases with advancing age, and the findings may or may not be symptomatic.

Palmer[23] described the most widely used system for the classification of TFCC lesions. Class I lesions represent the traumatic injuries: IA, central perforation; IB, avulsion from the ulna; IC, avulsion from the distal attachment sites to the lunate and/or triquetrum; and ID, avulsion from the distal radius (Fig. 7.13). Avulsion of the TFCC from the radius and ulna may be of an osseous nature in the form of avulsion fractures.

Class II lesions relate to degeneration: IIA, TFCC degeneration; IIB, TFCC degeneration accompanied by chondromalacia of the ulna or lunate; IIC, TFCC perforation accompanied by chondromalacia of the ulna or lunate; IID, TFCC perforation with LT ligament disruption accompanied by chondromalacia of the ulna or lunate; and IIE, all the findings of IID with associated osteoarthrosis.[23]

Triangular fibrocartilage degeneration first occurs at its thinner membranous portion. There is increased signal in both T1- and T2-weighted images. It is important to carefully evaluate the T2-weighted images, however, to distinguish mucoid degeneration from fluid within a tear that appears brighter. Defects and perforations of the TFC appear as a band of fluid signal intensity spanning the TFC in conventional MRI. Partial tears of the TFC are also encountered, frequently occurring on its ulnar surface. They probably relate to biomechanical factors during forearm rotation, which places more stress along the ulnar (i.e., proximal) surface than the carpal (i.e., distal) surface of the TFC.[24]

Direct MR arthrography is advantageous in evaluating persons with suspected TFC tears. Although it does not increase diagnostic sensitivity, it does improve the specificity.[25] Passage of the injected dilute gadolinium solution from the radiocarpal joint to the distal radioulnar joint is usually indicative of a TFC perforation. Magnetic resonance imaging is superior to conventional arthrography in its ability to characterize the nature of the perforation. Indirect MR arthrography can be utilized as well, although the literature has shown no definitive advantage of this method over conventional MRI in the diagnosis of TFC abnormalities.[18]

Ulnar Impaction Syndrome

Ulnar impaction syndrome is an entity that is also known by many other names including ulnocarpal abutment, ulnolunate impingement, and ulnocarpal loading. Its symptoms include pain, swelling, and limitation of motion.[26]

The pathophysiology of ulnar impaction syndrome is related to excessive load that is distributed across the ulnar aspect of the wrist. The underlying abnormality is an ulnar positive variance that also leads to a repetitive impaction of the ulna and the carpus. The sequela of this injury includes TFC and LT ligament tears, chondromalacia of the lunate or ulna, and localized synovitis. There are both primary and secondary causes of ulnar impaction syndrome.[27] Examples include a congenitally long ulna. Also, impacted radial fractures, radial growth arrest, and radial head resection are secondary causes of a disproportionately long ulna.[2]

Conventional radiographs serve as a first-line imaging modality for the evaluation of ulnar impaction syndrome. These are adequate in assessing ulnar variance and osteoarthrosis of the ulnocarpal articulation. Both standard MRI and MR arthrography enable assessment of the soft tissue findings of ulnar impaction syndrome (Fig. 7.14), specifically abnormalities of the LT ligament and TFC. Magnetic resonance is also more sensitive in the evaluation of chondromalacia of the lunate or ulna, offering more detailed information of the extent of cartilaginous damage.

Kienbock's Disease (Lunatomalacia)

This condition was first described by Kienbock in 1910, and has since been associated with his name. Symptoms include a stiff and painful wrist commonly occurring in young and active adults in their third or fourth decade of life. The exact etiology of this condition is unclear. Based on cadaveric studies, investigators have found that 32% of persons have a lunate blood supply that is derived from a solitary volar vessel.[28] It is believed that a stress fracture is the inciting event, leading to devascularization of the bone. An association with ulnar minus variance exists, and Kienbock's disease is four times more common in persons with ulnar minus variance.[29] Biomechanically this configuration subjects the lunate to greater compression and shear stresses, thereby increasing the risk of Kienbock's disease.

The classic radiographic findings include bone sclerosis sometimes associated with superimposed fracture lines. Advanced cases demonstrate osseous fragmentation and progressive collapse of the lunate. Secondary changes include SL ligament tears, radiocarpal osteoarthrosis, and proximal migration of the capitate. Magnetic resonance imaging can be beneficial because the early stages of osteonecrosis can be radiographically occult. There is global decreased signal intensity of the lunate on T1-weighted images accompanied by increased signal on T2-weighted images (Fig. 7.15) in the early stages of osteonecrosis, when it has the highest likelihood of being radiographically negative. There is variability in the MRI findings, particularly in the advanced stages of the disease. The staging system for Kienbock's disease can be helpful in guiding the course of treatment. Treatment varies depending on the severity of disease. Options include immobilization, revascularization, radial shortening, and carpal fusion.[30]

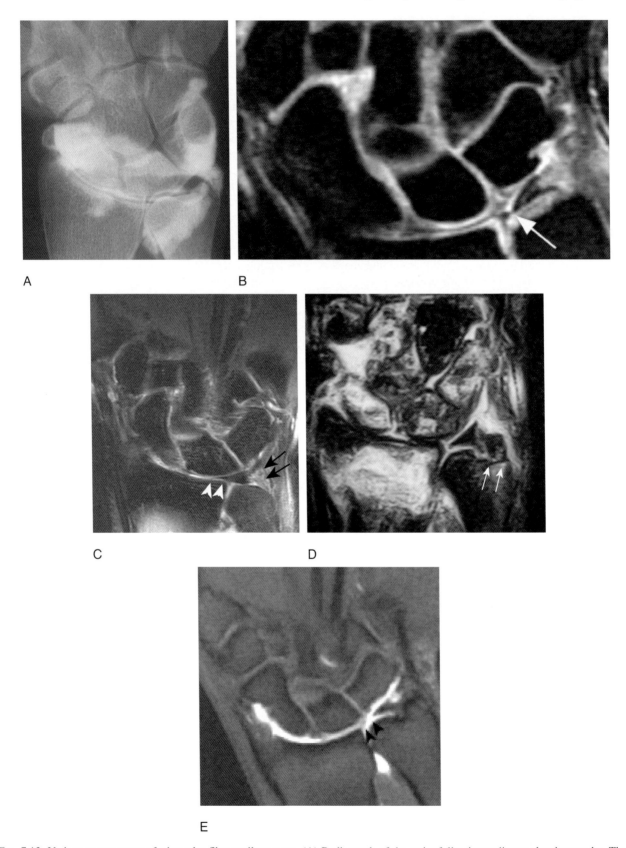

Fig. 7.13. Various appearances of triangular fibrocartilage tears. (A) Radiograph of the wrist following radiocarpal arthrography. There is abnormal passage of contrast from the radiocarpal compartment into the distal radioulnar joint through a torn triangular fibrocartilage. (B) Coronal T2 fat-suppressed MRI of the wrist. There is a central perforation of the triangular fibrocartilage, a Palmer IA injury. There is an alteration in the normal contour of the disk (white arrow). (C) Coronal T2 fat-suppressed MRI of the wrist. The triangular fibrocartilage

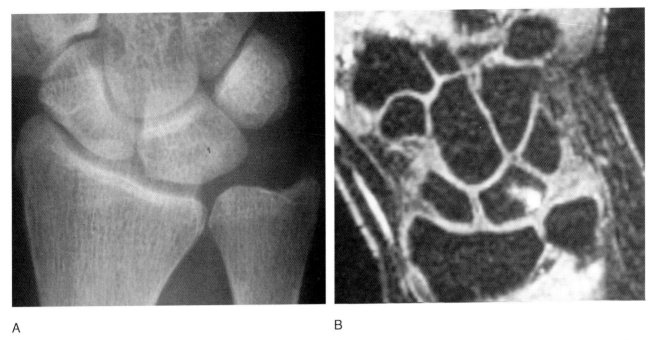

A   B

FIG. 7.14. Ulnar impaction syndrome. (A) Radiograph of the wrist. There is mild ulnar positive variance. Other findings of ulnocarpal abutment are radiographically occult. (B) Coronal T2 fat-suppressed MRI of the wrist. As seen on the plain film of the wrist, there is mild ulnar positive variance. Cystic change is noted at the articular surface of the lunate at its ulnar aspect. The articular cartilage is not well visualized, but the presence of cystic changes raises the possibility of underlying cartilage disease. Degenerative signal is noted within the triangular fibrocartilage with a possible focal perforation.

Carpal Tunnel Syndrome

This relatively common disorder is a cause of wrist pain and hand paresthesias in the distribution of the median nerve. It is the most common peripheral nerve entrapment syndrome. It has gained notoriety as an occupational injury associated with the repetitive motion of typing on a computer keyboard. However, this disorder is not isolated to computer users. It can be seen in athletes such as gymnasts and lacrosse players who repetitively flex and extend their wrists.[2] Weight-lifters can experience the same phenomenon, as their lumbrical muscles hypertrophy, diminishing the space available to the remainder of the structures within the carpal tunnel.[2]

The carpal tunnel measures approximately 6 cm in length extending from the proximal wrist to the middle of the palm. The concavity of the carpus forms the dorsal aspect of the tunnel, which then is sealed volarly by the transverse carpal ligament or flexor retinaculum, extending from the scaphoid and trapezial ridge to the hook of the hamate. The median nerve assumes its normal position just superficial to the flexor digitorum superficialis tendon of the index or middle finger.[3]

The causes of carpal tunnel remain idiopathic in many cases. When they are identified, they can be classified into two basic categories: (1) those leading to a diminished carpal tunnel volume, such as masses or displaced fractures; and (2) those leading to a hypertrophy of the structures native to the carpal tunnel, such as radial or ulnar bursitis from rheumatoid arthritis.[31]

Four major MRI findings have been associated with carpal tunnel syndrome, and are best evaluated in the axial imaging plane: (1) increased size of the median nerve best assessed at the level of the pisiform where it is normally flat; (2) flattening of the median nerve distally at the level of the hamate;

FIG. 7.13. (continued) has shifted radially overlapping the distal radial articular surface (white arrowheads). This overlap is only possible when there has been an avulsion of the triangular fibrocartilage (TFC) from its ulnar attachment, a Palmer IB injury. The region of high signal (black arrows) was interpreted as a tear. (D) Coronal T2 fat-suppressed MRI of the wrist. This is the osseous variant of the Palmer IB lesion. There is an avulsion injury to the ulnar aspect of the wrist. Instead of injury to the ulnar attachment of the TFC, the failure occurs at the base of the ulnar styloid with a fracture (white arrows). There is minimal radial displacement of the fracture fragment. The patient also had a fracture of the distal radius. (E) Coronal T1 fat-suppressed MRI of the wrist following radiocarpal arthrography. There is abnormal communication of the intraarticular gadolinium within the radiocarpal compartment with the distal radioulnar joint. The triangular fibrocartilage has pulled away from its radial attachment (black arrowheads), a Palmer ID injury. The intraarticular gadolinium fills this gap.

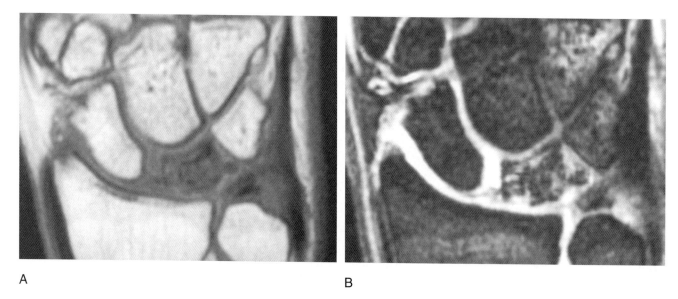

FIG. 7.15. Kienbock's disease. Coronal T1- (A) and fat-suppressed T2-weighted (B) images of the wrist. MRI demonstrates signal alterations in the marrow of the lunate bone compatible with Kienbock's disease. There is low signal on the T1-weighted image with relatively high signal on the T2-weighted image. The lunate contour abnormality suggests early fragmentation. There is also a detachment of the SL ligament from its scaphoid attachment.

(3) palmar bowing of the flexor retinaculum, the MR correlate to the increased pressure within the carpal tunnel; and (4) increased median nerve signal intensity in T2-weighted images[3,31] (Fig. 7.16). Magnetic resonance imaging is not routinely performed for the evaluation of the carpal tunnel syndrome, but it is valuable in assessing secondary causes such as mass lesions or radial and ulnar bursitis. Evaluation of the wrist following release of the flexor retinaculum is another indication for MRI, particularly when symptoms persist or recur. Fibrosis or regrowth of the flexor retinaculum can correlate with a recurrence of symptoms. Other causes include persistent median neuritis, excessive adipose tissue, or ganglion cysts and neuromas.[32]

Guyon's Canal Syndrome

Ulnar nerve entrapment occurs at the wrist in Guyon's canal (distal ulnar tunnel), although this is less frequent than entrapment of the ulnar nerve at the cubital tunnel of the elbow. The pisiform, hamate, flexor retinaculum, and hypothenar muscles form the floor of Guyon's canal. The volar

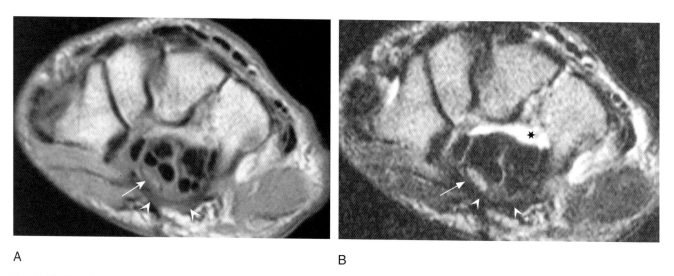

FIG. 7.16. Carpal tunnel syndrome. Axial T1-weighted (A) and fat-suppressed T2-weighted (B) images of the wrist. At the level of the hamate, there is abnormal flattening and increased signal of the median nerve (white arrow). The flexor retinaculum is bowed (white arrowheads). Fluid is present within the ulnar bursa (asterisk).

carpal ligament, palmaris brevis muscle, and portions of the palmar fascia form its roof.[33] This fibro-osseous tunnel extends for a distance of 4 cm from the pisiform to the origin of the hypothenar muscles just distal to the hamulus. As ulnar neurovascular bundle pass through the tunnel, it is circumferentially surrounded by fat. The ulnar nerve is particularly vulnerable to compression by space-occupying lesions within Guyon's canal. Ganglia, lipomas, displaced fractures, and anomalous muscles are potential causes of nerve entrapment. Ulnar artery pseudoaneurysms or aneurysms, manifestations of "hypothenar hammer syndrome" associated with the use of jackhammers, can also cause nerve conduction abnormalities.[34]

De Quervain's Tenosynovitis

Inflammatory changes can affect the flexor and extensor tendon sheaths. De Quervain's tenosynovitis refers to an inflammatory condition of the first dorsal extensor compartment involving the abductor pollicis longus and extensor pollicis brevis tendon sheaths. The clinical presentation is pain localized to the radial aspect of the wrist radiating from the proximal forearm along the radial styloid toward the thumb. Soft tissue swelling and tenderness are present. This condition is associated with racquet sports, golf, and activities involving repetitive radial and ulnar deviation of the wrist.

Traditionally, de Quervain's tenosynovitis has been a clinical diagnosis. However, awareness of the MR features is important with the increasing number of wrist MR examinations being performed. Fluid or high signal is present within a distended tendon sheath, reflecting inflammatory changes. It is frequently associated with tendinosis. The involved tendons demonstrate an increased caliber and signal intensity. Most often these changes are exclusive to the first dorsal extensor compartment.[35] If many other tendons are affected, other etiologies should be considered.

Extensor Carpi Ulnaris Tendinosis and Tenosynovitis

The extensor carpi ulnaris (ECU) tendon, the only tendon of the sixth dorsal extensor compartment, frequently demonstrates changes of tendinosis and tenosynovitis. It is the second most common site of tenosynovitis of the upper extremity following, de Quervain's tenosynovitis. Extensor carpi ulnaris tendinosis presents with pain along the dorsal surface of the ulna sometimes accompanied by crepitus. This condition is commonly seen in athletes involved in sports with repetitive wrist motion. The pain is exacerbated by wrist motions involving pronation-supination and ulnar deviation including tennis and golf. The injury relates to repetitive stress rather than a single traumatic event.[36]

The ECU tendon extends through a longitudinal osseous groove in the dorsal aspect of the distal ulna. It is stabilized by both the extensor retinaculum and the "linea jugata," connecting the ulnar styloid with the antebrachial fascia. Normally the tendon appears as a longitudinally oriented structure with low signal intensity in both T1- and T2-weighted images. Transaxial images demonstrate the tendon as an ovoid dark structure. The ECU tendon has increased caliber and signal intensity when affected by tendinosis (Fig. 7.17). Concurrent tenosynovitis may be present.

Extensor carpi ulnaris tendinosis and tenosynovitis can occur alone or in combination with ECU tendon subluxation or dislocation. A congenitally flat or convex ECU tendon groove is an additional predisposing factor for tendon displacement.[37] The ECU tendon has inherent instability during pronation and supination of the wrist, demonstrating a shift in location away from the osseous groove during supination of the wrist. Tendon dislocation occurs when the reinforcing structures including the extensor retinaculum and linea jugata are disrupted.[38] If ECU tendon instability is suspected, MR examination of the wrist can be performed in both pronation and supination of the forearm.

Intersection Syndrome

The tendons of the first dorsal extensor compartment, the abductor pollicis longus and extensor pollicis brevis, cross obliquely over the tendons of the second dorsal extensor compartment, the extensor carpi radialis longus and brevis tendons, at the level of the distal forearm just distal to their musculotendinous junction. An overuse syndrome has been described at this intersection affecting persons engaged in activities involving repetitive flexion and extension of the wrist. These persons include rowers, weight-lifters, secretaries, carpenters, and even rice harvesters in Thailand. Since its original description by Velpeau in 1841, it has been known by many alternative names including "oarsmen's wrist," "bugaboo wrist," and "squeaker's wrist."[39–41] The designation intersection syndrome was first introduced by Dobyns and has become the preferred term for this condition.[13]

Clinical symptoms of intersection syndrome include pain, tenderness, and swelling located 4 to 8 cm proximal to Lister's tubercle at the site of tendon intersection. In severe cases, crepitus is described with both motion and palpation of the wrist. Two theories have been proposed to describe the pathophysiology of this syndrome. One relates to the underlying friction between the tendons of the two compartments at the point of intersection.[42] A second theory postulates that there is tenosynovial constriction of the intersecting tendons causing proximal swelling.[43]

When intersection syndrome is suspected as the underlying cause of wrist pain, the MRI protocol should include the distal forearm in the field of view. A routine wrist MR examination may not include this anatomic area. The MR findings of intersection syndrome include peritendinous edema and tenosynovial fluid emanating from the intersection (Fig. 7.18). The normal ovoid-shaped appearance of the tendons may be lost, and they appear enlarged and rounded.

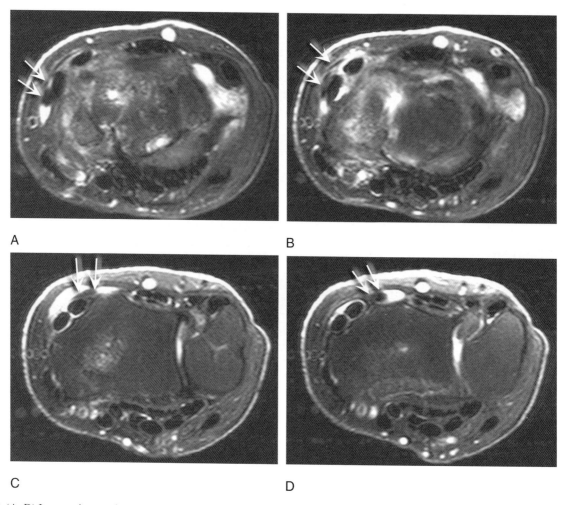

FIG. 7.17. (A–D) Intersection syndrome. Sequential axial T2 fat-suppressed MRI of the wrist. Focal tenosynovial fluid is noted in the tendons sheaths of the first and second dorsal extensor compartment (arrows) as the tendons of the first compartment cross over the dorsal surface of the second compartment. No abnormalities of the tendons are identified (A., most distal image; D, most proximal image).

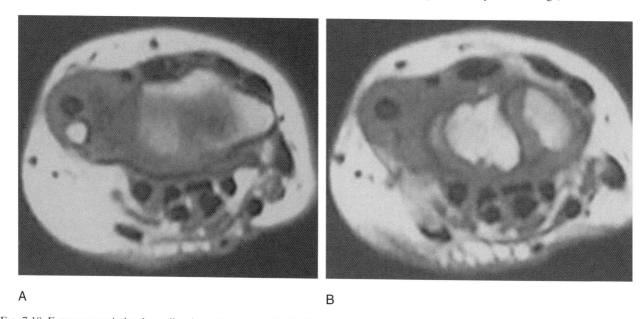

FIG. 7.18. Extensor carpi ulnaris tendinosis and tenosynovitis. (A,B) Two axial T1-weighted images of the wrist. There is enlargement of the extensor carpi ulnaris tendon with a central region of increased signal intensity consistent with tendinosis. The rind of intermediate signal surrounding the tendon correlates to tenosynovial fluid on other imaging sequences

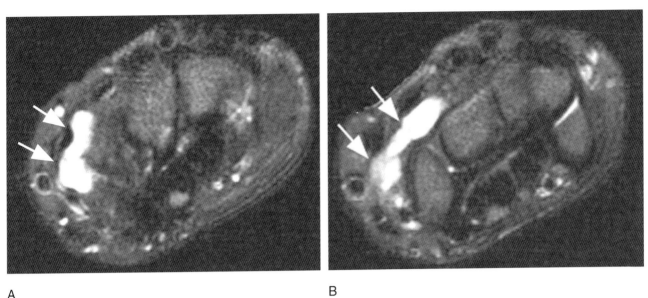

A

B

FIG. 7.19. Ganglion cyst. (A,B) Two axial T2 fat-suppressed MR images of the wrist. A lobulated, cystic mass is located at the dorsal aspect of the wrist, adjacent to the extensor tendons and also the lunotriquetral ligament. Its signal characteristics are identical to simple fluid

A second lesser known intersection syndrome may also occur. At the level of the radiocarpal joint, there is an intersection of the tendons in the second and third dorsal extensor compartments. The extensor pollicis longus tendon, the lone tendon of the third dorsal extensor compartment, courses superficially over the extensor carpi radialis longus and brevis tendons, the tendons in the second dorsal extensor compartment. The pathophysiology of this type of intersection syndrome is probably similar to the classic intersection syndrome. Magnetic resonance features include the accumulation of tenosynovial fluid and a loss of the normal ovoid morphology of tendons.

Ganglion Cysts

A ganglion is described as viscous cystic masses occurring in proximity to joints or tendon sheaths. Ganglion cysts account for approximately 70% of the soft tissue masses of the hand and wrist. Most occur in middle-aged persons, and they may or may not be symptomatic. These cysts occur with higher frequency along the dorsal surface of the wrist, often near the dorsal intercarpal and scapholunate ligaments. When symptomatic, they can produce pain or pressure due to distention and inflammatory changes. Direct communication with the adjacent articulation may be demonstrated

with MR arthrography. Ganglions are low in signal intensity on T1-weighted images and high in signal intensity on T2-weighted images with signal characteristics identical to those of fluid (Fig. 7.19). They may sometimes appear septated. Intravenous gadolinium administration confirms the presence of a fluid-filled mass, with only a thin, peripheral rind of enhancement.

It is hypothesized that ganglion cysts form in response to internal derangements of the wrist. Studies have linked wrist ganglia to ligamentous injuries in up to 30% of cases.[44] When ganglia are identified, a thorough search for ligamentous abnormalities can yield additional findings.

Conclusion

This section examined the considerations when requesting an MR examination of the wrist. Although most MR examinations of the wrist are performed with a routine protocol, the examination can be tailored to specific purposes when the specific clinical question is known beforehand. Masses are assessed more completely with intravenous gadolinium administration, and ligamentous injuries can be investigated with MR arthrography. The wrist is a complicated joint with many pathologic conditions. Magnetic resonance imaging is an excellent modality for the investigation of these entities.

B. Orthopedic Perspective: Wrist Injuries

Matthew Meunier and Joshua N. Steinvurzel

Scapholunate Ligament Injuries

Wrist sprains are common in sports injuries, particularly falls on an outstretched hand. There can often be acute swelling and considerable discomfort. In most cases radiographs should be obtained to look for fractures, with special attention to the distal radius and carpus. Diastasis of the scapholunate space of greater than 3 mm is a classic finding on plane radiographs, famously known as the "Terry Thomas" or "Leon Spinks" sign, depending on your frame of reference, and represents complete rupture of the scapholunate ligament.[45] Other signs can include an increase in the scapholunate angle, the "V" sign described by Taleisnik, the signet ring sign, and the DISI deformity.[46] In the cases where there is diastasis but no fixed instability, films of the contralateral wrist are required to confirm asymmetry, and if this is present, MRI is not needed. A clenched-fist view is often obtained to look for dynamic instability. In cases where there are exam findings consistent with scapholunate injury but no fixed or dynamic diastasis, MRI both without and then with contrast is our preferred evaluation. Arthrography has also been used but lacks the ability of MRI to evaluate surrounding structures or the morphology of the ligament.

Treatment of incomplete injuries can sometimes be limited to a period of cast immobilization followed by a gentle protected range of motion. Complete ruptures can be treated acutely with surgical repair and are usually immobilized for approximately 8 weeks following repair and then protected for an additional 4 to 6 weeks. Late presentations are not infrequent and can be difficult to treat. The results of delayed repair are inconsistent and often result in continued wrist pain. If injuries are missed, there is a classic pattern of degenerative arthrosis known as the SLAC wrist[47] (Fig. 7.20), which ultimately requires a salvage procedure with a limitation of motion.

One caveat with these injuries is that, particularly in contact sports such as football or rugby, there can be significant trauma to the wrist that can be missed by inexperienced physicians. Perilunate dislocation and perilunate fracture dislocations do occur and can be missed if there is not a significant index of suspicion (Fig. 7.21). These are significant injuries, and they require prompt surgical attention for any chance at an acceptable recovery.[48]

Triangular-Fibrocartilage Complex Injuries

Ulnar deviation and wrist extension injuries can often lead to ulnar-sided wrist pain and can be difficult to fully diagnose. Strain of the extensor carpi ulnaris is a common outcome from this mechanism, as is a sprain of the lunotriquetral interval, the distal radioulnar joint, or the TFCC. The TFCC has a complex anatomy including the fibrous disk, the meniscal homologue, the palmar and dorsal distal radioulnar ligaments, and the ulnotriquetral and ulnolunate ligaments. The function of the TFCC is complex and involves stability of the distal radioulnar joint during rotation of the forearm.[49]

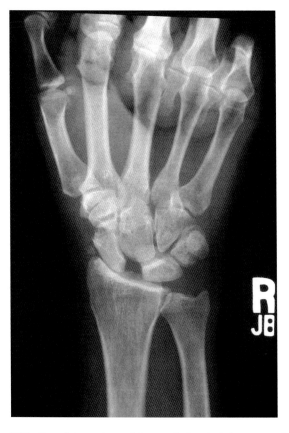

Fig. 7.20. Complete rupture of the scapholunate interosseous ligament with diastasis of the joint

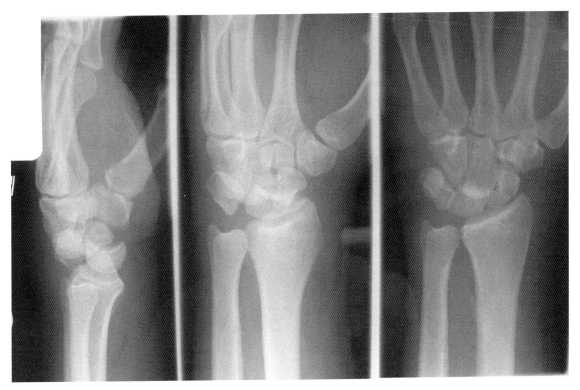

FIG. 7.21. Transscaphoid perilunate fracture dislocation of the wrist sustained during a rugby game. This injury was initially diagnosed as a "wrist sprain"

Physical exam usually shows tenderness over the distal aspect of the ulnar head. In addition there is often pain with forced wrist extension–ulnar deviation or with attempted forearm rotation against resistance, particularly attempted pronation. Nonoperative evaluation includes wrist arthrography and MRI. Arthrography is less expensive but it lacks anatomic specificity. Magnetic resonance imaging, particularly with intraarticular contrast, can delineate the size, location, and morphology of TFCC tears and has become the study of choice prior to surgical treatment.[50] If conservative measures such as splinting, icing, activity modification, and antiinflammatory modalities fail, then surgical evaluation is considered. Arthroscopy is the treatment of choice, and if there has been an acute injury along the periphery of the TFCC, then repair is often feasible. Since the vascularity of the TFCC is limited to the periphery, central tears are often irreparable and are treated with debridement.[49]

Carpal Fractures

Falls on an outstretched hand are common in sports and are a common mechanism for many wrist injuries. The majority of these injuries are sprains, which require little more than supportive care and protected mobilization; however, occasionally fractures occur. Of the carpal fractures, scaphoid fractures are by far the most frequent, approximately 80% in most series.[51] The mechanism is a fall on an outstretched hand with the carpus hyperextended and the forearm pronated. It most commonly occurs in a young male. Older athletes tend toward distal radius fractures. Diagnosis is again based on symptoms, exam findings, and radiographs. Most patients present with significant pain on the radial aspect of the wrist, although swelling may not be that significant. Tenderness is usually elicited at the "anatomic snuffbox," which corresponds to the waist of the scaphoid and is the triangular space delineated by the dorsoradial distal radius, and the first and the third dorsal compartments. The standard frontal, oblique, and lateral views are obtained, along with a scaphoid-specific view with the wrist held in ulnar deviation to extend the proximal row and fully expose the scaphoid. Most fractures are evident at the time of injury; however, it is well known that some patients will show no fracture on initial films but ultimately prove to have a scaphoid fracture. In the patient in whom a fracture is suspected but not seen on initial films, the classic teaching has been to immobilize the patient for 3 weeks and then do repeat films out of plaster. This allows the process of resorption at the fracture site to occur and allows the fracture to become apparent.[52] As surgery has become more frequent, the earlier diagnosis of these injuries has become more important, and so alternative diagnostic tools are used. Initially, triple-phase bone scanning was the preferred tool; however, this indicates only increased metabolic activity and lacks anatomic specificity. Magnetic resonance imaging is currently preferred for early diagnosis of occult scaphoid fractures, and can be ordered almost immediately.[53]

The initial management is thumb spica splinting, and there has been some debate as to whether long arm or short arm casting is required, or whether surgery is the optimal treatment, particularly in a young active population. For fractures with no displacement, healing with immobilization occurs approximately 95% of the time and in approximately 8 to 12 weeks. In these cases operative fixation may decrease the time to union.[54] Two other variants warrant mention. Distal scaphoid fractures most commonly involve the tubercle and can often be treated with gentle mobilization and protection during sports. If they remain symptomatic, the distal fragment is excised. Proximal injuries have a much higher complication rate. As few as 20% heal with simple immobilization, and so surgical treatment is recommended in the acute setting for optimal results.

Although the scaphoid is by far the most frequently injured of the carpal bones, other carpal injuries do occur. Falls on an outstretched hand can cause dorsal triquetral impaction injuries. In themselves these are not typically serious; however, the dorsal radiocarpal ligament attaches to the triquetral fracture and untreated injuries can lead to a volar wrist instability pattern. Surgery is rarely indicated for these injuries, but a period of immobilization of approximately 1 month is often recommended. Patients can also present with pain over the ulnar side of the wrist, particularly with deep palpation or grip. If there is a history of impact sports such as golf or baseball, then suspicion should be given to fractures of the hamate hook. The most common history is of a miss-hit golf shot or baseball swing with pain over the ulnar base of the palm.

Occasionally symptoms of ulnar neuritis can occur, and very occasionally patients present with loss of flexion at the small finger distal interphalangeal joint. A high index of suspicion is required for these injuries, and diagnosis with conventional radiography can be difficult. The standard three views of the wrist rarely show hamate hook fractures, and so a carpal tunnel view is often ordered, although this too is rarely diagnostic (Fig. 7.22) There has been some debate about the preferred study for these suspected injuries. Bone scintigraphy localizes metabolic activity but not anatomy. Computed tomography scan, however, enables an excellent assessment of the bony injury, and MRI enables an assessment of surrounding structures and should show signal characteristics of a fracture of the hamate hook (Fig. 7.23). Some patients present with numbness and tingling in the ulnar nerve distribution, localized to the region of Guyon's canal, and some even present with acute ruptures of the flexor digitorum profundus tendon to the small finger secondary to the fracture. An MRI enables assessment of other potential etiologies for these symptoms.

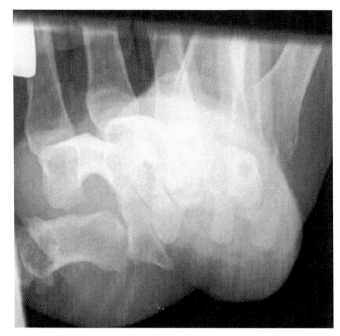

FIG. 7.22. Carpal tunnel view demonstrating a fracture at the base of the hamate hook

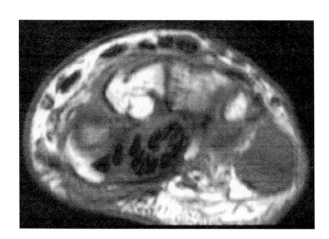

FIG. 7.23. MRI of the same hamate hook fracture

References

1. Berquist T. Anatomy. In: Berquist T, ed. MRI of the Hand and Wrist. Philadelphia: Lippincott, 2003;1–32.
2. Resnick D. Wrist and hand. In: Resnick D, Kang SK, eds. Internal Derangement of Joints. Philadelphia: Elsevier and Saunders, 1997;387–472.
3. Kim S, Choi J, Huh Y, et al. Role of magnetic resonance imaging in entrapment and compressive neuropathy—what, where, and how to see the peripheral nerves on the musculoskeletal magnetic resonance image: part 2. Upper extremity. Eur Radiol 2007;2:509–522.
4. Aguiar RO, Gasparetto EL, Escuissato DL, et al. Radial and ulnar bursae of the wrist: cadaveric investigation of regional anatomy

with ultrasonographic-guided tenography and MR imaging. Skeletal Radiol 2006; 35:828–832.

5. Palmer AK, Werner FW. The triangular fibrocartilage complex of the wrist—anatomy and function. J Hand Surg 1981;6:153–162.

6. Pfirrmann C, Zanetti M. Variant, pitfalls and asymptomatic findings in wrist and hand imaging. Eur J Radiol 2005;56: 286–295.

7. Robinson G, Chung T, Finlay K, Friedman L. Axial oblique MR imaging of the intrinsic ligaments of the wrist: initial experience. Skeletal Radiol 2006;35:765–773.

8. Breitenseher MJ, Metz VM, Gilula LA, et al. Radiographically occult scaphoid fractures: value of MR imaging in detection. Radiology 1997;203:245–250.

9. Dobyns JH, Linscheid RL. Fractures and dislocations of the wrist. In: Rockwood CA Jr, Green DP, eds. Fractures in adults, 3rd ed. Philadelphia: Lippincott, 1984:411–509.

10. Goldfarb CA, Yin Y, Gilula LA, et al. Wrist fractures: what the clinician wants to know. Radiology 2001;219:11–28.

11. Smith DK, Gilula LA, Amadio PC. Dorsal lunate tilt (DISI Configuration): sign of scaphoid fracture displacement. Radiology 1990;176:497–499.

12. Resnick, D, Goergen TG. Physical injury: concepts and terminology. Bone and joint imaging. In: Resnick D, Kransdorf MJ, eds. Philadelphia: Elsevier and Saunders, 2005:789–830.

13. McNally EG, Goodman R, Burge P. The role of MRI in the assessment of scaphoid fracture healing: a pilot study. Eur Radiol 2000;10:1926–1928.

14. Cerezal L, Faustino A, Canga A, et al. Usefulness of gadolinium-enhanced MR imaging in the evaluation of the vascularity of scaphoid nonunions. AJR 1999;174:141–149.

15. Cohen M. Fractures of the carpal bones. Hand Clin 1997;13: 587–599.

16. Daunt N. Magnetic resonance imaging of the wrist: anatomy and pathology of interosseous ligaments and the triangular fibrocartilage complex. Curr Probl Diagn Radiol 2002;31:158–176.

17. McAlinden PS, Teh J. Imaging of the wrist. Imaging 2003;15: 180–192.

18. Haims AH, Schweitzer ME, Morrison WB, et al. Internal derangement of the wrist: indirect arthrography versus unenhanced MR imaging. Radiology 2003;227:701–707.

19. Watson HK, Kao S. Degenerative disorders of the carpus. In: Lichtman DM, Alexander AH, eds. The Wrist and Its Disorders, 2nd ed. Philadelphia: WB Saunders, 1997:583–591.

20. Schmitt R, Froehner S, Coblenz G, et al. Carpal instability. Eur J Radiol 2006;10:2161–2178.

21. Dobyns JH, Linscheid RL, Macksoud WS. Proximal carpal row instability—nondissociative. J Hand Surg [Br] 1994;19: 763–773.

22. Mikic ZD. Age changes in the triangular fibrocartilage of the wrist joint. J Anat 1978;126:367–384.

23. Palmer A. Triangular fibrocartilage disorders: injury patterns and treatment. J Arthrosc Rel Surg 1990;6:125–32.

24. Kang HS, Kindynis P, Brahme SK, et al. Triangular fibrocartilage and intercarpal ligaments of the wrist: cadaveric study with gross pathologic and histologic correlation. Radiology 1992;181: 401–404.

25. Zanetti M, Bram J, Hodler J. Triangular fibrocartilage and intercarpal ligaments of the wrist: Does MR arthrography improve standard MRI? J Magn Reson Imaging 1997;7:590–594.

26. Friedman SL, Palmer AK. The ulnar impaction syndrome. Hand Clin 1991;7:295–310.

27. Deitch, MA, Stern PJ. Ulnocarpal abutment. Hand Clin 1998;14:251–263.

28. Lee ML. The intraosseous arterial pattern of the carpal lunate bone and its relation to avascular necrosis. Acta Orthop Scand 1963;33:43–55.

29. Hulten O. Uber anatomische variationen der handgelenkknochen. Acta Radiol Scand 1928;9:155.

30. Lichtman DM, Gaenslen ES, Pollock GR. Keinbock's disease and idiopathic necrosis of carpal bones. In: Lichtman DM, Alexander AH, eds. The Wrist and Its Disorders, 2nd ed. Philadelphia: WB Saunders, 1997:329–346.

31. Mesgarzadeh M, Schneck C, Bonakdarpour A, et al. Carpal tunnel: MR imaging. Part II carpal tunnel syndrome. Radiology 1989;171:749–754.

32. Wu HT, Schweitzer ME, Culp RW. Potential MR signs of recurrent carpal tunnel syndrome: initial experience. J Comput Assist Tomogr 2004;28:860–864.

33. Grundberg AB. Ulnar tunnel syndrome. J Hand Surg [Br] 1984;9:72–74.

34. Liskutin J, Dorffner R, Resinger M, et al. Hypothenal hammer syndrome. Eur Radiol 2000;10:542.

35. Glajchen N, Schweitzer ME. MRI features of de Quervain's tenosynovitis of the wrist. Skeletal Radiol 1996;25:63–65.

36. Carneriro RS, Fontana R., Mazzer N. Ulnar wrist pain in athletes caused by erosion of the floor of the sixth dorsal compartment. Am J Sports Med 2005;33:1910–1913.

37. Allende C, LeViet D. Extensor carpi ulnaris problems at the wrist-classification, surgical treatment and results. J Hand Surg 2005;30B:265–272.

38. Montalvan B, Parier J, Brasseur JL, et al. Extensor carpi ulnaris injuries in tennis players: a study of 28 cases. Br J Sports Med 2006;40:424–429.

39. de Lima JE, Kim HJ, Alberotti F, et al. Intersection syndrome: MR imaging with anatomic comparison of the distal forearm. Skeletal Radiol 2004;33:627–631.

40. Palmer DH, Lane-Larsen CL. Helicopter skiing injuries: a case report of "bugaboo forearm." Am J Sports Med 1994;22:148–149.

41. Dobyns JH, Sim FH, Linscheid RL. Sports stress syndrome of hand and wrist. Am J Sports Med 1978;6:236–254.

42. Howard N. Peritendinitis crepitans. J Bone Joint Surg [Br] 1937;19:447–459.

43. Grundberg AB, Reagen, DS. Pathologic anatomy of the forearm: intersection syndrome. J Hand Surg 1985;10:299–302.

44. El Noueam KI, Schweitzer ME, Blasbalg R, et al. Is a subset of wrist ganglia the sequela of internal derangements of the wrist joint? MR imaging findings. Radiology 1999;212:537–540.

45. Mayfield JK, et al. Carpal dislocations: pathomechanics and progressive perilunar instability. J Hand Surg 1980;5A: 226–241.

46. Lavernia CJ, et al. Treatment of scapholunate dissociation by ligamentous repair and capsulodesis. J Hand Surg 1992;17A: 354–359.

47. Watson HK, Ballet FL. The SLAC wrist: scapholunate advanced collapse pattern of degenerative arthritis. J Hand Surg 1984;9A:358–365.

48. Hildebrand KA, et al. Dorsal perilunate dislocations and fracture-dislocations: questionnaire, clinical, and radiographic evaluation. J Hand Surg 2000;25A:1069–1079.

49. Palmer AK, Werner FW. The triangular fibrocartilage complex of the wrist—anatomy and function. J Hand Surg 1981;6A: 153–162.
50. Potter HG, et al. The utility of high-resolution magnetic resonance imaging in the evaluation of the triangular fibrocartilage complex of the wrist. J Bone Joint Surg 1997;79A:1675–1684.
51. Smith DK, et al. The effects of simulated unstable scaphoid fractures on carpal motion. J Hand Surg 1989;14A:283–291.
52. Cooney WP, Scaphoid fractures: current treatments and techniques. Instr Course Lect 2003;52:197–208.
53. Fowler C, et al. A comparison of bone scintigraphy and MRI in the early diagnosis of the occult scaphoid waist fracture. Skeletal Radiol 1998;27(12):683–687.
54. Bond CD, et al. Percutaneous screw fixation or cast immobilization for non-displaced scaphoid fractures. J Bone Joint Surg 2001;83A:483–488.

8
Hand and Fingers

A. Radiologic Perspective: Magnetic Resonance Imaging of the Hand and Fingers

Nicolas Theumann

Techniques

Magnetic resonance imaging (MRI) of the hand and fingers has benefited from the use of dedicated surface coils, which allow a fine depiction of the intricate anatomy of these structures, owing to high spatial resolution images as well as an excellent soft tissue contrast. Optimization of numerous imaging techniques and approaches is important in today's cost-conscious environment.[1,2] Any number of imaging methods, either alone or in combination, can be used to evaluate the hand and fingers. These techniques include routine radiography, scintigraphy, diagnostic ultrasonography, computed tomography (CT) scanning, arthrography, and MRI. In this chapter, the role of MRI is addressed, and MR techniques are discussed. The evaluation of the hand and fingers with MRI is optimized by a high-field (>1.0 tesla [T]) system. The role of MRI has continued to evolve as innovations have expanded in pulse sequencing and high-resolution imaging, including MR arthrography, angiographic techniques, and 3.0-T imaging.[3,4] Recent studies have demonstrated that MRI has significant usefulness and has impact on clinical decision making in a significant number of patients. Hobby et al.[5] demonstrated that magnetic resonance (MR) studies have changed the clinical diagnosis.

Dedicated surface coils are fundamental to achieving high-resolution images. In some clinical situations, simultaneous imaging of both hands and fingers may be required, for which a dedicated knee coil or head coil may be used. Depending on the specific lesion sought, it is always better to place the patient in the magnet in the prone position, with the arm (or both arms) extended over the head, to be centered in the main magnetic field. In general, the prone position with arm extended is less well tolerated, eventually resulting in image degradation due to patient motion, but in general the time necessary to perform the study is short enough for the patient to remain quiet. For the examination of masses, or in patients with point tenderness, taping a fat-containing capsule on the skin at the site of the suspected abnormality is helpful. Also, in certain clinical situations, a stress position at the time of imag-

ing may provide additional information. Magnetic resonance imaging of the hand and fingers is usually accomplished in one or more of the three basic planes (coronal, sagittal, and transverse), according to the anatomy of each finger.

On some occasions, when the patient cannot hold the hand above the head, a supine position with the hand at the side is possible. This is generally more comfortable for the patient. Once the hand and fingers are well positioned, foam pads or bolsters should be used to reduce motion and improve comfort. When a motion study is required, motion control devices can be used to optimize position changes. The coil selection varies with the clinical indication and position required. To achieve high spatial resolution, a small field of view (FOV) of 4 to 10 cm is routinely employed. The image matrix should be 256 to 512 with 1- to 3-mm-thick sections. Smaller sections (0.6 to 1 mm) are used for volume acquisitions and three-dimensional (3D) studies.[6] In general, one acquisition is sufficient. Most imaging examinations of the hand and fingers are performed at 1.5 T. However, experience with 3.0-T magnets is increasing. The primary advantage of extremity imaging at 3.0 T lies in the increased signal-to-noise ratio (SNR) at 3.0 T, compared with lower strength fields. The SNR increases linearly with field strength. This allows a significant improvement in spatial resolution without increasing acquisition time, providing more detailed anatomic imaging of the small structures.

Pulse sequences are numerous; in general a combination of T1- and T2-weighted images is used. High resolution and optimal image quality are essential. Three-dimensional volume acquisitions, using gradient echo images, allow very thin slices (0.6 to 1 mm), which are necessary to identifying the fingers' anatomic structures. The selection of image sequences and planes varies with clinical indication. At the level of the fingers, pathologic lesions and joint fluid have a high intensity on T2-weighted sequences. The same is true for fast spin echo (FSE) T2-weighted sequences. The FSE sequences can be performed more quickly and are less degraded by motion artifacts. The use of the fat-suppression technique with the FSE sequences aids in the detection of bone marrow and soft tissue abnormalities. In any examination, all three planes should be included in the imaging protocols. Gadolinium has gained popularity due to T1 shortening and the relative lack of side effects, but it is not routinely used for hand and fingers imaging. However, the application continues to expand, using intravenous gadolinium for enhancing pathology and angiographic techniques.[7] In most cases, precontrast T1- and T2-weighted images are obtained. Postcontrast T1-weighted images are obtained with fat suppression. Pre- and postcontrast sequences are usually performed in the same planes to permit comparison. The use of MR arthrography is not very common at the level of the hand and fingers. Direct MR arthrography is useful to confirm palmar plate lesions or to better depict all the small structures of the different finger joints.[8]

Magnetic resonance angiography may be performed without intravenous gadolinium.[4] Phase contrast (PC) and time of flight (TOF) techniques are performed without intravenous gadolinium but, at the level of the fingers, contrast enhanced, 3D angiographic techniques have become increasingly popular in recent years.[9] A rapid acquisition data set avoids the flow-sensitive issues seen with nonenhanced MR angiography techniques. The short acquisition time improves the image quality and reduces venous filling, thereby allowing easier interpretation.[4] New 3D sequences allow us to perform these sequences in less than 1 minute. These techniques can also be applied to a bilateral investigation of the two hands and wrists (with the use of a larger FOV) of about 20 cm. In our institution, we use the precontrast 3D sequence, which allow us to subtract postcontrast images, resulting in greater vessel details as described by Lee et al.[4]

Normal Anatomy

Thumb Carpometacarpal Joint

The thumb requires dexterity and precision to handle fine objects with stability, and strength to counteract a force applied by the fingers when grasping. Large loads are imparted through this carpometacarpal joint, so it has a complex and strong ligamentous system that can withstand axial loading and yet has a low mobility. The tendons on the thenar muscles encase these ligaments. There are four main ligaments that contribute to the stability of the carpometacarpal joint of the thumb.[10]

The dorsal radial ligament, which arises from the dorsal and radial aspect of the trapezium, inserts onto the adjacent portion of the thumb's metacarpal base. This ligament is reinforced by the abductor pollicis longus tendon. The posterior oblique ligament runs from the dorsal ulnar tubercle of the trapezium to the ulnar tubercle of the thumb's metacarpal base. The intermetacarpal ligament runs from the radial base of the index metacarpal to the ulnar aspect of the thumb metacarpal base. The anterior oblique ligament is a short thick band with fibers running from the palmar tubercle of the trapezium to insert into the base of the thumb metacarpal. The

ligament is composed of two bands, a superficial component (SAOL) and a deeper component (DAOL). The SAOL arises from the palmar tubercle of the trapezium and inserts broadly into the ulnar tubercle of the thumb metacarpal base, close to the joint capsule, creating a capsular recess. It lies immediately deeper to the thenar eminence but superficially to the deep component and blends with the capsule. It is taut at the extreme of joint motion, especially with extension. The DAOL inserts adjacent to the articular margin of the trapezium and the thumb metacarpal. It is intraarticular and lies close to the center of the joint. It is shorter than the SAOL and therefore becomes taut first, preventing ulnar subluxation. Owing to its location, the DAOL probably serves as a pivot point for the thumb's carpometacarpal (CMC) joint. The anterior oblique ligament therefore acts as the primary stabilizer of the CMC assisted by the ulnar collateral ligament, which runs in the similar direction, though with a different attachment.

Common Carpometacarpal and Intermetacarpal Joints

The anatomy of the tendons and ligaments of the common carpometacarpal (CCMC) joint and the second to the fifth intermetacarpal (IMC) joints is quite complex and differs from the anatomy of the first ray.[11] Although injuries of the CCMC joints and the second to fifth IMC are relatively uncommon, their detection is important as they can result in significant functional disability of the hand. At the level of the second to fifth IMC and CCMC joints, six CCMC ligaments, three IMC ligaments, and four tendinous insertions in the metacarpal bases are found.

Common Carpometacarpal Ligaments

The dorsal CCMC ligaments are thick and attached to the dorsal aspect of the carpal bones of the second row. No separation between these ligaments is visible. They extend to the dorsal aspect of the second to the fifth metacarpal bases. They are seen only in the sagittal plane and better visualized with MR arthrography than with MRI (100% versus 91%).[8] The palmar CCMC ligaments are arranged symmetrically with a dorsal ligament between the palmar aspect of the carpal bones of the second row and the palmar aspect of the metacarpal bases. These ligaments are very thin and blend with the joint capsule. They are not well visualized either with MRI or MR arthrography (0% versus 22%). The pisometacarpal ligament (PMS) is a thin and elongated fibrous structure of low signal intensity in all sequences. In all cases, it arises from the distal aspect of the pisiform and extends to the palmar aspect of the bases of the fourth and fifth metacarpal bones. It crosses through the concavity along the ulnar aspect of the hook of the hamate. It is always visualized with either MR arthrography or MRI. The radial collateral ligament arises from the dorsoradial aspect of the trapezoid and extends distally to the dorsoradial aspect of the second metacarpal bone, proximal to the insertion of the tendon of the extensor carpi radialis longus muscle. The ulnar collateral ligament extends from the dorsoulnar aspect of the hamate to the dorsoulnar aspect of the fifth metacarpal bone, proximal to the insertion of the extensor carpi ulnaris tendon. The capitate-third metacarpal ligament arises from the distal ulnar aspect of the capitate and extends distally to the base of the third metacarpal bone. They are well visualized with MR arthrography and MRI. These three ligaments are the best visualized in the coronal plane and are always visualized as low signal intensity linear structures.

Intermetacarpal Ligaments

The dorsal IMC ligament is a thin fibrous ligament that extends transversally from the base of the second metacarpal bone to the base of the fifth metacarpal bone. It has low signal intensity in all sequences. Most of the time it is visible with MRI and MR arthrography, the length of this ligament is significantly shorter between the second, the third, and the fourth metacarpal bones than between the fourth and fifth metacarpal bones (8.7 and 8.6 versus 11.1 mm).[11]

The palmar IMC ligament is more proximal than the dorsal one. It extends between the palmar aspects of the metacarpal bases and is always visible with MRI and MR arthrography in the axial plane. The interosseous IMC ligament complex includes anterior and posterior bands that are found between each metacarpals bases. The complex extends perpendicularly to the main axes of the wrist, distally to the collateral articular facet. The anterior band arises from the bases of the second, third, and fifth metacarpal bones, about 5 mm distally to the CCMC articular surface, at the level of the palmar IMC ligament. The anterior band runs distally and dorsally, attaching to the adjacent metacarpal bone. The posterior band arises from the base of the second, the third, and the fifth metacarpal bones, at the level of the dorsal IMC ligament. It runs distally and palmary inserts in the adjacent metacarpal neck. These ligaments have a V-shaped configuration, whose apex is at the third metacarpal bone, in the second IMC space, and at the fourth metacarpal bone, in the third IMC space. For the last IMC space, the V-shaped configuration is never seen and the ligament complex appears as loose soft tissue between both metacarpal bases. The anterior and posterior bands have intermediate to low signal intensity in all sequences. The axial plane is the best to allow visualization of these ligaments.

Musculotendinous Structures of the Carpometacarpal Joints

Four tendons insert in the metacarpal basis: (1) The flexor carpi radialis (FCR) tendon inserts in the proximal palmar aspect of the second metacarpal bone. (2) The extensor carpi radialis longus tendon is attached to the dorsoradial aspect of the base of the second metacarpal bone, distally to the insertion of the radial collateral ligament. (3) The extensor carpi radialis brevis tendon inserts in the radial side of the dorsal aspect of the base of the third metacarpal bone. (4) The extensor carpi ulnaris tendon inserts in the ulnar prominence of the base of the fifth metacarpal bone. All four tendons insertions are visible as low signal intensity structures in axial planes.

Metacarpophalangeal Joint of the Thumb

The metacarpophalangeal (MCP) joint of the thumb is a condylian joint that includes two axes. The lateral stability is formed on both sides (ulnar and radial) by two ligaments: a main collateral ligament, which arises from both sides of the metacarpal head and runs distally to the base of the proximal phalanges, and an accessory ligament, which arises from a common proximal attachment with the main ligament and runs distally on both sides of the palmar plate. The palmar plate includes two sesamoid bones, a medial and a lateral one. The palmar plate gives the anteroposterior stability of the joint. The main collateral ligaments are tightened in flexion and relaxed in extension, and the accessory ligaments are relaxed in flexion and tightened in extension, as is the case for the MCP joint of the long fingers.[12]

On the ulnar sides, there is an extension of the aponeurosis of the abductor pollicis brevis to the extensor pollicis longus. This extension runs over the ulnar side of the joint capsule, as an extensor hood of the extensor pollicis longus tendon. It is important to retain this extension; of the Stener lesion is an interposition of the aponeurosis between the distal tear of the main ulnar collateral ligament and its distal insertion.

Metacarpophalangeal Joints of the Fingers

Although uncommon, the injuries of the MCP joints of the fingers necessitate accurate diagnosis, because a loss of function of even one MCP joint can seriously impair the overall hand function. To ensure appropriate treatment, the identification of the damaged structures at the time of injury is essential. High spatial resolution due to advances in MRI technology allows the visualization of important intra- and periarticular structures of small joints such as the MCP joints, with standard clinical equipment. Detailed knowledge of the normal anatomy remains essential to the analysis of the MR images of this area.

Capsule and Cartilage

On MRI, depiction of the proximal and distal attachment of the capsule necessitates intraarticular injection of a contrast agent. These attachments are best seen on the sagittal T1-weighted spin-echo MR arthrographic images of the fingers in an extended position. The visualization of the chondral surface is better after intraarticular injection of a contrast agent compared with visualization with standard spin echo MRI.[8] Fast gradient recalled echo images should be performed instead of standard spin echo images to visualize MCP joint cartilage when no intraarticular contrast is injected.

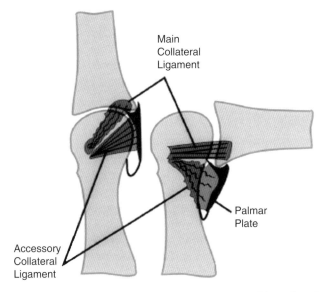

FIG. 8.1 Drawing of the collateral ligament complex. The main collateral ligament is relaxed in extension and taut in flexion, and the accessory collateral ligament is taut in extension and more relaxed in flexion. (From Theumann et al.,[8] with permission).

Ligaments

The ligaments are situated on the radial and ulnar side of each joint, blending with and reinforcing the capsule. The collateral ligaments include two distinctive bands, which represent the main collateral ligaments and the accessory collateral ligaments. The main collateral ligaments are taut in flexion and relaxed in extension (Fig. 8.1). They arise in depressions on the radial and ulnar sides of the metacarpal heads and extend distally toward the base of the proximal phalanges (Fig. 8.2). The transverse MRI of the joint in flexion enable the most complete analysis of the attachments of the main collateral ligaments and their body. The coronal sequences enable good visualization of the proximal and distal attachments of the main collateral ligaments. When extended, the main collateral ligaments have intermediate signal intensity. The accessory collateral ligaments arise in the same depression as the main collateral ligaments, but in a more palmar location. Their proximal attachments are not separable. They extend in a palmar direction and are firmly attached to the palmar plate. The accessory collateral ligaments are taut in extension and more relaxed in flexion (Fig. 8.1). Transverse MRI in extension enables the best visualization of their attachments and body.

The palmar plate is a thick and dense structure at the palmar aspect of the MCP joints, in the intervals between the accessory collateral ligaments to which they are connected. The palmar plate is firmly inserted into the palmar base of the proximal phalanx. A central distal recess can be seen between two strong attachments. The palmar plate gets thinner proximally into a membranous capsule. A groove is found on the palmar aspect of the palmar plate containing the flexor tendons and the tendon sheaths, which are held to the side of the groove by the A1 pulley.

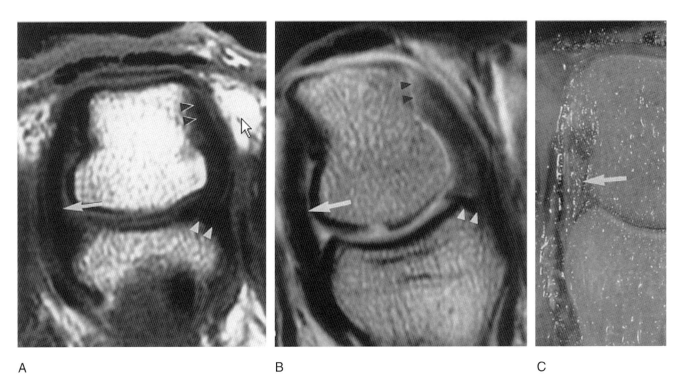

A   B   C

FIG. 8.2. Transverse views of the metacarpophalangeal (MCP) joint of the third finger in flexion, with anatomic correlation. T1-weighted spin echo conventional MR image (A), MR arthrogram (B), and the corresponding anatomic section (C) show the proximal attachments (black arrowheads), distal attachments (white arrowheads), and taut body (arrow) of the main collateral ligament. (From Theumann et al.,[8] with permission).

The deep surface of the palmar plate forms part of the articular surface for the head of the metacarpal bone. Transverse MRI in extension enables the best visualization of the axial extent of the palmar plate (PP), the deep transverse metacarpal ligament (DTML), and the A1 pulley attaching to the PP.

Sagittal MRI of the joints, either in extension or flexion, enable the best delineation of the shape of the body of the palmar plate, its distal attachment, and the recess. The sagittal plane remains the best way for visualization of this structure. The deep transverse metacarpal ligament consists of a short, wide, flattened band that connects the palmar plate of the second to the fifth MCP joints. The lumbrical muscles and the digital vessels are located on the palmar aspect of the DTML. The interosseous muscles and tendons are located on the dorsal aspect of the DTML. Transverse MRI proves to be the only technique to enable analysis of these ligaments, which are much better seen with the finger extended than flexed.

The main collateral ligaments have a primary role in stabilizing the MCP joints in all modes of joint alignment and especially in flexion.[13] When the MCP joint is extended, the angle of the main collateral ligament relative to the constant magnetic induction field is unpredictable, and the magic angle effect is maximized and can possibly cause an increase of signal intensity and consequently diminish visualization. There are interesting pictures showing the radial collateral ligaments, which are usually thicker than the ulnar collateral ligaments.[8] The accessory collateral ligaments prevent palmar displacement of

the proximal phalanges.[14] The palmar plate prevents hyperextension and dorsal subluxation of the MCP joints.[15] The DTML allows dorsal and palmar mobility as well as limited rotation but they limit medial and lateral mobility.[16]

Extensor Hood

The sagittal bands are thin; they extend from the common extensor tendons to the junction of the palmar plate and the DTML and course between the interosseous tendons and the main collateral ligament (Fig. 8.3). The central digits have a palmar soft tissue confluence on each side, consisting of sagittal bands, palmar plates, the A1 pulley, and the DTML. Magnetic resonance imaging of the fingers in extension is the best way to analyze the sagittal bands. The transverse fibers form a triangular lamina, distal to the sagittal bands. These transverse fibers are also better seen in the axial plane. The extensor muscle of the index finger, the extensor muscle of the little finger, and the corresponding tendons represent a part of the extensor complex of the index and little fingers. A fibrous connection of the extensor hood contains the proper and common extensor tendons. Transverses images are required to see the fibers.

Muscles and Tendons

The digital flexor tendon sheaths begin at the level of the metacarpal neck and continue to the distal insertion of the tendon

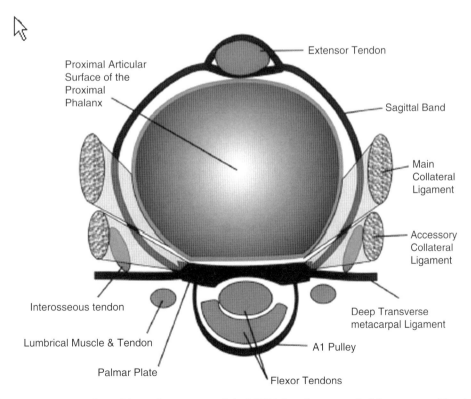

FIG. 8.3. Drawing illustrates transverse view of the main structures of the MCP joint after removal of the metacarpal head. (From Theumann et al.,[8] with permission).

of the deep flexor muscle of the fingers. The tendons of the superficial flexor muscles of the fingers and of the deep flexor muscle of the fingers reside in the sheaths, which are maintained against the palmar plate by the A1 pulley, which is attached to the junction of the palmar plate and the DTML. Transverse MRI, in extension, is the best way to evaluate the tendon sheaths and the A1 pulley. The interosseous muscles and tendons are dorsal to the DTML and insert into the proximal phalanges, with fibers continuing to the extensor hood. Again, transverse images provide the best visualization of these tendons. The lumbrical muscles are in a palmar location in relation to the DTML, they cross to the radial side of the corresponding MCP joint, and they then insert into the digital extensor mechanism. The interosseous and lumbrical muscles and tendons provide stabilization of the MCP joints in full extension.[17] At the level of the MCP joint, transverse MRI is the best way to evaluate these structures.

Pulley System of the Fingers

Normal finger flexion is a complex fine motor action that requires the integrity and orchestration of a number of delicate structures that are centered around the flexor tendon system. One of the most important, the pulley system, composed of focal thickened areas of the flexor tendon sheaths, is of paramount biomechanical importance in flexion, not only for accurate tracking of the tendon but also to maintain the apposition of tendons and bones across the joints and provide a fulcrum to elicit flexion and extension.[18,19] Loss of all or part of the flexor tendon pulley system has a substantial effect on digital motor performance because of the system's role in maintaining the angle of approach of the flexor tendon to its insertion and as a retinacular restrainer.[20]

Anatomic and Biomechanical Considerations

The flexor synovial sheath is composed of visceral and parietal elements that extend from the metacarpal bone to the distal interphalangeal joints and are overlaid by a series of retinacular structures at five specific points along the tendon sheaths (Fig. 8.4). There are retinacular structures, which are focal and well-defined areas of thickening of the tendon sheaths, referred to as the annular pulley system. Additional crossing fibers between the components of the annular pulley system are referred to as the cruciate pulley system. In general, the length of each pulley varies in direct proportion to the lengths of the digit, and the thickness is directly proportional to the length of the pulley.[18]

The first annular pulley (A1) begins in the region of the palmar plate of the MCP joint and extends to the level of the base of the proximal phalanx. The second annular pulley (A2) arises from the volar aspect of the proximal part of the proximal phalanx and extends to the junction of the proximal two thirds and the distal third of the proximal phalanges. The third pulley (A3) is small and extends over the region of the proximal interphalangeal joint. The forth pulley (A4) is in the

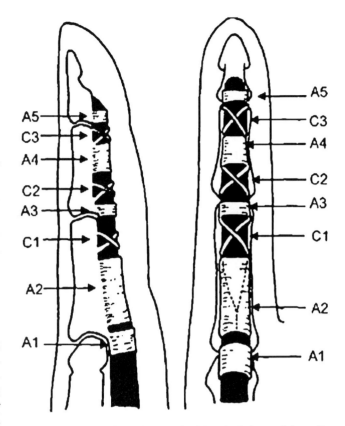

FIG. 8.4. Sagittal (left) and coronal (right) depictions of the pulley system of a typical flexor tendon (black areas) of the finger: fibro-osseous annular pulleys (A2, A4), palmar plate annular pulleys (A1, A3, and A5), and cruciate pulleys (C1, C2, and C3). Dotted lines represent the division of the flexor digitorum superficialis tendon into two bands at this level. (From Theumann et al.,[20] with permission).

midportion of the middle phalanx, and the fifth pulley (A5) is in the region of the distal interphalangeal joint.

The first cruciate pulley (C1) is located between A2 and A3, the second (C2) between A3 and A4, and the third (C3) between A4 and A5. The annular pulleys are of biomechanical importance in preventing tendon excursion during digital flexion, whereas the cruciate pulleys provide the necessary flexibility for approximation of the annular pulley at flexion while maintaining the integrity of the flexor sheaths. The primary function of the flexor pulley system in the fingers is to convert the available linear translation and force in the muscle tendon unit into rotation and torque at the finger joint. Loss of all or part of the flexor tendon pulley system may have a significant effect on digital performance. Studies have shown that the A2 pulley is the strongest, followed by A1 and A4 pulleys.[18,21,22] The pattern of injury follows the progressive and predictable pattern: disruption begins at the distal part of the A2 pulley and progresses from partial to complete rupture, which is followed by involvement of the A3, A4, and, in rare situations, the A1 pulley.

Transverse planes have proved to be the best to depict the insertion of the pulley into adjacent bone. The A3 and A5 pulleys are difficult to see on MRI, because of their small size and lack of osseous insertion.

Neurovascular Anatomy

The neurovascular anatomy of the hand and fingers is complex. The vascular anatomy is important for soft tissue injuries, fracture healing, and avascular necrosis. Nerve compression has numerous causes, so it is essential to understand neurovascular and related anatomy in the hand and fingers. The vascular anatomy can be demonstrated with conventional sequences and image planes or with MR angiography.[6] The vascular supply to the hand can be divided into extrinsic and intrinsic. The extrinsic supply is derived from branches of the radial, ulnar, and anterior interosseous arteries. The radial and ulnar arteries form the margins of three dorsal and palmar arcades.[23] The most proximal arcades lie palmar and dorsal to the radiocarpal joint. The second arcades are palmar and dorsal to the intercarpal joints, and the most distal arcades are at the dorsal basal and deep palmar arches. Distal to the palmar arch, the common digital arteries extend to the level of the MCP joints, where they branch to send proper digital arteries along the margin of each digit.[6] The intrinsic vascular supply is critical for bone healing and involves distal branches of the extrinsic vessels that supply the osseous structures of the wrist.

The median and the ulnar nerves, distal to the flexor retinaculum and the Guyon's canal, divide into small branches. These small branches are difficult to identify, even when thin axial MR sections are obtained.[24]

Flexor and Extensor Tendons

The muscles and tendons that cross the wrist originate at the elbow or proximal forearm. The muscles of the forearm are largely responsible for the flexion and extension of the wrist and the fingers. There are also multiple intrinsic muscles of the hand, which will be described further. If we consider all the tendons that have attachments at the level of the hand and fingers, we note the following:

- The abductor digiti minimi takes its origin on the pisiform and inserts distally at the medial aspect of the base of the proximal phalanx of the little finger.
- The flexor digiti minimi brevis originates from the hook of hamate and the flexor retinaculum and runs distally to the medial side of the base of the proximal phalanx of the little finger.
- The opponens digiti minimi originates distally from the hook of the hamate and the flexor retinaculum and runs distally to the medial border of the fifth metacarpal.
- The abductor pollicis longus inserts distally at the basis of the first metacarpal.
- The abductor pollicis brevis takes its origin on the flexor retinaculum and tubercles of scaphoid and trapezium and inserts distally on the lateral side of the thumb's proximal phalanx base.
- The flexor carpi radialis originates from the medial epicondyles of the humerus and inserts distally at the palmar aspect of the base of the second metacarpal bone.

- The flexor carpi ulnaris has two heads, humeral and ulnar; they insert distally on the pisiform and continue by two bands to the hook of the hamate bone and to the palmar aspect of the base of the fifth metacarpal bone.
- The flexor digitorum superficialis originates from the medial epicondyles of the humerus and the anterior aspect of the ulna and radius. The flexor digitorum profundus originates from the anterosuperior two-thirds of the ulna and interosseous membrane. They run distally through the carpal tunnel and are surrounded by a common tendon sheath.[25] Each tendon of the flexor digitorum superficialis splits into two slips at the level of the proximal phalanges to allow the passage of the profundus tendon. The flexor digitorum superficialis tendons spiral down to insert on the palmar aspect of the middle phalanges, and the flexor digitorum profundus tendon inserts on the palmar aspect of the distal phalanx base.
- The adductor pollicis muscle has two heads: a transverse and an oblique one. The oblique head originates from the base of the second and third metacarpals, capitate, and adjacent carpals. The transverse head originates from the anterior surface of the third metacarpal body. The adductor pollicis tendon inserts distally on the medial side at the base of the proximal phalanges of the thumb.
- The flexor pollicis longus originates from the anterior surface of the radius and adjacent interosseous membrane and inserts distally on the base of the distal phalanx of the thumb.
- The flexor pollicis brevis originates from the flexor retinaculum and tubercles of the scaphoid and trapezium and runs distally to the lateral side of the base of the proximal phalanx of the thumb.
- The opponens pollicis originates from the flexor retinaculum and tubercles of scaphoid and trapezium and inserts distally on the lateral side of the first metacarpal.

Normal finger flexions require the integrity of the pulley system, which was described above. The flexor pulley system is important in maintaining rotation and torque at the finger joints. The major function of the pulley is to stabilize the flexor tendon during finger flexion and thereby avoid radial displacement or volar "bow stringing." Transverse planes offer an optimal visualization of the pulleys and the tendon sheaths. Sagittal planes offer the best visualization of the entire length of the tendon and the possible retraction in case of complete rupture.

Considering the extensor tendons that have attachments at the level of the hand and fingers, we note the following:

- The extensor digitorum originates from the lateral epicondyles of the humerus. It inserts distally in the medial four-digit extensor expansion. The extensor expansion inserts to the dorsal aspect of the middle phalanx via the central band and to the dorsal aspect of the base of the distal phalanx via the lateral bands.
- The extensor carpi radialis brevis tendon inserts at the dorsal aspect of the base of the third metacarpal.
- The extensor carpi radialis longus tendon inserts at the dorsal aspect of the base of the middle metacarpal.

- The extensor carpi ulnaris tendon inserts distally at the base of the fifth metacarpal.
- The extensor digiti minimi is in the fifth compartment of the extensor retinaculum and extends distally to the dorsal aspect of the fifth digit's middle phalanx.
- The extensor indicis originates from the posterior surface of the ulna and interosseous membrane and insert distally on the extensor expansion of the second digit.
- The extensor pollicis brevis tendon runs in the first compartment of the extensor retinaculum and inserts at the thumb's proximal phalanx base.
- The extensor pollicis longus tendon runs in the third compartment of the extensor tendon at the level of the wrist and inserts distally in distal phalanx base of the thumb.

Finger extension involves simultaneous action of both extrinsic and intrinsic extensor muscles. Extrinsic muscles originate in the elbow and forearm and include the following: extensor digitorum, extensor indicis, and extensor digiti minimi. The primary function of these muscles is the extension of the MCP and interphalangeal joints. The intrinsic muscles that originate and insert within the hand are the lumbrical and interosseous muscles.

The function of these intrinsic muscles is primarily to extend the interphalangeal joints and secondarily to contribute to the flexion of the MCP joints. These groups of extrinsic and intrinsic muscles are coordinated by a series of stabilizing retinacular structures, which facilitates the balance of transmission of muscular force. These structures are found in the dorsum of the carpus (extensor retinaculum), the hands (intertendinous connections), and the fingers (extensor hood, retinacular and triangular ligaments). The dorsum of the hand features greater (than palmar) anatomic variability because of tendinous multiplicity and the presence of connections between the different tendons. In most cases, there is more than one tendon in each finger, between the wrist and the MCP joints.[26] The most frequent distribution pattern is as follows: a single extensor indicis tendon located ulnar to the extensor digitorum tendon of the index finger in the MCP joint, a single extensor digitorum tendon for the index finger, a single thick extensor digitorum tendon for the middle finger, a double extensor digitorum tendon for the ring finger, no extensor digitorum tendon for the little finger, and a double extensor digiti minimi tendon for the little finger.

Awareness of the variation and the multiplicity of the extensor tendons of the dorsum of the hand is crucial for adequate assessment of hand lesions but, although both axial and coronal MRI may demonstrate this multiplicity, it is extremely difficult to precisely identify the muscle group corresponding to each tendinous structure.[27]

Near the MCP joints, the extensor tendons are interconnected in the dorsum of the hand by intertendinous connections. These connections create a space between finger extensor tendons, redistribute their force, coordinate finger extension, and stabilize the MCP joints.[28] They also prevent independent extension of the fingers, although this is also due to the distance of the common muscle belly. From a clini-

cal point of view, they are very important because they can act as a bridge, masking tendinous lesions and because of potential snapping related to their subluxation at the MCP joint.[27]

With MRI in the axial plane, the intertendinous connection characteristically appears as a tendinous structure, located between the extensor tendons between the second and fifth fingers, adjacent to the MCP joints. Distally, when the extensor tendon reaches the MCP joint, it links with the sagittal bands, one of the main elements of the extensor hood. Distal to the sagittal bands, the transverse and oblique fibers appear as an initial contribution of the intrinsic muscles to the extensor mechanism. The intrinsic muscles include the lumbrical and interosseous groups. There are four lumbrical muscles, which originate in the deep flexor muscles of the fingers, at the level of the middle palmar region of the hand. The four lumbrical muscles reach the MCP joint at its radial aspect and run palmar to the deep transverse metacarpal ligament and act as flexors of the MCP joints and, in a distal position, as extensors of the interphalangeal joints.

There are seven interosseous muscles, three palmar and four dorsal. The three palmar muscles take their origin at the second, fourth, and fifth metacarpals. The first of these muscles is located on the ulnar side of the metacarpal, whereas the two others are located on the radial side. They act as adductors of the fingers as well as MCP joints' flexors, and interphalangeal joints' extensors. The four dorsal interosseous muscles originate at the adjacent metacarpals. These muscles are the adductors of the fingers, just like the interosseous palmar muscles, and they act as flexors of the MCP joints and extensors of the interphalangeal joint.[29] At MRI the lumbrical muscles may be easily identified on axial sections. They are located at the palm, next to the deep flexor tendons, from which they originate. The most dorsal interosseous muscles appear in the intermetacarpal spaces.

Distal to the MCP joint, the extrinsic and intrinsic tendons blend into the dorsal apparatus and are circumferentially distributed over the dorsum of the fingers (Fig. 8.5). The extrinsic extensor tendon constitutes a central and lateral band of the slips.[29] The intrinsic tendons also provide medial fibers to form the central slip. This central slip inserts on the base of the middle phalanx. The lateral slips emerge with the intrinsic tendon, forming the conjoint tendons. The conjoint tendons pass over the dorsal zone of the middle phalanges, to converge distally and form the terminal tendon, which is then inserted in the dorsum of the base of the distal phalanges. Axial MRI is the best to visualize all of this dorsal apparatus, and sagittal MRI is the best to follow the tendons on their entire length.

There are some pitfalls for MRI of the tendons. The compact parallel arrangement of fibers and low water content account for the homogeneous intensity of tendons on all magnetic resonance pulse sequences.[30] However, there are some exceptions to this general role. Intrasubstance, hyperintensity can be seen in normal tendons, owing to the magic angle effect, a phenomenon that occurs on low echo time (TE) sequences, in tendons that have a 55-degree orientation to the magnetic field.[31] The magic angle

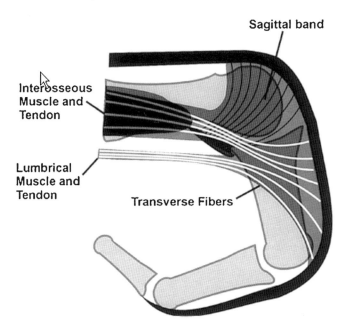

Sagittal band

Interosseous Muscle and Tendon

Lumbrical Muscle and Tendon

Transverse Fibers

FIG. 8.5. Drawing of the extensor hood. The sagittal bands are located above the joint line, and the transverse fibers of the lumbrical and interosseous tendons are more distal, over the proximal phalanx. (From Theumann et al.,[8] with permission).

effect is common in wrist tendon and is most frequently observed on the flexor pollicis longus (FPL) tendon, as it courses in the distal aspect of the carpal tunnel and in the palm.[32] The absence of additional pathologic features and the presence of high signal on short TE images without signal alteration on other pulse sequences are highly suggestive of the magic angle effect. A small amount of physiologic fluid, often seen within the synovial sheaths, can also cause T2 hyperintensity around extensor tendons, which is not indicative of tenosynovitis.[33] Sometimes, striation and heterogeneous signal can be noted in the abductor pollicis longus because of the presence of multiple slips that can simulate longitudinal split tears. This appearance can be the result of fat interposition between the tendinous fascicles and should not be misinterpreted as pathologic. Finally, the position of the wrist in neutral, pronation, or supination at the time of the MRI examination will modify the alignment of the extensor carpi ulnaris tendon at the level of the ulnar styloid groove.[34] The position of the fingers in flexion may also allow a 55-degree angulation with the main magnetic field and give hyperintense signal in flexor tendons at the level of the fingers.

Pathology

Traumatic Lesions

Common Carpometacarpal and Intermetacarpal Joints

The injuries of the CCMC joints and the second to fifth IMC joints are relatively uncommon. Injuries to the IMC and CCMC can result when a large torsional force is applied. Common

carpometacarpal (CCMC) dislocation most commonly results in dorsal displacement of the metacarpal base.[35] The most common single-digit CCMC dislocation involves the small finger, followed by the index and ring fingers. The evaluation of ligamentous and tendinous injuries of the CCMC and IMC joints has, to date, been limited to standard radiography.[11]

Carpometacarpal Joint of the Thumb

Trauma to the carpometacarpal joint of the thumb eventually results in a spectrum of ligamentous injury, dependent on the rate and direction of the loading force.[36] The anterior oblique ligament is the most common ligament injured, followed by the dorsoradial ligament.[10] The assessment of the carpometacarpal joint injuries of the thumb is based on a clinical examination supplemented by radiographs. The patient commonly presents with focal tenderness and pain deep to the thenar eminence, following dislocation, and ligamentous instability can be difficult to diagnose clinically, particularly when there is pain, swelling, and hematoma. Radiographs may demonstrate soft tissue swelling and occasional avulsion of a fragment of bone from the thumb's metacarpal base (Bennett's fracture) but, in the absence of a fracture, they will be normal. Stress views may show a loss of anatomic alignment, providing indirect information about ligament stability. Magnetic resonance imaging has the ability to diagnose the degree of ligamentous injury and differentiate avulsions from partial tear (Fig. 8.6). In the case of a complete tear, MRI can confirm the clinical findings as well as identifying concomitant pathologies such as chondral injuries, occult fractures, and intraarticular bony fragments or interposed soft tissue. This information could help in surgical planning. When patients are treated conservatively, MRI can be used to monitor healing and resolution of a hematoma and to evaluate ligament quality and joint stability before returning to normal activity. The superficial component of the anterior oblique ligament is the most common site for either complete or partial tears.[10] The dorsoradial ligament is the next most common injury with tearing, occurring exclusively on the trapezial side. The anterior oblique ligament is a primary stabilizer of the thumb's carpometacarpal joint and thus dislocation results in injury to this structure, which has implications for joint stability and secondary osteoarthritis.[10]

Metacarpophalangeal Joint of the Thumb

The most frequently requested MRI examination for the MCP of the thumb is to diagnose a potential rupture of the ulnar collateral ligament (UCL) of the thumb. A rupture of the UCL of the thumb is one of the most frequently occurring ligament injuries of the hand.[37] When left untreated, the injury may lead to a loss of pinch grip strength, instability, pain, and later osteoarthritis.[38] Skiing and cycling accidents and falling on the hands are common causes of this injury.[39] The trauma mechanism is hyperabduction, and often also hyperextension of the MCP joint of the thumb. For treatment of fresh and unstable UCL ruptures, early repair of the insertions of the ligaments has been advocated with fixation of the bony

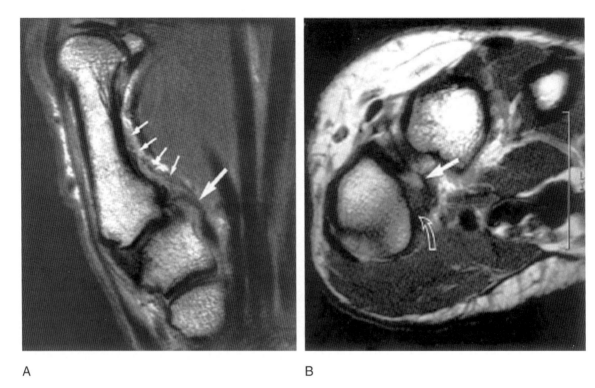

A   B

FIG. 8.6. A 25-year-old platform diver following injury to the thumb carpometacarpal joint. (A) Coronal fast spin echo (FSE) T2 image showing high-grade partial tearing of the anterior oblique ligament (straight arrow) with periosteal stripping (small arrows) from the base of the thumb metacarpal. (B) Axial FSE T2 image showing the periosteal stripping (open curved arrow) and the torn anterior oblique ligament (straight arrow). (From Connell et al.,[10] with permission).

avulsion if present.[40] This rupture occurs more often at the distal insertion. An uninjured UCL lies beneath the adductor aponeurosis. After a total rupture, the proximal part of the ligament may be located superficial to the adductor aponeurosis. In these cases, successful healing is not possible, as the ruptured ends of the ligament are in contact with one another. This is the so-called Stener lesion,[41] which should be treated operatively, as should an unstable lesion.[42]

When the UCL rupture is primarily diagnosed and correctly treated, the results are good. Unfortunately, this lesion is sometimes primarily missed. The longer the time before ligament reconstruction, the worse the result.[43] Magnetic resonance imaging has been shown to be a reliable method for primary diagnosis of UCL lesions and their classification into either Stener or non-Stener lesions[44] (Fig. 8.7). In cases of subacute disruption of the UCL, MRI can verify the UCL rupture, but typing the lesion as either a Stener or a non-Stener is not always possible.[42]

Traumatic Lesion of the Metacarpophalangeal Joints of the Fingers

Traumatic lesions of the MCP joints of the fingers are uncommon compared with those of the thumb. The index and small fingers are injured, mainly during twisting force. The clinical diagnosis is obvious when the tear is extensive and involves the collateral ligaments, the dorsal capsule, or the palmar

plate. In these cases, spontaneous laxity of the injured finger may be depicted, sometimes with associated rotational disturbance. However, the diagnosis is often missed initially, when there is an isolated lesion of a collateral ligament. Residual pain may persist for months. Clinical testing of stability of the MCP joint of the middle and fourth fingers is difficult, because valgus and varus stress tests are not possible.[45]

There are classically three grades of joint sprain: (1) no instability indicates a sprain with continuous collateral ligaments; (2) a discrete instability and firm end point indicates a partial tear of collateral ligaments; and (3) a gross instability without a firm end point is indicative of a complete tear of the collateral ligaments.[46]

The treatment of collateral ligament lesions type 1 and 2 is conservative, with immobilization for 3 weeks in a cast and rehabilitation in the case of a type 1 lesion; type 2 lesions are treated with immobilization that lasts 3 weeks longer. The treatment for a type 3 lesion is conservative if possible (6 weeks) or surgery.

Magnetic resonance imaging is useful to help to decide on a course of treatment. Conservative treatment with a cast is possible only when the free margins of the torn ligament are very close to each other. If the gap is significant, surgery should be performed. Association with another joint structure lesion could be an additional argument for surgery. Thus, it is clinically impossible to assess whether a patient should or should not undergo surgery.[47] In chronic posttraumatic disability of

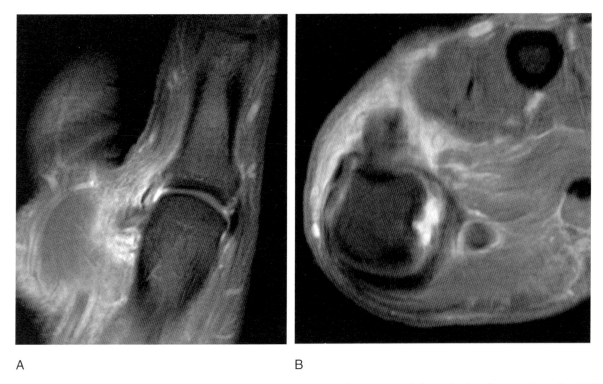

A   B

FIG. 8.7. Stener lesion. A 32-year-old patient following ski injury to the thumb metacarpophalangeal joint. Coronal (A) and axial (B) T1-weighted fat saturated enhanced images showing a Stener lesion with proximally retracted torn ulnar collateral ligament with respect to the adductor pollicis aponeurosis.

the MCP joints, MRI appears useful in delineating abnormalities of the collateral ligaments and the palmar plates, which represent the sites of 80% of injuries in large series.[47] Accurate imaging of the MCP joint may be obtained with a commercial phase array coil. The smallest possible field of view (4 cm) is necessary to analyze this thin element. Only the axial plane with the MCP joint in a flexed position is useful to demonstrate the whole course of the main collateral ligament. The images of the MCP joint in a flexed position also facilitate assessment of the stability of the extensor tendon at the level of the metacarpal head (Fig. 8.8).

Axial T2-weighted images are less accurate than T1-weighted images in the depiction of collateral ligament tears because of the decreased signal-to-noise ratio. In the case of chronic lesions, owing to the presence of scar tissue, the soft tissue contrast in T2-weighted images is also poor. The presence of fluid in chronic ligament tears is also uncommon. Intravenous injection of gadolinium increases the signal intensity and contrast of the images and is helpful in the depiction of small ligament tears. In one of our series of collateral ligament injuries, MRI accurately depicted associated lesions in 40% of cases. The most common associated lesions were of the sagittal band. Lesions on the radial side were the most common. The palmar plate is rarely injured at the level of the MCP joint, compared with the level of the proximal interphalangeal joint.[47] The palmar plate is stretched in extension and a distal avulsion can occur during hyperextension of the joint.

A small hematoma in the palmar aspect of the MCP joint may be noted. Manipulation or even skin pressure is painful. A bone avulsion of the palmar aspect of the base of the proximal phalanx may be depicted on lateral radiographs.[48] A proximal avulsion is less common and is present only in cases of an associated tear of the accessory collateral ligament. Injury of the palmar plate is often missed clinically and results in antalgic flexion with painful stiffness. In cases of palmar plate rupture, arthrography may show leakage of contrast agent into the flexor tendon sheaths.[49] Palmar plate injuries heal easily and are associated with very little disability. A synovial recess is normally present at the distal insertion of the palmar plate and must not be misdiagnosed as a distal avulsion of the palmar plate with MRI (Fig. 8.9). However, the diagnosis of a complete tear of the palmar plate with an associated ligament tear may necessitate surgical intervention. Proximal interphalangeal (PIP) and distal interphalangeal (DIP) lesions are similar to those seen at the level of the MCP. Better resolution is mandatory to delineate the structures and lesions at these levels (Fig. 8.10).

Tendon Injuries

Tendon injuries are often secondary to repetitive trauma or overuse.[34] Overstretching from excessive tensile strains results in the rupture of tendon fibers. Tendon injuries can be grouped into six categories: tendinosis, peritendinitis, tenosynovitis,

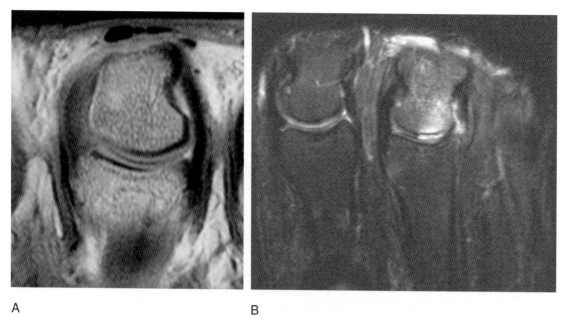

A   B

FIG. 8.8. Main collateral ligament tear of the MCP joint. MRI of the third MCP joint in flexed position. (A) Axial MR arthrography image demonstrating normal main collateral ligaments of the MCP joint in a specimen. (B) Axial T1-weighted fat saturated enhanced image showing a distal complete tear of the main ulnar collateral ligament.

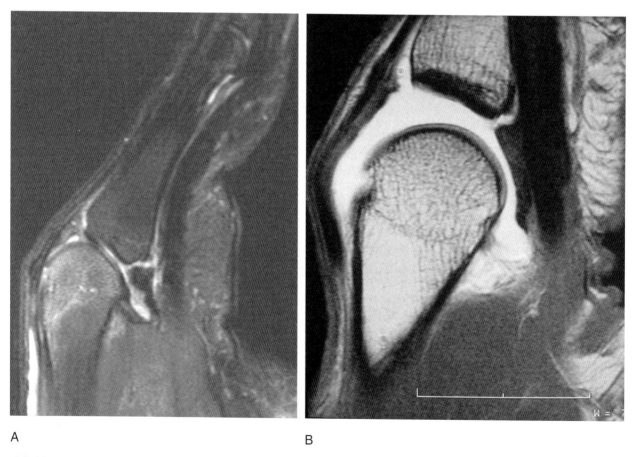

A   B

FIG. 8.9. Distal tear of the palmar plate. MRI of the palmar plate in a third MCP joint. (A) Sagittal T1-weighted fat saturated enhanced image showing an avulsion at the distal insertion of the palmar plate that is too large to represent a synovial recess. Note that the palmar plate is retracted. (B) Sagittal MR arthrography image demonstrating normal distal recess of the palmar plate in a specimen.

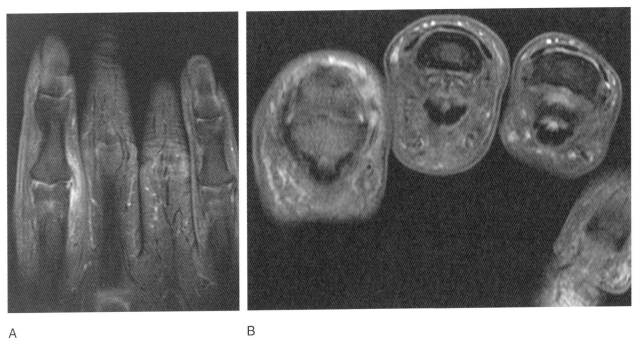

FIG. 8.10. Collateral ligament tear of the proximal interphalangeal (PIP) joint. MRI of the second PIP joint. T1-weighted fat saturated enhanced images, coronal in extended position (A) and axial in flexed position (B) showing a proximal complete tear of the ulnar collateral ligament.

entrapment, rupture, and instability. These conditions often coexist and overlap with the clinical, gross anatomic, and histologic manifestations, which complicates MRI diagnosis. There are several types of tendinosis and tendon degeneration, including fibromatosis (hypoxic), lipoid, and myxoid.[50] The MRI characteristics of tendinosis include the fusiform shape of the focal area of increased tendon width associated with increased intrasubstance signal on T1-weighted or proton density images. T2 hyperintensity is noted when severe degeneration is present. Peritendinitis and tenosynovitis are caused by inflammatory or mechanical irritation of the peritenon and tendon sheaths, respectively. Magnetic resonance imaging reveals fluid accumulation within the tendon sheaths, synovial proliferation, or scarring. Stenosing tenosynovitis occurs when synovial proliferation and fibrosis lead to scar formation around the tendon, with subsequent entrapment and even rupture. Areas of intermediate to low signal in soft tissues around the tendon are seen in all MRI sequences. Tendon ruptures can be acute or chronic, and partial or complete. Ruptures usually occur in previously diseased tendons. In the hand and fingers, repetitive minor trauma may be caused by bony prominences that are secondary to fracture, deformity, or degenerative osteophytes. Acute tendon ruptures often demonstrate areas of increased T2-weighted hyperintensity, owing to the presence of edema and hemorrhage. In chronic tendon ruptures, scar tissue formation appears in MRI as areas of low signal intensity on all pulse sequences. Partial ruptures can be depicted on T1- or T2-weighted images as intrasubstance sig-

nal intensity similar to that seen in advanced tendinosis. Complete rupture is depicted as complete disruption of the tendon fibers. Fluid, hemorrhage, or scar tissue can fill in the gap, depending on the age of the tear. Tendon dislocations are easily detected on MRI, especially in the axial plane (Fig. 8.11).

Closed ruptures of the digital flexor tendons are uncommon compared to flexor tendon laceration. Most often chronic conditions that result in weakening of tendons are typically present, such as osteoarthritis or posttraumatic deformation.

Flexor tendon ruptures are classified, based on location, according to the system of International Committee of Tendon Injuries.[32] Zone 1 extends from the distal insertion of the flexor digitorum profundus (FDP) tendon to the distal insertion of the flexor digitorum superficialis (FDS) tendon. Zone 2 extends from the distal insertion of the FDS tendon to the distal palmar fold. At this level, the FDP and FDS tendons course together in the narrow fibro-osseous digital canal. Zone 3 extends from the proximal part of the A1 pulley (distal palmar fold) to the distal part of the flexor retinaculum. At this level, the lumbrical muscles originate from the FDP tendons. Additional zones concern the carpal and forearm levels. The thumb has three separates zones: T1 extends from the A2 pulley to the FPL tendon insertion, T2 extends between the A1 and A2 pulleys, and T3 extends between the trapezium and the A1 pulley.

"Jersey finger" is the most frequent type of flexor digitorum tendon rupture and involves distal avulsion of the FDP and FDS from their insertion into the distal and middle phalanges, respectively. Proximal retraction of the torn tendon classically

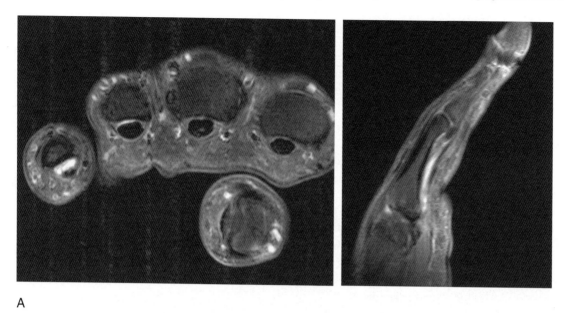

A

FIG. 8.11. Flexor tendon tear. MRI of the fifth finger. T1-weighted fat saturated enhanced images in the axial plane at the level of the proximal phalanx (A) and a sagittal plane showing flexor digitorum profundus tendon tear and absent tendon in the digital canal (B).

stops just at the level of the digital canal. Magnetic resonance imaging has proved useful for displaying the zones of ruptures on the proximal and distal tendons, and it accurately measures the gap between the torn tendon ends.[32] The gap size is considered a determinant factor in treatment decision making. If the gap is greater than 3 cm, a tendon graft is preferred to primary tendon repair. Assessment of the integrity of the adjacent tendon before performing a tendon graft is well accomplished by using MRI.[51] Also, MRI helps to locate the proximal end of the tendon, which, in some cases, may displace between the adjacent tendons or even refract to the palm. In case of rupture, peritendinous enhancement is noted, suggesting the presence of synovitis. The tendons themselves show thickening and signal abnormalities, due to tendinopathy.

Extensor tendon injuries are also common because of their poorly protected anatomic location. Because the excursion of the extensor tendons over the fingers is less than that of the flexors, preservation of their length is far more critical to restoring the normal tendon balance.[52] The relationship between the location of injury and the outcome is an important concept. The type of injury, deformity, and surgical outcome will be different according to the affected anatomic regions. As a result, the categorical classification of tendon injuries into anatomic zones is crucial to the diagnostic process.

The zones are identical to those described before for flexor tendons. Injuries at zone 1 (DIP joint) may provoke disruption of the terminal extensor tendon, which is dorsally and superficially located at this level. This type of lesion is called a mallet finger and is characterized by a deficit of DIP joint extension. A mallet finger injury may be open but more often is closed. The mechanism of the closed injury is most commonly a sudden, effortful flexion of the DIP joint in an extended digit.

This results in the rupture of the terminal extensor tendon or avulsion of a bone fragment at its insertion. The most common treatment is closed splinting with the DIP joint in extension.

In zone 2 (middle phalanx), injuries are usually secondary to laceration. A simple laceration can transect all of the dorsal apparatus. If less than 50% of the tendon width is cut, the treatment involves routine wound care and splinting, followed by active motion. Injuries involving more than 50% of the tendon width should be primarily repaired.[53]

In zone 3 (PIP joint), injuries may cause disruption of the central slip with eventual development of a boutonniere deformity, secondary to flexion of the PIP joint and hyperextension of the DIP joint. Initial treatment should be splinting the PIP joint in extension. Surgical indications are a displaced avulsion fracture, associated instability of the PIP joint, and chronic symptomatic cases.[54]

In zone 4 (proximal phalanges), injuries are usually partial since, at this level, the dorsal apparatus is circumferentially distributed over the dorsum of the fingers and simple injuries seldom result in a complete laceration. The lacerated tendon does not retract appreciably because of the interconnections and due to the presence of retinacular ligaments.[27]

In zone 5 (MCP), injuries are almost always open and commonly secondary to a human bite. These injuries most often occur with the joint in flexion, and the laceration in the extensor tendon may be proximal to the dermal injury. Primary tendon repair is indicated. Oblique laceration may include the sagittal band and may lead to subsequent subluxation or dislocation of the extensor tendon. Tearing of the sagittal band and a subsequent subluxation and dislocation of the extensor mechanism may also occur as a consequence of a closed injury, secondary to a blow forcing the finger into flexion or after forced flexion and ulnar deviation of the finger.[55] In chronic untreated cases, the patient presents with a history of multiple episodes of pain and swelling over the MCP joint with a snapping sensation in the fingers. Treatment of the sagittal band disruption, in most cases, is surgical repair.[55]

Magnetic resonance imaging is useful to show tendinous disruptions, complete or partial tears, and their precise locations. It is particularly useful in the evaluation of extensor or flexor apparatus injuries, as clinical examination is not always unequivocal, especially in the acute phase. Diagnosis of a partial tear with MRI is based on the presence of areas of increased signal intensity in a portion of the tendon on T1- and T2-weighted images (Fig. 8.12). A complete tendon tear appears as an area of discontinuity with fraying and irregularities at both ends of the ruptured tendon. In addition, evaluation of the tendinous gap is very important, particularly in the proximal areas, where the frequency of retraction is higher, thus avoiding inappropriate surgical maneuvers. In lesions of the articular zones, it is crucially important to evaluate possible lesion extension to the supporting ligamentous structures and to the capsular articular ones, which represents an indication for surgical repair.[55]

Traumatic Lesions of the Pulley

Traumatic lesions of the pulley system are frequently associated with rock climbing. The hands are used as tools for ascending a wall of rock face. Depending on the type of climbing technique required, the entire body weight is placed on the finger, with a considerable overload. As a result, high-stress forces are exerted at the interphalangeal joints, the flexor tendons, and the finger flexor pulley system for extended periods of time. Based on recent series, approximately 75%

of the elite and recreational sport climbers are reported to have injured their upper extremities, and up to 30% of them have specific signs of flexor pulley system rupture with loss of strength across the full range of motion of the fingers, and decreased range of motion.[56] From clinical findings, it may be difficult to distinguish overuse syndromes related to excessive training and climbing exercises and exposure to chronic stresses from tears of the flexor tendon pulley system. Many injured athletes with minor bow-stringing do not seek medical attention in cases of persistent pain and soft tissue swelling in the affected fingers, with the risk of developing fixed flexion contractures of the PIP joint and secondary osteoarthritis.[57]

Regarding pulley injuries, physiologic studies demonstrated that the A5 (4 mm) annular pulley, the A2 pulley (mean length, 16-3 mm), which attaches directly to the bone of the proximal phalanges, and the A4 pulley (mean length 5.8 mm), which attaches to the bone of the middle phalanx, are the broadest, the most important, and able to resist palmar displacement of the flexor tendons.[58] The A2 pulley is the strongest, and the A4 has the greatest stiffness.[20,22] Among rock climbers the A2 pulley tears more commonly than the A4, and its rupture may occur alone or in association with the A3 pulley, whereas the A1 pulley always remains intact.[59] In these high-level professional climbers presenting with significant flexor tendon bow stringing, the ruptured pulleys can be reconstructed to restore efficient biomechanical characteristics of the flexor apparatus. Free tendon or retinaculum grafts are used for digital pulley reconstruction, placing the graft in the same location as the native pulley.[60] After operation, patients are usually free of pain and able to return to climbing at their preinjury levels. Patients who are treated conservatively or who refuse surgery usually tape their fin-

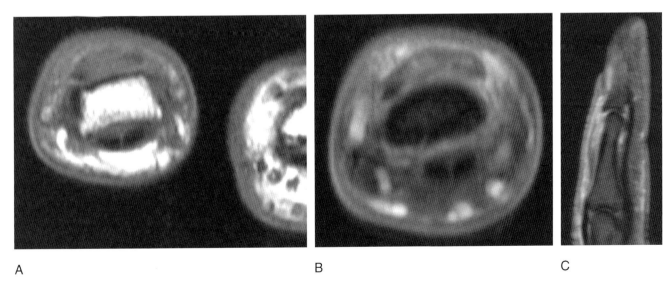

A   B   C

Fig. 8.12. Extensor tendon partial tear. MRI of the fifth finger. (A) T1-weighted axial image. (B) T1-weighted fat saturated enhanced images on the axial plane at the level of the proximal phalanx. (B) The sagittal plane showing heterogeneity and hyperintensity of the terminal tendon at its insertion on the base of the distal phalanx.

gers between the joints to reinforce the flexor tendon pulley system and avoid worsening of existing lesions.[59]

Complete acute rupture of a pulley is easily investigated by ultrasound (US). The advantages of US are dynamic examinations performed at rest and during resisted flexion, and a higher spatial resolution. Overall, US has proved to be 98% sensitive, 100% specific, and 99% accurate in the diagnosis.[61] Alternatively, incomplete pulley rupture is more difficult to diagnose since it causes only mild or absent tendon displacement. In this case, the affected pulley appears swollen and hypoechogenic,[62] and is more difficult to see with US, but this is very well depicted by MRI.

Compared with US, MRI gives a better delineation of the pulley attachments into the bony cortex of the phalanges. In suspected annular pulley tears, an appropriate MRI technique includes positioning the finger in extension and forced flexion: the patient has to push the fingertips on the surface of the tuft.[63] The protocol consists of T1- and T2-weighted spin echo sequences in axial and sagittal planes. Correlation with adjacent normal fingers should be performed to confirm the diagnosis during the analysis of findings. Direct visualization of the pulley tear is diagnostic

(Fig. 8.13). When not visualized, there are indirect MRI criteria for complete annular pulley tears, mainly related to the grade and location of tendon dislocation: bow-stringing, extending: a) from the base of the proximal phalanx to the PIP, indicates rupture of the A2 pulley; b) from the base of the proximal phalanx to the distal area of the PIP indicates a combined A2 and A3 pulley tear; c) and from the base to the middle third of the intermediate phalanx indicates a A4 pulley tear. In an incomplete A2 pulley tear, the bow-stringing does not reach the base of the proximal phalanx. Additional signs of pulley rupture include synovial effusion, cysts, and local soft tissue edema and hematoma.[59]

Tumoral Lesions

Tumors and tumor-like lesions of the hand are more frequently benign tumour-like lesions rather than true neoplastic diseases.[6,64] Different imaging methods including plain film, US, CT, and MRI can be performed.[65]

Plain films must be obtained in all patients since they are extensive and panoramic. Ultrasound, if performed by an experienced operator, can accurately assess the internal structure of

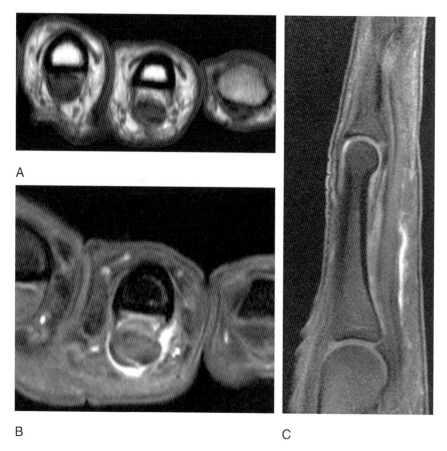

A

B

C

FIG. 8.13. A2 pulley rupture. MRI of the annular finger. (A) T1-weighted axial image. (B) T1-weighted fat saturated enhanced images in axial plane at the level of the proximal phalanx and (C) sagittal enhanced image. Note the discontinuity of the A2 pulley, the inflammation around the intact flexor tendon and the tendon separation from the phalanx.

the mass and the relation with adjacent nerves and vessels. Moreover, US color Doppler can assess the internal vascularity. Because of its multiplanar capability and excellent tissue contrast, MRI has now superseded CT in the assessment of the extension of the mass. Magnetic resonance imaging is an important method for assessing disorders of the musculoskeletal tissues. It is particularly sensitive to bone marrow involvement and is highly effective in detecting and characterizing a wide variety of soft tissue conditions. Advances in surface coil technology with higher spatial resolution increase the usefulness of MRI in the evaluation of joint disease. However, CT remains the method of choice in evaluating bone involvement of soft tissue tumors and small bone tumors such as osteoid osteoma. When a malignant tumor is considered, thoracoabdominal CT or bone scintigraphy is essential to evaluate the presence of metastatic lesions.

Bone Tumors

Bone tumors of the hand and fingers are uncommon.[65] However, benign tumors and tumor-like conditions occur more frequently than malignant neoplasm.[66,67] Table 8.1 summarizes the most common benign and malignant bone lesions in the hand and fingers.[67–70] As a general rule, clinical findings and standard radiography allow an accurate diagnosis of the majority of bone tumors located in the hand and fingers. Computed tomography scanning remains the best modality for assessment of bone destruction, whereas MRI can evaluate bone marrow involvement and tumor extension in the adjacent soft tissues.

However, when a malignant tumor is suspected, exhaustive presurgical evaluation and diagnostic biopsy are warranted. Due to their superficial location, malignant tumors of the hand and fingers can be early diagnosed and treated successfully if they are considered in the differential diagnosis.[71]

TABLE 8.1. Most common bone tumors in the hand (percentage of each tumor in the hand).

Benign	
Enchondroma	54%
Giant cell tumor	12%
Intraosseous ganglia	8.5%
Osteoid osteoma	6%
Aneurysmal bone cyst	6%
Osteochondroma	4%
Osteoblastoma	4%
Chondromyxoid fibroma	4%
Exostosis	3%
Fibrous dysplasia	3%
Benign vascular tumor	2.5%
Malignant	
Malignant vascular tumor	6%
Malignant fibrous histiocytoma	3%
Chondrosarcoma	2%
Metastasis	0.5%
Osteosarcoma	0.4%
Firbrosarcoma	0.2%

Source: Theumann and Drape,[65] with permission.

Enchondromas

Enchondroma is the most common benign bone tumor in the hand and fingers. About 40% of these tumors involve the hand.[71] Most of them are detected incidentally on routine plain films or after pathologic fractures. When the lesion becomes symptomatic without fracture, malignant degeneration should be considered and evaluated.[6] Radiographically, radiolucent well-defined medullar lesions, containing thin orbicular, tiny punctuated and scattered calcifications of the cartilage matrix, are observed. Magnetic resonance features of enchondroma are lobular high signal intensity on T2-weighted spin echo sequences, and isointense signal on T1-weighted sequences in comparison with the muscles. Cortical destruction and soft tissue involvement are useful features that indicate on aggressive tumor. Enhancement after injection of gadolinium is not specific.

Chondroblastoma of the hand is extremely rare. Clinical and some imaging findings are similar to those of enchondroma, although chondroblastoma affects more commonly the epiphysis rather than the diaphyses and may present with a large area of bone marrow and soft tissue edema, which is very well depicted on MRI examination. Local recurrence after surgical removal and malignant degeneration can occur.[72]

Giant Cell Tumors

These tumors represent about 5% of benign bone tumors.[73] They are usually observed in young patients and originate from the epiphysis and can expand into the metaphysis and diaphysis. Local aggressive behavior explains the high rate of recurrence after surgery. Radiographically, a pure lytic lesion in the metaphysis and epiphysis is observed. It can extend to the subchondral bone. The margins are well or poorly defined. Magnetic resonance imaging adds little to the diagnosis, but its features may show areas of low signal intensity on T2-weighted images, suggesting the presence of hemosiderin deposition.[74]

Aneurysmal Bone Cysts

Aneurysmal bone cyst is rarely seen about the hand.[75] The most common locations are the phalanges and metacarpal bones followed by carpal bones. Plain film demonstrates a lytic lesion, which often causes expansion of the involved bone. Septations are common. Magnetic resonance imaging shows a well-defined, lobulated, septated lesion with multiple fluid-fluid levels.[76] Fluid-fluid levels are not specific for aneurysmal bone cyst, however, similar features have been described in other benign and malignant lesions.

Intraosseous Ganglions Cysts

These cysts appear commonly as small, well-circumscribed, oval lytic lesions, bordered by a sclerotic ring on plain film of the wrist and hand. Internal mucous content is present at MRI (low to intermediate signal on T1- and high signal on T2-weighted images).[77]

Malignant Tumors

Malignant bone tumors are rare. However, metastases of the hand are more frequent than primary bone tumors. The phalanges are more commonly involved than the metacarpal bones and bones of the wrist. Radiographically, metastases appear as nonspecific lytic aggressive lesions. Plain film and MRI are the best imaging methods to evaluate tumor extension and relation with surrounding structures. However, currently, MRI has not been found to be useful for histologic differentiation of malignant bone lesions.

Soft Tissue Tumors

Soft tissue tumors are more frequent than bone tumors in the hand and wrist.[47] The majority of soft tissue masses are benign (Table 8.2).[78] Radiographs may demonstrate vascular calcifications, localized soft tissue masses, and adjacent bone changes. Magnetic resonance imaging with its multiplanar capability and excellent soft tissue contrast remains the method of choice. Ultrasound still remains an effective examination if performed by an experienced radiologist.

Soft Tissue Benign Tumors

Ganglia Cyst. Wrist ganglia represent the most common soft tissue masses of the hand and wrist. They are painless, lobulated masses, filled with mucous fluid and lined by a fibrous wall, located close to the tendon sheath or joint capsule.[78,79] The most common site of ganglion cysts is the distal interphalangeal joint. Ganglia can communicate with the adjacent joint cavity by a one-way valve, which allows the synovial fluid to move from the joint into the cyst. However, they may enlarge or resolve spontaneously. Magnetic resonance imaging demonstrates a well-defined lesion with low signal intensity on T1- and high signal intensity on T2-weighted images.[80] Thin peripheral enhancement is noted after gadolinium injection. Complicated (hemorrhagic) ganglia may cause variation in signal intensity.

Giant Cell Tumor of the Tendon Sheath. Giant cell tumor of the tendon sheath (GCTTS) is the second most common soft tissue mass in the hand and fingers.[81] It is a localized villo-

nodular tenosynovitis.[78] There are two forms of GCTTS. The local form (nodular tenosynovitis) presents as a nodular mass typically in the hand and fingers; the diffuse form, located near larger joints of the wrist, represents an extraarticular extension of pigmented villonodular synovitis.[82] Characteristic pathologic findings include a loose connective tissue with multinucleated giant cells and hemosiderin inclusions. Bone erosion can occur. Magnetic resonance imaging shows isointense signal compared to muscle on T1- and heterogeneous intensity on T2-weighted sequences. Diffuse hemosiderin deposits are well seen with T2* sequences. A diffuse heterogeneous enhancement is noted on T1-weighted sequences after intravenous gadolinium injection (Fig. 8.14).

Lipoma. Lipoma is the fifth most frequent benign tumor of the hand and fingers (5%).[82] The most frequent benign tumors are ganglion cysts, giant cell tumors of the tendon sheath, epidermoid cysts, and hemangiomas. Clinically, soft tissue lipomas in the hand and wrist do not differ from lipomas encountered in other locations. Magnetic resonance imaging shows high signal on both T1- and T2-weighted imaging and can accurately depict the extension of the lesion. Although there may be fine septations or a lobulated appearance, the remainder of the tumor is fat.

There are variations of intermuscular or intramuscular lipoma, lipoma of the tendon sheaths, and neural fibrolipoma.[84] Intramuscular lipomas may infiltrate between muscle fibers, showing irregular margins compared with well-defined margins of benign lipomas and can extend along tendons. Nerve fibrolipoma is a slow-growing tumor (hamartoma), predominantly present during early adulthood. The most common nerve involved is the median nerve (80%). Carpal tunnel syndrome is the most common clinical sign.[85] Magnetic resonance imaging shows serpiginous structures, hypointense on T1- and T2-weighted images, corresponding to the fibrous component embedded in adipose tissue (high signal on both sequences).[86]

Vascular Tumors or Malformations. Hemangioma is the fourth most common benign soft tissue lesion of the hand and fingers (7%).[87] Hemangioma may contain nonvascular elements, such as fatty tissue, smooth muscle, fibrous tissue, and bone. Hemangiomas are usually classified according to vessel size as cavernous (large vessel) or capillary (small vessels).[88] Though skin and subcutaneous lesions are easily diagnosed at physical examination, deep hemangioma requires an additional imaging method for proper evaluation.[87]

Radiographs reveal rounded regular calcifications within the mass, corresponding to phleboliths contained in the low-flow vessels. Ultrasound with color Doppler easily demonstrates the vascular origin of the mass. Magnetic resonance imaging also shows characteristic features. Serpiginous low signal intensity structures, within regions of high signal intensity on T1-weighted images, are characteristics. The lesions are diffusely hyperintense on T2-weighted sequences. Phlebolites are seen as round areas of low signal intensity (flow void artifacts).[88]

TABLE 8.2. Most common soft tissue tumors in the hand (percentage of each tumor in the hand).

Benign	
Intraosseous ganglia	NA
Glomus tumor	52%
Giant cell tumor of the tendon sheath	44%
Hemangioma	12%
Nodular fascititis	11%
Lipoma	6%
Malignant	
Epithelioid sarcoma	32%
Malignant fibrous histiocytoma	0.2%
Fibrosarcoma	4%
Extraskeletal chondrosarcoma	18%

Source: Theumann and Drape,[65] with permission.

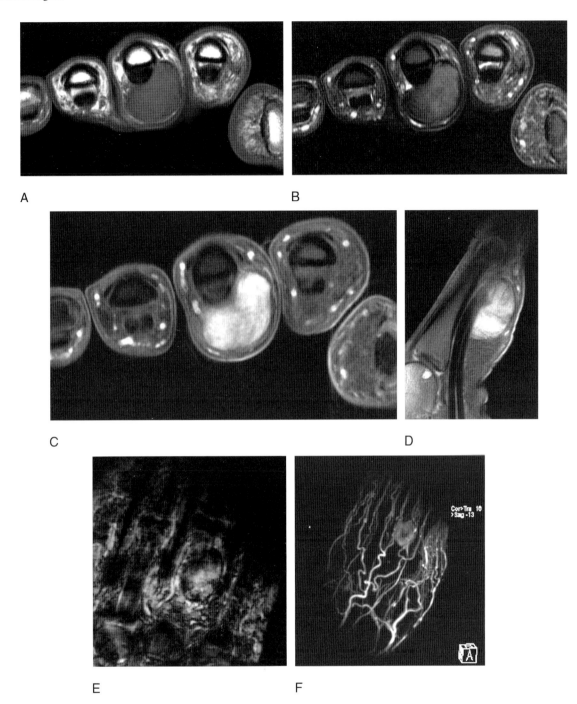

FIG. 8.14. Giant cell tumor of the tendon sheath. MRI of the third finger. (A) Axial T1-weighted. (B) Axial T2 fat saturated. (C,D) Axial and sagittal T1-weighted fat-saturated enhanced images. (E) MR angiography of the hand in arterial phase. Note the central isointensity in T1- and T2-weighted images with a strong enhancement after intravenous contrast injection. Note the peripheral hypointensity corresponding to the hemosiderin deposit. (F) MR angiography confirms the hypervascularization of the tumor.

Magnetic resonance imaging remains an excellent method to evaluate the size of the lesion, its margin, and its relationship with surrounding structures. Magnetic resonance angiography confirms the vascular nature and may reveal the feeding vessels of the lesion.

Glomus Tumors. Glomus bodies are present in the dermis throughout the body, but they are most evident in the digits of the hand and foot.[89,90] They are arteriovenous anastomoses responsible for thermoregulation. They present as afferent artery and tortuous arteriovenous anastomoses collecting veins and a neurovascular system that regulates flow through the anastomoses.[90] The glomus tumors are very small hamartomas of the neuromyoarterial apparatus (<1 cm). They can occur anywhere in the body but most are located in the fingertips, usually beneath the fingernails. Most lesions occur in 30- to 50-year-olds. Clinical diagnosis is often difficult and may be delayed for up to 5 years.[91] Glomus tumors represent about 1.5% to 5% of all hand tumors.[92] The lesions may be painful, often exacerbated by changes in temperature. Detection and accurate localization is critical, as a complete resection is mandatory to relieve symptoms.[93] Radiographs can demonstrate smooth bone erosions.[93] Magnetic resonance imaging and MR angiography have an important role in detecting and characterizing glomus tumors.[92] Lesions are well defined and hypointense on T1 and hyperintense on T2. They reveal homogeneous high enhancement after intravenous gadolinium injection.[90,93] Surgical excision remains the best treatment for glomus tumors. Recurrence is common (5% to 50%).[90] In the postsurgery situation, MRI has proven to be a useful method to differentiate scar tissue from tumor recurrence.[90]

Nerve Tumor. Neurofibromas and schwannomas are rare in the hand and fingers. Multiple neurofibromas can be found in von Recklinghausen's disease. Schwannomas present as a fusiform mass and more commonly affect the ulnar nerves.[1] Benign nerve tumors show isointensity to muscles on T1- and hyperintensity on T2-weighted images.[1] The "split fat" sign is a sign representing the peripheral rim of fat signal intensity surrounding the lesion. The target sign (seen in neurofibromas) is a low central region with high peripheral signal intensity on T2-weighted sequences, corresponding to central fibrosis and surrounding myxomatous tissue.[6]

Soft Tissue Malignant Tumors

Soft tissue sarcomas of the hand are uncommon.[94] Malignant sarcomas show bone erosions and sometimes matrix calcifications on plain films. Magnetic resonance imaging enables the best assessment of tumor extension. Though differentiation between benign and malignant lesions on MRI remains difficult, internal irregularity is the most specific criteria in the diagnosis of a malignant tumor.[73] Sarcomas are typically poorly marginated. They are hypointense on T1- and inhomogeneously hyperintense on T2-weighted sequences. They show irregular enhancement after intravenous gadolinium injection. Necrotic areas, which do not enhance, may be noted. Dynamic MR sequences can help in the diagnosis of sarcomas when the enhancement curve fulfills neoangiogenesis criteria such as early enhancement and washout. Magnetic resonance imaging also remains the best imaging method for the detection of recurrence. Demonstration of local nodules with enhancement after gadolinium injection is the best criterion of local recurrence.

Desmoid tumors are locally aggressive benign lesions. The presence of longitudinal low signal intensity (corresponding to fibrous tissue) within a heterogeneous mass should suggest the diagnosis. The vascularization of desmoid tumor with dynamic MR sequences shows an early strong enhancement as malignant tumors.[95]

Inflammatory Diseases

Magnetic resonance imaging is able to detect bone, cartilage, and soft tissue changes, including synovial inflammation, earlier than can radiographs.[96,97] Early studies also indicate that MRI may be useful for evaluating treatment response, especially in patients with rheumatoid arthritis.[98] A closed approach, with dedicated wrist coils and small fields of view, is essential to provide the needed image quality that provides a global view of the entire spectrum of lesions about the hand and wrist. In our institution, we perform MRI in cases of inflammatory disease with the patient in the supine position with both hands over the head in a knee coil.[97] Conventional T1-weighted sequences provide excellent anatomic detail and can demonstrate early bone erosions. The T2-weighted sequences with fat saturation demonstrate joint effusion and bone marrow edema. T1-weighted sequences with fat saturation and after intravenous injection of gadolinium enable detecting subtle inflammation of the synovial tissues. Contrast-enhanced studies are more accurate at depicting early bone erosions, articular changes, and synovial inflammation than are conventional MRI studies.[99]

Rheumatoid Arthritis

Magnetic resonance imaging has been most commonly employed to evaluate early changes, treatment response, and disease activity in patients with rheumatoid arthritis.[97,99] Magnetic resonance imaging is more sensitive than clinical evaluation for detection of early synovial inflammation.[100] Early detection of rheumatoid changes is important to optimize therapy.[99] Contrast-enhanced MRI demonstrates synovial inflammation, pannus, erosions, and marrow edema before radiographic changes become evident. A recent study demonstrated erosions in 45% of patients with rheumatoid arthritis of less than 4 months' duration. Radiographs demonstrated erosions in only 15%.[101] At the level of the wrist, the capitate and the ulnar side of the radiocarpal joint appeared to be involved early with synovial inflammation. Erosions were evident on MRI in 74% of patients by 1 year.[102] In addition to typical changes seen on radiographs, extensor tendinosis is common in patients with rheumatoid arthritis (50%). Therefore, there is an increased incidence of tendon rupture, which can be easily evaluated using MRI. Magnetic resonance angiography sequences are very useful to show hypervascularization mapping of both hands (Fig. 8.15). Magnetic resonance imaging is also useful for evaluating the response to therapy, measuring active synovial inflammation and pannus volume and defining remission.[103] The dynamic enhancement technique is useful for demonstrating active synovial enhancement and synovial volumes. Patients with active disease have more rapid synovial enhancement and increased synovial tissue and pannus volume. This is well

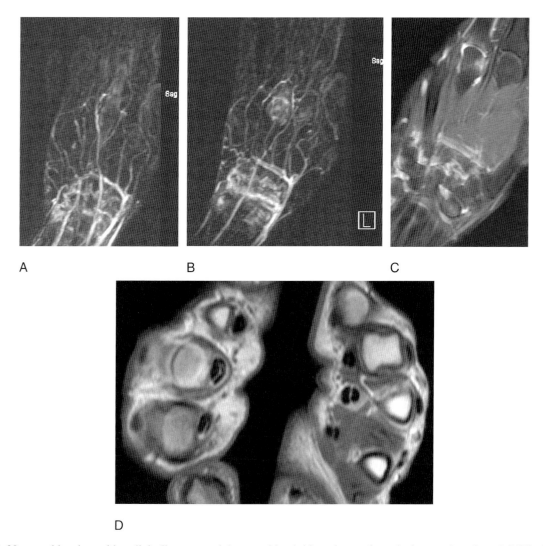

FIG. 8.15. A 29-year-old patient with a clinically suspected rheumatoid arthritis and normal standard x-rays (not shown). MRI of both hands placed over the head of the patient in a knee coil. MR angiography of the left (A) and right (B) hands. Note the hypervascularization at the level of the carpal rows, the tendon sheaths of third left flexor tendon sheath and third right MCP joint. (C) Coronal T1-weighted fat-saturated enhanced image of the right hand shows enhanced synovium of the carpus and the third MCP joint. (D) Axial T1-weighted enhanced image of both hands at the level of the MCP joints shows enhanced synovium and tenosynovium of both third rays. No erosions were noted.

demonstrated at the level of the wrist, but can be applied to the finger MRI studies or global hand studies.[97]

Gout

Clinical evaluation, laboratory data, and, after 6 to 8 years, radiographs, are generally adequate for diagnosis and management of patients with gout. Magnetic resonance imaging is not commonly used. Although changes appear earlier and the extent of disease is more clearly depicted,[104] patients with gout also have an increased incidence of avascular necrosis of carpal bones. Magnetic resonance imaging is the technique of choice for diagnosis and follow-up in patients with avascular necrosis. The osteonecrosis is not described at the level of the fingers. Tophi are typically of intermediate signal intensity on T1-weighted images. On T2-weighted images, the signal intensity may be increased or decreased. The

latter is obviously dependent on the extent of calcifications and fibrosis in this chronic process. Contrast enhancement of tophi is typically uniform or discretely heterogeneous (Fig. 8.16).

Other Arthropathies

The role of MRI in the evaluation of other arthropathies is less clearly defined, although bone and soft tissue changes can be defined earlier with MRI than with radiographs.[105] However, there are few studies of significance compared to those in rheumatoid arthritis. Magnetic resonance imaging has been used to confirm symmetrical synovitis in the wrist in patients with polymyalgia rheumatica. Patients with sausage digit associated with psoriasis and seronegative spondyloarthropathies have also been studied.[105] The primary purpose for MRI in this setting is to evaluate the degree of flexor tendon involvement.

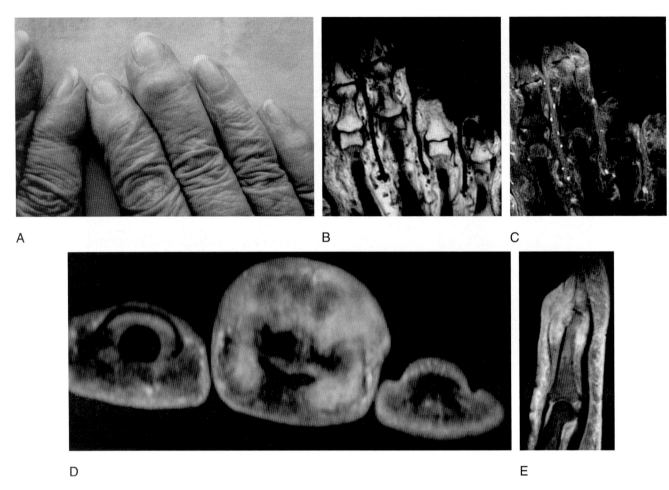

FIG. 8.16. A 68-year-old patient with a gout. (A) Clinical appearance of the DIP joints. Coronal T1-weighted (B), coronal (C), axial (D), and sagittal (E) T1-weighted fat-saturated enhanced images. Note the intermediate signal intensity of the tophi on the T1-weighted images. There is a strong heterogeneous enhancement around the tophus on enhanced images. Enhancement is dependent on the extent of calcifications and fibrosis in this chronic process.

Also, MRI is useful to determine the extent of involvement in patients with myositis and periarticular soft tissue changes in other connective tissue disorders.

Infections

As in the wrist, infection in the hand and fingers may involve the soft tissues (muscles, cutaneous, and subcutaneous tissues, tendon sheaths, fascia, and nail beds), bones, and joints. Infections may be isolated or involve multiple sites. Onset may be acute (pain, swelling, and erythema) or insidious, depending on the organism and the clinical setting.[106] It can result from hematogenous spread, spread from a contiguous site, or direct implantation (puncture wound or bite), or it may occur secondary to previous surgery.[107] Bone, joints, and soft tissue infections may all occur via these routes. However, most soft tissue infections are related to trauma, specifically puncture wounds and skin disorders. Hematogenous spread to the soft tissues of the hand and wrist occurs less frequently. The site of involvement varies with the source of contamination. Patients with trauma surgery, in which spread occurs from a contiguous site,

will have infection involving the adjacent bone, joint, or soft tissue. In the hand, infection may spread along the fasciae, tendon sheaths, or lymphatics. Hematogenous osteomyelitis may involve different sites, depending on the patient age, clinical conditions, and organisms involved. In infants (0 to 1 year of age), the metaphyseal vessels may penetrate the growth plate. In children (1 to 16 years of age), the vessels do not penetrate the growth plate. In adults, with the growth plate closed, the vessels penetrate the closed physis.[107] Therefore, the epiphysis may be involved in infants and adults, which results in the joint space being involved more frequently. In children, the metaphysis is most commonly involved without extension to the epiphysis. The joint space is therefore affected less frequently, depending on the location of the capsular attachment.

Early diagnosis and treatment of osseous infection is essential to avoid irreversible bone and soft tissue loss. Imaging plays an important role in patient management. Routine radiographs should be obtained initially in patients with suspected osteomyelitis. Radiographic changes may be nonspecific in the early stages. Localized soft tissue swelling and distortion of soft tissue or fat planes may be the only findings. Bone changes are

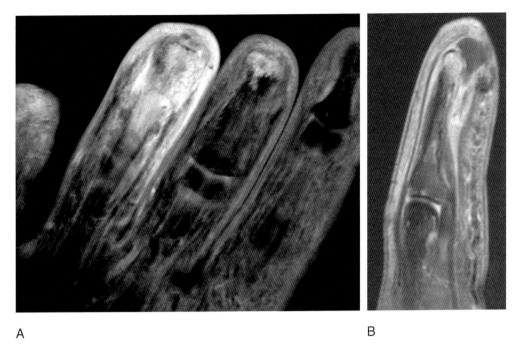

A   B

FIG 8.17. Osteomyelitis and an abscess of the tip of the finger. Coronal T2-weighted fat saturated (A) and sagittal T1-weighted fat saturated (B) enhanced images. Note the hypersignal intensity of the distal phalanx and the collection at the tip of the finger. There is soft tissue involvement around the distal phalanx. (From Theumann et al.,[11] with permission).

typically found in the metaphyseal regions of the tubular bones. However, bone destruction is typically not appreciated until 30% to 40% of the involved region is destroyed. This may take 10 to 14 days to be detected on radiographs.[108] Therefore, the extent of bone and soft tissue involvement is frequently underestimated on radiographs. Computed tomography and radioisotope studies can provide important information, but MRI is particularly suited to evaluate osteomyelitis due to superior tissue contrast and multiple image plane capabilities. Anatomic detail is superior to that of radionucleic studies, and subtle bone and soft tissue changes are more easily appreciated in comparison with CT. As noted earlier, CT may be superior for evaluation of thin cortical bone and sequestra.[107]

T1-weighted sequences offer excellent anatomic details and provide excellent contrast between the high signal intensity fatty marrow and low signal intensity areas of infection. Fat saturated T2-weighted sequences demonstrate areas of infection as high signal intensity compared with the suppressed signal of marrow fat, low signal cortical bone, and intermediate muscle intensity.[109] Magnetic resonance imaging with intravenous injection of gadolinium is also very useful and showed a high sensitivity (100% compared to 69% for isotope studies) for distinguishing bone and soft tissue involvement.[110] The gadolinium-enhanced images are very sensitive and provide high confidence for detection of bone and soft tissue changes (Fig. 8.17). However, other inflammatory or neoplastic changes may create similar abnormalities. Biopsy and aspiration may still be required to isolate the offending organism.[107] Lack of enhancement with gadolinium effectively excludes infection. Abscesses may appear later in the disease.

Typical MRI features are an area of isosignal intensity in T1 with peripheral enhancement, and the center appears heterogenously hyperintense in T2 sequences.

Infective Arthritis

Infectious arthritis is generally monoarticular in the hand but typically extends from one compartment to another at the level of the wrist.[106] Monoarticular involvement in the hand is useful in differentiating infections from other inflammatory arthropathies. Early detection is essential to prevent cartilage and bone loss with resulting deformities and loss of joint function. The role of MRI in evaluating joint space infections is becoming more clearly defined. Early bone and soft tissue changes and joint fluid are easily defined.[110] Bone erosions and cartilage loss can also be detected with MRI. However, even with intravenous gadolinium enhancement, the changes may not differentiate infections from other inflammatory arthropathies. Isolated joint involvement may still be the most useful feature.[107,111] Common features are joint effusions, synovial thickening, bone erosions, marrow edema, and synovial enhancement after intravenous gadolinium. Bony erosions and marrow edema are the most useful features supporting infection but are not specific.[112]

Acknowledgments. I thank my secretary, Mrs. F. Hermenjat for her work on this manuscript; our MRI technologist, Mrs. S. Behzad, for her efficiency in performing examinations of fingers; and my colleague Dr. D. Guntern, for reading the manuscript.

B. Orthopedic Perspective: Hand Injuries

Matthew Meunier

Mallet Finger

Mallet finger is one of the injuries commonly described as "jammed finger." The specific mechanism of injury is forced hyperflexion of the DIP joint. The anatomy of the injury is the loss of the insertion of the terminal tendon into the dorsal aspect of the distal phalanx. Sometimes patients have pain with palpation at the base of the distal phalanx. Extensor lag or "drooping" finger is the definitive exam finding. A secondary swan-neck deformity may develop due to the subsequent concentration of extension forces at the PIP joint following the disruption of the terminal tendon insertion. Radiographs are needed for diagnosis, mostly to evaluate for possible fracture. Usually these films show normal bony anatomy with flexion at the DIP joint. Occasionally radiographs show a fracture of either the base of the distal phalanx or shaft of the distal phalanx. In addition, the DIP joint can either subluxate or even dislocate (Figs. 8.18 and 8.19).

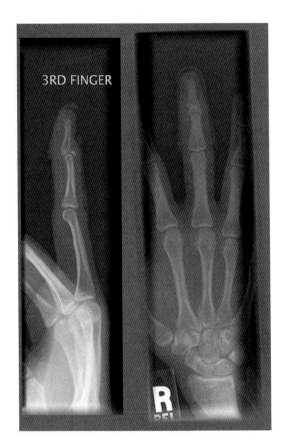

FIG. 8.19. Bony mallet finger of the long finger.

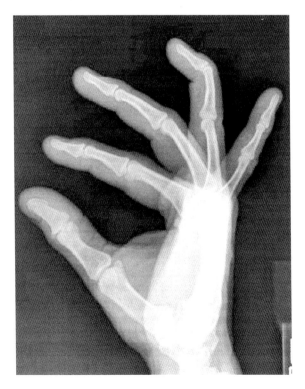

FIG. 8.18. Soft tissue mallet finger of the ring finger.

Mallet finger injuries are evident from the DIP flexion deformity and positive radiographs and do not require further workup. The treatment is a minimum of 6 weeks of extension splinting at the DIP and can usually be accomplished with a removable splint. There are numerous options including dorsal or volar foam-coated aluminum or orthoplast splints as well as pre-made plastic sheaths for the DIP joint.[113] Occasionally percuataneous pinning of the DIP joint is performed.[114] In cases in which a fracture is present there is some debate about the appropriate treatment. Closed splinting is usually successful in cases in which there is less than 50% involvement of the joint surface and in which there is no subluxation of the joint.[115] In cases in which either of these two deformities are present, surgical correction can be performed, and reduction and pinning of both the joint surface as well as the DIP joint are often required. If left untreated, the forces of the extensor mechanism are now concentrated at the PIP joint and can ultimately lead to a "swan-neck" deformity or hyperextension at this joint.

Flexor Digitorum Profundus Avulsion

Avulsion of the flexor digitorum profundus (FDP) tendon occurs when the patient attempts to grip against an eccentric load, such as attempting to hold an opposing player's jersey as he is running away. The injury is seen in football and rugby players most commonly, but any sport in which grip against an eccentric load is required, such as rock climbing, can generate this injury. The injury occurs most commonly in the ring finger (75%).[116] Patients usually present with pain and swelling in the flexor sheath, ecchymosis, and an inability to flex the DIP joint. The proximal portion of the FDP tendon can often be localized to a painful mass either at the midportion of the middle phalanx (the chiasma of the flexor superficialis or distal edge of the A4 pulley), the distal edge of the A2 pulley, or in the palm. Anatomically the injury is usually an avulsion of the FDP tendon from the bony insertion and may even include part of the distal phalanx. Failure of the tendon may also occur in the tendon substance itself. Leddy and Packer[116] classified the injury and radiographs that are required for the classification. Type I injuries retract into the palm, type II to the PIP joint, and type III to the level of the A4 pulley. Retraction is limited by an impinging bony fragment, the vinculae, or the lumbrical muscle, and although the tendon may curl up on itself, it rarely retracts beyond the mid-palm. Physical exam and radiographs are again usually all that is required for diagnosis and classification. Occasionally fracture of the middle phalanx is present and represents an additional injury rather than part of the mechanism of the profundus avulsion. Magnetic resonance imaging is rarely indicated, although occasionally a pulley rupture may also be present and MRI can help with this diagnosis. The treatment is reinsertion of the flexor digitorum profundus tendon. If the rupture is either from bone, or within less than 1 cm from the bony insertion, the bone edge is freshened and the tendon is reinserted. Current suture anchor designs are not sufficient for fixation for the postoperative rehabilitation,[117] and so the most common technique is tying the repair sutures over a dorsal button that is removed at 6 weeks. If the rupture is more than 1 cm from the bony insertion, advancement will lead to the quadregia effect, and primary repair of the tendon is advocated. The goal of any tendon repair is to achieve a repair of sufficient strength to allow dynamic postoperative therapy. The outcome from these injuries is often worse than from a simple laceration due to the associated hematoma and ecchymosis with resultant scarring. They often require a subsequent tenolysis.

Pulley Ruptures

Occasionally a patient presents with pain and swelling over the proximal or middle phalanx of the finger following a con-

traction against a load, such as with rock climbing. Patients often hear or feel a pop with loss of flexion of the DIP joint and occasionally loss of extension at the PIP joint. Blocking of the middle phalanx in extension will allow DIP motion, in contrast to avulsions of the FDP tendon in which there will be a lack of DIP joint flexion, even with blocking. Clinically the diagnosis is closed pulley rupture. Ruptures of the A2, A3, and A4 pulleys are described. Diagnosis is suspected on clinical grounds. Magnetic resonance imaging is quite useful for confirming the diagnosis. The pulleys themselves do not enhance well; however, the tendon can be seen separated from the underlying phalanx, particularly if the digit is in flexion (Fig. 8.20). Ruptures are classified into four grades: grade I is a strain of the pulley, grade II is a complete rupture of the A4 or partial rupture of the A4, grade III is a single rupture of the A4, and grade IV is a rupture of A4 combined with another pulley. The treatment for grades I through III is often protection of the pulley with a ring splint and gentle mobilization. The treatment for grade IV ruptures and failed closed treatment of the lesser grades is reconstruction of the pulley with a graft, usually derived from either the palmaris longus or the extensor retinaculum and a rehabilitation

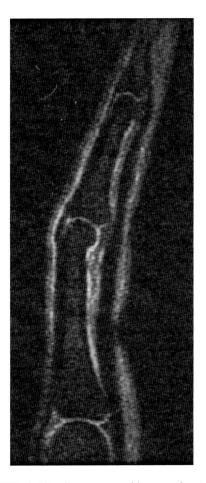

FIG. 8.20. MRI of A2 pulley rupture with separation of the flexor tendon from the proximal phalanx.

program to enhance tendon gliding.[118] Simple pulley repair is rarely effective.

Central Slip Injury, Fracture, or Soft Tissue Trauma

Another of the injuries in the "jammed finger" spectrum is a hyperflexion of the middle phalanx against an extension load. This can result in pain at the dorsal aspect of the PIP joint and a loss of extension at this joint. The classic exam finding is a positive Elson test, with the appearance of active DIP joint extension when the PIP joint is held in flexion.[119] This is due to the loss of the tethering effect that the central slip has on the lateral bands.[120] Radiographs are required, preferably prior to examination, as nondisplaced fractures can be displaced through active motion. In addition, joint subluxation does occasionally occur with this injury and is frequently treated inadequately with simple immobilization. Evaluation of the injury is mostly clinical, with conventional radiographs; however, in some cases MRI can be helpful. For cases with a purely soft tissue injury, immobilization of the PIP joint in extension, with active DIP joint flexion will allow the lateral bands to maintain their normal position and also allow the central slip to stay reduced distally. If there is a large bony fragment, or if the joint is subluxated, then surgical repair with fixation of the fracture, reduction of the joint, and repair of the central slip is indicated (Fig. 8.21). In these cases pinning of the joint for 6 weeks replaces the PIP joint splint. Distal interphalangeal joint motion should continue during this time. If this injury is untreated, or missed, the triangular ligament will ultimately stretch, and the lateral bands will remain subluxated volar to the axis of rotation for the PIP joint. At this point attempted extension at the PIP joint will actually result in flexion at the interphalangeal joint with hyperextension at the DIP joint, creating the boutonniere deformity. If caught early

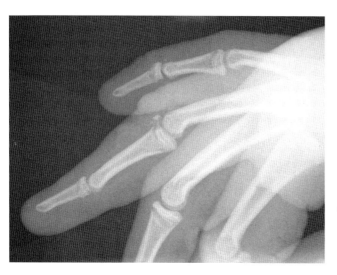

FIG. 8.21. Avulsion fracture of the central slip, with concomitant subluxation of the PIP joint.

and when the deformity is still flexible, extension splinting for the PIP joint with active DIP joint flexion is the preferred treatment. Once a fixed deformity is present, reconstruction is difficult and does not often lead to satisfactory results.[121]

Proximal Interphalangeal Joint Sprain or Dislocation

A common injury, particularly in contact sports, is dislocation or sprain of the interphalangeal joints. Simple dislocations are usually obvious, even without conventional radiographs, and are often treated directly, either by the patients themselves or associated staff on the field. Subsequent evaluation is necessary to determine the presence or absence of associated fractures as well as the adequacy of reduction. Although the collateral ligaments are by definition torn, these injuries are usually stable following reduction, and treatment is aimed at recovery of motion. Irreducible dislocations are also quite evident clinically and usually indicate interposed tissue. Irreducible dislocations require operative reduction and removal of interposed material. Following a successful reduction, protected motion is the treatment of choice. Typically the finger is kept blocked at 30 degrees of flexion for 1 to 2 weeks while the patient tries to regain full flexion. After this initial period of immobilization, extension is advanced by 10 degrees a week until full extension is achieved. If the finger is stable in extension, our preferred treatment is to forgo the period of immobilization and progress directly to protected motion to limit the risk of subsequent stiffness. If this is the case, hyperextension is to be avoided, as this is often the unstable position. In addition, some patients are unstable in even the neutral position of the interphalangeal joint and require immobilization in 30 to 45 degrees of flexion to achieve a stable reduction.

Sprains of the interphalangeal joints are also quite common and encompass injuries to the collateral ligament and to the volar plate. Collateral ligament injuries represent either a varus or valgus load, and volar plate injuries are usually due to hyperextension of the PIP joint. Volar plate injuries may be purely soft tissue or may have a small avulsion fracture from the base of the middle phalanx (Fig. 8.22). This represents the insertion of the volar plate and serves as a marker for the soft tissue injury. Most sprains heal with gentle range of motion; however, the joint can frequently remain swollen for 3 months or more.[122] Gross instability in either direction is not likely to heal and so if the joint remains subluxated or angulated on plain films, then repair of the ligament with pinning of the joint is usually required. Of note, conventional films should be evaluated carefully in these injuries as impaction fractures of the base of the middle phalanx can often be missed (Fig. 8.23). If a fracture is present, then surgical treatment with elevation of the joint surface is required. Late reconstruction of these fractures is difficult and often unsatisfactory. The PIP joint, like the elbow, tends to get stiff in flexion, and so with

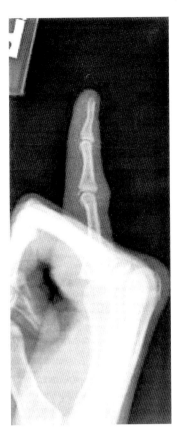

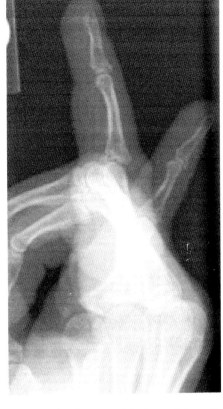

FIG. 8.22. A small bony fleck from the palmar aspect of the middle phalanx, representing an avulsion injury related to the volar plate of the PIP joint.

FIG. 8.23. An impaction fracture of the base of the middle phalanx with subluxation of the middle phalanx dorsally. This injury can be thought of as similar to the tibial plateau fracture.

a volar plate injury the goal is to both preserve flexion and regain extension.

If a sprain does not heal, the PIP joint will remain unstable to a varus or valgus load.[123] Exam findings are usually a painful soft endpoint to loading rather than gross instability. Stability should be checked in slight flexion to decrease the stabilizing force of the joint morphology. Magnetic resonance imaging can be helpful in determining the condition of the collateral ligament. Even with instability, surgical treatment is rarely required; however, if primary repair seems feasible, this is preferred; otherwise graft reconstruction of the collateral ligament is required.

Digital Fractures

Fractures are common injuries in athletes' hands, particularly in athletes involved in contact sports; note that this chapter is not a definitive survey of digital fractures. Fractures may also be a component of many sports injuries in the hands and may complicate the treatment of some injuries. Mallet fingers, volar plate injuries, and sprains can often have an associated small avulsion fracture at the level of the base of the middle or distal phalanx. Distal phalanx fractures are usually tuft inju-

ries and represent a crush injury to the tip of the finger. They are sometimes associated with nailbed injuries, and removal of the nailplate and repair of the nailbed is sometimes needed. While the nailbed is often repaired promptly, these fractures are rarely treated surgically in the acute setting. Occasionally they remain symptomatic and are treated with excision of the fragment.

Transverse fractures of the distal phalanx are also often associated with nailbed injuries and not infrequently are open injuries with avulsion of the nail plate from its proximal attachment. These need to be treated with operative irrigation and debridement and reduction of the phalanx and nail bed repair (Fig. 8.24). Mallet fractures have been discussed earlier, and again, the stability of the joint and the reduction of the dorsal fragment are the important parameters.

Middle and proximal phalanx fractures can range from intraarticular injuries of the head of the phalanx to shaft fractures to avulsion injuries at the collateral ligament insertion (Fig. 8.25). As with any long bone fracture, joint integrity and mechanical alignment are of paramount importance. In the fingers the extensor tendons can accommodate approximately 3 mm of bony shortening before their function is affected.[124] Diaphyseal fractures are often unstable with attempted closed treatment, and operative fixation allows for both definitive

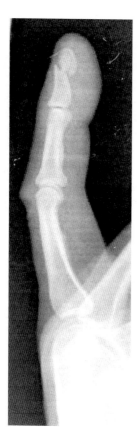

FIG. 8.24. Transverse fracture of the distal phalanx. This injury also has an injury to the sterile matrix of the nailbed, and requires operative treatment.

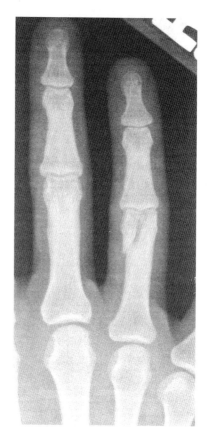

FIG. 8.25. Intraarticular fracture of the head of the proximal phlanx.

reduction and early mobilization. One particularly difficult fracture is at the base of the proximal phalanx. The fracture is often intraarticular and often creates an apex volar angulation deformity. Surgical treatment of these injuries is challenging because there is often very little bone stock for fixation and the joint itself gets stiff following surgery. In addition, rotation is a key parameter in finger injuries, and this cannot be adequately assessed purely on radiographs with a thorough clinical examination also required. One quick examination tool to assess rotational deformity is to have the patient make bilateral gentle fists and compare finger overlap to that on the noninjured side. Rotation of approximately 5 degrees in the metacarpal leads to a 5-mm overlap of the injured finger on the neighboring nail plate.[125] Metacarpal fractures also represent a challenge with regard to assessing rotation and need to be evaluated clinically as well as radiographically. Shortening of simple fractures with acceptable alignment tends to be limited by the transverse metacarpal ligament and can often be treated closed. Fractures with a rotational malalignment or with a significant angulation at the fracture should be operatively reduced and stabilized. As with any fracture, the goal of treatment is to achieve a stable reduction with restoration of articular congruity and mechanical alignment to allow a return to full mobility and function. One advantage of surgical

fixation is an earlier return to motion. Diagnosis is usually easily made with conventional radiographs.

Metacarpophalangeal Joint Sprains and Dislocations

Sprains and dislocations of the MCP joints are common sports injuries, with the injury of the ulnar collateral of the thumb MCP joint (gamekeeper's or skier's thumb) the most common. The true gamekeeper's thumb is an attritional rupture of the ulnar collateral ligament. Patients often complain of pain at the ulnar aspect of the thumb MCP joint along with weakness, particularly when attempting to pick up large heavy objects with the affected hand. Skier's thumb is an acute disruption of the same ligament at its insertion. As the thumb dislocates radially, the adductor hood is brought distally and volarly due its attachment to the base of the proximal phalanx. The ulnar collateral ligament ruptures from the phalangeal base as the thumb dislocates and its reduction to the base of the proximal phalanx is prevented by the adductor hood as the thumb reduces. Acute presentations often show considerable laxity with no endpoint to valgus testing, but delayed presentation may not be as clear and a soft end-point may be noted.

The classic lesion noted on exam is the Stener lesion, a palpable mass over the ulnar aspect of the MCP joint, which represents the displaced end of the ulnar collateral ligament. In these cases MRI is not often required; however, in delayed presentations or those with an equivocal exam, it can be quite helpful in defining the injury. Testing in both full extension and 30 degrees of flexion has been recommended, and stress films in these positions are advocated. An increase in laxity to greater than 30 degrees of valgus instability or an increase of 15 degrees compared to the opposite side is consistent with complete rupture, and the Stener lesion is present approximately 80% of the time.[126] In cases in which the clinical exam is somewhat equivocal, MRI can be a useful adjunct to diagnosis, particularly if there is a possibility of nonoperative treatment. Complete ruptures rarely heal well without surgical intervention, particularly in the case of the Stener lesion, which represents the displaced stump of the ulnar collateral ligament. The ideal situation allows for secure repair of the ligament to the volar plate and distal insertion of the ligament. In delayed cases there is poorly defined ligamentous tissue and reconstruction may be required. Following repair or reconstruction, immobilization for approximately 6 weeks in a thumb spica cast is standard to allow for soft tissue healing before motion is started.

Other digits will also sustain collateral ligament injuries, particularly the ulnar aspect of the index finger, both the radial and ulnar sides of the long finger, and the radial aspect of the small finger. The mechanism is usually a sudden valgus moment. Evaluation is similar to thumb injuries with an increase in laxity of more than approximately 15 degrees compared to the opposite side strongly suggestive of a complete rupture. Radiographs are useful to evaluate for fractures, and in equivocal cases MRI can be quite beneficial in diagnosing complete ruptures. Commonly the collateral ligament is avulsed from its origin rather than its insertion in contrast to the presentation in the thumb. Treatment with buddy taping and avoidance of valgus stress to the joint is often successful; however, some patients require operative stabilization. Following repair, immobilization is often required for approximately 6 weeks, although particularly compliant patients can be started on early protected motion.

Rarely, the MCP joint dislocates completely and shows the characteristic deformity on exam. These are almost always limited to border digits, with the thumb, index, and small finger MCP joints being by far the most frequent. If initial attempts at closed reduction, usually undertaken on the playing field, are unsuccessful, radiography is required. These injuries can frequently be irreducible. The head of the metacarpal is trapped between the lumbrical radially, the flexor tendon ulnarly, the palmar fascia proximally, and the natatory ligament distally.[127] In addition, the volar plate is entrapped within the joint, further preventing reduction of the joint. Continued traction and manipulation will be unsuccessful and operative reduction is required. Both dorsal and palmar incisions are described; however, a thorough knowledge of the anatomy is essential for a successful outcome.[128]

References

1. Anderson MW, Kaplan PA, Dussault RG, Degnan GG. Magnetic resonance imaging of the wrist. Curr Probl Diagn Radiol 1998;27(6):187–229.
2. Berquist TH, Kimberly K. Magnetic resonance imaging techniques. In: Berquist TH, ed. MRI of the hand and wrist. Philadelphia: Lippincott Williams & Wilkins, 2003:33–44.
3. Girgis WS, Epstein RE. Magnetic resonance imaging of the hand and wrist. Semin Roentgenol 2000;35(3):286–96.
4. Lee VS, Lee HM, Rofsky NM. Magnetic resonance angiography of the hand. A review. Invest Radiol 1998;33(9):687–98.
5. Hobby JL, Dixon AK, Bearcroft PW, et al. MR imaging of the wrist: effect on clinical diagnosis and patient care. Radiology 2001;220(3):589–93.
6. Berquist TH. MRI of the musculoskeletal system, 4th ed. In. Philadelphia: Lippincott Williams & Wilkins, 2001.
7. Winterer JT, Scheffler K, Paul G, et al. Optimization of contrast-enhanced MR angiography of the hands with a timing bolus and elliptically reordered 3D pulse sequence. J Comput Assist Tomogr 2000;24(6):903–8.
8. Theumann NH, Pfirrmann CW, Drape JL, Trudell DJ, Resnick DI. MR imaging of the metacarpophalangeal joints of the fingers: part I. Conventional MR imaging and MR arthrographic findings in cadavers. Radiology 2002;222(2):437–45
9. Connell DA, Koulouris G, Thorn DA, Potter HG. Contrast-enhanced MR angiography of the hand. Radiographics 2002;22(3):583–99.
10. Connell DA, Pike J, Koulouris G, van Wettering N, Hoy G. MR imaging of thumb carpometacarpal joint ligament injuries. J Hand Surg [Br] 2004;29(1):46–54.
11. Theumann NH, Pfirrmann CW, Chung CB, Antonio GE, Trudell DJ, Resnick D. Ligamentous and tendinous anatomy of the inter-metacarpal and common carpometacarpal joints: evaluation with MR imaging and MR arthrography. J Comput Assist Tomogr 2002;26(1):145–52.
12. Lamb DW, Angarita G. Ulnar instability of the metacarpophalangeal joint of thumb. J Hand Surg [Br] 1985;10(1):113–4.
13. Minami A, An KN, Cooney WP, 3rd, Linscheid RL, Chao EY. Ligament stability of the metacarpophalangeal joint: a biomechanical study. J Hand Surg [Am] 1985;10(2):255–60.
14. Smith RJ, Peimer CA. Injuries to the metacarpal bones and joints. Adv Surg 1977;11:341–74.
15. Kraemer BA, Gilula LA. Anatomy affecting the metacarpal and phalangeal bones of the hand. In: Gillula L, ed. The traumatized Hand and Wrist: Radiographic and Anatomic Correlation. Philadelphia: WB Saunders, 1992:65–100.
16. Dubousset JF. Finger rotation during prehension. In: Tubiana R, ed. The Hand, vol 1. Philadelphia: WB Saunders, 1981:202.
17. Craig SM. Anatomy of the joints of the fingers. Hand Clin 1992;8(4):693–700.
18. Idler RS. Anatomy and biomechanics of the digital flexor tendons. Hand Clin 1985;1(1):3–11.
19. Lin GT, Amadio PC, An KN, Cooney WP. Functional anatomy of the human digital flexor pulley system. J Hand Surg [Am] 1989;14(6):949–56.

20. Hauger O, Chung CB, Lektrakul N, et al. Pulley system in the fingers: normal anatomy and simulated lesions in cadavers at MR imaging, CT, and US with and without contrast material distention of the tendon sheath. Radiology 2000;217(1):201–12.

21. Marco RA, Sharkey NA, Smith TS, Zissimos AG. Pathomechanics of closed rupture of the flexor tendon pulleys in rock climbers. J Bone Joint Surg [Am] 1998;80(7):1012–9.

22. Lin GT, Cooney WP, Amadio PC, An KN. Mechanical properties of human pulleys. J Hand Surg [Br] 1990;15(4):429–34.

23. Cooney WP. Vascular neurologic anatomy of the wrist. In: Cooney W, Linchaid R, Dobyns J, eds. The Wrist: Diagnosis and Operative Treatment. St. Louis: Mosby, 1998:106–23.

24. Maurer J, Bleschkowski A, Tempka A, Felix R. High-resolution MR imaging of the carpal tunnel and the wrist. Application of a 5-cm surface coil. Acta Radiol 2000;41(1):78–83.

25. Strauch B, de Moura W. Digital flexor tendon sheath: an anatomic study. J Hand Surg [Am] 1985;10(6 pt 1):785–9.

26. Mestdagh H, Bailleul JP, Vilette B, Bocquet F, Depreux R. Organization of the extensor complex of the digits. Anat Clin 1985;7(1):49–53.

27. Clavero JA, Golano P, Farinas O, Alomar X, Monill JM, Esplugas M. Extensor mechanism of the fingers: MR imaging-anatomic correlation. Radiographics 2003;23(3):593–611.

28. von Schroeder HP, Botte MJ. Functional anatomy of the extensor tendons of the digits. Hand Clin 1997;13(1):51–62.

29. Zancolli E, Cozzi EP. Extensor apparatus of the digit. In: Zancolli E, ed. Atlas of surgical anatomy of the hand. New York: Churchill Livingstone, 1992:147–216.

30. Beltran J, Noto AM, Herman LJ, Lubbers LM. Tendons: high-field-strength, surface coil MR imaging. Radiology 1987;162(3):735–40.

31. Erickson SJ, Cox IH, Hyde JS, Carrera GF, Strandt JA, Estkowski LD. Effect of tendon orientation on MR imaging signal intensity: a manifestation of the "magic angle" phenomenon. Radiology 1991;181(2):389–92.

32. Drape JL, Tardif-Chastenet de Gery S, Silbermann-Hoffman O, et al. Closed ruptures of the flexor digitorum tendons: MRI evaluation. Skeletal Radiol 1998;27(11):617–24.

33. Timins ME, O'Connell SE, Erickson SJ, Oneson SR. MR imaging of the wrist: normal findings that may simulate disease. Radiographics 1996;16(5):987–95.

34. Bencardino JT. MR imaging of tendon lesions of the hand and wrist. Magn Reson Imaging Clin North Am 2004;12(2):333–47, vii.

35. Bloom M, Stern PJ. Carpo-metacarpal joints of the fingers, their dislocation or fracture dislocation. Orthopedic Rev 1983;12:77–82.

36. Strauch RJ, Behrman MJ, Rosenwasser MP. Acute dislocation of the carpometacarpal joint of the thumb: an anatomic and cadaver study. J Hand Surg [Am] 1994;19(1):93–8.

37. Diao E, Lineticum ND. Game-keeper thumb. Curr Opin Orthop 1996;7:10.

38. Boyes JH. Bunnel's Surgery of the Hand, 5th ed. Philadelphia: Lippincott Williams & Wilkins, 1970.

39. Posner MA, Retaillaud JL. Metacarpophalangeal joint injuries of the thumb. Hand Clin 1992;8(4):713–32.

40. Dray J, Eaton R. Dislocation and ligament injuries in the digit. In: Green D, ed. Operative Hand Surgery. New York: Churchill-Livingstone, 1993:767.

41. Stener B. Displacement of rupture in a collateral ligament of the metacarpophalangeal joints of the thumb. J Bone Joint Surg [Br] 1962;44:879.

42. Lohman M, Vasenius J, Kivisaari A, Kivisaari L. MR imaging in chronic rupture of the ulnar collateral ligament of the thumb. Acta Radiol 2001;42(1):10–4.

43. Helm RH. Hand function after injuries to the collateral ligaments of the metacarpophalangeal joint of the thumb. J Hand Surg [Br] 1987;12(2):252–5.

44. Haramati N, Hiller N, Dowdle J, et al. MRI of the Stener lesion. Skeletal Radiol 1995;24(7):515–8.

45. Riederer S, Nagy L, Buchler U. Chronic post-traumatic radial instability of the metacarpophalangeal joint of the finger. Long-term results of ligament reconstruction. J Hand Surg [Br] 1998;23(4):503–6.

46. Schubiner JM, Mass DP. Operation for collateral ligament ruptures of the metacarpophalangeal joints of the fingers. J Bone Joint Surg [Br] 1989;71(3):388–9.

47. Theumann NH, Pessis E, Lecompte M, et al. MR imaging of the metacarpophalangeal joints of the fingers: evaluation of 38 patients with chronic joint disability. Skeletal Radiol 2005;34(4):210–6.

48. Zemel NP. Metacarpophalangeal joint injuries in fingers. Hand Clin 1992;8(4):745–54.

49. Gilbert A. Palmar fibrocartilage lesions. In: Brüser P, Gilbert A, eds. Finger Bone and Joint Injuries. London: Martin Dunitz, 1999:241–4.

50. Jozsa L, Balint BJ, Reffy A, Demel Z. Hypoxic alterations of tenocytes in degenerative tendinopathy. Arch Orthop Trauma Surg 1982;99(4):243–6.

51. Boyes JH, Stark HH. Flexor-tendon grafts in the fingers and thumb. A study of factors influencing results in 1000 cases. J Bone Joint Surg [Am] 1971;53(7):1332–42.

52. Minamikawa Y, Peimer CA, Yamaguchi T, Banasiak NA, Kambe K, Sherwin FS. Wrist position and extensor tendon amplitude following repair. J Hand Surg [Am] 1992;17(2):268–71.

53. Rockwell WB, Butler PN, Byrne BA. Extensor tendon: anatomy, injury, and reconstruction. Plast Reconstr Surg 2000;106(7):1592–603; quiz 1604, 1673.

54. Massengill JB. The boutonniere deformity. Hand Clin 1992;8(4):787–801.

55. Aronowitz ER, Leddy JP. Closed tendon injuries of the hand and wrist in athletes. Clin Sports Med 1998;17(3):449–67.

56. Logan AJ, Makwana N, Mason G, Dias J. Acute hand and wrist injuries in experienced rock climbers. Br J Sports Med 2004;38(5):545–8.

57. Bollen SR, Gunson CK. Hand injuries in competition climbers. Br J Sports Med 1990;24(1):16–8.

58. Rohrbough JT, Mudge MK, Schilling RC. Overuse injuries in the elite rock climber. Med Sci Sports Exerc 2000;32(8):1369–72.

59. Martinoli C, Bianchi S, Cotten A. Imaging of rock climbing injuries. Semin Musculoskelet Radiol 2005;9(4):334–45.

60. Seiler JG 3rd, Leversedge FJ. Digital flexor sheath: repair and reconstruction of the annular pulleys and membranous sheath. J South Orthop Assoc 2000;9(2):81–90.

61. Klauser A, Frauscher F, Bodner G, et al. Finger pulley injuries in extreme rock climbers: depiction with dynamic US. Radiology 2002;222(3):755–61.

62. Martinoli C, Bianchi S, Nebiolo M, Derchi LE, Garcia JF. Sonographic evaluation of digital annular pulley tears. Skeletal Radiol 2000;29(7):387–91.

63. Gabl M, Rangger C, Lutz M, Fink C, Rudisch A, Pechlaner S. Disruption of the finger flexor pulley system in elite rock climbers. Am J Sports Med 1998;26(5):651–5.

64. Butler E, Hamell J, Seipel R, et al. Tumors of the hand. A 10-year survey and report of 437 cases. Am J Surg 1960;100:293–302.

65. Theumann N, Drape JL. Imaging of tumors and tumor-like lesions of the hand and fingers. In: Egloff DV; Federation of European Societies for Surgery of the Hand. London and New York: Taylor & Francis, 2004:15–26.

66. Alam F, Schweitzer ME, Li XX, Malat J, Hussain SM. Frequency and spectrum of abnormalities in the bone marrow of the wrist: MR imaging findings. Skeletal Radiol 1999;28(6):312–7.

67. Campanacci M. Bone and Soft Tissue Tumors. New York: Springer-Verlag, 1999.

68. Dahlin D, Unni K. Bone Tumors: General Aspect and Data on 8542 Cases, 4th ed. Springfield, IL: Charles C Thomas, 1986.

69. McCullough C, Thomine J-M. Tumeurs osseuses de la main. In: Tubiana R, ed. Chirurgie de la Main. Paris: Masson, 1995:732–52.

70. Wilner D. Radiology of Bone Tumors and Allied Disorders. Philadelphia: WB Saunders, 1982.

71. Bogumill G. Tumors of the wrist. In: Lichtmann D, ed. The Wrist and Its Disorders. Philadelphia: WB Saunders, 1988:373–84.

72. Garcia J, Bianchi S. Diagnostic imaging of tumors of the hand and wrist. Eur Radiol 2001;11(8):1470–82.

73. Manaster BJ, Doyle AJ. Giant cell tumors of bone. Radiol Clin North Am 1993;31(2):299–323.

74. Aoki J, Tanikawa H, Ishii K, et al. MR findings indicative of hemosiderin in giant-cell tumor of bone: frequency, cause, and diagnostic significance. AJR Am J Roentgenol 1996;166(1):145–8.

75. Fuhr S, Herndon J. Aneurysmal bone cyst involving the hand. A review and report of two cases. J Hand Surg [Am] 1979;4:152–9.

76. Hudson T. Fluid-fluid levels in aneurysmal bone cysts. A CT feature. AJR 1984;141:1001–4.

77. Tanaka H, Araki Y, Yamamoto H, Yamamoto T, Tsukaguchi I. Intraosseous ganglion. Skeletal Radiol 1995;24(2):155–7.

78. Leclercq C, Glicenstein J. Tumeurs des parties molles de la main. In: Tubiana R, ed. Chirurgie de la Main. Paris: Masson, 1995:753–72.

79. Razemon J. Les kystes du poignet. In: Tubiana R, ed. Chirurgie de la Main. Paris: Masson, 1995:627–33.

80. Blam O, Bindra R, Middleton W, Gelberman R. The occult dorsal carpal ganglion: usefulness of magnetic resonance imaging and ultrasound in diagnosis. Am J Orthop 1998;27(2):107–10.

81. Ushijima M, Hashimoto H, Tsuneyoshi M, Enjoji M. Giant cell tumor of the tendon sheath (nodular tenosynovitis). A study of 207 cases to compare the large joint group with the common digit group. Cancer 1986;57(4):875–84.

82. Goodman HJ, Richards AM, Klaassen MF. Use of magnetic resonance imaging on a large lipoma of the hand: a case report. Aust N Z J Surg 1997;67(7):489–91.

83. Dooms GC, Hricak H, Sollitto RA, Higgins CB. Lipomatous tumors and tumors with fatty component: MR imaging potential and comparison of MR and CT results. Radiology 1985;157(2):479–83.

84. Amadio PC, Reiman HM, Dobyns JH. Lipofibromatous hamartoma of nerve. J Hand Surg [Am] 1988;13(1):67–75.

85. Silverman TA, Enzinger FM. Fibrolipomatous hamartoma of nerve. A clinicopathologic analysis of 26 cases. Am J Surg Pathol 1985;9(1):7–14.

86. Miller TT, Potter HG, McCormack RR Jr. Benign soft tissue masses of the wrist and hand: MRI appearances. Skeletal Radiol 1994;23(5):327–32.

87. Theumann NH, Bittoun J, Goettmann S, Le Viet D, Chevrot A, Drape JL. Hemangiomas of the fingers: MR imaging evaluation. Radiology 2001;218(3):841–7.

88. Berquist T, Kransdorf M. Tumors and tumor-like lesions. In: Berquist T, ed. MRI of the Hand and Wrist. Philadelphia: Lippincott Williams & Wilkins, 2003.

89. Greenspan A, McGahan JP, Vogelsang P, Szabo RM. Imaging strategies in the evaluation of soft-tissue hemangiomas of the extremities: correlation of the findings of plain radiography, angiography, CT, MRI, and ultrasonography in 12 histologically proven cases. Skeletal Radiol 1992;21(1):11–8.

90. Theumann NH, Goettmann S, Le Viet D, et al. Recurrent glomus tumors of fingertips: MR imaging evaluation. Radiology 2002;223(1):143–51.

91. Boudghene FP, Gouny P, Tassart M, Callard P, Le Breton C, Vayssairat M. Subungual glomus tumor: combined use of MRI and three-dimensional contrast MR angiography. J Magn Reson Imaging 1998;8(6):1326–8.

92. Drape JL, Idy-Peretti I, Goettmann S, Guerin-Surville H, Bittoun J. Standard and high resolution magnetic resonance imaging of glomus tumors of toes and fingertips. J Am Acad Dermatol 1996;35(4):550–5.

93. Dalrymple NC, Hayes J, Bessinger VJ, Wolfe SW, Katz LD. MRI of multiple glomus tumors of the finger. Skeletal Radiol 1997;26(11):664–6.

94. Weiss S, Goldblum J. Enzinger and Weiss' Soft Tissue Tumors, 4th ed. St. Louis: Mosby, 2001.

95. Kasakowa Y, Okoda K, KHashimoto M, et a. Extra-abdominal desmoid tumor of the hand: a case report and review of the literature. Tokyo J Exp Med 1999;189:163–79.

96. Disler DG, Recht MP, McCauley TR. MR imaging of articular cartilage. Skeletal Radiol 2000;29(7):367–77.

97. Theumann N, Berner IC, Dudler J. [Interest of magnetic resonance imaging in rheumatoid arthritis]. Rev Med Suisse 2005;1(10):670–3.

98. Tonolli-Serabian I, Poet JL, Dufour M, Carasset S, Mattei JP, Roux H. Magnetic resonance imaging of the wrist in rheumatoid arthritis: comparison with other inflammatory joint diseases and control subjects. Clin Rheumatol 1996;15(2):137–42.

99. Cimmino MA, Bountis C, Silvestri E, Garlaschi G, Accardo S. An appraisal of magnetic resonance imaging of the wrist in rheumatoid arthritis. Semin Arthritis Rheum 2000;30(3):180–95.

100. Sugimoto H, Takeda A, Hyodoh K. Early-stage rheumatoid arthritis: prospective study of the effectiveness of MR imaging for diagnosis. Radiology 2000;216(2):569–75.

101. McQueen FM, Stewart N, Crabbe J, et al. Magnetic resonance imaging of the wrist in early rheumatoid arthritis reveals a high prevalence of erosions at four months after symptom onset. Ann Rheum Dis 1998;57(6):350–6.

102. McQueen FM, Stewart N, Crabbe J, et al. Magnetic resonance imaging of the wrist in early rheumatoid arthritis reveals progression of erosions despite clinical improvement. Ann Rheum Dis 1999;58(3):156–63.

103. Ostergaard M, Hansen M, Stoltenberg M, Lorenzen I. Quantitative assessment of the synovial membrane in the rheumatoid wrist: an easily obtained MRI score reflects the synovial volume. Br J Rheumatol 1996;35(10):965–71.

104. Popp JD, Bidgood WD Jr, Edwards NL. Magnetic resonance imaging of tophaceous gout in the hands and wrists. Semin Arthritis Rheum 1996;25(4):282–9.

105. Berquist T. Arthropathies. In: Berquist TH, ed. MRI of the Hand and Wrist. Philadelphia: Lippincott Williams & Wilkins, 2003.

106. Resnick D. Bone and Joint Imaging, 2nd ed. Philadelphia: WB Saunders, 1996.

107. Berquist T. Infections. In: Berquist TH, ed. MRI of the Hand and Wrist. Philadelphia: Lippincott Williams & Wilkins, 2003.

108. Boutin RD, Brossmann J, Sartoris DJ, Reilly D, Resnick D. Update on imaging of orthopedic infections. Orthop Clin North Am 1998;29(1):41–66.

109. Morrison WB, Schweitzer ME, Bock GW, et al. Diagnosis of osteomyelitis: utility of fat-suppressed contrast-enhanced MR imaging. Radiology 1993;189(1):251–7.

110. Beltran J, McGhee RB, Shaffer PB, et al. Experimental infections of the musculoskeletal system: evaluation with MR imaging and Tc-99 m MDP and Ga-67 scintigraphy. Radiology 1988;167(1):167–72.

111. Bonakdar-pour A, Gaines VD. The radiology of osteomyelitis. Orthop Clin North Am 1983;14(1):21–37.

112. Graif M, Schweitzer ME, Deely D, Matteucci T. The septic versus nonseptic inflamed joint: MRI characteristics. Skeletal Radiol 1999;28(11):616–20.

113. Crawford GP. The molded polyethylene splint for mallet finger deformities. J Hand Surg 1984;9A:231–7.

114. Casscells SW, Strange TB. Intramedullary wire fixation of mallet finger. J Bone Joint Surg 1969;51A:1018–9.

115. Wehbe MA, Schneider LH. Mallet fractures. J Bone Joint Surg 1984;66A:658–69.

116. Leddy JP, Packer JW. Avulsion of the profundus tendon in athletes. J Hand Surg 1977;2:66–9.

117. Silva MJ, et al. The effects of multiple-strand suture techniques on the tensile properties of repair of the flexor digitorum profundus tendon to bone. J Bone Joint Surg 1998;80A:1507–14.

118. Schöffle VR, Schöffle I. Injuries to the flexor pulley system in rock climbers: Current concepts. J Hand Surg 2006;31A:647–54.

119. Elson RA. Rupture of the central slip of the extensor hood of the finger. A test for early diagnosis. J Bone Joint Surg 1986;68B:229–31.

120. Burton RI, Eaton RG. Common hand injuries in the athlete. Orthop Clin North Am 1973;4:809–38.

121. Burton RI, Melchior JA. Extensor tendons—late reconstruction. In: Green's Operative Hand Surgery, 4th ed. New York: Churchill Livingston, 1999.

122. Wray RC, et al. Proximal interphalangeal joint sprains. Plast Reconstr Surg 1984;74:101–7.

123. Morgan WJ, Slowman LS, Acute hand and wrist injuries in athletes: evaluation and management. J Am Acad Orthop Surg 2001;9:389–400.

124. Low CK, et al. A cadaver study of the effects of dorsal angulation and shortening of the metacarpal shaft on the extension and flexion force ratios of the index and little fingers. J Hand Surg 1995;20B:609–13.

125. Opgrande JD, Westphal SA. Fractures of the hand. Orthop Clin North Am 1983;14(4):779–92.

126. Heyman P, Gelberman RH, Duncan K, et al. Injuries of the ulnar collateral ligament of the thumb metacarpophalangeal joint. Biomechanical and prospective clinical studies on the usefulness of valgus stress testing. Clin Orthop Rel Res 1993;292:165–71.

127. Kaplan EB. Dorsal dislocation of the metacarpophalangeal joint of the index finger. J Bone Joint Surg 1957;39A:1081–6.

128. Bohart PG, et al. Complex dislocations of the metacarpophalangeal joint. Clin Orthop Rel Res 1982;164:208–10.

9
Hip

A. Radiologic Perspective: Magnetic Resonance Imaging of the Athlete with Hip and Groin Pain

Cheryl A. Petersilge

As magnetic resonance (MR) has become increasingly more popular for assessment of hip and groin pain, our knowledge of the many pathologic conditions affecting the hip and pelvis has grown. Magnetic resonance has contributed significantly to our understanding of sports-related injuries as well as to underlying conditions such as femoroacetabular impingement, which can lead to pain and limited range of motion.

Localization of pain originating from the hip or pelvis is clinically difficult. Patients present with nonspecific complaints of hip pain, groin pain, pelvic pain, and even medial knee pain. As discussed in the previous chapter, the differential diagnosis includes internal derangements of the hip, femoroacetabular impingement, loose bodies, bursitis, stress injuries and stress fractures, musculotendinous injuries, tendon avulsions, sports hernias, as well as nerve injury, arthritis, and infection. The site of injury may be the hip joint, the symphysis pubis, the sacroiliac joint, the many sites of tendon origin and insertion, as well as the anterior abdominal wall and inguinal canal. The athletes most at risk for these injuries are those engaged in sports such as soccer, ice hockey, and track—sports that involve kicking, sprinting, and pivoting.

Imaging Anatomy

Joint

The hip is a ball-and-socket joint, a joint structure that enables a wide range of motion. The acetabulum is a spherical structure with an inferiorly oriented opening, the acetabular notch. The articular cartilage of the acetabular surface has an inverted-horseshoe configuration and resides at the outer margin of the joint. The central portion of this horseshoe is filled with fibrofatty pulvinar. The entire femoral head is covered with articular cartilage except for a small area on the center of the head known as the fovea capitus.

The joint capsule of the hip is much thicker than other joint capsules. Like other joints capsule it has several regions of focal thickening. These correspond to the extrinsic ligaments of the hip and include the longitudinally oriented pubofemoral, iliofemoral ligaments anteriorly, and the ischiofemoral ligament posteriorly. Similarly, the zona orbicularis represents a group of circularly oriented capsular fibers along its deep surface at the femoral head–neck junction. Anteriorly and posteriorly the joint capsule inserts at the base of the labrum, creating a small perilabral sulcus (perilabral recess) between the joint capsule and labrum. Superiorly the joint capsule inserts several millimeters above the base of the labrum, creating a more prominent superior perilabral recess. The hip joint communicates with the iliopsoas bursa in 14% of individuals via a deficiency between the pubofemoral and iliofemoral ligaments.[1] A posterior outpouching between the ischiofemoral ligament and the zona orbicularis creates the obturator externus bursa.[2]

The transverse ligament bridges the acetabular notch and at the margins of the notch this ligament merges with the labrum. The ligament serves to complete the deficiency of the osseous socket created by the acetabular notch. A sulcus may be created at the anteroinferior and posteroinferior margins of the joint where the transverse ligament and labrum join. This labroligamentous sulcus may be mistaken for a detachment. The ligamentum teres connects the transverse ligament and the femoral head. It attaches to the fovea capitus of the femoral head. The artery of the ligamentum teres, a minor blood supply, courses through the ligament. Lined by synovium, the ligamentum teres is considered an extraarticular structure. The role of the ligamentum teres is not well understood.

Labrum

The acetabular labrum projects laterally from the acetabular rim and deepens the acetabular socket. The labrum aids in distribution of the weight-bearing forces through the joint by maintaining a joint fluid layer between the articular cartilage of the femur and head, and by preventing lateral translation of the femur.[3–5] The labrum is composed of fibrocartilaginous tissue and dense connective tissue.[6,7] Histologically, three separate layers are identified within the labrum: a randomly oriented fibrocartilaginous layer at the articular surface, a central lamellar layer of collagen, and a circumferentially oriented layer along the capsular surface.[6,8,9] The labrum is a relatively avascular structure, resulting in a limited ability to repair itself.[6,10–12] The labrum is innervated, and damage directly to

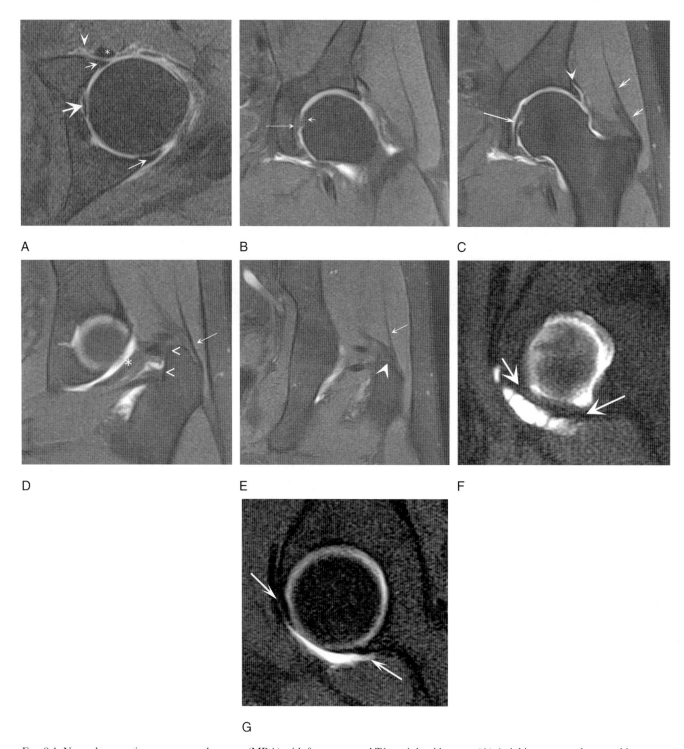

FIG. 9.1. Normal magnetic resonance arthrogram (MRA) with fat suppressed T1–weighted images. (A) Axial image reveals several important features of the joint. Minimal filling of the iliopsoas bursa (arrowhead) is seen along the medial aspect of the iliopsoas tendon (asterisk). Anterior and posterior labra (small arrows) with small perilabral recesses are present. The cross section of the ligamentum teres is seen (large arrow). (B–E) Coronal images from anterior to posterior reveal the fibrofatty pulvinar (long arrow in B) and the fovea capitus of the femoral head (short arrow in B). The larger superior perilabral sulcus is seen (arrowhead in C). The long axis ligamentum teres is visible (long arrow in C). The insertions of the gluteus minimus onto the anterior facet of the greater trochanter (shorts arrows in C) and gluteus medius tendons onto the lateral (long arrow in D and E) and superoposterior facets (long arrow in E) of the greater trochanter are easily identified. The attachment of the piriformis and obturator internus to the inner aspect of the greater trochanter can be seen ("<"s in D). (F,G) Sagittal images from medial to lateral depict the transverse ligament as it spans the acetabular notch (arrows in F) and the anterior and posterior perilabral recesses (arrows in G).

this structure plays a role in pain generation.[13] Pertinent MR arthrographic anatomy is demonstrated in Figure 9.1.

The acetabular labrum is typically triangular in shape, and this is the dominant shape in 66% to 94% of asymptomatic and presumably normal labra.[14–16] The thickest portion of the labrum is superior and posterior, and it is widest along the anterior and superior portions of the joint.[7,15,17–19] Rounded, blunted, and absent labra have been described.[14] A consistent constellation of findings including an absent anterior labrum accompanied by a blunted anterosuperior labrum has been observed in 10% to 14% of individuals.[15,16] Because of the consistency of this pattern it is believed to represent an anatomic variant rather than a pathologic finding.[7,20] With advancing age, labral morphology becomes increasingly variable, with a decreasing percentage of triangular labra.[14,16]

The most common pattern of signal intensity within the labrum is low signal intensity on all magnetic resonance imaging (MRI) sequences. This pattern of signal intensity has been reported in up to 44% to 56% of asymptomatic hips.[14,16] However, a spectrum of increased internal signal has been observed in the asymptomatic labrum. The incidence of this increased internal signal increases with increasing age.[14,16] Signal variations are more common in men and within the superior and anterior labrum.[14–16] Variations include intermediate signal on T1-weighted and proton-density weighted images in 58% of asymptomatic labra, and 37% of asymptomatic labra have intermediate signal on T2-weighted sequences.[15] Bright signal may be seen on T2-weighted images in up to 15% of patients.[15] This internal signal may be globular, linear, or curvilinear, and may extend to the margins of the labrum. This extension to the labral margin is one reason that differentiation of normal and abnormal labra is difficult without the benefit of intraarticular contrast material. Many factors may contribute to this internal signal. There may be extension of the osseous rim into the labral substance.[7,21] Fibrocartilaginous bundles within the labral base are also contributory.[21] In one anatomic study there was poor correlation between degeneration and this intrasubstance signal; however, in another study an increasing incidence of intrasubstance signal correlated with increasing age, suggesting a degenerative component.[16,21]

The relationship between the acetabular labrum and articular cartilage is a subject of controversy. A separation between the articular cartilage and the labrum at the posterior aspect of the joint, the posterior labrocartilaginous cleft, has been identified as a normal variant occurring in 22.6% of hips.[22] Whether an anterior labrocartilaginous cleft is a normal variant or a pathologic finding is unclear.

When this cleft occurs at the anterosuperior aspect of the joint and the margins of the adjacent cartilage and labrum are smooth, the attachment of the labrum to the acetabular rim is intact, and no other abnormalities are seen within the joint, this cleft is believed to represent an anterior labrocartilaginous cleft that is an anatomic variant.[6,8,23] An example of such a cleft is presented in Figure 9.2. This conclusion is based on several different pieces of evidence. In cadaveric studies this

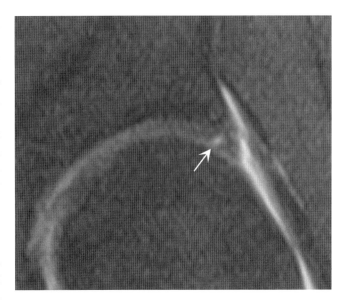

FIG. 9.2. Labrocartilaginous cleft. On this fat-suppressed T1-weighted image with intraarticular contrast, a collection of contrast is located between the articular cartilage and labrum (arrow). Its margins are smooth and it is at the anterosuperior corner of the joint. The attachment of labrum to the acetabular rim is intact. The remainder of the joint is unremarkable (not shown).

cleft was identified in four of 74 (5%) fetal specimens and 19 of 24 (79%) adult specimens (age range 23 to 77 years).[6,8] In one clinical study this finding was identified in three of 46 (6.5%) asymptomatic hips.[15] A similar finding was identified in 19% of 54 cadaver hips with an average age of 78 years.[12] These data imply that there is an underlying incidence of this cleft of 5% to 6.5%, and the incidence increases with increasing age. This situation seems analogous to the case of a type I superior labrum anterior to posterior (SLAP) lesion in the shoulder, with an increasing incidence of asymptomatic tears with age.

Evidence to support the absence of a normal cleft at this site includes histologic studies in which the articular cartilage and labrum are intimately related without an intervening cleft.[7,19,21] In one additional cadaveric study and two other clinical studies, no cleft/sulcus was identified in symptomatic hips, although those study populations were small.[20,22,23] However with a proposed incidence of 5% to 6.5%, these patient populations may have been too small to conclusively rule out such a normal variant. In an arthroscopic study of 56 patients, evidence of attempted healing was identified within defects at the articular cartilage labral interface in 41 patients.[24] These data would suggest that the anterior labrocartilaginous cleft is pathologic. In two separate cadaveric studies of elderly specimens, 89% of tears found in 74% of hips were at the anterosuperior margin.[7,19] This high incidence of labral pathology in these elderly specimens calls into the question the significance of the findings and again suggests a situation analogous to a type I SLAP lesion of the shoulder.

Symphysis Pubis and Anterior Abdominal Wall

The symphysis pubis is a cartilaginous articulation between the bodies of the pubic bones. The articular margins are lined with hyaline cartilage, and a central fibrocartilaginous disk is present within the articulation. With advancing age a cleft may develop within this disk. The superior pubic ligament reinforces the joint superiorly. The arcuate pubic ligament provides support inferiorly. Intersecting fibers from the adductor longus and brevis muscles and from the rectus femoris muscle strengthen the joint anteriorly and this relationship is visible in Figure 9.3.

A number of muscles originate and insert onto the pubis and pubic rami. The muscles of concern in the production of groin pain include the gracilis, the adductor longus of the adductor compartment of the thigh, the rectus abdominus, and the conjoined tendon (of the transverses abdominus and internal oblique muscles) of the anterior abdominal wall. The gracilis tendon originates from the anterior margin of the symphysis and spans the entire length of the inferior pubic ramus. The adductor longus muscle originates from the medial aspect of the superior pubic ramus while the adductor brevis muscle is located deep to the longus and originates from the inferior pubic ramus lateral to the gracilis muscle.

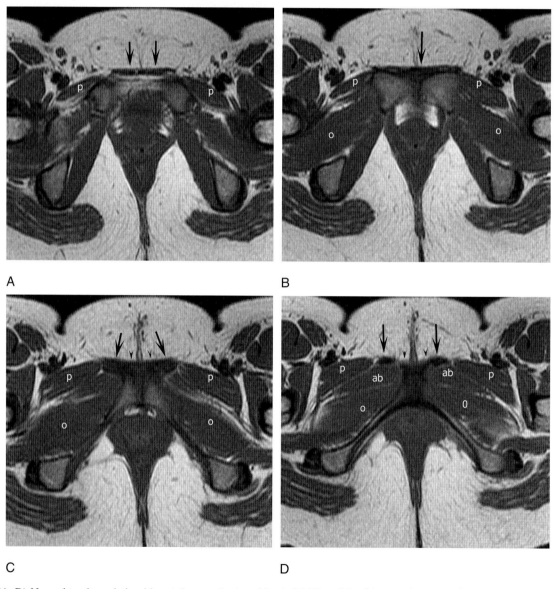

Fig. 9.3. (A–D) Normal tendon relationships at the symphysis pubis. Axial T1-weighted images from superior to inferior demonstrate the origins of the rectus abdominus muscles from the superior aspect of the superior pubic rami (arrows in A) and the intersection of rectus abdominus and adductor muscle fibers anterior to the symphysis pubis (arrow in B). The adductor longus tendon (long arrows in C, D) and gracilis tendon (arrowheads in C, D) origins are identified more inferiorly. The pectineus (p), adductor brevis (ab), and obturator externus (o) muscles are also visible.

The rectus abdominus muscles originate from the superior border of the superior pubic ramus and the symphysis pubis. The conjoined tendon inserts lateral to the rectus abdominus muscle origin. A complex relationship of the fascia of the muscles of the anterior abdominal wall exists, leading to the creation of the inguinal canal.

Marrow

In general, marrow conversion from hematopoietic marrow to adipose marrow progresses from distal to proximal, and thus the marrow of the proximal femoral metaphysis is one of the last sites in the appendicular skeleton to undergo conversion.[25–27] Red marrow persists in this location until the mid-30s in men and the mid-50s in women.[28] Even in the absence of disease, patients with demand for extra hematopoietic marrow may have persistent red marrow in the proximal femur. This includes fit adults, menstruating women, smokers, and obese patients.[29,30]

Marrow conversion in the axial skeleton, and thus the pelvis, lags behind the appendicular skeleton, and hematopoietic marrow will persist longer in the pelvis than the femur.[26,31,32] Four stages of marrow conversion within the pelvis have been described, beginning in infancy and continuing to early adulthood.[31] In all stages, the marrow of the acetabuli and anterior ileum is typically higher in signal than the rest of the pelvis on T1-weighted images, and this pattern may be seen as early as age 2 years.[31] Increasing heterogeneity throughout the pelvis is observed during marrow conversion.[32] With this conversion, adipose marrow accumulates along the anterior iliac wings and near the sacroiliac joints, although hematopoietic marrow may persist around the sacroiliac joints as age progresses.[26,31,32]

Muscles, Tendons, and Bursa

The pelvis and proximal femur are the sites of origin and insertion for many muscles that are frequently injured. These attachment sites involve various anatomic regions where muscles may be injured in isolation or in common patterns involving both soft tissue and osseous abnormalities. These sites include the anterior aspect of the pelvis where injuries involve the insertions of the anterior abdominal wall musculature, the origins of the adductors of the thigh, and the obturator muscles. The hamstring tendons (semimembranosus, semitendinosus, biceps femoris) and the ischial tuberosity are another anatomic region. The lateral hip includes the gluteal musculature, the external rotators of the hip, and associated bursa. There are multiple apophyses of the pelvis that are prone to avulsion injuries as discussed later in this chapter. The sacroiliac (SI) joint, sacrum, and other bones of the pelvis may also be injured. A detailed discussion of the anatomy of these sites is beyond the scope of this text, and the reader is referred to any one of the many anatomy and imaging anatomy textbooks available.

Imaging Protocol

Noncontrast Examination

There are two basic tenets that must be kept in mind when evaluating the patient with hip, groin, or pelvic pain. The first is that pain is difficult to localize in this anatomic region, and thus a screening examination of the entire pelvis should be performed in all patients. This screening is easily performed with a short-tau inversion recovery (STIR) sequence, which provides great sensitivity and the ability to cover this large anatomic area with a single acquisition. The field of view (FOV) for this sequence ranges from 32 to 44 cm depending on patient size. Slice thicknesses of 5 to 8 mm are used to cover the entire pelvis from the symphysis pubis through the entire sacrum. T1-weighted images may be useful to help with defining anatomy. They are particularly helpful in locating the pubic rami on the STIR sequence.

The second tenet is that small FOV images must be acquired to adequately evaluate abnormalities. Use of surface coils and phased array coils optimizes signal to noise. Imaging parameters include a FOV of 14 to 26 cm, slice thicknesses of 3 to 5 mm, and a matrix of 192–256 × 256. There is greater variability in the use of sequences in the hip than there is for other joints. Ideally, the protocol should be tailored based on the screening examination. A protocol that nicely complements the coronal screening examination in many instances includes fluid-sensitive sequences of the painful side in the axial and sagittal plane, with T1-weighted imaging in the oblique axial plane. The oblique axial plane is prescribed off a coronal image along the long axis of the femoral neck (Fig. 9.4).

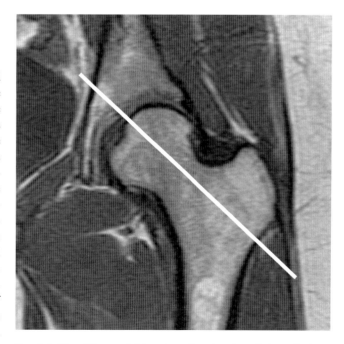

FIG. 9.4. The oblique axial imaging plane is oriented along the long axis of the femoral neck.

This plane has also been called the oblique sagittal plane. Structures that should be covered include the hip joint, the tendons of the greater tuberosity, and the hamstring tendons.

If the screening examination or physical and clinical examination reveals abnormality in the symphyseal region, images should be centered over this region. Fluid-sensitive axial and coronal small FOV images are most useful. The FOV ranges from 18 to 30 cm and a slice thickness of 3 to 5 mm should be used. Imaging of this area with the patient prone often eliminates subtle motion artifacts. Intravenous contrast material has no significant role in evaluation of the injured athlete.

Magnetic Resonance Arthrography

Magnetic resonance arthrography (MRA) with its accompanying joint distention is preferred for the assessment of the intraarticular structures of the hip and should be an integral part of the evaluation of the hip with mechanical symptoms. It is essential for evaluation of the acetabular labrum. The reported sensitivity is 91% to 92%, specificity 71% to 100%, and accuracy 88% to 92%.[20,33,34] Evaluation of the articular cartilage is extremely difficult due to its thin nature in the hip. The joint distention of arthrography greatly aids in the detection of cartilage abnormalities, although detection of abnormalities remains less than ideal even with dedicated cartilage sequences. Reported accuracy for detection of cartilage lesions is 50% to 84%.[35–38]

The joint distention for MRA is typically performed with a dilute gadolinium solution (0.2 mmol/L of gadopentetate dimeglumine). For low-volume practices this dilution may be achieved by mixing 0.1 cc of gadopentetate dimeglumine with 20 cc of normal saline. Mixing 15 cc of that solution with 5 cc of iodinated contrast is helpful for confirming intraarticular injection; 2 to 3 mL of 1% lidocaine may be added to the injection. Pain relief following the intraarticular injection of lidocaine provides additional evidence of an intraarticular source of pain.[35] However, the lack of pain relief does not eliminate the joint as the source of pain. The capacity of the hip joint is 8 to 20 cc.[23,36] Placing the hip in flexion and slight internal rotation increases joint capacity.

A combination of T1-weighted images with and without fat saturation is employed. The use of fat saturation improves the detection of abnormal contrast distribution, while the use of T1-weighted images without fat suppression provides assessment of the marrow and aids in defining anatomy. A screening examination of the pelvis is recommended for all MRAs to help identify potential associated injuries outside the joint. Recommended imaging parameters include FOV of 14 to 26 cm, slice thicknesses of 3 to 5 mm for spin echo sequences and 1.5 mm for gradient echo sequences, and a matrix of 192–256 × 256.

In order to completely cover the entire hip joint and visualize the entire labrum, imaging should be performed in multiple imaging planes. A typical imaging protocol for MRI includes fat-suppressed T1-weighted coronal, sagittal, and oblique axial images, T1-weighted axial images of the hip, and screening STIR images of the entire pelvis. The oblique axial plane has become a critical component of MRA. This imaging plane is oriented along the long axis of the femoral neck. It bisects the joint and provides an excellent cross section of the joint especially the labrum. It is also valuable for assessment of the alpha angle described in the discussion on impingement (see below). Radial imaging has also been employed for optimizing coverage of the joint and may be used with or without joint distention.[39–43] With radial imaging, images are planned from the center of the femoral head. In several, 4-mm slice-thickness images are obtained at 15-degree (range, 10 to 22.5 degrees) increments rotating around the center point of the femoral head. Some investigators believe that the acetabular labrum can be adequately assessed without the addition of intraarticular contrast.[44] Studies that compared MRI without joint distention with MRA, however, showed that sensitivity and accuracy increased from 8% to 30% to 90% to 92% (sensitivity) and 36% to 91% (specificity) for the detection of labral pathology.[33,34]

Osseous Injury

In the athletic population common osseous injuries include stress injury as well as apophyseal avulsions in the younger population. Stress injury is the result of abnormal forces acting on normal bone (fatigue injury or fracture) or normal forces acting on abnormal bone (insufficiency fracture). Fatigue injuries dominate in the athletic population and may be seen in both the mature and immature skeleton. These injuries typically develop over time, and are the result of chronic repetitive injury to the skeleton. For this discussion the term *stress injury* is used to encompass both fatigue injury and fatigue fracture.

Avulsion injuries, on the other hand, are usually associated with a single event with sudden onset of pain. In the immature skeleton the weak link in the bone–tendon unit is the growth plate, and failure occurs at this site when subjected to distraction by a sudden muscle contraction. The repetitive stresses of a demanding training program may lead to weakening of the apophysis predisposing to this injury.[45] In the mature skeleton the counterpart to this injury is myotendinous damage, which is discussed in greater detail later in this chapter and in the chapter on muscle injury. When an avulsion injury is seen in the mature skeleton, it is most often pathologic in nature.[46–48]

A variety of other osseous injuries are uncommonly seen in the athlete but should always be considered especially when more common causes of the pain have been excluded. The entities include osteochondral injuries of the femoral head, thigh splints, and transient subluxation of the hip. There are those injuries that occur commonly and that are typically diagnosed clinically such as the hip pointer. This injury is the result of a direct blow to the iliac crest. If symptoms are unusual, the patient may be imaged. Bone marrow edema and soft tissue edema may be seen over the anterior aspect of the iliac crest. There are also entities that are not necessarily a direct result of athletic activity but that may produce pain in the athletic population such as transient osteoporosis of the hip.

Avulsion Injuries

The ischial tuberosity and the anterior superior iliac spine are the most common sites of avulsion.[45,49–52] These injuries are commonly seen in gymnasts and soccer players.[45] Magnetic resonance imaging is rarely the primary diagnostic test for identification of avulsion injuries. These injuries are typically recognized on radiographs with separation of the apophysis from pelvis. Ill-definition of the adjacent physeal margins with accompanying osteopenia may be present. New bone formation between the apophysis and the donor site develops in subacute injuries. This early new bone formation is immature, and if the patient is imaged at this time the aggressive appearance may raise concern for neoplasm.[50,53] A detailed clinical history as well as knowledge of the common sites of avulsion as well as recognition of this radiographic appearance helps prevent unnecessary intervention. Follow-up radiographs demonstrating maturation of the new bone help confirm this diagnosis, especially in equivocal cases. In chronic or remote avulsion the new bone seen is mature and is usually readily identified as an old avulsion.

In some cases, however, the avulsion does not result in significant apophyseal displacement, and the injury is not recognized radiographically. When these patients are evaluated by MR, the findings include growth plate widening with hyperintense signal on fluid-sensitive images. Edema may be present in the adjacent bone, periosteum, and tendon origin as seen in Figure 9.5. A hematoma at the site is an uncommon finding. On MR images the avulsed fragment may be difficult to identify if it is small. In more severe cases a gap secondary to tendon retraction may be seen and the retracted tendon fibers may be lax or wavy. When an avulsed fragment is not appreciated or when there is no gap or tendon laxity the MR findings may be misinterpreted for an aggressive lesion.[51,54] Again correlation between clinical history and the site of abnormality will help establish the diagnosis. Radiographs, if not previously obtained, may also be useful.

Stress Injuries

The pelvis and proximal femur are uncommon sites of stress injury to bone accounting for less than 10% of stress injuries in a study of 320 athletes.[55] These injuries are most commonly seen in runners and military recruits and occur more frequently in women.[56,57] In a study of pelvic and proximal femoral stress injuries in 340 patients, 60% of the injuries occurred in the proximal femur and 40% were located in the pelvis (Fig. 9.6).[57] A slightly different distribution with an even greater percentage of proximal femur injuries has been observed when military recruits were evaluated.[58] Within the

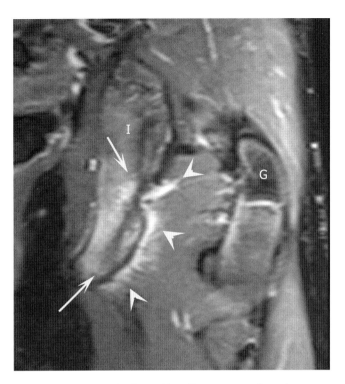

FIG. 9.5. Ischial apophysis avulsion. Intraosseous edema is present along the entire length of the ischial apophysis (long arrows) and extensive edema is present in the adjacent musculature (arrowheads). The apophyseal fragment is nondisplaced. I, ischium; G, greater trochanter.

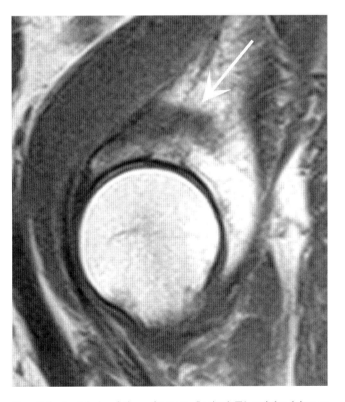

FIG. 9.6. Acetabular fatigue fracture. Sagittal T1-weighted image demonstrates ill-defined linear low intensity signal (arrow) within the supraacetabular ileum.

pelvis 49% of injuries occurred in the inferior pubic ramus, 41% in the sacrum, 4% in the superior pubic ramus, 4% in the ileum, and 1% in the acetabulum.[57] The presence of more than one stress injury has been documented in up to 24% of patients, and 16% of those injuries were bilateral.[56,57] The absence of symptoms referable to all sites of injury suggests that some stress injuries may be asymptomatic, and this conclusion has been supported by several researchers.[57–59] These asymptomatic injuries tended to be bone marrow edema without a visible fracture line. Despite the lack of symptoms, these injuries should be treated. In the pelvis and hip it is unlikely that the bone marrow edema is simply the result of excessive stress without damage such as might be anticipated in marathon runners.[60]

Stress injury to bone represents a spectrum of osseous abnormality of increasing severity from fatigue injury to fatigue fracture to complete fracture.[61] Magnetic resonance is the imaging modality of choice for identification of these injuries when radiographic examination is unrevealing.[62] Up to two thirds of femoral neck fractures may be radiographically occult, and sacral fractures are rarely seen on radiographs.[63,64] A continuum of abnormality is seen on MRI. In the earliest stage, fatigue injury, focal areas of bone marrow edema, low on T1-weighted images and bright on fluid-sensitive sequences, are seen. Pubic fatigue injury is illustrated in Figure 9.7. The edema may extend to involve the periosteum and the adjacent muscles.[57] Fatigue fractures are recognized by the presence of low signal lines (fatigue lines) within the areas of edema. Extension of the fracture line through the cortical surfaces indicates completion of the fracture. Differentiation between fatigue injury and fatigue fracture is clinically significant as symptoms persist for a longer period of time in patients with fatigue fracture.[65]

Once a stress injury is identified and appropriate therapy is instituted, MR findings will resolve. In one study, 70% of patients with femoral neck fatigue fractures had resolution of edema on STIR images at 3 months and 90% had resolution by 6 months. Clinical symptoms may persist beyond the resolution of edema on STIR images.[66] In this study, at the time of follow-up MRI a focal area of persistent T1-weighted low signal was identified along the medial femoral neck in 50% of patients.[66] This MR appearance correlated with the finding of focal sclerosis on plain films. Bright T1 signal surrounding this area of sclerosis may be identified and is likely fat marrow surrounding the healing fracture. In one case bright signal on STIR images developed in the fatigue line, likely representing granulation tissue.

Femoral Stress Injuries

The most common site of stress injury in the femur is the femoral neck. In a study of 340 patients 67% of femoral injuries occurred in the femoral neck, 32% in the proximal shaft, and 1% in the femoral head.[57] In another study of 185 stress injuries of the femur, 50% occurred in the femoral neck.[65] Two different types of stress fractures of the femoral neck with very different sequelae have been described. These fractures are tensile injuries and compression injuries.[67] The more common compression injuries occur along the medial aspect of the basicervical neck as seen in Figure 9.8. Tensile injuries are transversely oriented relative to the femoral neck and occur along the superior aspect of the neck at the head neck junction as seen in Figure 9.9. Tensile injuries are at greater risk than compressive injuries for the development of a complete fracture. These injuries are more common in the elderly but are not

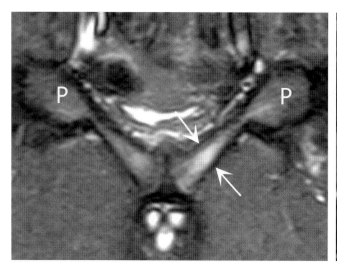

A

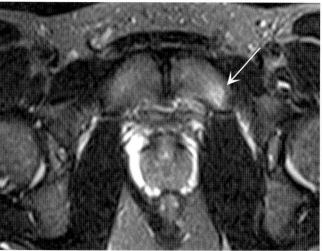

B

FIG. 9.7. Fatigue injury. Fat-suppressed turbo T2-weighted coronal (A) and axial (B) images demonstrate subtle focal bone marrow edema (arrows) within the left superior pubic ramus at the site of the patient's symptoms. P, superior pubic rami.

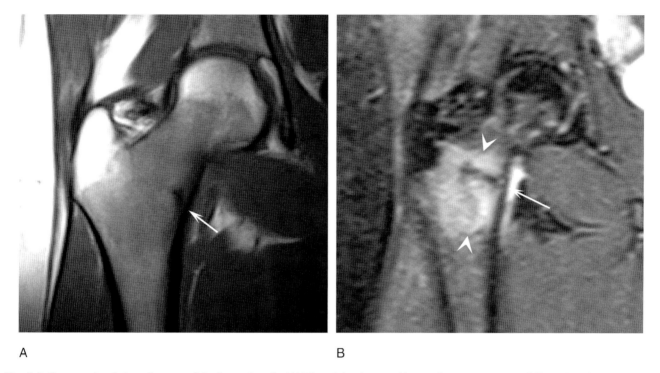

A   B

FIG. 9.8. Compressive fatigue fracture of the femoral neck. (A) T1-weighted coronal image demonstrates a small linear low signal intensity line along the medial aspect of the base of the neck (arrow). The edema is difficult to distinguish from the adjacent hematopoietic marrow. (B) On the screening STIR image at the same slice position the fracture line appears much more extensive (arrow) and the edema is more conspicuous (arrowheads).

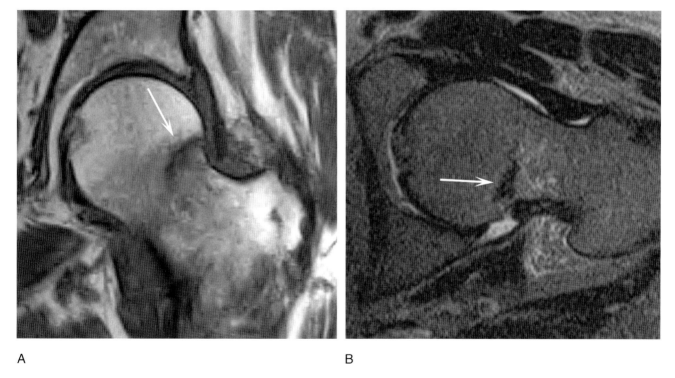

A   B

FIG. 9.9. Tensile stress fracture of the femoral neck. The fracture line (arrow) is located along the superolateral aspect of the subcapital region. An incomplete fracture line is visible on both T1-weighted coronal (A) and T2-weighted axial (B) images and is accompanied by minimal edema.

unique to that population, and thus represent both fatigue and insufficiency fractures. Completion of the fracture is a significant complication usually requiring surgical treatment and potential development of avascular necrosis.

Fatigue injury with bone marrow edema occurs in only 57% of patients with stress injuries of the femur, while a fatigue fracture with a visible fracture line occurs in 22% to 43%.[57,65] In at least one study of military recruits, the presence of a femoral stress fracture (at any site in the femur) was associated with an increased risk of additional fatigue fractures, and 25% of patients with a femoral fatigue fracture developed a second fatigue fracture within 1 year.[68]

Subchondral fractures of the femoral head are typically identified in elderly women and thus represent insufficiency fractures. However, these injuries have been reported in military recruits and thus are a rare form of fatigue fracture.[69] Whenever bone marrow edema is seen within the femoral head in a patient at risk, a detailed search of the subchondral bone should be made to identify this rare injury.

Sacral Stress Injuries

Patients with sacral stress injuries often present with low back pain, and the initial diagnostic evaluation may be directed toward the detection of disk disease.[70,71] Rarely visible on radiographs, these injuries have been underdiagnosed.[71] In these stress injuries the pattern of bone marrow edema is vertically oriented and linearly shaped.[71] On MR images, most sacral stress injuries are accompanied by a visible fracture line that is typically present in the first and second sacral segments (22 of 28 [79%]).[56,57,71] This pattern is different from insufficiency fracture, which parallels the sacroiliac joint.[56] The signal alterations on fluid-sensitive sequences in these stress injuries have been reported to resolve within 6 weeks of the initiation of therapy. In more severe cases the low signal on T1-weighted images resolved and was replaced by hyperintense T1-weighted signal, consistent with adipose marrow, which returned to normal at 5 to 6 months.[56] There are conflicting reports regarding the clinical resolution of symptoms. In one report of 31 patients, resolution of symptoms occurred within 6 weeks,[56] while in another study the pain persisted for over 6 months.[70]

Osteochondral Injuries

Osteochondral injuries of the femoral head have been identified. The MRI appearance of these injuries includes irregularity of the articular cartilage with small subchondral lesions that are low on T1-weighted images and demonstrate increased signal on T2-weighted images. These injuries are typically located in the anterosuperior aspect of the femoral head and may be accompanied by a joint effusion.[72] The mechanism of this injury has not yet been established. Proposed mechanisms include transient subluxation of the hip and high-energy impaction.[72] Whenever a focal area of subchondral signal

abnormality is seen in the athlete, the overlying articular cartilage should be scrutinized.

Subluxation of the Hip

Subluxation of the hip joint is an underrecognized disorder that results from rapid stopping and pivoting or from falling on a flexed knee in American football.[73,74] Posterior subluxations are more common than anterior subluxations. On MRI, the posterior acetabular lip fracture with its associated soft tissue and osseous edema is visible. An impaction injury on the femoral head may also be seen.[73] Anteriorly, disruption of the iliofemoral ligament is seen.[74]

Transient Osteoporosis of the Hip

This entity is a poorly understood condition that produces hip pain and MR findings of bone marrow edema.[75] Though initially described in women in the third trimester of pregnancy, it is more common in middle-aged men. The presenting complaint is spontaneous onset of hip pain without an inciting injury. The symptoms in this condition usually last for 4 to 12 months and represent a self-limited process.[76–78] Additional joints may become involved, including the opposite hip and the knees. With the involvement of additional joints, the entity is known as regional migratory osteoporosis

Radiographs are negative initially, but between 5 and 16 weeks after the onset of symptoms osteopenia is visible.[77] An MR examination demonstrates bone marrow edema, low on T1-weighted images and bright on fluid-sensitive sequences, involving the femoral head with variable extension into the femoral neck and intertrochanteric region. This pattern is seen in Figure 9.10.[76–78] Acetabular edema may also be present. A joint effusion is a consistent finding. An inconsistent feature is sparing of the subchondral bone of the femoral head, seen in 22.6% of 42 patients in one study between the 14th and 17th week after the onset of symptoms.[77] The joint space is maintained. The MR appearance is nonspecific and has been termed the bone marrow edema pattern.

The differential diagnosis of the bone marrow edema pattern includes transient migratory osteoporosis, bone contusion, subchondral fracture, avascular necrosis, infection, and neoplasm. There is little overlap in the patients at risk for these various entities, and clinical correlation often aids the establishment of a diagnosis. The possibility of a subchondral fatigue fracture of the femoral head should be considered in patients in whom a diagnosis of transient osteoporosis is entertained.[78] It is unclear whether this fracture is the cause of, or the result of, the osteoporosis, or if these entities are even distinct.[77,78]

In the past it has been proposed that transient osteoporosis of the hip is the early stage of avascular necrosis. Subsequent studies have demonstrated that transient osteoporosis of the hip is a separate entity from avascular necrosis.[13,79] The two can be differentiated by the presence of the double line sign in

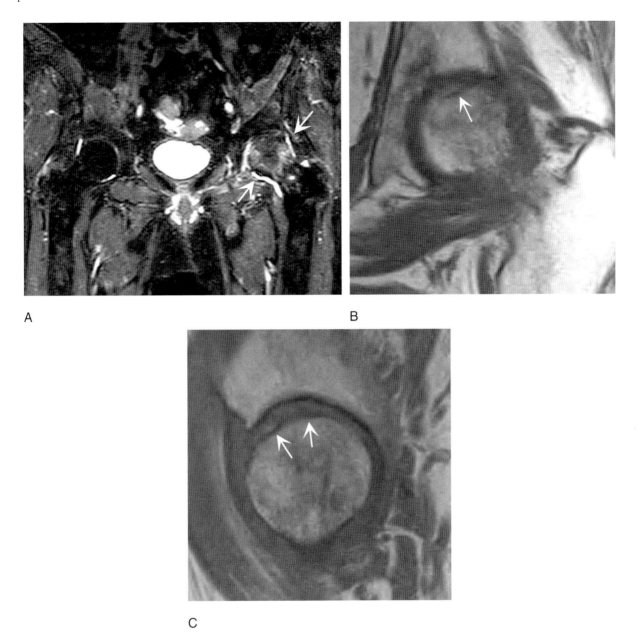

FIG. 9.10. Bone marrow edema pattern secondary to femoral head stress fracture. (A) The screening STIR coronal examination reveals diffuse bone marrow edema of the left femoral head accompanied by a joint effusion (arrows). (B) T1-weighted coronal image demonstrates a subtle low signal line (arrow) of the subchondral bone. (C) Sagittal T1-weighted depicts subtle foci of collapse of the articular surface of the femoral head (arrows).

patients with avascular necrosis. The crescentic subchondral fracture of avascular necrosis occurs within the area encompassed by the double line sign. Additionally, there will be clinical progression of symptoms in avascular necrosis.[80]

Thigh Splints

Thigh splints result from chronic repetitive stress at the insertion of the adductor longus and brevis muscles onto the femur.[81,82] These patients may present with hip, groin, or thigh pain. Abnormalities occur along the posteromedial aspect of the femoral diaphysis just above the midportion of the diaphysis as illustrated in Figure 9.11. Radiographic changes if present include focal periosteal new bone formation. Magnetic resonance findings include edematous signal along the periosteal surface of the femur in a linear orientation that may be accompanied by cortical or marrow edema.[81,82] The presence of cortical and marrow edema raises the possibility of progression to osseous stress injury.[81] Because this area of abnormality is outside

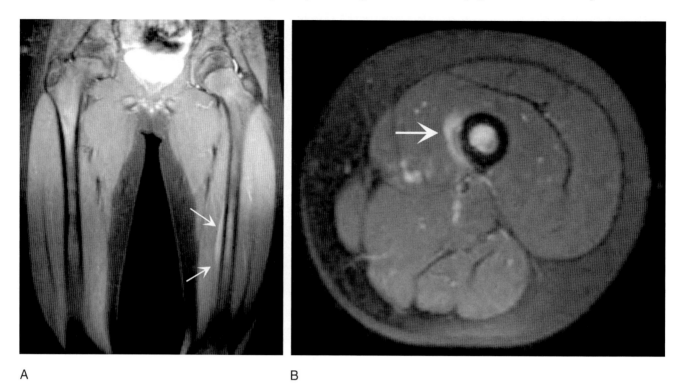

A   B

FIG. 9.11. Thigh splints. Fat-suppressed T2-weighted coronal (A) and axial (B) images reveal diffuse edema along the posteromedial periosteal surface of the femur at the insertion of the vastus medialis muscle (arrows).

the field of view of the typical screening examination, in the face of a normal study for hip or groin pain one should consider imaging the proximal thigh.

Soft Tissue Injuries

Common soft tissue abnormalities of the hip and pelvis, exclusive of internal derangement, include hamstring myotendinous injuries followed by rectus femoris myotendinous injuries.[73,83] Additional injuries related to the soft tissues of the hip and pelvis included the greater trochanteric pain syndrome related to the tendons and bursa of the external rotators of the thigh and hip abductors, the iliopsoas syndrome, and snapping hip.

Hamstring Injuries

The hamstring tendons consist of the tendons of the semimembranosus, semitendinosus, and the long head of the biceps femoris muscles. These powerful hip extensors and knee flexors originate from the ischial tuberosity via a conjoined tendon. Because they cross two joints, they are at increased risk for injury, and the hamstring muscles are one of the most frequently injured muscle groups. Hamstring injuries are commonly seen in athletes involved in sprinting and jumping activities.

In a series of 179 hamstring injuries Koulouris and Connell[83] found 21 (12%) occurred at the proximal bone–tendon unit, 154 (86%) occurred in the muscle belly, and four (2%) occurred distally. In their study of 60 athletes, Connell et al.[84] identified injuries at the musculotendinous junction in 52.4%, at the myofascial junction in 35.7%, and at the bone tendon junction in 7.1%. In two other studies, one of 37 athletes and one of 15 athletes with hamstring injuries, no proximal injuries were identified, and in a third study of 22 athletes 20 sustained proximal attachment hamstring injuries.[85–87] Only proximal bone–tendon injuries are considered in this discussion

In the skeletally immature athlete, injury at the bone–tendon unit results in avulsion of the ischial tuberosity. Magnetic resonance findings include displacement of the apophysis from the pelvis, edema, or hematoma within the gap; edema in the adjacent ischial body and within the apophysis tendon laxity often results. Chronic disability may result from this injury, including decreased athletic performance, as well as symptoms related to the displaced bone fragment and potential hypertrophic new bone formation.[52] A separation of greater than 2 cm has been suggested as an indication for surgery in this injury.[52]

In adults, injuries at the proximal bone–tendon junction include complete and partial tears of the tendons. A complete tear is evident in Figure 9.12. In their study Koulouris and Connell[83] found that at the proximal bone–tendon unit avulsion of all three tendons is most common, followed by avulsion of the

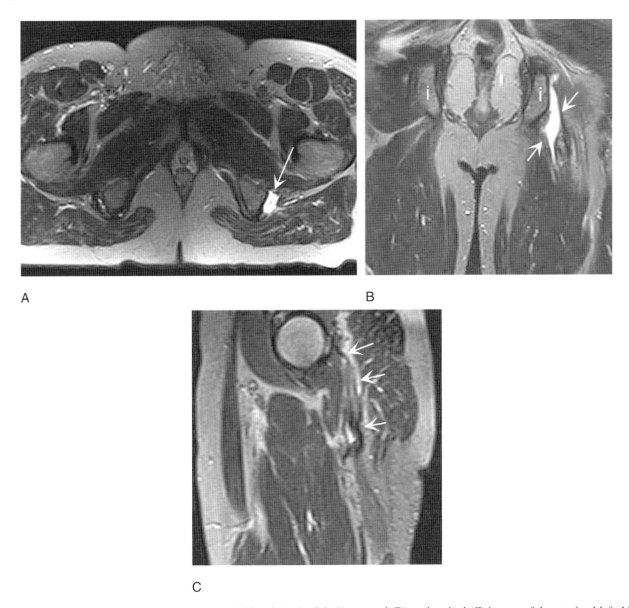

Fig. 9.12. Hamstring tendon rupture. Fat suppressed T2-weighted axial (A), coronal (B), and sagittal (C) images of the proximal left thigh depict a gap in the left hamstring tendons at their origin from the ischial tuberosity (arrows in A, B). The wavy, minimal retracted tendon fibers are apparent on the sagittal image (arrows in C). i, ischium.

biceps femoris tendon and semitendinosus tendon, followed by isolated biceps femoris avulsion. Partial tears are less common than complete avulsions, and most typically involve the biceps femoris muscle. Several other studies also confirm the finding that the biceps femoris is the most commonly involved tendon, followed by the semitendinosus muscle.[84–86] Tendon avulsions are recognized by a gap between the tendon margin and the ischial tuberosity with edema and hematoma within the gap. Edematous changes may also be seen within the tendon margin and along the muscle belly. Long axis images aid in defining the extent of retraction of the tendon margins. Partial tendon avulsion is recognized by a transversely oriented fluid-filled cleft within the tendon. Magnetic resonance

imaging characterization of hamstring injuries may provide prognostic information regarding the amount of time lost from training or competition.[84,87,88] Findings associated with longer absences from athletic activities include complete tendinous or myotendinous disruption, and hematoma.[88]

Greater Trochanteric Pain Syndrome

The greater trochanteric pain syndrome is pain over the lateral aspect of the hip that is attributable to trochanteric bursitis and abnormalities within the gluteus medius and minimus tendons.[89–91] The mechanism of injury is not well delineated but is hypothesized to be altered gait, hyperadduction of the hip, and friction between the iliotibial band and the gluteus medius and minimus tendons.[91] Abnormalities of the greater trochanteric tendons typically occur in the elderly patient population, especially women but have been seen in athletes such as runners, weightlifters, and those who participate in step aerobics.[92–94]

In the past this diagnosis was usually established clinically by point tenderness over the greater trochanter along the lateral aspect of the hip. The patients were typically treated with a steroid injection. Most patients responded to this injection, and further assessment was not warranted. With the increasing use of MR, however, those patients who do not respond to treatment are undergoing imaging evaluation. Other patients are being imaged because of atypical pain or to explore the possibility of pain referred to the hip joint.

The gluteus medius and minimus tendons have been dubbed the rotator cuff of the hip. The accompanying bursae include the subgluteus maximus (trochanteric bursa), and the subgluteus medius, and the minimus bursa.[95–97] The pathology of this region is similar to pathology within the rotator cuff of the shoulder. As with the rotator cuff of the shoulder the abnormalities range from tendinopathy to full-thickness tears.[89,91,98] Abnormalities of these tendons typically involve the gluteus medius tendon initially and may be accompanied by extension into the gluteus minimus tendon. Involvement of both tendons

is evident in Figure 9.13. Radiographs are nonspecific but may reveal a focal area of soft tissue calcification or ossification just above the greater trochanter and irregularity of the superior margin of the greater trochanter.[89,90]

On MR examination, tendinosis manifests as tendon thickening with bright signal on fluid-sensitive sequences and intact tendon fibers. Findings of partial- and full-thickness tears include partial or complete disruption of tendon fibers. Most tears occur at the tendon insertion rather than at the musculotendinous junction.[98] Bright signal is present within the defect on T2-weighted images. Retraction may accompany full-thickness tears. The gluteus medius tendon may appear elongated.[99] In long-standing cases atrophic changes are present within the muscle. The gluteus medius tendon is most commonly involved, and it may be accompanied by gluteus minimus pathology. The prevalence of tears vs. tendinosis varies with clinical studies.[89,91,98]

Inflammation within the trochanteric bursa frequently accompanies tendon abnormalities. Bursal inflammatory changes are apparent as lower signal on T1-weighted images and bright signal on T2-weighed images. The clinical significance of bursal fluid alone is indeterminate since it is frequently identified in an asymptomatic hip.[99] In symptomatic hips bursal fluid was not commonly seen in the absence of tendon abnormalities.[98]

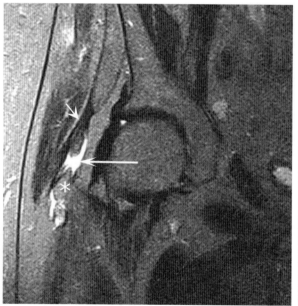
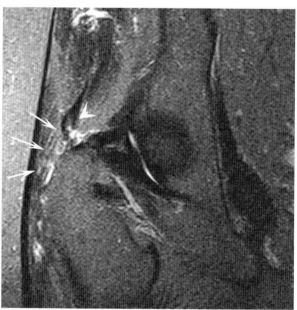

A   B

FIG. 9.13. Gluteal tendon injury. Fat-suppressed T2-weighted coronal images along the anterior (A) and posterior (B) margins of the greater tuberosity. Anteriorly the gluteus minimus tendon (short arrows in A) is partially torn along its deep surface. Fluid within the tear extends into the subgluteus minimus bursa (long arrow in A). The gluteus medius tendon is completely torn and retracted with a large gap (arrows in B). The retracted tendon margin is thickened with intrasubstance tear (arrowhead in B)*, greater trochanter.

Iliopsoas Bursitis and Tendinosis

The iliopsoas bursa is the largest bursa in the human body. It is located on the posterior surface of the iliopsoas tendon anterior to the hip joint and pectineal eminence. It is bounded medially by the femoral neurovascular structures. Inferiorly the bursa extends to the lesser trochanter and superiorly it extends for a variable distance into the pelvis. In its normal state the bursa is collapsed.

Abnormalities of the iliopsoas bursa are typically associated with direct trauma, chronic overuse, or intraarticular abnormalities of the hip, especially rheumatoid arthritis.[100] These abnormalities have a predilection for women.[100] Symptoms are often the result of compression of adjacent structures, although patients may present with an asymptomatic mass or limitation of hip motion.[101,102] The association with intraarticular pathology is a result of a direct communication between the hip and bursa in 14% of individuals.[1] Due to this communication between the hip joint and the bursa, the bursa may become distended whenever a joint effusion is present.[102,103] To recognize that the pain may originate in the tendon, the bursa, or both, the term *iliopsoas syndrome* has been proposed.[100]

Chronic overuse may lead to symptomatic bursitis and tendonitis. Overuse results from the motion of flexion and extension of the hip and is the result of either forceful stretching or friction during motion as discussed in the snapping hip syndrome (see below). Injuries are seen in rowers, runners, and dancers. This condition may or may not be associated with the snapping hip. However, MR changes within the iliopsoas tendon are uncommon and are consistent with tendinopathy as seen at other sites. Disruption of the tendon has not been described in the athletic population, although spontaneous rupture of the iliopsoas tendon has been described in the elderly population.[104]

Abnormalities within the bursa are readily recognized. On MRI the distended bursa will appear as a sausage-shaped fluid collection medial to the tendon. An enlarged bursa may also be seen along the lateral tendon margin.[102] The bursa wall is typically thin but may be thickened. Contrast enhancement of the wall suggests inflammation and is a frequent finding.[102]

Snapping Hip

The patient with snapping hip syndrome presents with complaints of an audible or palpable snap, which typically occurs in dancers and athletes such as runners.[105] External and internal as well as intraarticular forms of snapping hip have been described.[106] The intraarticular causes of snapping hip include labral tears, loose bodies and other entities such as synovial osteochondromatosis. These entities are discussed in greater detail below (see Internal Derangement). The internal and external forms of snapping hip are the result of a tendon that "snaps" over an osseous excrescence during normal motion. The external form of snapping hip is a result of the iliotibial band or gluteus maximus tendon snapping over the greater trochanter. The diagnosis of this form of snapping hip is made clinically, and imaging is typically not performed. If MR is performed, trochanteric bursitis, edema in the region of the iliotibial band, or thickening of the posterior aspect of the iliotibial or the anterior aspect of the gluteus maximus muscle may be identified.[106]

The internal form of snapping hip is the result of the iliopsoas tendon snapping over the femoral neck, the lesser trochanter, or the iliopectineal eminence. Findings on MR examination are nonspecific, and the examination may be normal. The iliopsoas bursa may be enlarged from fluid, inflamed synovium, or a combination of both. The tendon is typically normal, although findings of tendinopathy may be apparent.[107] More useful imaging examinations include iliopsoas bursography and dynamic sonography. These examinations allow direct visualization of the tendon during motion. Confirmation of the diagnosis is achieved by observation of an abrupt "snap" of the tendon as it moves from lateral to medial as the hip is extended and internally rotated from a position of flexion, abduction, and external rotation.[105,108] Therapeutic injection of the bursa may be useful to confirm this diagnosis and to provide temporary pain relief.

Internal Derangement

Our understanding of the multifactorial conditions contributing to internal derangements of the hip has undergone significant maturation in the past 10 to 15 years. At the time that MR arthrography of the hip was gaining popularity, we looked at labral pathology as an isolated entity similar to a meniscal tear in the hip.[11,24,35,109–115] These tears were identified as a cause of hip pain. They were frequently identified in young adults with hip pain and usually were not associated with any significant event. Cartilage defects frequently were associated with labral tears and were perceived as companion abnormalities.[11,12] The presence of a labral tear was thought to be a factor in the development of osteoarthritis.

In parallel with our exploration of the significance of labral tears, the concept of femoroacetabular impingement was undergoing development and refinement. Femoroacetabular impingement is the result of a wide spectrum of anatomic abnormalities within the hip that lead to abnormal contact between the femoral head and neck during motion of the hip.[110,116–122] Impingement results in the labral tears and cartilage defects that had been well recognized but not fully explained. The triad of abnormalities including abnormal head–neck morphology, anterosuperior cartilage damage, and anterosuperior labral pathology is extremely common, occurring in 88% of patients with symptoms of impingement.[123] This damage to the acetabular labrum and cartilage leads to alterations in the mechanics of the joint, further increasing damage to the joint. This damage culminates in osteoarthritis. Thus we now recognize that labral pathology is one phase in a sequence of abnormalities and events that culminate in osteoarthritis. To appropriately treat the labral pathology, the underlying anatomic abnormality must be addressed.[116] The presence of osteoarthritis, the end stage of this process, indicates a poor outcome for any surgical intervention.[9,124]

While labral pathology is most commonly the result of impingement, it may result from an isolated injury to the hip. Hip dislocations may also result in injury to the acetabular labrum.[125–128] With transverse acetabular fractures the labrum may also be injured.[129] The damaged or displaced labral fragment may prevent anatomic reduction and should always be considered when reduction is not satisfactory.

Impingement

Femoroacetabular impingement is most commonly the result of anatomic alteration within the hip joint, although it may occasionally be seen in patients with normal anatomy with a superphysiologic range of motion. Impingement is more commonly seen in active individuals rather than sedentary persons.[119] For discussion purposes, impingement is divided into two types: cam impingement and pincer impingement. In reality, however, both mechanisms are commonly present in a single hip.[117] Intervention in these patients is directed toward restoration of the normal anatomy.[116,130]

The anatomic alterations underlying impingement may be secondary to another insult to the hip including developmental dysplasia, Legg-Calvé-Perthes disease, slipped capital femoral epiphysis, as well as posttraumatic and postoperative deformities.[115,118,121,131–137] Most cases of impingement, however, are due to more subtle changes within the femoral head and neck or acetabulum.

Cam Impingement

The cam mechanism of impingement is the result of an abnormal femoral head–neck relationship. It is more common than pincer impingement and is typically seen in young active males. Conditions underlying cam impingement include decreased femoral anteversion, abnormal femoral head–neck offset, shallow taper between the femoral head and neck, nonspherical femoral head, a femoral neck "bump" or osseous excrescence, pistol grip deformity, and generalized enlargement of the femoral head (coxa magna).[119,130,138,139] Radiographs are extremely useful in identifying many of these anatomic alterations.[140] The alpha angle has been described to quantify the abnormal head neck relationship (Fig. 9.14).[122]

In this form of impingement osseous excrescences or enlargement of the femoral neck prevent the normal movement of the femur within the acetabulum, most commonly with flexion, internal rotation, and adduction. With this action the abnormal head–neck junction does not "clear" the acetabulum. The anterior aspect of the neck, where most structural abnormalities occur, impinges on the anterosuperior acetabular rim. The abnormal portion of the neck acts as a wedge that is driven between the articular cartilage and labrum, leading to separation of these two structures.[117] The primary damage

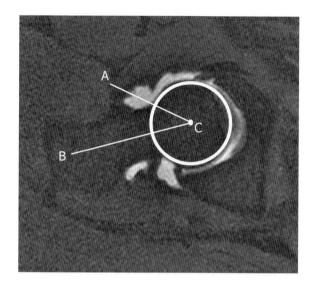

FIG. 9.14. The alpha angle. This angle is used for identifying an abnormal femoral head neck relationship. It is constructed by identifying the center (C) of the femoral head. A circle is draw around the circumference of the femoral neck. A line is then drawn along the long axis of the femoral neck through point C (line BC). Next a line is drawn from point C to the point where the femoral neck and the circle meet (line AC). The angle ACB should be less than 50 degrees.

on the acetabular side of the joint is to the articular cartilage.[117] The cartilage damage begins at the margin of the joint and progresses more centrally (outside to inside delamination) as the injury progresses. As this delamination continues the articular cartilage is torn from the labrum and initially the labrum maintains a stable attachment to the rim.[117]

Pincer Impingement

The pincer mechanism of impingement is not as commonly seen as the cam mechanism. The pincer mechanism most typically occurs in middle-aged women who are active. It also occurs during flexion and internal rotation. In this type of impingement the underlying anatomic condition resides at the acetabular rim. The acetabular rim in these cases extends more laterally with over-coverage of the femoral head. The over-coverage is most commonly isolated to the anterosuperior aspect of the joint. This condition may be seen with excessive acetabular retroversion, protrusio acetabuli, and coxa profunda.[110,141,142] When the femoral head rotates within the acetabulum, the neck impinges on the overextended acetabulum. The primary site of damage in this condition is the labrum. It is caught or "pinched" between the femoral neck and the acetabular rim, and the damage is usually intrasubstance tearing of the labrum.[117] Articular cartilage damage is secondary. The articular cartilage damage, while more extensive from anterior to posterior than cam impingement, does not extend as deeply into the joint.[117] Countercoup injuries are frequently observed with this type of impingement with the contact anteriorly acting as a lever that drives the head posteriorly.[117]

Labral Tears

Labral pathology encompasses both labral intrasubstance tears and detachments, and in the literature the term *labral tears* commonly encompasses both of these abnormalities. Detachments are more common than intrasubstance tears.[12] Most labral pathology occurs in the anterior and anterosuperior aspect of the joint.[7,9,11,12,19,20,23,24,33,38,114,124,143] Less commonly involved are the posterosuperior and anteroinferior portions of the labrum. Posteroinferior pathology is not commonly seen. Posterior lesions are typically the result of trauma or dysplasia.[11,12] The tear extends beyond one quadrant in up to 32% of cases, and this extension correlates with arthroscopically unstable tears.[7,11,19,144] Tears at multiple separate sites may be seen in 6.9% of patients.[11] In cases with anterior and posterior tears the sequence of events is hypothesized to be anterior damage first leading to instability and hinging of the femoral neck along the anterior rim driving the head into the posterior aspect of the joint, as seen with pincer impingement.[11]

Magnetic resonance arthrography is the ideal tool for detection of labral pathology. A fragment may or may not be displaced. Labral detachments involve separation of the labral from the acetabular rim and are identified by contrast material interposed between the labrum and the rim as seen in Figure 9.15.[23,33] Detachments may be complete or partial, with or without a displaced fragment as demonstrated in Figure 9.16. Labral tears are identified by the presence of intrasubstance contrast material.[23,33] As shown in Figure 9.17, tears and detachments may occur in the same labrum. Up to 90% of labral pathology is in the form of a detachment.[7,20,24]

A staging system for tears based on MR arthrography findings has been developed by Czerny et al.[20] This staging system combines features of the perilabral recess and the presence of intrasubstance contrast. Any obliteration of the perilabral sulcus is considered abnormal. An arthroscopic classification system for labral pathology has been described. Labral tears may be longitudinal and peripheral, and radial fibrillated or flap tears.[114] In Lage et al.'s[114] study of 267 patients with 37 labral tears, 56.8% of tears were radial flap, 21.6% radial fibrillated, 16.2% longitudinal peripheral, and 5.4% were unstable. At least one study has concluded that the Czerny classification system does not correlate with the arthrographic staging system.[144] Further work in this area will be needed to develop terminology that correlates MRA with the arthroscopic appearance

Evaluation of every MR arthrogram of the hip should include scrutiny of the articular cartilage. The articular cartilage of the hip is relatively thin compared to the knee, and defects may require a detailed inspection to be identified. Evaluation is further hampered by the contact between the two articular surfaces. Cartilage defects are identified by the presence of the bright signal of contrast within the less intense cartilage layer. Cartilage damage may present as signal changes within the cartilage without a defect. Subchondral signal changes may direct attention to the over-

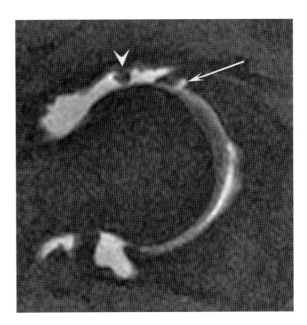

FIG 9.15. Partial detachment. Contrast material tracks between the labrum and the acetabular rim along the anterior margin of the joint (arrow) on this fat suppressed T1-weighted with intraarticular contrast. An air bubble is noted (arrowhead).

lying cartilage as these signal changes are often the result of cartilage abnormalities.

Associated Abnormalities

A host of associated abnormalities are seen in patients with labral tears and impingement. Osseous metaplasia within the labrum is a frequent finding especially in patients with pincer impingement.[9,145] Hypertrophy of the labrum is commonly seen in association with development dysplasia.[136,146] Os acetabuli, once believed to be accessory ossicles of the hip, now are attributed greater significance. They are likely fatigue fractures of the acetabular rim, a result of the chronic stress generated by contact between the femur and acetabulum.[134] They are another imaging indicator of impingement.

Synovial Herniation Pits, and Fibrocystic Changes of the Femoral Neck

Synovial herniation pits on the femoral neck were once believed to be benign lesions that, while typically asymptomatic, occasionally enlarged or became symptomatic.[147–149] These defects were identified in 5% of the patient population. These defects are now believed to be a direct result of the impingement process and thus a radiographic and MR indicator of impingement.[110,123,150] In association with the impingement process they are known as fibrocystic changes of the femoral neck (Fig. 9.18). Typically located on the anterior aspect of the femoral neck distal to the physeal scar, these lesions are recognized as well-defined rounded areas of varying size. The lesions are of

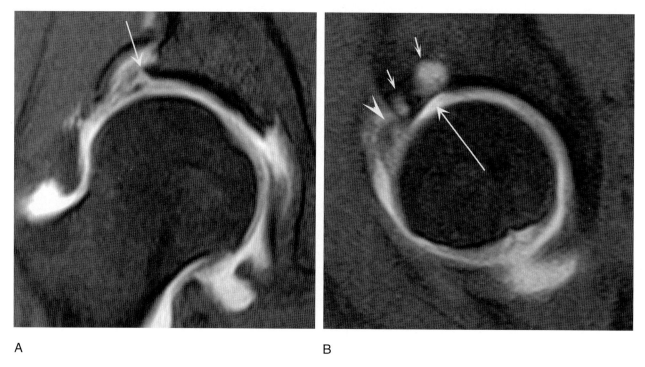

A   B

Fig. 9.16. Complete labral detachment. Fat suppressed T1-weighted coronal (A) and sagittal (B) images demonstrate complete separation of the labrum from the acetabulum (arrow in A). The labrum is hypertrophied with intrasubstance tearing (arrowhead in B). Uncovering of the lateral aspect of the femoral head is present, consistent with mild dysplasia. Extensive cartilage loss is present adjacent to labral injury (long arrow in B) with accompanying subchondral signal changes and cyst formation (short arrows in B).

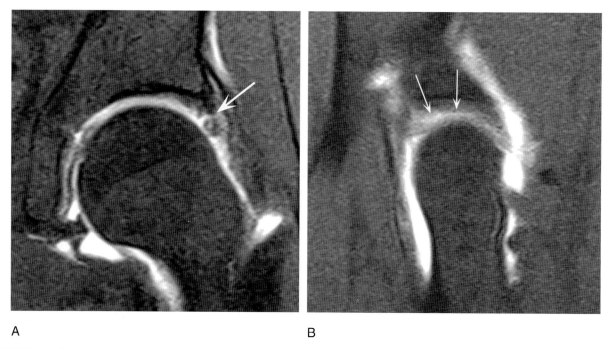

A   B

Fig 9.17. Partial labral detachment and intrasubstance tear. Fat suppressed T1-weighted coronal (A) and sagittal (B) images reveal a partial detachment (arrows) of the labrum. The extent along the superior aspect of the joint is well seen on the sagittal image. On the coronal image a small intrasubstance tear is present and the articular cartilage adjacent to the labrum is irregular consistent with damage.

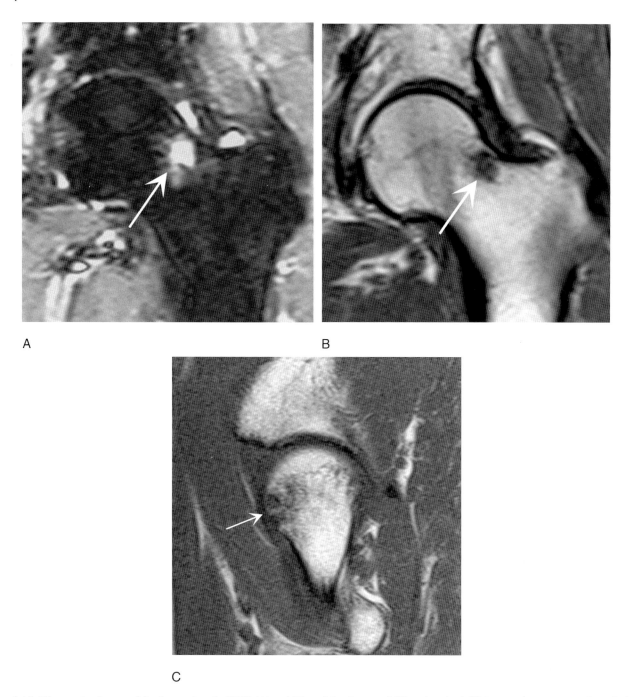

FIG. 9.18. Fibrocystic change of the femoral neck. STIR (A) and T1-weighted coronal (B) and sagittal (C) images demonstrate a large lesion in the anterosuperior aspect of the femoral neck (arrow).

lower signal on T1-weighted images with bright signal on fluid-sensitive sequences.[151] Occasionally the T2-signal will also be low. The MR characteristics reflect the mixed fibrous and cystic changes. A low signal intensity rim is consistent with the thin sclerotic border.

Paraarticular Cysts

Paraarticular cysts of the hip may accompany labral abnormalities.[20,33,35,123,152–156] More commonly seen in patients with developmental dysplasia, these cysts are not limited to that patient population. They are commonly found in the posterosuperior aspect of the joint.[155] Recognition of a cyst on a nonarthrographic study should prompt a search for labral pathology. These cysts may be completely soft tissue in nature but may extend into bone.[152] In other cases they may extend into the pelvis.[156,157]

Rupture of the Ligamentum Teres

The function of the ligamentum teres is unknown. It reaches maximal tension in flexion, adduction, and external rotation.[158]

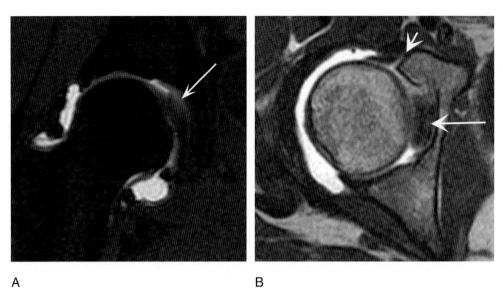

A   B

FIG. 9.19. Ligamentum teres injury. Fat-suppressed T1-weighted coronal (A) and axial (B) images after the intraarticular administration of contrast demonstrate thickening of the ligamentum teres adjacent to the fovea capitus (arrow in A) and enlargement of the cross section of the ligament on the axial image (arrows in B). These findings are associated with partial tears of the ligament.

The significance of injury to the structure is also unknown; however, disruption of the ligamentum has been associated with pain.[158,159] As with tears of other ligaments, injury to this ligament may result from a wide variety of trauma that may result in partial or complete disruption.[10,158] Complete disruption is commonly the result of a violent force such as occurs during severe football or hockey injury or may be associated with abnormal mechanics such as in dysplasia.[158,159] Complete disruption may occur as an avulsion injury with an attached bone fragment as or a ligamentous disruption. Partial tears may also occur as shown in Figure 9.19.[160]

Chronic Groin Pain

A multifaceted interaction of forces across the anterior aspect of the pelvis can lead to both acute and chronic injury involving the anterior structures of the pelvis. Acute injuries are typically well delineated and respond nicely to treatment. The causes of chronic groin pain are more complex, and imaging features and clinical implications of these conditions more intricate.[161] The structures implicated in chronic groin pain include the symphysis pubis, the pubic rami, the adductor tendon origins, the insertions of the anterior abdominal wall musculature, and the inguinal canal. Abnormalities of the hip, sacroiliac joint, musculature of the back, and abnormalities of the lower extremity contribute to abnormal stresses across the anterior pelvis.[63,162,163] Injuries to this area result from sprinting, twisting, and kicking activities, and are especially common in soccer players, rugby players, runners, Australian-rules football play-

ers, and hockey players. The injuries are more common in men than in women.

The abnormalities of chronic groin pain tend not to be isolated, but rather multiple abnormalities are typically present, reflecting the complex interrelationship among these structures.[164,165] There is likely a continuum of injury with initial damage to one of the supporting structures leading to instability at the symphysis, followed by evidence of ongoing damage at the symphysis and eventual appearance of the sequelae of damage to the symphysis. Imaging may occur at any time in this cycle, and since the inciting force continues with continuation of athletic activity, the cycle may repeat itself with overlap of various stages of injury.

Symphysis Pubis

The symphysis pubis often demonstrates radiographic and MRI abnormalities in both symptomatic and asymptomatic athletes. The term *osteitis pubis* is frequently used when referring to the radiographically abnormal symphysis pubis. This term may be confusing since clinically it is often used to describe a condition that includes a combination of pubic bone marrow edema and chronic groin pain.

The radiographic changes of osteitis pubis include narrowing or widening of the joint, movement greater than 2mm which may only be evident on flamingo views (views with weight bearing on a single leg), mild beaking (<3mm), osteopenia or sclerosis, erosions, osteophytes, and cyst formation. Frequently identified in the athletic population at risk for groin injury, these radiographic abnormalities do not have a significant correlation with current groin pain.[2,162,166–168] There is an association with a history of groin pain.[168] These changes are best interpreted as the result of chronic repetitive stress to the symphysis pubis or may be the sequelae of a more significant injury.

Pubic Bone Marrow Edema

At MRI bone marrow edema adjacent to the symphysis pubis is a common finding in both the symptomatic and asymptomatic athletic populations. Pubic bone marrow edema has been detected in 37% to 61% of asymptomatic athletes.[167–169] The significance of this finding in the asymptomatic population is unknown.[167] Magnetic resonance findings in the asymptomatic athlete that correlated with a history of groin pain and tenderness included bone marrow edema greater than 2 cm in length, cyst formation, symphyseal fluid, symphyseal beaking greater than 3 mm, and joint irregularity (Fig. 9.20).[168] These changes are likely the result of a previous injury that is no longer symptomatic. Non–activity-related causes of an abnormal symphysis such as infection should always be considered.

When associated with ongoing symptoms the condition is known as the clinical form of osteitis pubis (traumatic osteitis pubis) or pubic bone stress injury.[163] The injury is believed to be the result of ongoing insult to the supporting structures of the symphysis including the adductor and gracilis muscles and the anterior abdominal wall.[2,170]

Diffuse pubic bone marrow edema, located adjacent to the symphysis and contacting the subchondral bone, should be considered distinct from unilateral or bilateral focal bone marrow edema within a pubic ramus distant from the symphysis pubis. This finding is consistent with pubic ramus stress injury, which may be a precursor of stress fracture. In their study, Slavotinek et al.[167] found linear hyperintense subchondral signal changes on T2-weighted images with linear low signal adjacent in 31% asymptomatic individuals at the start of the season. The authors were able to demonstrate a relationship among preseason groin pain, linear hyperintense subchondral signal on T2-weighted images, pubic bone tenderness, and eventual training restriction.[167]

The intraarticular disk of the symphysis may also be abnormal. Extrusion of the intraarticular disk of the symphysis is common, and typically occurs posteriorly and may be seen superiorly (Fig. 9.21).[171] The central cleft of the intraarticular disk, a common finding, is identified as a bright line on fluid-sensitive sequences. Extension of this bright line to the right or left of midline along the inferior border of the pubis indicates the presence of a secondary cleft that correlates with symphyseal injection findings.[172,173] The secondary cleft is either within the adductor tendons or along the adjacent fascial planes, indicating injury to those structures.

Adductor Tendon Abnormalities

Injuries related to the adductor muscles include avulsions and tenoperiosteal and musculotendinous injuries. Musculotendinous injuries are recognized by bright intramuscular signal on fluid-sensitive sequences. These injuries respond well to treatment and typically to do not contribute to chronic problems. Avulsion and tenoperiosteal injuries are more likely to contribute to chronic groin pain. The gracilis syndrome entails avulsion of the gracilis tendon from the symphysis and adjacent pubis.[174] This avulsion may be accompanied by a small fleck of bone from the inferior medial border of the pubis.[174] Adductor longus tenoperiosteal injuries are recognized by bright signal on fluid-sensitive sequences at the tendon origin from the pubic ramus. As contributors to stability at the symphysis pubis, abnormality within these tendons may or may not be associated with changes of osteitis pubis or pubic bone marrow edema.

Abdominal Wall Abnormalities and Sportsman's Hernia

Abnormalities of the anterior abdominal wall associated with groin pain include hernias, injuries to the rectus abdominus insertion, abnormalities of the conjoined tendon, inguinal hernia, posterior inguinal wall deficiency, as well as tears of the external oblique aponeurosis leading to nerve entrapment.[174–176] In one study of 189 athletes, symptoms were attributable to hernias in 50%, and this should be one of the first diagnostic considerations in patients with groin pain.[164,177] While most hernias should be identifiable on physical examination, all are not. Some hernias are only apparent with straining, as in athletic activity, and in their

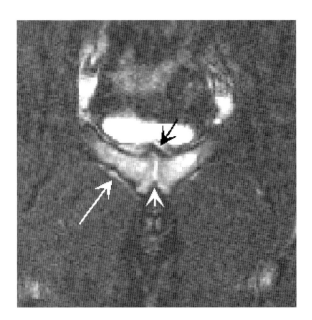

FIG. 9.20. Abnormal symphysis pubis and adductor tendons. STIR coronal image reveals extensive edema within both superior pubic rami. Bright signal is present within the intraarticular disk (short white arrow). Subtle edema tracks along the adductor tendon origins (long arrow). Beaking of the superior aspect of the symphysis is present (black arrow).

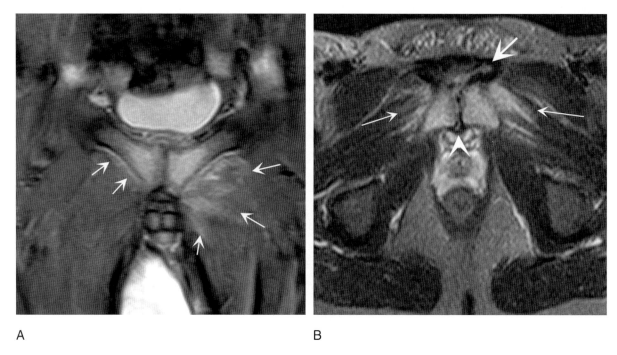

A   B

FIG. 9.21. Abnormal symphysis pubis and adductor tendons. T2-weighted coronal (A) and fat-suppressed T2-weighted axial (B) image demonstrate extensive edema within the superior pubic rami accompanied by extensive edema within the adductor musculature (arrows in A, long arrows in B), especially on the left. Abnormal signal is present with the origin of the left adductor longus tendon (short arrow in B). Posterior extrusion of the symphysis is noted (arrowhead in B).

earliest stages are evident only as abdominal musculofascial abnormalities.[170] These earliest stages of hernia formation have been dubbed the sportsman's hernia. This condition is the most likely cause of pubalgia, which is defined as groin pain with an inconclusive physical examination.[178] Magnetic resonance imaging findings of the sportsman's hernia include rectus abdominus muscle edema, rectus atrophic changes, generalized thinning of the fascial layers of the anterior abdominal wall, focal bulge of the anterior abdominal wall, and widening of the anteroposterior (AP) diameters of the inguinal canal.[170] Additional findings include edema within the pubic bones, and within the adductor and obturator muscle group.[170,179] The use of dynamic MRI may contribute to identification of the sportsman's hernia.[180]

B. Orthopedic Perspective: Hip Magnetic Resonance Imaging

Carlos A. Guanche

Painful hips in the young and middle-aged patient impose a diagnostic challenge. Approximately 2.5% of all sports-related injuries are located in the hip region, and this figure increases to 5% to 9% of high school athletes.[181] With improved imaging modalities and an increasing capacity to treat intraarticular pathology, more treatments have become available. Arthroscopic treatment of intraarticular and extraarticular lesions of the hip continues to expand. As a result, our awareness of many hip problems has increased. We now have more definitive answers for the active patient without radiographic evidence of degenerative joint disease, and less commonly must formulate vague diagnoses such as generalized hip sprains, strains, or tendonitis. One of the most important developments in the management of these injuries has been the expanding armamentarium of imaging modalities.

When a pathologic process alters the function of the homeostatic chemical and mechanical forces within a joint, articular cartilage breakdown can occur and joint deterioration may follow. This is especially important in the hip, as it often sees loads of up to five times body weight. It is therefore important to have a sense of the specific indications for further imaging in anticipation of surgical intervention since the majority of intraarticular pathology does not respond well to conservative treatment.

The orthopedic literature is vague and generally poor in its delineation of the history, physical examination findings, and treatment of hip pathologies, with the exception of arthritis. Of late, an expansion of knowledge in this area has occurred, most likely as a result of the expanding armamentarium that allows minimally invasive surgery about the hip. With this in mind, this section discusses the current understanding of the history and physical examination findings as they relate to the pathologies being treated in many individuals.

History

As with any other area of the body, the history is important in determining the necessary physical examination maneuvers that will help in making a variety of diagnoses. A patient who develops an insidious onset of stiffness and pain superimposed on an acute event that significantly increases symptomatology is different from one without a prodromal phase who suffers an injury. In addition, significant congenital problems may have some bearing on the symptomatic pathology, and it is important to discuss them at the time of the initial examination.

The important factors in the history that impact the need for various imaging modalities include the presenting injury and its mechanism of injury. In events where significant energy has been dissipated, such as a motor vehicle accident, the likelihood of a fracture is high. Conversely, in twisting and minimal contact injuries, the likely etiology of the acute symptoms is probably a labral tear, and thus standard radiography is of little value.

Another factor that impacts the need for further imaging is lack of motion, or more precisely stiffness. In cases where the onset has been gradual and not associated with significant trauma, the most likely diagnosis is arthritis. In cases, where significant trauma has occurred in the recent past, the possibility of an acute soft tissue injury is more likely, and this impacts the imaging modality likely to be employed.

Locking or mechanical symptoms are another group to consider with regard to the imaging modality of choice. In situations where the event is acute and associated with a trauma, the possibility of a subluxation or dislocation must be considered. Where radiographs are positive for loose bodies, a computed tomography (CT) scan may be of more value than an MRI (Fig. 9.22). Conversely, in cases where mechanical symptoms are present yet no radiographic confirmation is found, the likely next step is an MRI. In most situations an intraarticular gadolinium enhanced arthrogram should be employed to maximize the likelihood of delineating the entire pathology that is present (Fig. 9.23).

Finally, the sport that caused the problem is also important. Many athletes in sports requiring repetitive twisting and cutting maneuvers are predisposed to specific pathologic entities about the hip.[182] In those cases, a combination of imaging modalities may be required to delineate the entire problem. It is not unusual for a higher level athlete to have a combination of bony impingement, acetabular version abnormalities, and significant labral and chondral surface abnormalities—all of which are important with respect to the overall diagnosis, treatment, and outcome of surgical procedures performed in that joint (Fig. 9.24).

Physical Examination

The physical examination of a painful hip has been limited historically in its ability to differentiate among intraarticular pathologies. In most cases, the workup and examination has

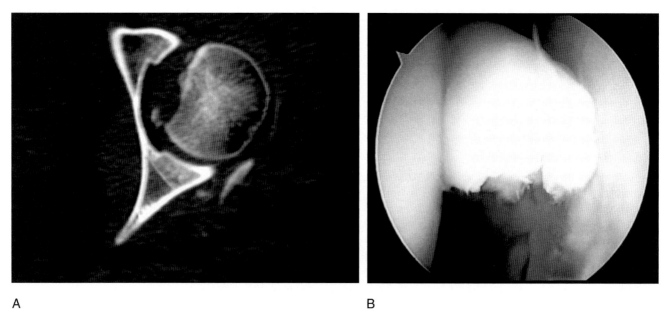

A   B

FIG. 9.22. (A) Computed tomography (CT) scan of a patient with a history of a traumatic hip dislocation, depicting a loose body within the joint. (B) Arthroscopic visualization of loose body.

been limited to the diagnosis of synovitis, infection, and arthritis, without much regard to other entities. Recently, a concerted effort has been made in the delineation of other problems, all of which have relevance to the state-of-the-art treatment of intraarticular problems, namely hip arthroscopy. Obviously, the ability to image the hip with high-resolution magnets and

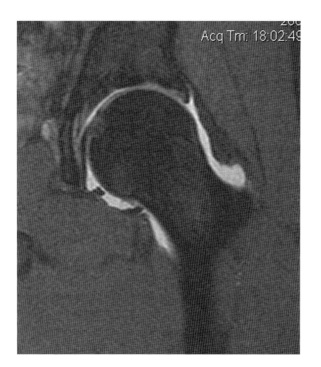

FIG. 9.23. MRI image (T2-weighted) with gadolinium arthrogram depicting a labral tear as well as a chondral flap of the weight-bearing acetabulum.

the development of algorithms for exact imaging sequences have helped push the diagnosis and treatment of many entities to a higher level of diagnostic acumen.

A series of diagnostic maneuvers has been delineated in order to determine the likely intraarticular problem that is being evaluated. With that in mind, the obvious first steps include an evaluation for muscular atrophy and limb-length discrepancy. These are potentially congenital factors that may be significant in the overall problem being treated. In addition, an obvious soft tissue contracture, especially in flexion, will impact the treatment of many entities about the hip.

As with any other joint examination, focal areas of tenderness are sought. Pain over the greater trochanter may be indicative of trochanteric bursitis, while anterior groin pain to palpation may be indicative of either a hernia or a muscle injury. In general, intraarticular injuries do not cause any focal superficial pain to palpation and, in fact, many patients complain of a deep-seated pain in the groin. A common sign that has been documented in the literature is the C-sign.[183] The typical patient cups the affected hip with the thumb over the posterior aspect of the joint and the long finger over the anterior portion of the hip (Fig. 9.25).

Following the determination of muscular symmetry, rotation is assessed. It is important to begin with the patient in the seated position and assess internal and external rotation in both hips (Fig. 9.26). Following this maneuver, the patient is positioned supine and again assessed for internal and external rotation with the legs in neutral flexion (Fig. 9.27). The degree of external rotation in this position is important with respect to instability. Greater than a 15-degree difference in external rotation (with the symptomatic side being greater) indicates an

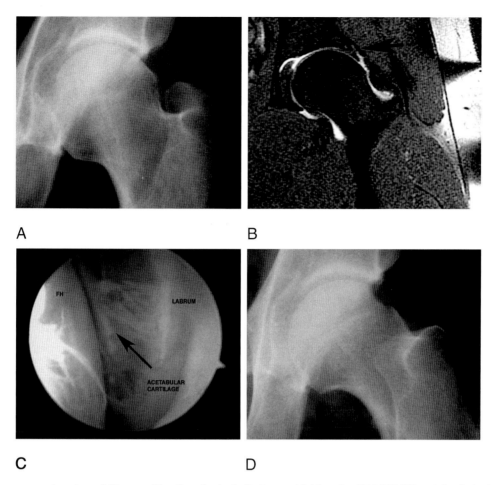

FIG. 9.24. (A) Anteroposterior view of 19-year-old college basketball player with hip pain. (B) MRI (T2-weighted) depicting a labral tear (arrow) as well as a femoral neck impingement lesion. (C) Arthroscopic view of patient with view of significant chondral delamination of the acetabular weight-bearing dome. (D) Postoperative AP view of the hip depicting the proximal femoral neck resection area at the head and neck junction. FH, Femoral head.

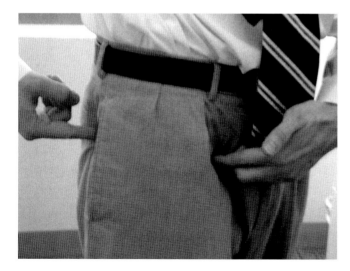

FIG. 9.25. The C-sign. Rather than cup the joint with one hand, patients with smaller hands will reach to the back with one hand and to the front with the other, and state that the pain is somewhere between these two points.

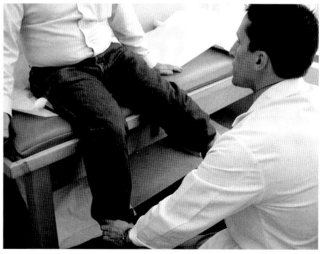

FIG. 9.26. The seated examination of internal rotation of the hips. It is important to determine the motion on the presumably normal contralateral side.

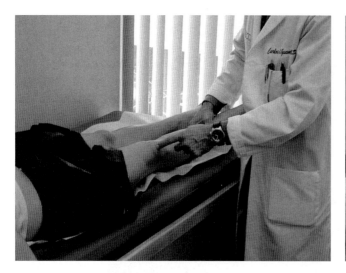

FIG. 9.27. Supine external rotation test. The patella can be used as a guide to indicate the amount of external rotation. Both sides should be assessed.

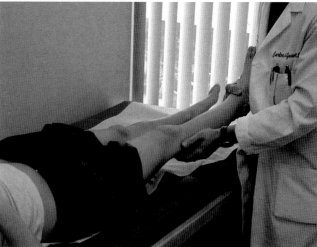

FIG. 9.28. Axial distraction of the extremity. The examiner stands at the foot of the table and pulls on the extremity at the ankle, while encouraging relaxation from the patient. A sense of the ability to sublux the femoral head out of the joint is obtained.

element of anterior capsular laxity that will obviously impact further imaging modalities.

With respect to internal rotation (in either the supine or flexed position), any difference greater than 10 degrees (with the affected side being less) indicates either a capsular contracture or bony impingement. The quality of the endpoint in this examination maneuver is important, in that a hard endpoint is indicative of bony impingement while a soft endpoint is more prognostic of capsular or labral pathology. The degree of bony involvement dictates the need for further assessment of the bony anatomy, perhaps with a CT scan, which, in many cases includes a three-dimensional reconstruction to look for femoral and acetabular pathologies such as abnormal acetabular version or femoral offset.

The next diagnostic maneuver should be the application of axial distraction to both lower extremities to gain a sense of the inherent laxity within the joint (Fig. 9.28). A sense of apprehension by the patient or objective translation with reduction following release of the traction is indicative of hip instability.

A third maneuver that may further delineate anterior capsular laxity is that of anterior capsular stressing. To perform this maneuver, the patient is placed in the lateral decubitus position, with the affected side up. The affected leg is cradled by the examiner from behind and abducted about 45 degrees. With the other arm, the examiner applies an anteriorly directed force to the hip joint at the level of the greater trochanter (Fig. 9.29). A significant reproduction of the patient's pain or symptomatology is consistent with anterior capsular laxity. In addition, in patients with a predominantly anterior labral tear, mechanical symptoms may be reproduced.

While assessing the range of motion of the joint, the area should also be palpated for crepitus either with passive or active motion. As with other joints, crepitus is nonspecific and often not painful. However, its presence along with the exacerbation of pain with its generation will often indicate a mechanical etiology to the problem.

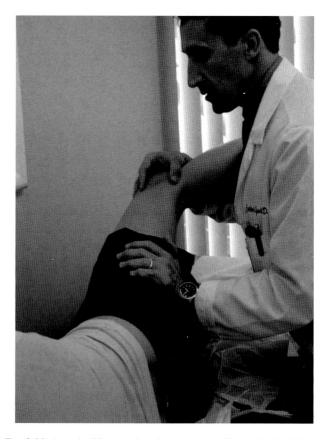

FIG. 9.29. Anterior hip apprehension maneuver. The patient's affected hip is above, while the examiner positions himself posteriorly. While one arm cradles the leg, the other is used to apply an anteriorly directed force to the hip over the greater trochanter.

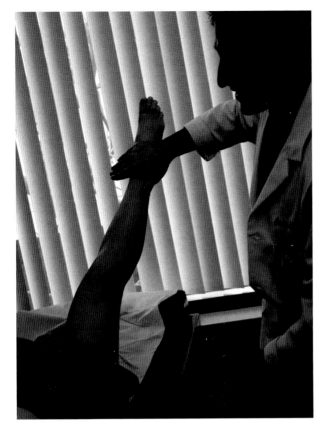

FIG. 9.30. Resisted straight leg raise. The patient is asked to hold the leg in the air, while the examiner forcefully pushes the leg down toward the table in an attempt to reproduce the patient's mechanical symptoms.

Finally, one maneuver that can reproduce the patient's mechanical symptoms and pain is that of the resisted straight-leg raise. This is performed with the patient supine and the affected leg raised in flexion. The examiner then forcefully pushes down on the extremity in an effort to push it down to the examining table[183] (Fig. 9.30). In patients with significant labral pathology, the pain that they typically experience with loading conditions is usually reproduced. It should be noted, however, that this is a very nonspecific maneuver that can be positive in many other pathologies such as arthritis and synovitis.

In a similar vein, the Thomas test correlated with surgical pathology.[184] This test is performed with bilateral hip flexion, followed by abduction and extension of the involved hip with a palpable or audible click, along with pain. A positive test has been correlated with a labral tear. Another test is the McCarthy maneuver: both hips are flexed while the affected hip is then extended, first in external rotation and then in internal rotation.[185] Hip extension in internal rotation stresses the anterior labrum and extension with external rotation elicits posterior pathology.

Specific Problems

To further delineate the management of hip injuries, the most commonly encountered pathologies are discussed in some detail. This serves to identify the necessary imaging modalities for definitive management of these entities. It is important to realize, however, that in many cases the obvious labral tear or loose body may simply be the secondary problem in any given hip. The treatment of the obvious pathology without treating the primary impingement, instability or capsular laxity may be a factor in a poor surgical outcome.

Labral Tears

The labrum is a rim of fibrocartilage that attaches to the base of the acetabular rim. It surrounds the perimeter of the acetabulum and is absent inferiorly where the transverse ligament resides. The labrum provides structural resistance to lateral motion of the femoral head within the acetabulum, enhances joint stability, and preserves joint congruity.[186] Similar to the meniscus, it also functions to distribute synovial fluid and provides proprioceptive feedback.[187]

A disruption of the acetabular labrum alters the biomechanical properties of the joint. The forces acting on the hip in the setting of a torn labrum often cause pain during sports participation in athletes. Patients with labral tears often present with mechanical symptoms, such as buckling, clicking, catching, or locking. Athletes may present with subtle findings, including dull, activity-induced, positional pain that fails to respond to rest. The most commonly reported cause of a traumatic labral tear is an externally applied force to a hyperextended and externally rotated hip.[188] However, a specific inciting event often is not identified, and the patient presents for evaluation after failed attempts at conservative management for groin pulls, muscle strains, or hip contusions.

Labral tears can be traumatic or acute, chronic, and in some cases degenerative in nature. The location of labral tears varies in population studies as a result of cultural differences, presumably. North American series have reported the vast majority of tears as being located anteriorly with acute tears resulting from sudden pivoting or twisting motions.[9] In contrast, in Asian populations, tears are more frequently found posteriorly and are associated with hyperflexion or squatting.[189]

Labral tears have been divided into four groups: radial flap tears, radial fibrillated tears, longitudinal peripheral tears, and mobile tears.[190] Radial flaps are the most common, followed by radial fibrillated, longitudinal peripheral, and mobile tears. In addition, degenerative tears have been subdivided based on location and the extent of the tear. Stage I degenerative tears are localized to one segment of an anatomic region, anterior or posterior. Stage II tears involve an entire anatomic region, and stage III tears are diffuse and involve more than one region (Fig. 9.31). The extent of the degenerative tear correlates to the degree of degenerative changes within the joint, with an increasing stage of degenerative labral tears correlating with erosive changes of the acetabulum or femoral head. The articular lesions are most often located adjacent to the labral tear, often at the labrochondral junction.[191]

Labral tears secondary to trauma generally are isolated to one quadrant depending on the direction and extent of the

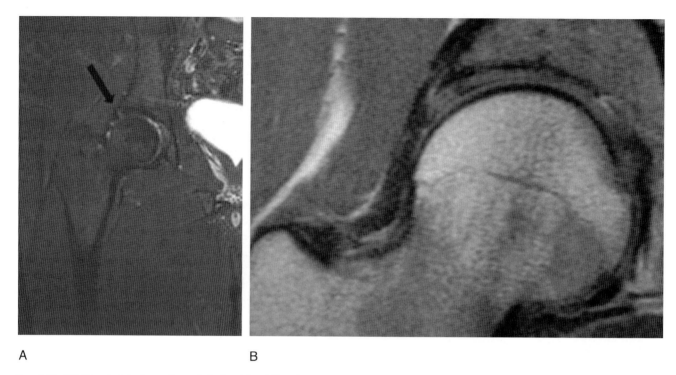

FIG. 9.31. (A) Simple labral tear (arrow) depicted in a T2-weighted study. (B) Complex labral tear depicted in a T1-weighted study.

trauma. For instance, patients with a known posterior sub-luxation or dislocations most frequently have posterior labral tears. If a bone fragment is avulsed as a result of a disloca-tion, the labral injury most often occurs on the capsular or peripheral region of the labrum and may be amenable to an arthroscopic repair.[192]

Idiopathic tears are often seen in athletic populations. Chronic, repetitive loading of the hip can subject the labrum to tensile and compressive forces and lead to tearing. Often, no specific injury is reported. The majority of patients partici-pate in sports requiring repetitive pivoting or twisting, such as football, soccer, basketball, or ballet. It has been theorized that recurrent torsional maneuvers subject the anterior portion of the articular–labral junction to recurrent microtrauma and eventual mechanical attrition.[192] It is this population that com-monly suffers from subtle instability of the hip; this entity, therefore, must be excluded in this group of patients.

The underlying cause of the labral injury should be delin-eated. There appear to be five common causes of labral tears: (1) trauma (2) laxity/hypermobility (3) bony impingement (4) dysplasia, and (5) degeneration.[193] The patient's characteris-tics, including age and activity, and radiographic and other imaging studies must be synthesized in order to determine the proper diagnosis. Isolated treatment of labral tears without addressing the primary factor will likely result in poor treat-ment outcomes.

Radiographs are often unremarkable when looking for a labral tear. Specific attention should be given to the superior neck, looking for subtle irregularities in the femoral head–neck

offset and decreased neck concavity compared to the contralat-eral side, which would suggest impingement (discussed later). Contrast-enhanced MRA is more sensitive than standard MRI at detecting intraarticular lesions of the hip.[194] In a compari-son of conventional MRI with MRA in the diagnosis of labral lesions, a sensitivity and accuracy of 80% and 65% for con-ventional MRI compared with 95% and 88% for MRA have been reported.[194] However, hip MRAs are not without frequent misinterpretation. One study found an 8% false-negative rate and a 20% false-positive interpretation of MRAs for all types of intraarticular pathology of the hip.[195] While MRAs offer a diagnostic advantage over conventional MRI for labral tears and other intraarticular pathology, their reported false-positive rate dictates cautious interpretation. Newer MRI modalities such as fast spin echo have improved the imaging capability of articular cartilage and may obviate the need for intraarticular gadolinium in the future.[196]

Magnetic resonance imaging may confirm the diagnosis, but the decision to proceed with operative intervention should be heavily weighted on refractory, mechanical symptoms. The majority of labral tears are treated by debridement; however, some tears are amenable to arthroscopic repair. Several studies have delineated the blood supply to the labrum and found blood vessels enter the labrum from the adjacent joint capsule, with the articular surface of the labrum having decreased vas-cularity.[197] Vascularity was detected in the peripheral one third of the labrum, while the inner two thirds are avascular, similar to the meniscus. Thus, peripheral tears have healing poten-tial, and repairs should be considered (Fig. 9.32). Repairable

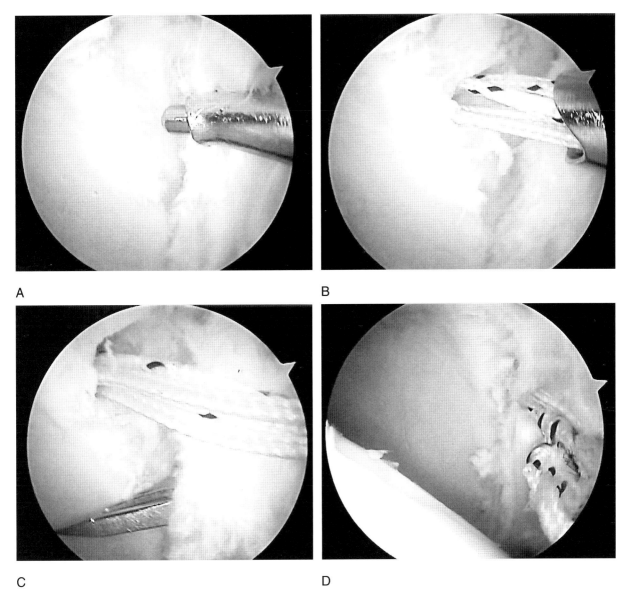

A   B

C   D

FIG 9.32. Steps involved in an arthroscopic labral repair of the hip. Patient is supine, and it is the left hip, visualized from the anterior portal while working through the anterolateral portal. (A) View of labral tear (to the right) and the exposed, decorticated bone with the anchor cannula in place. (B) Suture anchor in place. (C) Suture passing device being employed (lower portion) to pass suture through the labrum. (D) Completed labral repair.

peripheral tears, however, appear to be a rarity. McCarthy et al.[192] reported 436 consecutive hip arthroscopies performed over 6 years and treated 261 labral tears, all of which were located at the articular junction.

Loose Bodies

Loose bodies within the joint can cause pain and may mimic the snapping hip phenomenon. Anterior groin pain, episodes of clicking or locking, buckling, giving way, and persistent pain during activity suggest an intraarticular loose body. Loose bodies within the hip, whether ossified or not, have been correlated with locking episodes and inguinal pain.[198]

Loose bodies may occur as an isolated lesion following trauma or may present with many intraarticular lesions as seen in synovial chondromatosis. In cases of traumatic injury or dislocation, suspicion should be high for loose bodies to explain hip symptoms. Besides hip trauma, other diseases known to be associated with loose bodies include Perthes disease, osteochondritis dissecans, avascular necrosis, synovial chondromatosis, and osteoarthritis.[199–201] At this point, further imaging in the form of CT scanning versus MRI should be thoughtfully assessed depending on the most likely diagnosis. If the loose particles are more likely to be chondral or soft tissue, then MRI is more likely to yield useful diagnostic information. Although gadolinium-enhanced

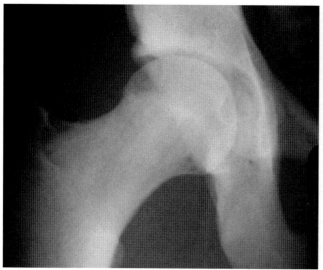

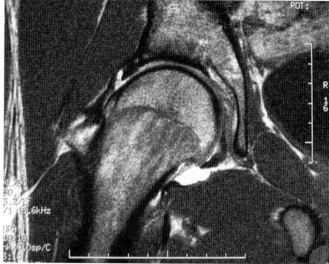

A   B

Fig. 9.33. A 47-year-old patient with mechanical symptoms in the hip. (A) AP radiograph depicting a femoral head–neck junction impingement lesion. (B) MRI (T1-weighted) depicting the soft tissue component of the impingement lesion as well as the degree of labral tearing.

MRA is currently the most promising imaging modality, it still has some limitations in reliably demonstrating chondral injuries, perhaps because of the static nature of the imaging study and the lack of hip joint distraction during the test. The use of cartilage-sensitive MRI for the detection of lesions, therefore, may be preferable,[202] although CT scans are highly sensitive for detection of suspected bony loose bodies and are more sensitive than MRI.[196]

Impingement

Femoral neck impingement against the acetabular labrum, femoroacetabular impingement (FAI), has been described as a structural abnormality of either the femoral neck or acetabulum that can lead to chronic hip pain and subsequent acetabular labral degenerative tears.[203] The repetitive microtrauma from the femoral neck abutting against the labrum produces degenerative labral lesions in the anterior-superior quadrant of the labrum. This mechanical impingement is believed to originate from either a "pistol grip" deformity of the femoral neck or a retroverted acetabulum (Fig. 9.33). Currently, evidence suggests that FAI may play a role in the cascade of hip osteoarthritis in some patients as a result of the structural proximal femoral head–neck abnormalities.[185,203–206] The typical patient is a middle-aged, athletic individual complaining of groin pain with activity. This often occurs during activities requiring hip flexion. Sports activities may cause symptoms, but often simple acts such as walking may aggravate the situation. Symptoms range from mild to severe and are often intermittent in presentation. The groin pain can become activity limiting, especially for athletes. Patients often have been seen by multiple physicians and have been given a wide range of diagnoses, such as a sports hernia, tendonitis, or synovitis (Fig. 9.34).

Impingement most often occurs at the extremes of motion. Abutment from the superior neck occurs in flexion, often with a variable degree of adduction and internal rotation. The repetitive trauma not only damages the labrum, but also can create adjacent chondral injuries (Fig. 9.35). One study noted that all patients treated operatively for impingement had labral lesions in the anterosuperior quadrant.[204] Furthermore, labral and cartilage lesions correlated with an absent anterolateral offset of the head–neck junction.

Although many patients will have been previously told that their hip radiographs are normal, subtle abnormalities may

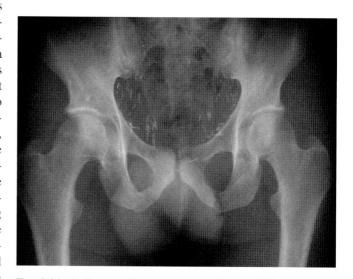

Fig. 9.34. A 43-year-old patient with a history of bilateral sports hernia repairs (note the multiple staples). Clinical examination and MRI of the hip delineated a labral tear and femoroacetabular impingement of the right hip. Note the lack of femoral offset as compared to the left hip.

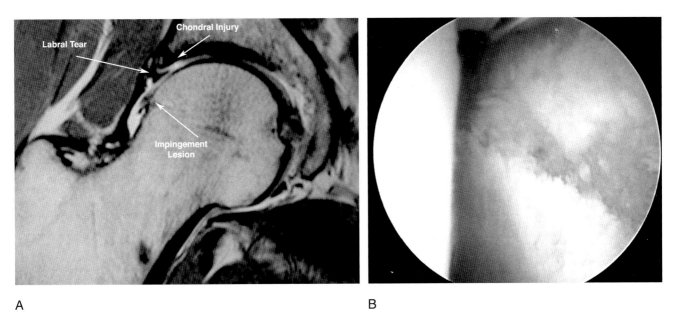

A   B

FIG. 9.35. Chondral delamination in a 25-year-old recreational athlete. (A) MRI image (T1-weighted) depicting the degree of chondral delamination that is apparent in many cases. (B) Arthroscopic view from the anterolateral portal showing the exposed subchondral bone (upper half of picture) following chondroplasty.

be present and should be suspected. An AP pelvis allows a gross comparison of both proximal femurs and acetabulae. The contour of the anterolateral neck should be compared to the unaffected side. A normal superior neck will have a distinctive concave appearance, with the concave contour takeoff at the head–neck junction through the neck–greater trochanter junction. A cross-table lateral radiograph is essential in addition to the AP radiograph. A properly taken cross-table radiograph demonstrates the appearance of the femoral neck, allowing for an additional view of the anterolateral neck (Fig. 9.36). Magnetic resonance arthrography detects labral pathology in addition to an assessment of the femoral head, neck, and acetabulum. In these cases, a CT scan

with three-dimensional reconstruction may add significant insight in the management of the bony anomalies causing the symptomatology (Fig. 9.37).

The employment of advanced imaging techniques such as delayed gadolinium-enhanced MRI of cartilage (dGEMRIC) may allow for the delineation of early and more subtle cartilaginous injuries.[207] This may further determine that earlier intervention in the form of arthroscopic or open resection of the offending bony injury may improve the outcome in these hips at risk.

Chondral Lesions

Articular surface lesions create an irregular contour of the joint surface and lead to abnormal intraarticular forces with motion and weight bearing, predisposing the patient to the development of progressive degenerative disease. Chondral injuries are found following trauma and have been associated with degenerative labral lesions as well as with early arthritic hips. McCarthy et al.[185] reported 74% of patients with a torn labrum had some degree of articular surface damage. In 80% of these patients, the labral and articular lesions occurred in the same quadrant. They also found an association among labral tears, the severity of articular injury, and age. The frequency and severity of cartilage lesions increased with age, and 24% of chondral injuries were observed arthroscopically in patients younger than 30 years of age compared to 81% of patients with chondral lesions in patients older than 60.

In many patients with acetabular chondral injuries and degenerative labral tears, there exists an element of degenerative arthritis. It is critical to assess plain radiographs for this factor. To that end, the first imaging study that should be done in patients with hip pain is a standing (or weight-bearing)

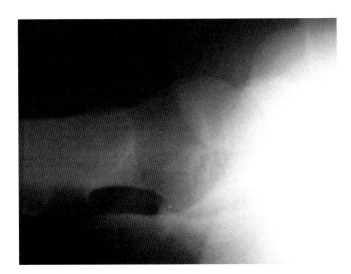

FIG. 9.36. Cross-table radiograph.

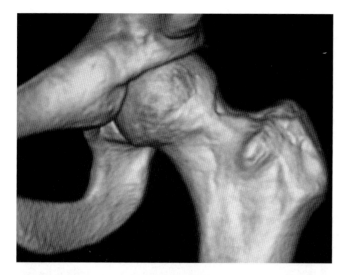

A

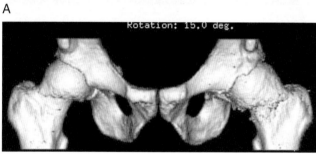

B

FIG. 9.37. CT scans with three-dimensional reconstructions. (A) Normal scan in a young athlete. (B) Abnormal bilateral hips in a 40-year-old former professional soccer player.

pelvic radiograph. A thoughtful assessment of the presence of narrowing of the joint should be undertaken as compared to the presumably normal contralateral hip.

Newer techniques may be available to assess the degree of chondral injury that is present. One such technique is dGEM-RIC. The basis for this tool is that the anionic molecule gado-pentetate[2-] (Gd-DTPA[2-]), if given time to penetrate cartilage tissue, will distribute in cartilage inversely to the concentration of negatively charged glycosaminoglycans (GAGs). These GAGs are typically decreased in concentration in normal articular cartilage with progression of degenerative changes. Thus, the concentration of Gd-DTPA[2-] will be relatively low in normal cartilage with abundant GAGs and will be relatively high in degraded cartilage from which GAGs have been lost.[207]

With the use of this technique, several studies have shown a direct correlation with the degree of GAG depletion within the articular cartilage of joints.[208] With the use of these techniques, it may be possible to identify a joint at risk or at the very least to stratify patients into categories that would be predictive with respect to outcome of invasive procedures.[207]

The arthroscopic debridement of patients with labral tears in the presence of degenerative joint disease or generalized

chondral pathology is generally poorer than in those with a normal articular surface.[208, 209] This is important to determine preoperatively since a patient with early arthritis is generally in a worse prognostic group than one with relatively normal cartilage. Unreasonable expectations with regard to outcome of patients undergoing hip arthroscopy can be obviated by thoughtfully discussing these expectations with the patient preoperatively.

Ligamentum Teres

The ligamentum teres is a triangular-shaped ligament arising from the posteroinferior region of the cotyloid fossa and inserting on the femoral head. It provides blood supply to the femoral head in children; however, its function in adults appears vestigial. Gray and Villar[210] suggest that the ligamentum teres injury causing symptoms without a history of traumatic hip dislocation may be more common than previously reported. The ligament becomes taut in flexion, adduction, and external rotation, and this has been a proposed mechanism for traumatic rupture.

Rupture of the ligament was the third most commonly encountered pathology during hip arthroscopy in another study.[212] In this analysis, 41 lesions of the ligamentum teres were found among 271 consecutive hip scopes. The lesions included 12 complete and 11 partial ruptures, while 18 ligaments were found to be hypertrophic or degenerative. Of the patients with traumatic injuries, 80% complained of mechanical symptoms. Preoperative diagnosis was made on imaging studies in only two of 23 cases. Eight lesions were isolated findings during arthroscopy, and 15 hips had additional pathology discovered during arthroscopy. All patients improved with arthroscopic debridement with an average preoperative hip score of 47 and postoperative score of 90 with more than a 1-year follow-up (Fig. 9.38).

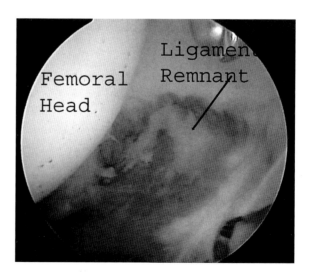

FIG. 9.38. Ligamentum avulsion in a 16-year-old dancer. Picture is of a left hip, visualized from the anterolateral portal.

Overall, ligamentum teres ruptures respond well to arthroscopic debridement. Ligamentum teres disruption has been known to occur with hip dislocations, and its occurrence following minor trauma and twisting injuries has been appreciated only in the past decade.[210,212] Twisting injuries often result in labral tears, so the clinician should consider ligamentum teres disruption as a potential source of pain after twisting injuries. The diagnosis of ligament tears remains elusive to imaging technology. This is an entity where a high index of suspicion should be maintained in the presence of mechanical symptoms and a history of trauma or twisting injury in order to make the diagnosis prospectively.

Capsular Laxity

Instability of the native hip is much less common than shoulder instability, but its presence can cause a significant amount of disability.[211] The hip relies less on the surrounding soft tissues for stability because it has a significant amount of inherent osseous stability. The labrum provides a great deal of stability at extremes of motion, especially flexion. With a torn or absent labrum, a great deal of force is transmitted through the capsule.[211] The capsule is very thick and robust in nearly all patients. The secondary development of capsular laxity may be due to the development of instability as a result of labral tearing. This can occur as either a single traumatic event or more likely form repetitive insult.

The labrum's ability to provide structural resistance to lateral and vertical motion of the femoral head within the acetabulum has been delineated by a poroelastic finite-element model.[186] It appears that the normal labrum helps to form a suction seal around the femoral head. With disruption of this ring, rotational instability or hypermobility of the hip can occur, leading eventually to symptomatic capsular laxity.[193]

Hip instability can be difficult to diagnose. Motions such as swinging a golf club or throwing a football often precipitate symptoms in active patients.[211] Similar to the shoulder, the causes of instability may be traumatic or atraumatic (due to cumulative microtrauma). The atraumatic or repetitive injury patients are often able to voluntary sublux or nearly dislocate the affected hip and may exhibit generalized ligamentous laxity. Some young patients may have an undiagnosed connective tissue disorders such as Ehlers-Danlos, Marfan, or Down syndromes. Bellabarba et al.[214] linked a group of atraumatic patients with idiopathic hip instability to subclinical capsular laxity from mild residual acetabular dysplasia. In the high-level athlete, the presentation of instability may be subtle, and a high degree of suspicion is necessary.

Traumatic dislocations of the native hip can also lead to capsular redundancy and clinical hip laxity. Liebenberg and Dommisse[215] described the development of capsular redundancy after recurrent anterior dislocation of the hip. They suggest that the presence of subclinical hip instability in these patients may results from a damaged capsulolabral complex.

The labrum may be torn and may not function as it did prior to the injury. Lack of the normal contribution of the labrum to stability requires the hip to rely more on the redundant hip capsule, thus stressing an already lax capsule, resulting in further instability.

One population subject to hip instability is the high-level or professional athlete. It has been recognized in sports requiring repetitive hip rotation with axial loading such as golf, figure skating, football, gymnastics, ballet, and baseball. A common injury pattern in athletes is labral degeneration combined with subtle rotational hip instability. This has been successfully treated by labral debridement and thermal capsulorrhaphy.[216] Early results of this procedure have yielded very positive results with 82% return to preinjury level of athletic competition.[182]

Synovial Plicae

In the knee, diagnosis and treatment of plica syndrome are well described.[217–219] Other joints, including the elbow, tibiotalar joint, and hip are also known to have synovial plicae that may become symptomatic, but few cases have been reported. Currently, six cases of symptomatic hip plicae have been reported in the literature.[220,221] Hip plicae have been described in cadavers and have been discovered in patients either through diagnostic arthroscopy or during arthrography.[220,221] Plicae are present as unusually large folds that are vulnerable to impingement between the articular surfaces. Repeated minor entrapments of a plica or one traumatic episode of entrapment can cause pain.

Patients may have a palpable click during the examination with passive motion. Plain films and nonenhanced MRI are likely to be reported as normal. Often, a gadolinium-enhanced MRA is obtained when there is the suspicion of a labral tear. Magnetic resonance arthrography can reveal an elongated ligamentous-like structure extending from the region of the femoral head–neck to a region of the hip capsule. Chondromalacia, if present, suggests repeated impingement from the plica on the articular surface has taken place.

Although plica syndrome of the hip seems to be rare, its true incidence may be underestimated. The presence of a symptomatically impinged hip plica should be considered in the differential diagnosis of recalcitrant hip pain. Suspicion of a hip plica that has failed conservative treatment should be treated with diagnostic arthroscopy. Debridement of the plica and thorough evaluation of the articular surfaces, looking in particular for associated chondromalacia from chronic plica impingement, will typically lead to symptom resolution.

Stress Fractures

A final area to consider with respect to hip injuries is that of stress fractures. Although stress fractures were described initially in military recruits and were clinically seen in these populations for many years, the incidence in the average civilian population has certainly exploded, perhaps as a result of the increased athletic participation level of the average person, especially as it relates to women participants.[222,223]

There is a distinction to be made in classifying these types of fractures into two different groups. The first is a fatigue fracture that occurs in normal bone when subjected to abnormal forces (such as the military recruit or marathon runner). The second subgroup is an insufficiency fracture where a fracture of abnormal bone subjected to normal forces occurs. This is typically seen in the elderly as well as other metabolically deficient persons, and will not be discussed in this chapter.

The most important principle in the diagnosis of a stress fracture is the clear association between the level of running (or other high-impact activity) and the likelihood of a fracture. This has been described as a dose-response relationship between the amount of training and the likelihood of injury.[224] The common denominator for all stress fractures is a change in the frequency, intensity, or duration of an activity to which the bone is unaccustomed.[225]

There also appears to be a predisposition for the development of stress fractures in females with rates as high as four to ten times higher than that of males.[224] Amenorrhea appears to be especially prevalent in endurance athletes with notable decreases in bone mineral density as compared those normally menstruating.[226] It is therefore important to obtain a complete menstrual and dietary history in the treatment of the female athlete with a potential stress fracture.[223]

The characteristic clinical presentation of a stress fracture depends, to some extent, on the area of the femur that is involved. The most confusing and dangerous are those of the femoral neck. The typical presentation of these injuries is activity-related groin pain that is relieved by rest, which brings to mind a rather large differential diagnosis.[222] In the more distal fractures, the pain may be more diffuse and typically is associated with more significant antalgia on presentation. Strenuous activity may intensify the pain to prohibit further athletic activity. Femoral shaft stress fractures, can present with symptoms that include anterior thigh pain, increasing with activity.[227] In some cases the patient presents with a complete fracture after having had minimal prodromal symptomatology.

Physical examination occasionally reveals tenderness to palpation but obviously depends on the level of the fracture. In general, the neck fractures would be difficult to palpate, and the pain is more diffuse. Limitation of the extremes of range of motion is often the only clinically obvious finding.[228] The other maneuvers that are typically employed with respect to hip pathology are useful in at least isolating the area of pathology. These maneuvers include log rolling of the extremity as well as a resisted (or active) straight leg raise. Other maneuvers that can be employed include percussion of the heel; however, this type of exam has not shown a high correlation with the present pathology.[229]

It is important to realize that a stress fracture can occur anywhere in the pelvis and femur, including the iliac wings (see Fig. 9.28).[229,230] The pubic stress fractures can present with diffuse hamstring spasm and adductor tightness and are not typically as dangerous with respect to likely displacement requiring surgical intervention. Likewise, iliac wing stress fractures can present with acute symptomatology, but are unlikely to cause significant residual once they heal.[229]

As a result of the variety of areas of stress fractures that can present with hip or groin pain, any imaging modality chosen should be carefully evaluated for its potential to delineate the cause of the problem as completely as possible. In many, if not most, situations, radiographs are normal at least in the first 2 to 4 weeks. There is a suggestion in the literature that up to 55% of stress fractures may never have positive radiographic findings.[223] Radiographs are typically good for the depiction of late changes such as cortical thickening or periosteal bone formation. Nonetheless, the standard of care would include AP pelvis view with a lateral view of the involved leg.

The use of bone scintigraphy has become commonplace in the diagnosis of stress fractures. The changes that accompany a stress fracture can be noted within 24 hours after the onset of pain in most healthy individuals.[231] However, in the older athlete and in patients with significant medical problems, the findings may lag for as much as 72 hours.[232] In the young patient, therefore, the use of bone scintigraphy with technetium-99 m methylene diphosphonate will yield a sensitivity of 93% to 100% and a specificity of 76% to 95% as compared with plain radiographs in the diagnosis of a stress fracture.[233] In addition, the study serves as a broad screening device for the rest of the pelvis and femur, should the diagnosis not be a femoral neck stress fracture.

More recently, the use of MRI has become more commonplace in the evaluation of these injuries. The characteristic findings of fatigue or insufficiency fractures on MRI include a decreased signal on T1-weighted images and increased signal on T2-weighted images as well as STIR sequences (see Fig. 9.29).[234] Although somewhat controversial, the findings are believed to represent edema secondary to microscopic trabecular fractures.[223]

The use of MRI in these injuries has been studied by several authors.[223] In most of the studies, MRI has been found to be superior as compared to radiographs and more importantly as compared to bone scintigraphy. The reason for the superiority has been the ability of MRI to delineate not only the acute findings of the stress fracture within the bone but also to help assess the soft tissues about the area of injury. In addition, the findings of edema and trabecular changes occur immediately as opposed to some of the metabolic events that need to take place before scintigraphy is positive.[232] The use of MRI, therefore, may supplant bone scintigraphy as the procedure of choice in the diagnosis of stress fractures.

The most important stress fracture to consider about the hip is that of the femoral neck. While the others are obviously important as well, the femoral neck fractures present a challenge with respect to diagnosis as well as treatment. While nondisplaced fractures have a relatively good prognosis with appropriate care, the treatment of the displaced fracture is a surgical emergency.[222,228] Expeditious open reduction and internal fixation is required to prevent further complications. Despite aggressive management, the prognosis in young patients is poor, with a prolonged period of non–weight-bearing and the potential to develop avascular necrosis in about 25% of cases up to 18 months after the fracture.[234]

Conclusion

Selecting the correct patient for an operative procedure and understanding the limitations of the currently available imaging studies is important for providing the patient with an appropriate diagnosis and treatment plan. A thorough synthesis of the history and physical examination is critical to establishing the proper diagnosis. Once the presumed pathology is identified, it is critical to maximize the yield from any given study by deciding the proper intervention(s) necessary. Individualizing each patient so that the most thorough assessment can be made with a minimum of interventions is ideal. This causes the least amount of inconvenience and discomfort to the patient, but also limits the expenses associated with treating these injuries.

The more common intraarticular injuries have certainly changed in their management in the last decade. For this reason, a more thoughtful assessment of each patient is critical to arrive at the proper diagnosis and more importantly to decide on the probability that surgical intervention would be of benefit. In addition, evolving imaging techniques are making it possible to identify problems earlier as well as allowing a possible stratification of patients based on physiologic parameters such as dGEMRIC.

References

1. Chandler SB. The iliopsoas bursa in man. Anat Rec 1934;58:235–240.
2. Robinson P, White LM, Agur A, et al. Obturator externus bursa: anatomic origin and MR imaging features of pathologic involvement. Radiology 2003;228:230–234.
3. Ferguson SJ, Bryant JT, Ganz R, et al. The acetabular labrum seal: a poroelastic finite element model. Clin Biomech 2000:15;463–468.
4. Ferguson SJ, Bryant JT, Ganz R, et al. The influence of the acetabular labrum on hip joint cartilage consolidation: a poroelastic finite element model. J Biomech 2000:33;953–960.
5. Ferguson SJ, Bryant JT, Ganz R et al. An in vitro investigation of the acetabular labrum seal in hip joint mechanics. J Biomech 2003;36;171–178.
6. Petersen W, Petersen F, Tillmann B. Structure and vascularization of the acetabular labrum with regard to the pathogenesis and healing of labral lesions. Arch Orthop Trauma Surg 2003;123:283–288.

7. Seldes RM, Tan V, Hunt J, et al. Anatomy, histologic features and vascularity of the adult acetabular labra. Clin Orthop Rel Res 2001:382;232–240.
8. Walker JM. Histological study of the fetal development of the human acetabulum and labrum: significance in congenital hip disease. Yale J Biol Med 1981:54;255–263.
9. Ito K, Leunig M, Ganz R. Histopathologic features of the acetabular labrum in femoroacetabular impingement. Clin Orthop Rel Res 2004;429;262–271.
10. Kelly B, Shapiro GS, Digiovanni CW, et al. Vascularity of the hip labrum: a cadaveric investigation. Arthroscopy 2005:21;3–11.
11. McCarthy JC, Noble PC, Schuck MR, et al. The role of labral lesions to development of early degenerative hip disease. Clin Orthop Rel Res 2001:393;25–37.
12. McCarthy J, Noble P, Aluisio FV, et al. Anatomy, pathologic features, and treatment of acetabular labral tears. Clin Orthop Rel Res 2003;406:38–47.
13. Kim YT, Azuma H. The nerve endings of the acetabular labrum. Clin Orthop Rel Res 1995;320:176–181.
14. Abe I, Harada Y, Oinuma K, et al. Acetabular labrum: abnormal findings at MR imaging in asymptomatic hips. Radiology 2000;216:576–581.
15. Cotten A, Boutry N, Demondion X, et al. Acetabular labrum: MRI in asymptomatic volunteers. J Comp Assist Tomogr 1998;22:1–7.
16. Lecouvet FE, Vande Berg BC, Malghem J, et al. MR imaging of the acetabular labrum: variations in 200 asymptomatic hips. AJR Am J Roentgenol 1996;167:1025–1028.
17. Keene GS, Villar RN. Arthroscopic anatomy of the hip: an in vivo study. Arthroscopy 1994;10:329–399.
18. Plotz CMJ, Brossman J, Schunke M, et al. Magnetic resonance arthrography of the acetabular labrum. Macroscopic and histological correlation in 20 cadavers. J Bone Joint Surg [Br] 2000;82–B:426–432.
19. Tan V, Seldes RM, Katz MA, et al. Contribution of acetabular labrum to articulating surface area and femoral head coverage in adult hip joints: an anatomic study in cadavera. Am J Orthop 2001;30;809–812.
20. Czerny C, Hofmann S, Urban M, et al. MR arthrography of the adult acetabular-labral complex: correlation with surgery and anatomy. AJR Am J Roentgenol 1999;173:345–349.
21. Hodler J, Yu JS, Goodwin D, et al. MR arthrography of the hip: improved imaging of the acetabular labrum with histologic correlation. Am J Roentgenol 1995;165:887–891.
22. Dinauer PA, Murphy KP, Carroll JF. Sublabral sulcus at the posteroinferior acetabulum: a potential pitfall in MR arthrography diagnosis of acetabular labral tears. AJR Am J Roentgenol 2004:183;1745–1753.
23. Petersilge CA, Haque MA, Petersilge WJ, et al. Acetabular labral tears: evaluation with MR arthrography. Radiology 1996;200:231–235.
24. Fitzgerald RH. Acetabular labrum tears: Diagnosis and management. Clin Orthop Rel Res 1995; 311:60–68.
25. Moore SG, Dawson KL. Red and yellow marrow in the femur: age-related changes in appearance at MR imaging. Radiology 1990; 175:219–223.
26. Ricci C, Cova M, Kang YS, et al. Normal age-related patterns of cellular and fatty bone marrow distribution in the axial skeleton: MR imaging study. Radiology 1990;177:83–88.

27. Waitches G, Zawin JK, Poznanski AK. Sequence and rate of bone marrow conversion in the femora of children as seen on MR imaging: are accepted standards accurate? Am J Roentgen 1994;162:1399–1406.

28. VandeBerg B, Lecouvet F, Moysan P, et al. MR assessment of red marrow distribution and composition in the proximal femur: correlation with clinical and laboratory parameters. Skeletal Radiol 1997;26:589–596.

29. VandeBerg BC, Malghem J, Lecouvet FE, et al. Classification and detection of bone marrow lesions with magnetic resonance imaging. Skeletal Radiol 1998;27:529–545.

30. Carlson DL, Mawdsley RH. Sports anemia: a review of the literature. Am J Sports Med 1986;1–4:109–112.

31. Dawson KL, Moore SG, Rowland JM. Age-related marrow changes in the pelvis: MR and anatomic findings. Radiology 1992;183:47–51.

32. Levine CD, Schweitzer ME, Ehrlich MS. Pelvic marrow in adults. Skeletal Radiol 1994;23:343–347.

33. Czerny C, Hofmann S, Kneehole A, et al. Lesions of the acetabular labrum: accuracy of MR imaging and MR arthrography in detection and staging. Radiology 1996;200:225–230.

34. Too Mayan GA, Holman WR, Major NM, et al. Sensitivity of MR arthrography in the evaluation of acetabular labral tears. AJR 2006;186:449–453.

35. Byrd JWT, Jones KS. Diagnostic accuracy of clinical assessment, magnetic resonance imaging, magnetic resonance arthrography, and intra-articular injection in hip arthroscopy patients. Am J Sports Med 2004;32:1668–1674.

36. Edwards DJ, Lomas D, Villar RH. Diagnosis of the painful hip by magnetic resonance imaging and arthroscopy. J Bone Joint Surg 1995;77–B:374–376.

37. Knuesel PR, Pfirrmann CW, Noetzli HP, et al. MR Arthrography of the hip: diagnostic performance of a dedicated water-excitation 3D double-echo steady-state sequence to detect cartilage lesions. AJR Am J Roentgenol 2004;183:1729–1735.

38. Schmid MR, Notzli HP, Zanetti M, et al. Cartilage lesions in the hip: diagnostic effectiveness of MR arthrography. Radiology 2003;226:382–386.

39. Chan YS, Lien LC, Hsu HL, et al. Evaluating hip labral tears using magnetic resonance arthrography: a prospective study comparing hip arthroscopy and magnetic resonance arthrography diagnosis. Arthroscopy 2005;21:1250J.

40. Horii M, Kubo T, Hirasawa Y. Radial MRI of the hip with moderate osteoarthritis. J Bone Joint Surg [Br] 2000;82–B:364–368.

41. Kubo T, Horii M, Harada Y, et al. Radial-sequence magnetic resonance imaging in evaluation of acetabular labrum. J Orthop Sci 1999;4:328–332.

42. Plotz CMJ, Brossmann J, von Knoch M, et al. Magnetic resonance arthrography of the acetabular labrum: value of radial reconstructions. Arch Orthop Trauma Surg 2001;121:450–457.

43. Siebenrock KA, Wahab KH, Werlen S, et al. Abnormal extension of the femoral head epiphysis as a cause of cam impingement. Clin Orthop Relat Res 2004;418:54–60.

44. Mintz D, Hooper T, Connell D, et al. Magnetic resonance imaging of the hip: detection of labral and chondral abnormalities using noncontrast imaging. Arthroscopy 2005;21;385–393.

45. Rossi F, Dragoni S. Acute avulsion fractures of the pelvis in adolescent competitive athletes: prevalence, location and sports distribution of 203 cases collected. Skeletal Radiol 2001;30:127–131.

46. Bertin KC, Horstman J, Coleman SS. Isolated fracture of the lesser trochanter in adults: an initial manifestation of metastatic malignant disease. J Bone Joint Surg [Am] 1984;66:770–773.

47. Bui-Mansfield LT, Chew FS, Lenchik L, et al. Nontraumatic avulsions of the pelvis. AJR Am J Roentgenol 2002;178:423–427.

48. Phillips CD, Pope TL Jr, Jones JE, et al. Nontraumatic avulsion of the lesser trochanter: a pathognomonic sign of metastatic disease? Skeletal Radiol 1988;17:106–110.

49. Fernbach SK, Wilkinson RH. Avulsion injuries of the pelvis and proximal femur. AJR Am J Roentgenol 1981;137:581–584.

50. Metzmaker JN, Pappas AM. Avulsion fractures of the pelvis. Am J Sports Med 1985;13:349–358.

51. Stevens M, El-Khoury G, Kathol M, et al. Imaging features of avulsion injuries. Radiographics 1999;19:655–672.

52. Sundar M, Carty H. Avulsion fractures of the pelvis in children: a report of 32 fractures and their outcome. Skeletal Radiol 1994;23:85–90.

53. Brandser EA, El-Khoury GY, Kathol MH. Adolescent hamstring avulsions that simulate tumors. Emerg Radiol 1995;2:273–278.

54. Yamamoto T, Akisue T, Nakatiani T, et al. Apophysitis of the ischial tuberosity mimicking a neoplasm on magnetic resonance imaging. Skeletal Radiol 2004;33:737–740.

55. Matheson GO, Clement DB, McKenzie DC, et al. Stress fractures in athletes. A study of 320 cases. Am J Sports Med 1987;15:46–58.

56. Ahovuo JA, Kiuru MJ, Visuri T. Fatigue stress fractures of the sacrum: diagnosis with MR imaging. Eur Radiol 2004;14: 500–505.

57. Kiuru M, Pihlajamaki H, Ahovuo J. fatigue stress injuries of the pelvic bones and proximal femur: evaluation with MR imaging. Eur Radiol 2003;13:605–611.

58. Milgrom C, Giladi M, Stein M et al. Stress fractures in military recruits. A prospective study showing an unusually high incidence. J Bone Joint Surg [Br] 1985;67:732–735.

59. Williams T, Puckett M, Dension G, et al. Acetabular stress fractures in military endurance athletes and recruits: incidence and MRI and scintigraphic findings. Skeletal Radiol 2002;31:277–281.

60. Hohmann E, Wortler K, Imhoff AB. MR imaging of the hip and knee before and after marathon running. Am J Sports Med 2004;32:55–59.

61. Yao L, Johnson C, Gentili A, et al. Stress injuries of bone: analysis of MR imaging staging criteria. Acad Radiol 1998;5: 34–40.

62. Waters PM, Millis MB. Hip and pelvic injuries in the young athlete. Clin Sports Med 1988;7:513–526.

63. Major N, Helms C. Pelvic stress injuries: the relationship between osteitis pubis (symphysis pubis stress injury) and sacroiliac abnormalities in athletes. Skeletal Radiol 1997;26:711–717.

64. Overdeck KH, Palmer WE. Imaging of the hip and groin injuries in athletes. Semin Musculoskeletal Radiol 2004;8:41–55.

65. Niva MH, Kiuru MJ, Haataja R, et al. Fatigue injuries of the femur. J Bone Joint Surg [Br] 2005;87:1385–1390.

66. Slocum KA, Gorman JD, Puckett ML, et al. Resolution of abnormal MR signal intensity in patients with stress fractures of the femoral neck. AJR Am J Roentgenol 1997;168:1295–1299.

67. Devas MB. Stress fractures of the femoral neck. J Bone Joint Surg [Br] 1965;47–B:728–738.

68. Giladi M, Milgrom C, Kashtan H, et al. Recurrent stress fractures in military recruits. One-year follow-up of 66 recruits. J Bone Joint Surg [Br] 1986;68:439–441.

69. Song WS, Yoo JJ, Koo KH, et al. Subchondral fatigue fracture of the femoral head in military recruits. J Bone Joint Surg [Am] 2004;86–A:1917–1924.

70. Johnson AW, Weiss CB Jr, Stento K, et al. Stress fractures of the sacrum: an atypical cause of low back pain in the female athlete. Am J Sports Med 29:498–508.

71. Major NM, Helms CA. Sacral stress fractures in long-distance runners. AJR Am J Roentgenol 2000;174:727–729.

72. Weaver CJ, Major NM, Garrett WE, et al. Femoral head osteochondral lesions in painful hips of athletes: MR imaging findings. AJR 2002;178:973–977.

73. Anderson K, Strickland S, Warren R. Hip and groin injuries in athletes. Am J Sports Med 2001;29:521–533.

74. Moorman CT III, Warren RF, Hershman EB, et al. Traumatic posterior hip subluxation in American football. J Bone Joint Surg [Am] 2003:85–A;1190–1196.

75. Wilson AJ, Murphy WA, Hardy DC, et al. Transient osteoporosis: transient bone marrow edema? Radiology 1988;167:757–760.

76. Bloem JL. Transient osteoporosis of the hip: MR imaging. Radiology 1988;167:753–755.

77. Malizos KN, Zibis AH, Dailiana Z, et al. MR imaging findings in transient osteoporosis of the hip. Eur J Radiol 2004;50:238–244.

78. Miyanishi K, Yamamoto T, Nakashima Y, et al. Subchondral changes in transient osteoporosis of the hip. Skeletal Radiol 2001;30:255–261.

79. Yamamoto T, Kubo T, Hirasawa Y, et al. A clinicopathologic study of transient osteoporosis of the hip. Skeletal Radiol 1999;28:621–627.

80. VandeBerg BE, Malghem JJ, Labaisse MA, et al. MR imaging of avascular necrosis and transient marrow edema of the femoral head. Radiographics 1993;13:501–520.

81. Anderson M, Kaplan P, Dussault R. Adductor insertion avulsion syndrome (thigh splints). AJR Am J Roentgenol 2001;177:673–675.

82. Anderson SE, Johnston JO, O'Donell RO, et al. MR imaging of sports-related pseudotumor in children: mid femoral diaphyseal periostitis at insertion site of adductor musculature. AJR Am J Roentgenol 2001;176:1227–1231.

83. Koulouris G, Connell D. Evaluation of the hamstring muscle complex following acute injury. Skeletal Radiol 2003;32:582–589.

84. Connell DA, Schneider-Kolsky ME, Hoving JL, et al. Longitudinal study comparing sonographic and MRI assessments of acute and healing hamstring injuries. AJR Am J Roentgenol 2004;183:975–984.

85. Brandser EA, El-Khoury GY, Kathol MH, et al. Hamstring injuries: radiographic, conventional tomographic, CT and MR imaging characteristics. Radiology 1995;197:257–262.

86. De Smet AA, Best TM. MR imaging of the distribution and location of acute hamstring injuries in athletes. AJR Am J Roentgenol 2000;174:393–399.

87. Slavotinek JP, Verrall JM, Fon GT. Hamstring injury in athletes: using MR imaging measurements to compare extent of muscle injury with amount of time lost from competition. AJR Am J Roentgenol 2002;179:1621–1628.

88. Pomeranz SJ, Heidt RS JR. MR imaging in the prognostication of hamstring injury. Work in progress. Radiology 1993;189:897–900.

89. Chung CB, Robertson JE, Cho GJ, et al. Gluteus medius tendon tears and avulsive injuries in elderly women: Imaging findings in six patients. AJR Am J Roentgenol 1999;173:351–353.

90. Karpinski MRK, Piggott H. Greater trochanteric pain syndrome. J Bone Joint Surg [Br] 1985;67–B:762–763.

91. Kingzett-Taylor A, Tirman P, Feller J, et al. Tendinosis and tears of the gluteus medius and minimus muscles as a cause of hip pain: MR imaging findings. AJR Am J Roentgenol 1999;173:1123–1126.

92. Clancy WG. Runner's injuries. 2. Evaluation and treatment of specific injuries. Am J Sports Med 1980;8:287–289.

93. Slawski DP, Howard RF. Surgical management of refractory trochanteric bursitis. Am J Sports Med 1997;25:287–289.

94. Yu JS, Habib PA. Common injuries related to weightlifting: MR imaging perspective. Semin Musculoskelet Radiol 2005;9:289–301.

95. Bunker TD, Esler CNA, Leach WJ. Rotator-cuff tear of the hip. J Bone Joint Surg [Br] 1997;79–B:618–620.

96. Kagan A. Rotator-cuff tear of the hip. J Bone Joint Surg [Br] 1998;80–B:182–183.

97. Pfirrmann CWA, Chung CB, Theumann NH, et al. "Greater trochanter of the hip" attachment of the abductor mechanism and a complex of three bursae-MR imaging and MR bursography in cadavers and MR imaging in asymptomatic volunteers. Radiology 2001;221:469–477.

98. Bird PA, Oakley SP, Shnier R, et al. Prospective evaluation of magnetic resonance imaging and physical examination findings in patients with greater trochanteric pain syndrome. Arthritis Rheum 2001;44:2138–2145.

99. Cvitanic O, Henzie G, Skezas N, et al. MRI diagnosis of tears of the hip abductor tendons (gluteus medius and gluteus minimus). AJR Am J Roentgenol 2004;182:137–143.

100. Johnston CAM, Wiley JP, Lindsay DM, et al. Iliopsoas bursitis and tendonitis: a review. Sports Med 1998;25:271–283.

101. Varma DGK, Richli WR, Charnsangavej C, et al. MR appearance of the distended iliopsoas bursa. AJR Am J Roentgenol 1991;156:1025–1028.

102. Wunderbaldinger P, Bremer C, Schellenberger E, et al. Imaging features of iliopsoas bursitis. Eur Radiol 2002;12:409–415.

103. Guerra J Jr, Armbruster TG, Resnick D, et al. The adult hip: an anatomic study. Part II: the soft-tissue landmarks. Radiology 1978;128:11–20.

104. Lecouvet FE, Demondion X, Leemrijse T, et al. Spontaneous rupture of the distal iliopsoas tendon: clinical and imaging findings. Eur Radiol 2005;15:2341–2346.

105. Schaberg JE, Harper MC, Allen WC. The snapping hip syndrome. Am J Sports Med 1984;12:361–365.

106. Allen WC, Cope R. Coxa saltans: the snapping hip revisited. J Am Acad Orthop Surg 1995;3:303–308.

107. Janzen DL, Patridge E, Logan M, et al. The snapping hip: clinical and imaging findings in transient subluxation of the iliopsoas tendon. Can Assoc Radio J 1996;47:202–208.

108. Vaccaro JP, Sauser DD, Beals RK. Iliopsoas bursa imaging: efficacy in depicting abnormal iliopsoas tendon motion in patients with internal snapping hip syndrome. Radiology 1995;197:853–856.

109. Altenberg AR. Acetabular labrum tears: a cause of hip pain and degenerative osteoarthritis. South Med J 1977;70;174–175.

110. Ganz R, Parvizi J, Beck M et al. Femoroacetabular impingement a cause for osteoarthritis of the hip. Clin Orthop Rel Res 2003:417;112–120.

111. Harris WH, Bourne RB, Oh I. Intra-articular acetabular labrum: a possible etiological factor in certain cases of osteoarthritis of the hip. J Bone Joint Surg 1979:61–A;510–514.

112. Hase T, Ueo T. Acetabular labral tear: arthroscopic diagnosis and treatment. Arthroscopy 1999;15:138–141.

113. Ikeda T, Awaya G, Suzuki S, et al. Torn acetabular labrum in young patients. J Bone Joint Surg [Br] 1988;70–13–16.

114. Lage LA, Patel JV, Villar RN. The acetabular labral tear: an arthroscopic classification. Arthroscopy 1996;12:;269–272.

115. Noguchi Y, Miura H, Takasugi S, et al. Cartilage and labrum degeneration in the dysplastic hip generally originates in the anterosuperior weight-bearing area: an arthroscopic observation. Arthroscopy 1999:15;496–506.

116. Beck M, Leunig M, Parvizi J, et al. Anterior femoroacetabular impingement. Part II. Midterm results of surgical treatment. Clin Orthop 2004;418:67–73.

117. Beck M, Kalhor M, Leunig M, et al. Hip morphology influences the pattern of damage to the acetabular cartilage: femoroacetabular impingement as a cause of early osteoarthritis of the hip. J Bone Joint Surg [Br] 2005;87:1012–1018.

118. Eijer H, Myers SR, Ganz R. Anterior femoroacetabular impingement after femoral neck fractures. J Orthop Trauma 2001;15:475–481.

119. Ito K, Minka MA II, Leunig M, et al. Femoroacetabular impingement and the cam effect: an MRI-based quantitative anatomical study of the femoral head-neck offset. J Bone Joint Surg [Br] 2001;83:171–176.

120. Leunig M, Beck M, Woo A, et al. Acetabular rim degeneration. Clin Orthop Rel Res 2003:413;201–207.

121. Leunig M, Podeszwa D, Beck M, et al. Magnetic resonance arthrography of labral disorders in hips with dysplasia and impingement. Clin Orthop 2004;418:74–80.

122. Notzli HP, Wyss RG, Stoecklin CH, et al. The contour of the femoral head-neck junction as a predictor for the risk of anterior impingement. J Bone Joint Surg [Br] 2002;84:556–560.

123. Kassarjian A, Yoon LS, Belzile E, et al. Triad of MR arthrographic findings in patients with cam-type femoroacetabular impingement. Radiology 2005;236:588–592.

124. Fargo LA, Glick JM, Sampson TG. Hip arthroscopy for acetabular labral tears. Arthroscopy 1999;15:132–137.

125. Dameron TB. Bucket-handle tear of acetabular labrum accompanying posterior dislocation of the hip. J Bone Joint Surg [Am] 1959;41:131–134.

126. Paterson I. The torn acetabular labrum A block to reduction of a dislocated hip. J Bone Joint Surg 1957:39–B;306–309.

127. Rashleigh-Belcher HJC, Cannon SR. Recurrent dislocation of the hip with a "Bankart-type" lesion. J Bone Joint Surg 1986;68–B:398–399.

128. Shea KP, Kalamchi A, Thompson GH. Acetabular epiphysis-labrum entrapment following traumatic anterior dislocation of the hip in children. J Pediatr Orthop 1986;6:215–219.

129. Leunig M, Sledge JB, Gill TJ, et al. Traumatic labral avulsion from the stable rim: a constant pathology in displaced transverse acetabular fractures. Arch Orthop Trauma Surg 2003:123;392–395.

130. Jager M, Wild A, Westhoff B, et al. Femoroacetabular impingement caused by a femoral osseous head-neck bump deformity: clinical, radiological, and experimental results. J Orthop Sci 2004;9:256–263.

131. Cooperman DR, Charles LM, Pathria M, et al. Post-mortem description of slipped capital femoral epiphysis. J Bone Joint Surg [Br] 1992;74–B:595–599.

132. Dorrell JH, Catterall A. The torn acetabular labrum. J Bone Joint Surg 1986;68–B:400–403.

133. Goodman DA, Feighan JE, Smith AD, et al. Subclinical slipped capital femoral epiphysis. J Bone Joint Surg [Am] 1997;79:1489–1487.

134. Klaue K, Durnin CW, Ganz R. The acetabular rim syndrome. J Bone Joint Surg 1991;73–B:423–429.

135. Leunig M, Casillas MM, Hamlet M, et al. Slipped capital femoral epiphysis Early mechanical damage to the acetabular cartilage by a prominent femoral metaphysis. Acta Orthop Scan 2000;71:370–375.

136. McCarthy JC, Lee J. Acetabular dysplasia: a paradigm of arthroscopic examination of chondral injuries. Clin Orthop Rel Res 2002:405;122–128.

137. Snow SW, Keret D, Scarangella S, et al. Anterior impingement of the femoral head: a late phenomenon of Legg-Calve-Perthes' disease. J Pediatr Orthop 1993;13:286–289.

138. Stulberg SD, Cordell LD, Harris WH, et al. Unrecognized childhood hip disease: a major cause of idiopathic osteoarthritis of the hip. In: The Hip. Proceedings of the Third Meeting of the Hip Society. St. Louis: CV Mosby, 1975:212–228.

139. Tonnis D, Heinecke A. Acetabular and femoral anteversion: relationship with osteoarthritis of the hip. J Bone Joint Surg [Am] 1999;81:1747–1770.

140. Beall DP, Sweet CF, Martin HD, et al. Imaging findings of femoroacetabular impingement syndrome. Skeletal Radiol 2005;34:691–701.

141. Reynolds D, Lucas J, Klaue K. Retroversion of the acetabulum: a cause of hip pain. J Bone Joint Surg [Br] 1999;81:281–288.

142. Siebenrock KA, Schoeniger R, Ganz R. Anterior femoro-acetabular impingement due to acetabular retroversion. J Bone Joint Surg [Br] 2003;85:278–286.

143. McCarthy JC, Busconi B. The role of hip arthroscopy in the diagnosis and treatment of hip disease. Orthopedics 1995;18:753–756.

144. Blankenbaker DG, De Smet AA, Keene JS. Abstracts of the Society of Skeletal Radiology: correlation of arthroscopic grading and localization of hip labral tears with MR arthrographic findings. Skeletal Radiol 2006;35:338.

145. Leunig M, Werlen S, Ungersbock A, et al. Evaluation of the acetabular labrum by MR arthrography. J Bone Joint Surg [Br] 1997;79–B:230–234.

146. Horii M, Kubo T, Inoue S, et al. Coverage of the femoral head by the acetabular labrum in dysplastic hips. Acta Orthop Scand 2003;74:287–292.

147. Crabbe JP, Martel W, Matthews. Rapid growth of femoral herniation pit. AJR Am J Roentgenol 1992;159:1038–1040.

148. Daenen B, Preidler KW, Padmanabhan S, et al. Symptomatic herniation pits of the femoral neck: anatomic and clinical study. AJR Am J Roentgenol 1997;168–149–153.

149. Pitt MJ, Graham AR, Shipman JH, et al. Herniation pit of the femoral neck. AJR Am J Roentgenol 1982;138:1115–1121.

150. Leunig M, Beck M, Kalhor M, et al. Fibrocystic changes at anterosuperior femoral neck: prevalence in hips with femoroacetabular impingement. Radiology 2005;236:237–246.

151. Nokes SR, Vogler JB, Spritzer CE, et al. Herniation pits of the femoral neck: appearance at MR imaging. Radiology 1989;172:231–234.

152. Haller J, Resnick D, Greenway G, et al. Juxtaacetabular ganglionic (or synovial) cysts: CT and MR features. J Comp Assist Tomogr 1989; 13:976–983.

153. Lagier R, Seigne JM, Mbakop A. Juxta-acetabular mucoid cyst in a patient with osteoarthritis of the hip secondary to dysplasia. Int Orthop 1984;8:19–23.

154. Magee T, Hinson G. Association of paralabral cysts with acetabular disorders. AJR 2000;174:1381–1384.

155. Schnarkowski P, Steinbach LS, Tirman PF, et al. Magnetic resonance imaging of labral cysts of the hip. Skel Radiol 1996; 25:733–737.

156. Yukata K, Arai K, Yoshizumi Y, et al. Obturator neuropathy cause by an acetabular labral cyst: MRI findings. AJR Am J Roentgenol 2005;184:S112–S114.

157. Sherman PM, Matchette MW, Sanders TG, et al. Acetabular paralabral cyst: an uncommon cause of sciatica. Skeletal Radiol 2003;32–90–94.

158. Gray AJ, Villar RN. The ligamentum teres of the hip: an arthroscopic classification of its pathology. Arthroscopy 1997;13:575–578.

159. Byrd JW, Jones KS. Traumatic rupture of the ligamentum teres as a source of hip pain. Arthroscopy 2004;20:385–391.

160. Armfield DR, Martin R, Robertson DD, et al. Abstracts of the Society of Skeletal Radiology: detection of partial tears of the ligamentum teres using MR arthrography of the hip. Skeletal Radiol 2006;35:319–348.

161. Fredberg U, Kissmeyer-Nielsen P. The sportsman's hernia—fact or fiction? Scand J Med Sci Sports 1996;6:201–204.

162. Martens MA, Hansen L, Muller JC. Adductor tendonitis and musculus rectus abdominis tendopathy. Am J Sports Med 1987;15:353–356.

163. Verrall GM, Hamilton IA, Slavotinek JP, et al. Hip joint range of motion reduction in sports-related chronic groin injury diagnosed as pubic bone stress injury. J Sci Med Sport 2005;8:77–84.

164. Lovell G. The diagnosis of chronic groin pain in athletes: a review of 189 cases. Aust J Sci Med Sport 1995;27:76–79.

165. Ekberg O, Persson NH, Abrahamsson P, et al. Longstanding groin pain in athletes. Sports Med 1988;6:56–61.

166. Fricker PA, Taunton JE, Ammann W. Osteitis pubis in athletes: infection, inflammation or injury? Sports Med 1991;12: 266–279.

167. Slavotinek JP, Verrall GM, Fon GT, et al. Groin pain in footballers: the association between preseason clinical and pubic bone magnetic resonance imaging findings and athlete outcome. Am J Sports Med 2005;33:894–899.

168. Verrall G, Slavotinek J, Fon G. Incidence of pubic bone marrow oedema in Australian rules football players: relation to groin pain. Br J Sports Med 2001;35:28–33.

169. Lovell G, Galloway H, Hopkins W, et al. Osteitis pubis and assessment of bone marrow edema at the pubic symphysis with MRI in an elite junior male soccer squad. Clin J Sport Med 2006;16:117–122.

170. Albers SL, Spritzer CE, Garrett WE JR, et al. MR findings in athletes with pubalgia. Skeletal Radiol 2001;30:270–277.

171. Gibbon W, Hession P. Disease of the pubis and pubic symphysis: MR imaging appearances. AJR Am J Roentgenol 1997;169:849–853.

172. Brennan D, et al. Secondary cleft sign as a marker of injury in athletes with groin pain: MR image appearance and interpretation. Radiology 2005;235:162–167.

173. O'Connell MJ, Powell T, McCaffrey NM, et al. Symphyseal cleft injection in the diagnosis and treatment of osteitis pubis in athletes. AJR Am J Roentgenol 2002;179:955–959.

174. Wiley J. Traumatic osteitis pubis: the gracilis syndrome. Am J Sports Med 1983;11:360–363.

175. Irshad K, Feldman LS, Lavoie C, et al. Operative management of "hockey groin syndrome" 12 years of experience in National Hockey League players. Surgery 2001;130:759–764.

176. Ziprin P, Williams P, Foster ME. External oblique aponeurosis nerve entrapment as a cause of groin pain in the athlete. Br J Surg 1999;86:566–568.

177. Malycha P, Lovell G. Inguinal surgery in athletes with chronic groin pain: the "sportsman's" hernia. Aust N Z J Surg 1992;62:123–125.

178. Taylor D, Meyers W, Moylan J, et al. Abdominal musculature abnormalities as a cause of groin pain in athletes: inguinal hernias and pubalgia. Am J Sports Med 1991;19:239–243.

179. Meyers WC, Foley DP, Garrett WE, et al. Management of severe lower abdominal or inguinal pain in high performance athletes. Pain (Performing athletes with abdominal or inguinal neuromuscular pain study group). Am J Sport Med 2000;28:2–8.

180. van den Berg JC, de Valois JC, Go PM, et al. Detection of groin hernia with physical examination, ultrasound, and MRI compared with laparoscopic findings. Invest Radiol 1993;34: 739–743.

181. DeAngelis NA, Busconi BD. Assessment and differential diagnosis of the painful hip. Clin Orthop 2003;406(1):11–18.

182. Philippon MJ. The role of arthroscopic thermal capsulorrhaphy in the hip. Clin Sports Med 2001;20:817–819.

183. Byrd JWT. Indications and contraindications. In: Byrd JWT, ed. Operative Hip Arthroscopy. New York: Thieme, 1998:69–82.

184. Fitzgerald RH Jr. Acetabular labrum tears: diagnosis and treatment. Clin Orthop Rel Res 1995;311:60–68.

185. McCarthy JC, Noble PC, Schuck MR, et al. The role of labral lesions to development of early hip disease. Clin Orthop 2001;393:25–37.

186. Ferguson SJ, Bryant JT, Ganz R, et al. The acetabular labrum seal: a poroelastic finite element model. Clin Biomech 2000;15: 463–468.

187. Kim YT, Azuma H. The nerve endings of the acetabular labrum. Clin Orthop 1995;320:176–181.

188. Mason JB. Acetabular labral tears in the athlete. Clin Sports med 2001;20:779–790.

189. Dorfmann H, Boyer T. Arthroscopy of the hip: 12 years of experience. Arthroscopy 1999;15:67–72.

190. Lage LA, Patel JV, Villar RN. The acetabular labral tear: an arthroscopic classification. Arthroscopy 1996;12:269–272.

191. McCarthy J, Noble P, Aluisio FV, Schuck M, Wright J, Lee JA. Anatomy, pathologic features, and treatment of acetabular labral tears. Clin Orthop 2003;406:38–47.

192. McCarthy J, Barsoum W, Puri L, et al. The Role of hip arthroscopy in the elite athlete. Clin Orthop 2003;406:71–74.

193. Kelly BT, Buly RL. Hip arthroscopy update. Hosp Special Surg J 2005;1:40–48.

194. Czerny C, Hofmann S, Urban M, et al. MR arthrography of the adult acetabular capsular-labral complex: correlation with surgery and anatomy. AJR Am J Radiol 1999;173: 345–349.

195. Byrd JWT, Jones KS. Prospective analysis of hip arthroscopy with 2–year follow-up. Arthroscopy 2000;16(6):58–587.

196. Connell DA, Potter HG, Wickiewicz TL. Noncontrast magnetic resonance imaging of superior labral lesions. 102 cases

confirmed at arthroscopic surgery. Am J Sports Med 1999;27: 208–213.

197. Kelly BT, Shapiro GS, Digiovanni CW, et al. Vascularity of the hip labrum: a cadaveric investigation. Arthroscopy 2005; 21:3–11.

198. Petersen W, Petersen F, Tillman B. Structure and vascularization of the acetabular labrum with regard to the pathogenesis and healing of labral lesions. Arch Orthop Trauma Surg 2003;123(6):282–288.

199. McCarthy JC, Busconi B. The role of hip arthroscopy in the diagnosis and treatment of hip disease. Orthopedics 1995;18: 753–756.

200. Holgersson S, Brattstrom H, Mogensen B et al. Arthroscopy of the hip in juvenile chronic arthritis. J Pediatr Orthop 1981;1:273–278.

201. Maurice H, Crone M, Watt I. Synovial chondromatosis. J Bone Joint Surg 1988;70B:807–811.

202. Murphy F, Dahlin D, Sullivan C. Articular synovial chondromatosis. J Bone Joint Surg 1962;44A:77–86.

203. Mintz DN, Hooper T, Connell D, et al. Magnetic resonance imaging of the hip: Detection of labral and chondral abnormalities using noncontrast imaging. Arthroscopy 2005;21:385–393.

204. Ganz R, Parvizi J, Beck M, et al. Femoroacetabular impingement: a cause for early osteoarthritis of the hip. Clin Orthop 2003;417:112–120.

205. Beck M, Leunig, Parvizi et al. Anterior Femoroacetabular impingement: part II: midterm results of surgical treatment. Clin Orthop 2004;418:67–73.

206. Lavigne M, Parvizi J, Beck M, et al. Anterior femoroacetabular impingement: part I: technique of joint preserving surgery. Clin Orthop 2004;413:61–66.

207. Ito K, Minka M, Leunig et al. Femoroacetabular impingement and the cam-effect. J Bone Joint Surg 2001;83B(2):171–176.

208. Kim YJ, Jaramillo D, Millis MB, et al. Assessment of early osteoarthritis in hip dysplasia with delayed gadolinium-enhanced magnetic resonance imaging of cartilage. J Bone Joint Surg 2003;85(A):1987–1992.

209. Bashir A, Gray ML, Hartke J, Burstein D. Nondestructive imaging of human cartilage glycosaminoglycan concentration by MRI. Magn Reson Med 1999;41:857–865.

210. Gray AJR, Villar RN. The ligamentum teres of the hip: An arthroscopic classification of its pathology. Arthroscopy 1997;13:575–578.

211. Byrd JWT, Jones KS. Traumatic rupture of the ligamentum teres as a source of hip pain. Arthroscopy 2004;20:385–391.

212. Santori N, Villar RN. Arthroscopic findings in the initial stages of hip osteoarthritis. Orthopedics 1999;22:405–409.

213. Kelly BT, Williams RJ, Philippon MJ. Hip Arthroscopy: Current indications, treatment options, and management issues. Am J Sports Med 2003;31(6):1020–1037.

214. Bellabarba C, Sheinkop MB, Kuo KN. Idiopathic hip instability. An unrecognized cause of coxa Saltans in the adult. Clin Orthop 1998;355:261–271.

215. Liedenberg F, Dommisse GF. Recurrent post-traumatic dislocation of the hip. J Bone Joint Surg 1969;51B:632–637.

216. Philippon MJ. Debridement of acetabular labral tears associated with thermal capsulorrhaphy. Oper Tech Sports Med 2002;10:215–218.

217. Dorchak JD, Barrack RL, Kneisl JS, Alexander AH. Arthroscopic treatment of symptomatic synovial plica of the knee: long-term follow-up. Am J Sports Med 1991;19:503–507.

218. Dupont JY. Synovial plicae of the knee: controversies and review. Clin Sports Med 1997;16:87–122.

219. Johnson DP, Eastwood DM, Witherow PJ. Symptomatic synovial plicae of the knee. J Bone Joint Surg 1993;75A:1485–1496.

220. Atlihan D, Jones DC, Guanche CA. Arthroscopic treatment of a symptomatic hip plica. Clin Orthop 2003;411:174–177.

221. Frich LH, Lauritzen J, Juhl M. Arthroscopy in diagnosis and treatment of hip disorders. Orthopedics 1989;12:389–392.

222. Blickenstaff LD, Morris JM. Fatigue fracture of the femoral neck. J Bone Joint Surg 1966;48A:1031–1047.

223. Shin AY, Gillingham BL. Fatigue fractures of the femoral neck in athletes. J Am Acad Orthop Surg 1997;5:293–302.

224. Jones BH, Harris JM, Vinh TN, et al. Exercise-induced stress fractures and stress reactions of bone: epidemiology, etiology, and classification. Exerc Sport Sci Rev 1989;17:379–422.

225. Anderson K, Strickland SM, Warren RF. Hip and groin injuries in athletes. Am J Sports Med 2001;29:521–533.

226. Drinkwater BL, Nilson K, Chestnut CH III, et al. Bone mineral content of amenorrheic and eumenorrheic athletes. N Engl J Med 1984;311:277–281.

227. McBryde AM Jr. Stress fractures in runners. Clin Sports Med 1985;4:737–752.

228. Fullerton LR Jr, Snowdy HA. Femoral neck stress fractures. Am J Sports Med 1988;16:365–377.

229. Atlihan D, Quick DC, Guanche CA. Stress fracture of the iliac bone in a young female runner. Orthopedics 2003; 26:729–30.

230. Iwamoto J, Takeda T. Stress fractures in athletes: review of 196 cases. J Orthop Sci 2003;8:273–278.

231. Greany RB, Gerber FH, Laughlin RL, et al. Distribution and natural history of stress fractures in U.S. Marine recruits. Radiology 1983;146:339–346.

232. Guanche CA, Kozin SH, Levy AS, et al. The use of MRI in the diagnosis of occult hip fractures in the elderly: a preliminary review. Orthopedics 1994;17:327–330.

233. Prather JL, Nusynowitz ML, Snowdy HA, et al. Scintigraphic findings in stress fractures. J Bone Joint Surg 1977;59A:869–874.

234. Aro H, Dahlstrom S. Conservative management of distraction-type stress fractures of the femoral neck. J Bone Joint Surg 1986;68B:65–67.

10
Knee

A. Radiologic Perspective: Magnetic Resonance Imaging of the Knee

Theodore T. Miller

In most radiology practices, the knee is the most commonly imaged joint in the appendicular skeleton. There is wide variation in the field strengths of clinical magnets (ranging from 0.2 to 3 tesla [T]), the configuration of the magnets (open or closed), the sequences (e.g., T1, T2, proton density, conventional spin echo, fast spin echo, gradient echo), and slice thicknesses used to image the knee, as well as a wide variety in the skill of the radiologist interpreting the images. All of these factors have bearing on the accuracy of the magnetic resonance (MR) examination[1] as well as the anecdotal usefulness of this modality to the referring physician. Nonetheless, Glynn et al.,[2] using Medicare data on reimbursements between 1993 and 1999, found a 145% increase in performance of magnetic resonance imaging (MRI) of the lower extremity and a 54.5% decrease in performance of diagnostic arthroscopy of the knee, suggesting an increasingly greater reliance by clinicians on MRI to provide diagnostic information. Similarly, Bryan et al.[3] found that the use of MRI in the diagnostic evaluation of patients with chronic knee complaints significantly reduced the need for surgery.

While careful physical examination is as accurate as MRI for tears of the menisci and rupture of the anterior cruciate ligament (ACL),[4–6] a survey of members of the ACL study group showed that 44% of respondents routinely order preoperative MR examinations for patients with suspected ACL injury and 51% order MR examinations for patients with suspected posterior cruciate ligament (PCL) injury.[7] In cases in which the physical examination is equivocal or multiple injuries are present, MRI does have a significant effect on surgical decision making,[8–11] and 63% of the respondents of the ACL study group order MR examinations for patients with multiple ligament injury.[7] The discerning use of MRI by orthopedic surgeons was described by both Sherman et al.[12] and Bernstein et al.,[13] who found that patients referred by nonorthopedic surgeons had a statistically significant higher rate of normal MR examinations than patients referred by orthopedic surgeons.

This chapter discusses the normal anatomy, mechanisms of injury, MRI appearances of injury, and, where appropriate, the postsurgical appearance of the structures in and around the knee joint.

Menisci

Anatomy

The menisci are crescent-shaped wedges of fibrocartilage whose purpose is to provide increased contact area between the rounded femoral condyles and flat tibial plateau, thereby providing increased stability to the femorotibial articulation, distributing axial load, absorbing shock, and distributing synovial fluid to nourish the adjacent hyaline articular cartilage of the condyles and plateau.

Looking down on the menisci, the lateral meniscus is C-shaped and is uniform in thickness and size in cross section throughout. The medial meniscus is slightly larger, less tightly curved, and the posterior horn is thicker and wider than the body and anterior horn. Thus, on sagittal images the anterior and posterior horns of the lateral meniscus are equal in size while the posterior horn of the medial meniscus is larger than that of the anterior horn. The blood supply of the meniscus comes from the joint capsule, but only the peripheral approximately 20% of the adult meniscus is vascularized, which has implications for the management of tears. The entire periphery of the medial meniscus is attached to the joint capsule. In contrast, the anterior horn and body of the lateral meniscus are entirely attached to the joint capsule, but the posterior horn is focally separated from the joint capsule and connected to it by superior and inferior popliteomeniscal fascicles, which form an oblique tunnel called the popliteal hiatus, through which runs the popliteus tendon (Fig. 10.1). In addition to their capsular attachment, the menisci are attached to the tibial plateau by fibrous bands at the roots of their anterior and posterior horns. The anterior horns of the menisci are also connected to each other by the transverse meniscal ligament, and the attachment site of this ligament on the meniscus can sometimes mimic a meniscal tear (Fig. 10.2).

The meniscofemoral ligaments of Humphry and Wrisberg are anatomically inconstant structures that run from the lateral aspect of the medial femoral condyle to the posterior horn of the lateral meniscus. The Humphry ligament lies anterior to the PCL, while the Wrisberg ligament is posterior to the PCL (Fig. 10.3).

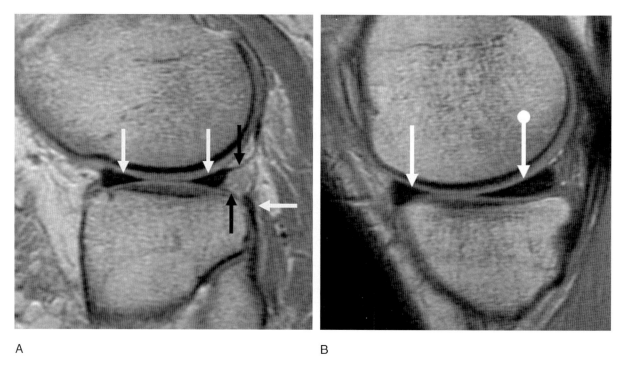

A   B

Fig. 10.1. Normal menisci. (A) Sagittal proton-density image of the lateral meniscus shows the anterior and posterior horns (vertical white arrows), which are similar in size and shape. The superior and inferior popliteomeniscal fascicles are seen (black arrows) as is the popliteus tendon (horizontal white arrow). (B) Sagittal proton-density image of the medial meniscus shows that the posterior horn (round tail arrow) is larger than the anterior horn (straight arrow).

These meniscofemoral ligaments, in concert with the menisco-popliteal fascicles, which connect the posterior horn of the lateral meniscus to the joint capsule, help to control motion of the posterior horn of the lateral meniscus during knee flexion.[14]

During knee flexion there is also mild rotation of the tibia relative to the femur; the flexion-extension motion occurs predominantly at the superior articular surface of the menisci, while the rotational movement occurs primarily at the inferior

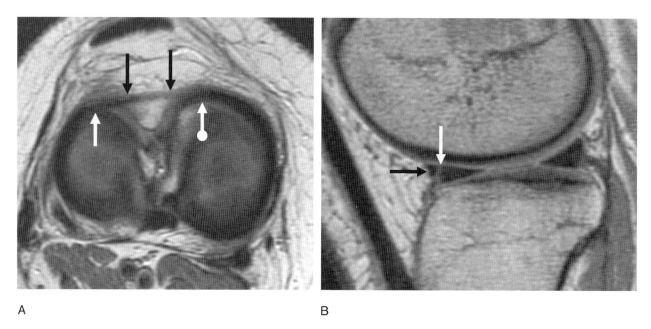

A   B

Fig. 10.2. Transverse meniscal ligament. (A) Axial T1-weighted image shows the transverse meniscal ligament (black arrows) connecting the anterior horn of the medial meniscus (round tail arrow) to the anterior horn of the lateral meniscus (straight white arrow). (B) Sagittal proton-density image through the lateral meniscus shows the cross section of the transverse meniscal ligament (black arrow) as it inserts on the anterior horn of the lateral meniscus. The space between the ligament and meniscus can mimic a tear (white arrow).

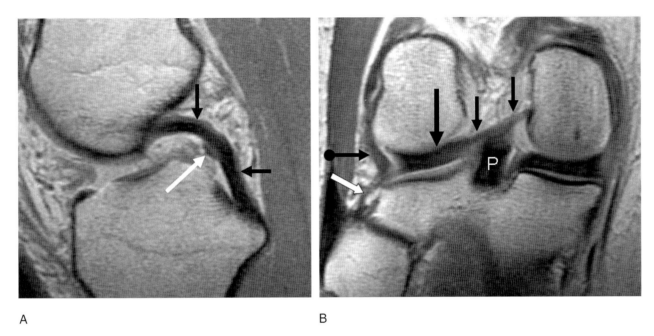

A   B

FIG. 10.3. Normal posterior cruciate ligament and meniscofemoral ligaments. (A) Sagittal proton-density image through the posterior cruciate ligament shows the uniformly low signal intensity and curved appearance of the posterior cruciate ligament (black arrows). The anterior meniscofemoral ligament of Humphry (white arrow) is present anterior to the posterior cruciate ligament. (B) Coronal proton-density image shows the longitudinal extent of the posterior meniscofemoral ligament of Wrisberg (short black arrows), as it attaches to the posterior horn of the lateral meniscus (long black arrow). The distal aspect of the posterior cruciate ligament is visualized (P). Also note the popliteofibular ligament (white arrow) extending from the fibular head to the popliteus tendon (round tail arrow).

articular surface. There are also different coefficients of friction between the femoral–meniscal surface and the tibial–meniscal surface, and all of these various forces and motions create shearing stress across the meniscus during normal knee activity. In addition, the medial joint capsule is less redundant than the lateral side and gives the medial meniscus less "play," and the medial meniscus has less posterior translation during flexion than the lateral meniscus,[15,16] and is therefore, in a sense, unable to "get out of the way" of the potentially crushing medial femoral condyle, a fact that is thought to be partly responsible for the higher incidence of tears of the medial meniscus.

A "discoid" meniscus, occurring in 4.5% to 13% of the population,[17,18] is a developmental abnormality of unknown etiology, in which the meniscus is slab-like instead of a crescent-shaped wedge. It is far more common on the lateral side,[19] and there are three types: (1) complete discoid, (2) incomplete discoid, and (3) Wrisberg-type discoid. The complete and incomplete forms maintain their capsular and anterior and posterior root attachments to the tibia, whereas the Wrisberg type lacks the posterior capsular and posterior root attachments but maintains its meniscofemoral ligament attachments.[20] The literature is controversial on whether the complete[21,22] or the incomplete[23,24] form is more common; the Wrisberg type is the least common.[20] The complete discoid meniscus is recognizable on both sagittal and coronal MRI as a rectangular block on every slice (Fig. 10.4), instead of looking like a wedge. One cannot use the number of imaging

slices in which the slab appears as the diagnostic criterion, since there is no standard slice thickness used by all imaging facilities. If the lateral meniscus has a wedge shape but the wedges are larger than the corresponding portions of the medial meniscus, then the lateral meniscus is considered an incomplete discoid. On sagittal images of the Wrisberg type, the popliteomeniscal fascicles are absent.[20] A discoid meniscus has a higher incidence of tear than a normal meniscus,[25] most often due to horizontal tears,[23,26] and occurring in 71% of discoid menisci in one large series.[18]

Meniscal flounce is the term used to describe the normal variation of a wavy or undulating free edge of the meniscus due to transient lack of tension across the free edge. It has a prevalence of less than 5% and involves the posterior horn of the medial meniscus.[27] Its presence is dependent on the position of the knee at the time of scanning, being most prominent in neutral position (the standard imaging position) and straightening out n maximal extension or mild flexion.[27]

Tears

The two imaging criteria for determining a meniscal tear are linear high signal intensity within the meniscus, which reaches the free edge or the superior or inferior articular surfaces, and abnormal meniscal morphology. The linear high signal should convincingly reach the articular surface on two or more consecutive slices in order to have 90% likelihood of truly being a tear; if the signal reaches the surface on only one image slice, the likelihood of tear

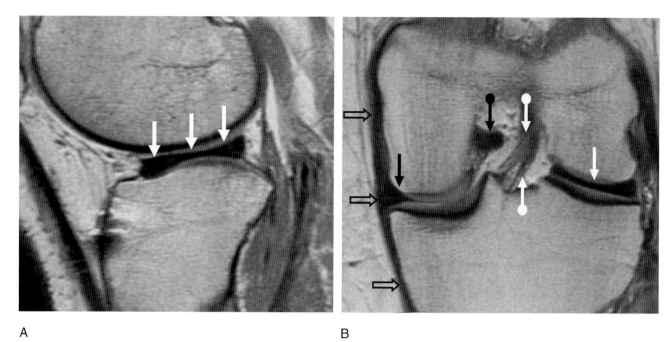

A   B

FIG. 10.4. Discoid meniscus. (A) Sagittal proton-density image through the lateral meniscus shows a rectangular slab of meniscal tissue (white arrows). (B) Coronal proton-density image of the same patient shows the large rectangular slap of discoid tissue (straight white arrow) compared to the normal wedge of the body of the medial meniscus (straight black arrow). Also note the normal striated appearance of the anterior cruciate ligament (white round tail arrows), the uniformly low signal intensity of the proximal aspect of the posterior cruciate ligament (black round tail arrow), and the medial collateral ligament (open black arrows). The distal aspect of the medial collateral ligament is not visualized on this image.

is 55% for the medial meniscus and only 30% for the lateral.[28] Early descriptions of abnormal signal within the meniscus used a grading system, in which grade I was a globular signal within the meniscus, grade II was a linear signal within the meniscus that did not reach an articular surface, and grade III was linear signal in the meniscus that did reach an articular surface.[29,30] Grades I and II signal represent intrasubstance degeneration and grade III signal is a tear, but many musculoskeletal radiologists no longer use this system, and instead just report that the meniscus is normal, has intrasubstance degeneration, or is torn. Some tears can be diagnosed only by recognizing the abnormal morphology of the meniscus, such as a truncated or abnormal shape, and not from the visualization of abnormal signal intensity within the meniscus.

The sensitivity and specificity of MRI for detection of meniscal tears generally ranges from 77% to 100%[31–33] on a 1.5-T scanner, with similar excellent performance at both low field strength (0.2 and 0.3 T)[34,35] and at 3 T,[36] but a wide variety of results can be found in both the radiology and orthopedic literature. In the presence of an acute tear of the ACL, the sensitivity for meniscal tears decreases, especially for tears of the posterior horn of the lateral meniscus, with De Smet and Graf[37] reporting a sensitivity of 94% for lateral meniscus tears without ACL injury, which dropped to 69% in the presence of an ACL tear, and Jee et al.[38] reporting only 57% sensitivity for lateral meniscus tears in the presence of a torn ACL.

Specific types of tears and their MRI appearances are as follows:

1. Radial tear: perpendicular to the free edge of the meniscus. The normal wedge-shaped meniscus may appear truncated, blunted, or even absent when the image slice is directly in the plane of the tear, and high signal intensity is present in the tear on images orthogonal to it[39] (Fig. 10.5). Magee et al.[39] found a 32% incidence of these tears in patients with new knee pain after prior partial meniscal resection.
2. Parrot-beak tear: similar to a radial tear, except that the plane of the tear is curved.
3. Bucket-handle tear: runs longitudinally along the length of the meniscus, and the inner rim flips into the intercondylar notch, while remaining attached to the anterior and posterior horns. The flipped fragment lies inferior and anterior to the PCL on a midline sagittal image,[40,41] giving the so-called double-PCL sign[42] (Fig. 10.6).
4. Flap tear: similar to a bucket-handle tear, except that the meniscal fragment is detached from the outer rim at one end.
5. Horizontal cleavage tear: horizontally oriented or shallowly oblique, most often involving the inferior articular surface of the meniscus.
6. Root tear: a full-thickness radial or vertical tear of the posterior horn of the meniscus near its root attachment to the tibia. This detaching of the posterior horn from its root may lead to extrusion of the meniscus because the meniscus is no longer able to withstand the hoop stress of axial loading,[43–45] and meniscal extrusion may predispose to degenerative arthritis (Fig. 10.7).

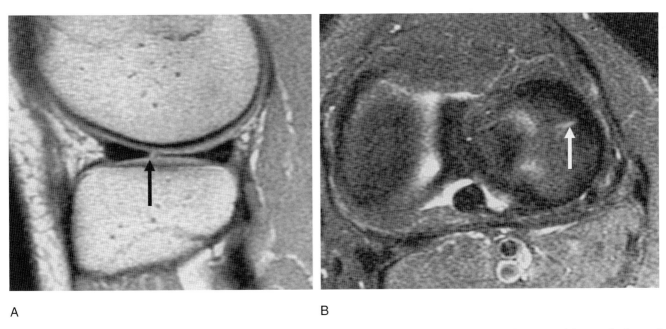

A   B

FIG. 10.5. Radial tear. (A) Sagittal proton-density image through the lateral meniscus shows blunting of the free edge of the anterior horn of the lateral meniscus (black arrow) and asymmetry in size of the anterior and posterior horns, all of which indicates a small radial tear. (B) Axial fat-suppressed T2-weighted sequence of the same patient shows the short high signal intensity tear (white arrow) oriented perpendicular to the lateral meniscus.

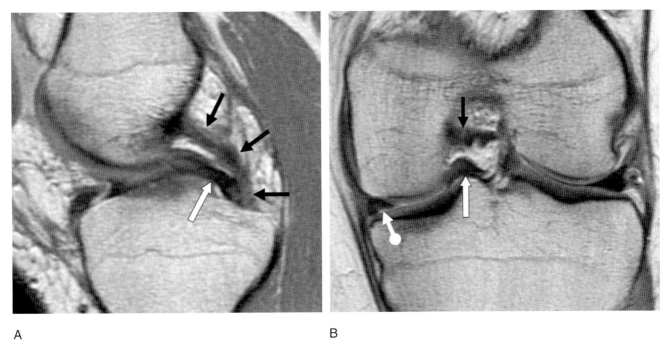

A   B

FIG. 10.6. Double posterior cruciate ligament sign of a bucket-handle tear of the medial meniscus. (A) Sagittal proton-density image through the intercondylar notch shows the low signal intensity displaced meniscal fragment (white arrow) paralleling the normal posterior cruciate ligament (black arrows). (B) Coronal proton-density image of the same patient shows the displaced meniscal fragment (straight white arrow) inferior to the posterior cruciate ligament (black arrow). The remaining outer rim of the medial meniscus (round tail arrow) has abnormal morphology and is smaller than the contralateral lateral meniscus.

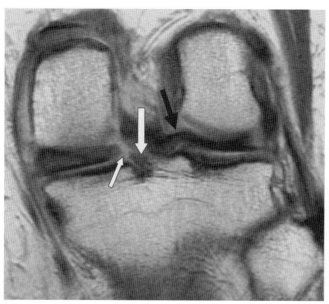

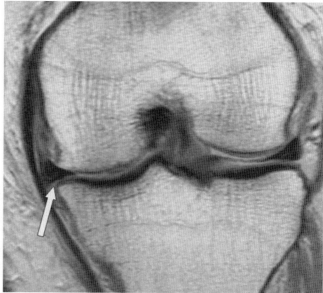

A   B

FIG. 10.7. Root tear and meniscal extrusion. (A) Coronal proton-density image shows a full-thickness tear (small white arrow) at the junction of the posterior horn of the medial meniscus and its root (large white arrow). Notice the intact root of the posterior horn of the lateral meniscus (black arrow). (B) Coronal proton-density image of the same patient shows extrusion of the body of the medial meniscus, overhanging the medial tibial plateau (white arrow). Note also the degenerative loss of articular cartilage overlying the medial femoral condyle compared to the contralateral lateral femoral condyle.

7. Complex tear: occurs in more than one plane, or several different types of tears occurring together.
8. Meniscocapsular separation: a vertically oriented tear, manifested as linear high signal intensity at the periphery of the meniscus.[46]

Tears may also be classified as degenerative or traumatic, based on configuration, history of an antecedent injury, and the presence of other acute injuries, such as cruciate ligament tears, or the presence of other degenerative findings, such as cartilage thinning and osteophytes. Vertical and longitudinal tears are considered traumatic, while horizontal cleavage tears are considered degenerative, but such a distinction seems artificial given that most people do not experience a single specific episode of injury, the ubiquity of degenerative changes, and the increasingly active lifestyle of older people. In addition, meniscal tears can be incidental, asymptomatic findings; Zanetti et al.[47] found a 36% prevalence of meniscal tears in asymptomatic knees, most often of a horizontal or oblique configuration, but other configurations were also found.

Tears of the popliteomeniscal fascicles are a form of meniscocapsular separation involving the posterior horn of the lateral meniscus. These tears are rare but often overlooked on MRI.[48,49] Since the normal popliteomeniscal fascicles are almost always routinely seen on sagittal MRI,[50] scrutiny should be paid to their absence or detachment. De Smet et al.[51] reported that an abnormal-appearing superior popliteomeniscal fascicle may also be a secondary sign of a tear of the posterior horn of the lateral meniscus itself.

The instability of a tear, and thus the need to repair or resect it, is best assessed by arthroscopic probing, but can be suggested on MRI if the tear is longer than 8 to 9 mm or more than 3 mm wide, if the tear is complex, or if the tear has high signal intensity on T2-weighted images.[52,53] A tear with an obviously displaced fragment such as a bucket-handle tear or a flap tear is unstable. When reporting a meniscal tear, one should describe the tear configuration (e.g., radial, horizontal cleavage, vertical, etc.), the length and location (e.g., meniscocapsular junction, peripheral 20%, inner 80%, free edge), the surface involved (e.g., free edge, superior/femoral articular surface, inferior/tibial articular surface), whether the tear is partial or full thickness (i.e., connecting the superior and inferior articular surfaces or transecting the entire substance of the meniscus), and the presence of a displaced fragment.

Sometimes a tear of the meniscus will allow joint fluid to be expressed through the tear and into the soft tissue adjacent to the meniscus, forming a meniscal cyst. One large study found an 8% incidence of cysts with meniscal tears,[54] with two thirds of the cysts occurring in the medial compartment. These cysts can be either intrameniscal or parameniscal[55] and can be large and multiloculated (Fig. 10.8), but in Campbell et al.'s[54] series only 15% were palpable. The most common type of tear associated with cysts is the horizontal cleavage tear,[56] but occasionally the original tear responsible for the cyst cannot be demonstrated because it has healed, leaving only the cyst. The cysts may dissect into the surrounding soft tissues, and erosion of adjacent bone by the cyst has been reported.[56]

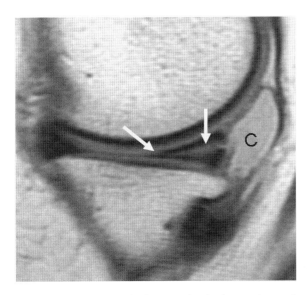

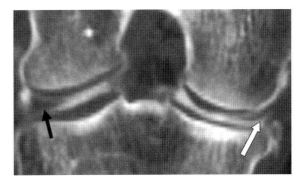

FIG. 10.9. Computed tomography (CT) arthrogram of meniscal tear. A coronally reformatted CT image after the intraarticular injection of contrast shows contrast in a vertical tear of the periphery of the body of the medial meniscus (white arrow). Note the normal low-density wedge appearance of the contralateral lateral meniscus (black arrow).

FIG. 10.8. Meniscal cyst. Sagittal proton-density image shows a large cyst (C) adjacent to the posterior horn of the medial meniscus. An oblique tear (white arrows) is visualized extending from the free edge of the meniscus into the cyst.

The cysts may occasionally be heterogeneous in appearance due to septations and hemorrhage.

For patients with contraindications to MRI, such as pacemakers or cerebral aneurysm clips, computed tomography arthrography (CTA) should be considered the second-line imaging modality after MRI because of the advent of helical and multidetector computed tomography (CT) and powerful computer processors that can reconstruct and reformat the large volume of CT data. After intraarticular injection of 20 to 40 cc of iodinated contrast, thin slices are performed in a helical fashion through the knee in the axial plane, with the data reformatted into the coronal and sagittal planes, thus resembling the planes of an MR examination. The normal low-density (dark) meniscus is outlined by the high-density (bright) contrast, and contrast insinuates itself into a tear. Thus, on the reformatted sagittal and coronal CT images, the high-density linear tear looks similar to that of the high signal intensity tear on MRI (Fig. 10.9). Reported sensitivities and specificities of this technique are 92% to 100% and 88% to 98%, respectively, even in the presence of ACL tears.[57–60]

Postoperative Meniscus

A challenging aspect of meniscal imaging is the evaluation of the postoperative meniscus. Because the peripheral 20% of a meniscus is vascularized, tears in this region can be repaired with the expectation that the tear will heal, whereas tears occurring in the avascular inner 70% to 80% of the meniscus do not heal and must be resected. However, even though repaired, the abnormal linear signal intensity that was formerly the peripheral tear may persist for years due to granulation tissue, and may mimic a re-tear on postoperative MRI.[61–66]

Similarly, after a tear of the avascular portion is trimmed and the meniscus is reshaped, the intrasubstance degenerative signal intensity that previously did not reach an articular surface may now abut the reshaped surface mimicking a new tear, a phenomenon called "signal conversion."[62] Thus, the overall accuracy of conventional MRI for evaluation of the postoperative meniscus is 66% to 82%.[62–64]

Magnetic resonance arthrography (MRA) and CTA have been advocated for evaluation of both of these scenarios, with a tear being present if contrast insinuates itself into the meniscus. Magnetic resonance arthrography has an accuracy of 88% to 92% for all postoperative menisci,[65,66] but is most useful for patients who have had meniscal resection of more than 25% or who have had meniscal repair.[65,67] Magee et al.[67] found that conventional MRI had only 52% sensitivity for meniscal tears in patients with greater than 25% resection, but that MRA had 100% sensitivity for this subgroup and that MRA was necessary to correctly evaluate all patients with meniscal repair who had persistent linear signal on the conventional MR images. Computed tomography arthrography has similar reported results.[68] Indirect MRA (a technique in which gadolinium contrast is injected intravenously and diffuses into the joint) has reported sensitivities of 83% to 91% and specificities of 78% to 100%,[69,70] but evaluation can be confounded by the fact that healing tears will enhance.[71] Having the preoperative MRI examination for comparison in order to see the original tear configuration can also be helpful, regardless of the postoperative imaging technique used.

The irreparably torn meniscus is often surgically removed, but because the menisci act as shock absorbers and distributors of axial load, extensive partial or complete meniscectomy can lead to degenerative arthritis. In such patients, meniscal allograft transplantation is sometimes performed to decrease the pain resulting from altered contact stress and forestall the progression of osteoarthritis. The surgical technique involves harvesting a cadaveric meniscus with either plugs of bone at the anterior and posterior meniscal root attachments or a single long bar of bone containing the root attachments; a trough is made in the tibial plateau of the recipient knee for the bone plugs or bony bar, and the bone is sutured to the plateau and the periphery of the transplanted meniscus is sutured to the host joint capsule.

Magnetic resonance imaging may be used to follow the transplanted meniscus, especially if the patient continues to complain of pain, swelling, or locking, and there is clinical concern for graft tear or failure. The transplanted allograft should be assessed for intrasubstance signal, frank tear, displacement or frank extrusion, and signal intensity along the transplant-capsular junction. Intrasubstance signal intensity correlates with mucoid degeneration and fibroblastic proliferation histologically,[72] which are features of degeneration, but Noyes et al.[73] believe that the transplanted meniscus undergoes a remodeling process accounting for the signal change but during which the meniscus is weakened. However, there are no studies of the preimplantation appearance of the graft and longitudinal series of the graft after implantation, to determine whether the signal is preexisting degeneration, developmental degeneration, or remodeling. Intrasubtance signal and mild meniscal displacement may be seen in patients who have both clinical improvement and persistent pain,[72–74] while frank tear, meniscal displacement more than 50% of its width, and high signal intensity at the capsular junction, indicating nonhealing, all suggest graft failure.[73] Potter et al.[72] found that patients with preoperative articular cartilage loss had poor clinical outcomes after transplant, which correlated with transplant fragmentation and extrusion. Similarly, Noyes et al.[73] found a higher rate of graft failure in patients with preexisting moderate knee arthrosis compared to patients with none or mild

arthrosis. The allograft may also gradually decrease in size, leading to its inability to function normally.[75]

Ligament Injury

Anterior Cruciate Ligament

Anatomy

The ACL provides restraint against anterior subluxation of the tibia, and is composed of an anteromedial bundle and a posterolateral bundle that twist on each other, thus providing reciprocal tautness as the knee ranges from extension to flexion. The ligament extends from the roof of the intercondylar notch to the tibial plateau anterior to the lateral tibial spine and has a straight course paralleling or slightly steeper than the intercondylar roof (called "Blumensaat's line" on lateral radiographs). On sagittal T2-weighted images the ligament has a linear striated appearance with intermediate signal intensity (Fig. 10.10). The anterior margin may occasionally have a darker and thicker appearance than the rest of the ligament, which may correspond anatomically to the anteromedial bundle.

Injury

An acutely ruptured ACL appears on sagittal MRI as either replacement of the normal linear striated appearance by an amorphous cloud-like appearance of high signal intensity, or as a discrete discontinuity of the ligament with fibers that do not course parallel to the intercondylar roof (Fig. 10.11), with

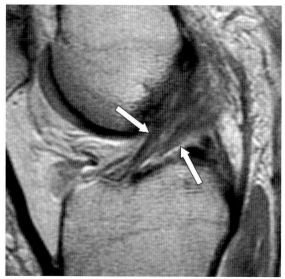
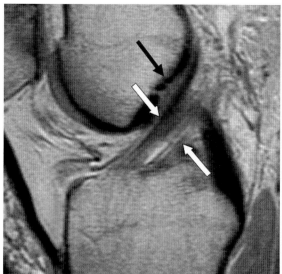

A   B

FIG. 10.10. Normal anterior cruciate ligament. (A) Sagittal proton-density image through the intercondylar notch shows the normal striated appearance of the anterior cruciate ligament (white arrows). Note that the anterior and posterior bundles are twisting on themselves. (B) Sagittal proton-density image of the same patient adjacent to the previous image shows the straight striated appearance of the ligament (white arrows). Its course is parallel or steeper than the cortex of the intercondylar roof (black arrow).

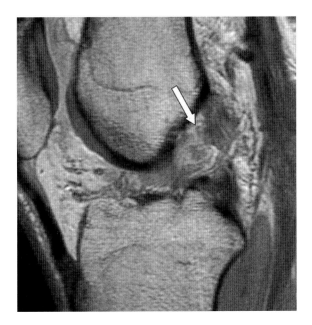

FIG. 10.11. Anterior cruciate ligament rupture. Sagittal proton-density image shows waviness and abnormal course of the fibers of the anterior cruciate ligament and frank discontinuity (arrow).

reports of 92% to 96% sensitivity and 89% to 99% specificity.[5,6,76] Rupture can also be assessed on T2-weighted axial images with a sensitivity of 92% and a specificity as high as 100% using the criteria of high signal intensity (representing edema and hemorrhage) in the expected location of the ACL or frank nonvisualization of the ligament in its expected location.[77] Using quantitative measurement of the ACL angle, Mellado et al.[78] and Murao et al.[79] found that an ACL angle of 45 degrees or less had 93% to 100% sensitivity and 84% to 100% specificity. Other authors have reported that the use of an oblique coronal sequence, oriented parallel to the plane of the ACL, can also increase the diagnostic accuracy of MRI.[80,81] Improved visualization of the ACL in the sagittal plane can also be obtained either by obliquing the sagittal plane along the course of the ligament based on the axial or coronal images or by doing straight sagittal images through the knee that has been externally rotated about 10 to 15 degrees. The distal stump may become displaced anteriorly, causing locking or a block to full extension, and appears either as a nodular mass in the anterior aspect of the intercondylar notch or a tongue-like free edge folded on itself.[82] A large hemarthrosis, best appreciated in the suprapatellar recess, usually accompanies an acute ACL rupture because of the well-vascularized nature of this ligament.

Partial tears of the ACL may appear as focal loss of the normal striated appearance that does not affect the entire diameter of this ligament, thus leaving some intact fibers on at least one imaging slice, or as increased signal intensity on T2-weighted images with mild swelling of the ligament,[83] but the reported performance for distinguishing partial tears from ruptures using the sagittal plane is only 40% to 75% sensitivity and 62% to 89% specificity in one study,[84] and as low as 19% accuracy in another.[85] Yao et al.[85]

found that posterior displacement of the posterior horn of the lateral meniscus and injury to the popliteus muscle were the most useful secondary signs for distinguishing rupture from partial tear. Pitfalls in the interpretation of acute ACL injury are cruciate ganglion cysts[86–88] and mucoid degeneration of the ACL,[89,90] both of which are chronic developments resulting from a remote trauma, but which can cause swelling of and abnormal signal intensity within an otherwise intact ACL, thus mimicking acute injury (Fig. 10.12).

In the patient who cannot undergo MRI, CTA should be considered the alternative imaging modality, with reformatting of the images into the sagittal and coronal planes. Using this technique, Van de Berg et al.[60] reported 90% sensitivity and 96% specificity. Sonographic evaluation of ruptured ACLs has been described but relies on indirect signs of injury, such as hematoma in the notch and a sonographic drawer sign, because the ACL cannot be visualized directly.[91,92]

Anterior cruciate ligament tears may be part of a larger injury pattern, such as "O'Donoghue's triad," consisting of ACL rupture, medial collateral ligament (MCL) injury, and tear of the medial meniscus. Remember, however, that the sensitivity of MRI for detecting meniscal tear in the setting of acute ACL rupture is diminished. The Segond fracture is a small vertically oriented fracture due to avulsion of the lateral joint capsule from the anterolateral aspect of the proximal tibia, just distal to the plateau, and is always associated with ACL rupture and often with tear of either the medial or lateral meniscus.[93–95]

In addition to the Segond fracture, there are other common types of bone injury associated with ACL rupture. The most common involves the combination of offset bone bruises in the weight-bearing portion of the lateral femoral condyle and poste-

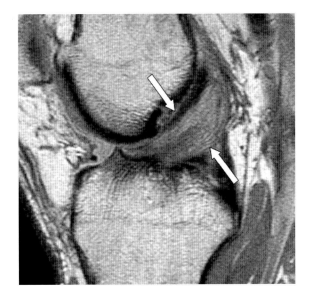

FIG. 10.12. Mucinous degeneration of the anterior cruciate ligament. Sagittal proton-density image shows generalized swelling of the anterior cruciate ligament (arrows) but its striated appearance is still present, and its fibers are continuous and parallel to the intercondylar roof.

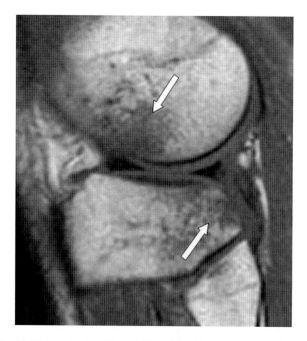

FIG. 10.13. Bone bruises. Sagittal T1-weighted image of the lateral aspect of the knee shows offset bone bruises (arrows) in the anterior aspect of the lateral femoral condyle and posterior aspect of the lateral tibial plateau, a secondary sign of rupture of the anterior cruciate ligament.

TABLE 10.1. Secondary signs of anterior cruciate ligament (ACL) tear.

1. Offset bone bruises in the weight-bearing portion of the lateral femoral condyle and posterior aspect of the lateral tibial plateau
2. Anterior "kissing" bone bruises in the anterior aspect of the tibial plateau and anterior aspects of the femoral condyles
3. Bone bruise or fracture in the posterior aspect of the medial tibial plateau
4. Lateral femoral notch sign
5. Buckling of the posterior cruciate ligament (PCL)
6. PCL line sign—a line drawn along the curve of the PCL on sagittal images does not intersect the femur within 5 cm of the distal aspect of the femur
7. Anterior subluxation of the tibia—a line drawn vertically along the posterior aspects of the femoral condyles is more than 7 mm from the posterior cortex of the tibial plateau
8. Uncovering of the posterior horn of the lateral meniscus—a line drawn vertically along the posterior cortex of the tibial plateau intersects the posterior horn of the lateral meniscus
9. Horizontal shearing tear of Hoffa's fat pad

rior aspect of the lateral tibial plateau (Fig. 10.13). This offset pattern of lateral bone bruises occurs as a result of external rotation of the femur on a fixed tibia and valgus angulation of the knee, as occurs in a cutting-type of running movement, allowing the posterolateral aspect of the tibial plateau to impact the weight-bearing portion of the lateral side of the lateral femoral condyle.[96] However, it should be noted that in children, this pattern of offset lateral bone bruises may not have an associated ACL tear, because of normal pediatric ligamentous laxity.[97,98] Bone bruises represent a spectrum of trabecular injury, but the overlying hyaline cartilage may also be injured, with histologic evidence of chondrocyte degeneration[99] and follow-up MR studies showing cartilage thinning over the site even after the bone bruise has resolved[100,101] (see below). "Kissing" bone bruises may occur in the anterior aspect of the tibial plateau and anterior aspects of the femoral condyles as a result of a hyperextension injury when the anterior aspects of the tibia and femoral condyles impact each other. A less common site of bone injury is the posterior aspect of the medial tibial plateau, consisting of bone bruise, impaction fracture, or small chip fracture due to avulsion of the semimembranosus tendon,[102] and this site of bone injury is almost always accompanied by tear of the periphery or meniscocapsular junction of the posterior horn of the medial meniscus.[103] These bony injuries are not only clues to the existence of an ACL tear, but also comorbid causes of pain.

Other secondary signs of ACL injury, though not injuries themselves, are anterior subluxation of the tibia relative to the femur with resultant uncovering of the posterior horn of the lateral meniscus (Fig. 10.10, and buckling of the PCL (Table 10.1).[104–106]

In skeletally immature patients the tibial attachment of the ACL is weaker than the ligament itself, and so ACL injuries may occur as tibial avulsions of the ACL rather than ruptures of the ligament. The avulsed fracture fragment, immediately anterior to the anterior tibial spine and sometimes involving it, can often be appreciated on radiographs, but CT scanning with sagittally reformatted images can better evaluate the amount of bony distraction.

A chronically ruptured ACL will be manifest as either nonvisualization of the ligament, angulation of the ligament (instead of a straight course) due to scarring and tethering, or will have a shallow orientation instead of paralleling the intercondylar roof[76,107,108] (Fig. 10.14). Occasionally, scarred remnants may mimic an intact ligament.[107] The associated findings of acute ACL injury such as large hemarthrosis and

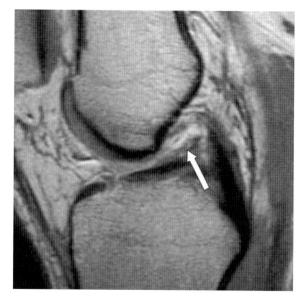

FIG. 10.14. Chronic rupture of the anterior cruciate ligament. Sagittal proton-density image through the intercondylar notch shows a small nubbin of anterior cruciate ligament remaining (arrow).

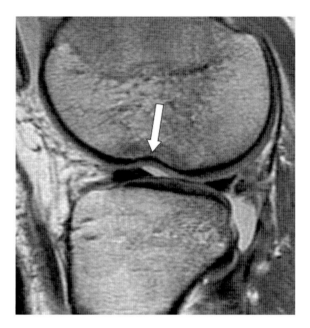

FIG. 10.15. Lateral femoral notch sign. Sagittal proton-density image of the lateral aspect of the knee shows a deepened condylopatellar sulcus (arrow), a secondary sign of injury to the anterior cruciate ligament.

bone bruises are typically not present with chronic ACL tear, though there may be anterior subluxation of the tibia and buckling of the PCL due to residual joint laxity. A deepened condylopatellar sulcus on the lateral femoral condyle, called the lateral femoral notch sign, is also an indication of chronic ACL insufficiency, but may also be seen in acute ACL injury due to traumatic impaction[109,110] (Fig. 10.15).

Anterior Cruciate Ligament Reconstruction

The ruptured ACL can be "reconstructed" using either a patellar tendon or a hamstring tendon. The patellar tendon graft is harvested from the central third of the patient's patellar tendon, taking a piece of patella and tibial tubercle on each end (called the bone–patellar tendon–bone graft). The hamstring tendon graft does not have any attached bone, and is usually doubled on itself to increase its strength and to mimic the normal double-bundled ACL. Tunnels are made in the femur and the tibia, through which the proximal and distal ends of the graft are secured. Proper positioning of the bone tunnels is necessary for isometric positioning of the graft; improper placement causes either persistent knee instability or graft impingement. The entrance of the femoral tunnel should be at the intersection of a line drawn along the posterior femoral cortex and a line drawn along the roof of the intercondylar notch on sagittal images, while on coronal images the femoral tunnel should be in the superolateral aspect of the intercondylar notch; the anterior margin of the tibial tunnel on sagittal images should be posterior to a line drawn along the roof of the intercondylar notch,[111,112] while on coronal images the

tunnel should be located between the tibial spines and angled inferomedially.

When the bone–patellar tendon–bone graft is used, fully threaded headless screws (called "interference" screws) are placed into each tunnel to hold the bony end of the graft against the inside of the bone tunnel so that it eventually fuses to the tunnel, thus providing a secure attachment for the graft. When the hamstring graft is used, the bone tunnels extend to the cortical surface of the femur and tibia, and the tendon is secured to the cortex with either staples or endobuttons.

The surgically reconstructed ACL is well visualized with MRI, regardless of the presence of interference screws, staples, or buttons. Bioabsorbable interference screws, made of either lactide-glycolide or polylactic acid, have a lower MR artifact profile than metal ones,[113,114] but even the dephasing artifact from the metal interference screws is usually not severe enough to preclude MRI of the reconstructed ligament. The intact functionally competent neoligament usually has a straight course but occasionally may be mildly bowed,[115,116] and it is more steeply oriented than the native ACL, averaging approximately 67 degrees from the plane of the tibial plateau compared to 51 degrees, respectively[117] (Fig. 10.16). Fujimoto et al.[118] stress that attention must also be paid to the course of the ACL graft in the coronal plane. In their study, the average angle of the native ACL in the coronal plane relative to the tibial plateau was 67 degrees, that of asymptomatic ACL grafts was 72 degrees, and that of ACL grafts that impinged the PCL was 79.5 degrees. This latter group also had no intervening space between the graft and the PCL on the coronal images.

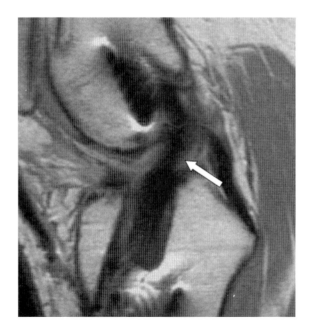

FIG. 10.16. Normal anterior cruciate ligament graft. Sagittal proton-density image shows the normal low signal intensity appearance of an anterior cruciate ligament graft (arrow). Note that its course is straight and steeper than the intercondylar roof.

The intact and functionally competent neoligament can have variable signal intensity, depending in part on the type of tendon graft used and the imaging time after placement. Some investigators have reported a temporal pattern of low signal intensity in the first few months after placement, with progressive development of high signal intensity on T1- or T2-weighted images with contrast throughout the intraarticular portion, peaking at about 1 year postplacement.[119,120] This high signal intensity is due to neovascularization of the graft, which occurs as part of a process called "ligamentization," which also includes development of type III collagen and changes in types and ratios of glycosaminoglycans.[121] Signal intensity gradually becomes low again by about 2 years after placement.[119,120] Other investigators, however, have reported persistent low signal intensity with both hamstring[122] and bone–patellar tendon–bone grafts.[123] Still others have reported longitudinal streaks of high signal intensity within the graft after 1 year,[116,124] and Horton et al.[115] reported three patients in their series with clinically normal grafts confirmed at second-look arthroscopy, one of whom had diffuse high signal intensity in the graft 56 months after graft placement and two of whom had focal high signal intensity an average of 46 months after graft placement. This variability in signal intensity in the normal graft decreases the usefulness of high signal intensity as an indicator of graft impingement or rupture.

Reasons for imaging the reconstructed ACL include assessment of graft impingement, graft rupture, or fibrosis. Impingement of the graft against the anterior aspect of the intercondylar notch may cause pain during extension, block to full extension, or even instability. This impingement may occur if the tibial bone tunnel is too anterior or if the notch is too small. Even though the tibial tunnel may be well depicted on MRI, the ability to interpret impingement is quite variable, with sensitivity of 32% to 83%, specificity of 52% to 100%, and poor interobserver agreement.[125] In addition, recortication of the notchplasty site and the development of an overlying layer of fibrocartilage after the ACL reconstruction can cause narrowing of an initially adequate notchplasty.[126] Notch impingement can cause high T2-weighted signal intensity in the distal two thirds of the intraarticular portion of the graft[122,123] (Fig. 10.17).

The patient with a ruptured graft usually complains of knee instability. Using conventional MRI and evaluating the graft in both the coronal and sagittal planes with such criteria as signal intensity, orientation, discontinuity, and thinning of the graft, Horton et al.[115] prospectively achieved only 50% sensitivity, 100% specificity, and 87.5% accuracy for rupture of the graft, and 0% sensitivity, 67% specificity, and 37.5% accuracy for partial tear. Retrospectively reviewing their data, they stress the evaluation of graft fiber continuity or complete graft discontinuity in the coronal plane and graft thickness in either plane as the most useful discriminators for graft rupture. Signal intensity was not helpful, with only 45% sensitivity and 59% accuracy for diagnosing tear (partial or full thickness) versus intact graft. They also found that secondary signs of

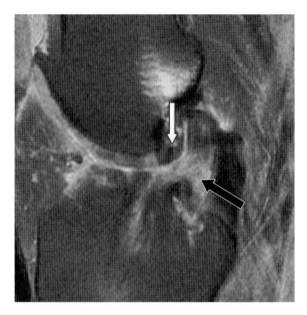

FIG. 10.17. Anterior cruciate ligament graft impingement. Sagittal proton-density image shows high signal intensity within the distal aspect of the anterior cruciate ligament graft (black arrow). The graft is impinged and displaced by an osteophyte arising from the anterior aspect of the intercondylar notch (white arrow).

ACL insufficiency, such as anterior tibial translation, uncovered posterior horn of the lateral meniscus, buckling of the PCL, and the PCL line, were not useful discriminators, in part due to only fair to moderate interobserver agreement for identifying these signs, and the fact that ACL reconstruction may not provide the same physiologic stability as a native ACL. Using MRA, McCauley et al.[125] improved both the sensitivity and specificity for graft rupture to 100% when the graft was discontinuous and contrast extended into the region of discontinuity.

The development of focal scar tissue in the anterior aspect of the intercondylar notch may act as a block to full extension after ACL reconstruction, and has been termed the "cyclops" lesion by orthopedic surgeons because it resembles an eye as they look at it arthroscopically. The cyclops lesion can be detected on MRI with 85% accuracy,[127] and appears as a nodular soft tissue mass of intermediate signal intensity on proton density and T2-weighted imaging anterior to the entrance of the tibial tunnel[127,128] (Fig. 10.18). The lesions are a histologic spectrum of fibrosis and fibrocartilage, and are believed to be a reactive process but they may not always be caused by graft impingement, since Bradley et al.[127] found no difference in tunnel placement or notch size between patients with and without these lesions.

In reconstructions using a hamstring and endobutton technique, Jansson et al.[124] reported that the diameter of the femoral and tibial bones tunnels increased by up to 33% in the first 2 years after placement, even though the knees were clinically stable and asymptomatic, whereas no such change occurred with patients who received bone–patellar tendon–bone graft.

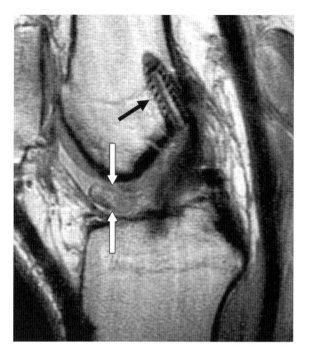

FIG. 10.18. Cyclops lesion. Sagittal proton-density image shows a normal appearing anterior cruciate ligament graft, but a large oval mass of fibrous tissue is present in the anterior aspect of the intercondylar notch (white arrows). Note the excellent visualization of the absorbable interference screw (black arrow).

In addition, regeneration of the hamstring tendon at the harvest site has been documented clinically[129] and experimentally.[130] In cases of bone–patellar tendon–bone graft, the patellar tendon harvest site may show postoperative changes for as long as 6 years after surgery, consisting of a persistent defect in the central third and increased width.[131] Lastly, reactive inflammatory edema has been noted in the marrow around lactide-glycolide interference screws but not around polylactic acid screws.[113]

Posterior Cruciate Ligament

Anatomy

The PCL is the primary restraint against posterior subluxation of the tibia. Although it is composed of an anterolateral and posteromedial bundle, similar to the ACL, the collagen fibers of the PCL are more tightly grouped, giving the normal PCL uniform low signal intensity on all MR pulse sequences and making it two to four times stronger than the ACL. On sagittal images the PCL has a gentle curve (see Fig. 10.3), and the meniscofemoral ligaments of Humphry and Wrisberg can occasionally be seen in cross section, anterior and posterior, respectively, to the PCL. The meniscofemoral ligaments originate on the medial side of the intercondylar notch, adjacent to the origin of the PCL, and insert on the root of the posterior horn of the lateral meniscus.

Injury

Injury of the PCL does not look the same as injury of the ACL. Both ruptures and partial-thickness tears may appear as generalized thickening and ill-definition of the ligament on MRI, with intermediate signal intensity on T1-weighted sequences and heterogeneous high signal intensity on T2-weighted sequences[132] (Fig. 10.16), and rupture can only be confidently distinguished from partial tear when there is frank ligamentous discontinuity[133] (Fig. 10.19). Avulsion of the distal aspect of the PCL from the tibia occurs in 10% of cases.[134]

The incidence of bone bruises associated with PCL tear was 83% in one series, but their pattern was more diverse and widespread than with ACL injury.[135] Injury of the PCL is often accompanied by injuries of the ACL, MCL, and the posterolateral stabilizers,[132,133] and the presence of a bone bruise in one location often indicates soft tissue injury in the contralateral portion of the knee.[135] In addition, an avulsion of the medial tibial plateau by the deep fibers of the MCL has been described in association with PCL tears, and has been termed a "reverse Segond" fracture.[136]

The injured PCL usually regains normal-appearing low signal intensity and continuity when it heals, but may still be functionally incompetent and allow tibial subluxation.[137–141] Surgical reconstruction of the ruptured PCL is not as common as the ACL, and there is disagreement among surgeons regarding the proper location of the femoral and tibial bone tunnels necessary for isometric positioning.[142] Location of the femoral tunnel may be more important to proper tensioning of the graft than the tibial tunnel but is technically more difficult to place correctly because of a lack of anatomic landmarks.[142]

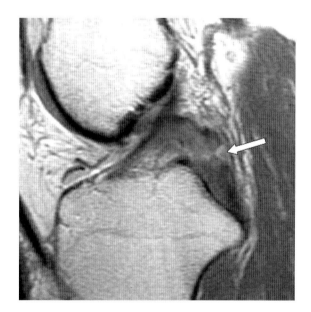

FIG. 10.19. Posterior cruciate ligament rupture. Sagittal proton-density image through the intercondylar notch shows swelling and signal heterogeneity of the posterior cruciate ligament with frank ligamentous discontinuity (arrow).

The patellar tendon graft also undergoes ligamentization as it does when used for ACL reconstruction, but its transformation is not as complete as an ACL reconstruction and its time course may be longer.[143] Mariani et al.[144] reported heterogeneous signal intensity in patellar tendon grafts lasting at least up to 1 year, and no correlation between the MR appearance of the graft and clinical status of the knee during this time period. After 3 years, however, the presence of abnormal signal intensity in the graft did correlate with changes in clinical stability.

Lastly, ganglion cysts may arise from the PCL and appear as discrete locular collections most often adjacent to the posterior surface of the ligament, as opposed to ganglion cysts of the ACL, which often can be traced into the fibers of the ligament itself.[87] Caution should be exercised in diagnosing a fluid-appearing collection behind the PCL as a cyst, since there is a normal capsular recess in which fluid may collect, but unlike a ganglion cyst fluid in the recess does not contact the proximal aspect of the PCL and can be traced into the posterior aspect of the medial femorotibial compartment of the knee.[145]

Medial and Posteromedial Stabilizers

Anatomy

The MCL is the primary restraint to valgus motion of the knee.[146] The ligament is composed of both superficial and deep components, corresponding to the second and third tissue layers of the medial side of the knee, respectively, described by Warren and Marshall,[147] with the first tissue layer representing deep crural fascia. The superficial and deep components may be separated by a thin layer of fat at the level of the joint line. Similarly, an anatomically inconstant bursa exists between the two components.[148] The superficial component of the MCL (also called the tibial collateral ligament[149]) is composed of vertically oriented collagen fibers that extend from the superior aspect of the medial femoral condyle to the proximal aspect of the tibial shaft. The posterior aspect of the superficial component blends with the deep component to form the posteromedial joint capsule, which also receives a branch of the semimembranosus tendon, thus forming a linear area of thickening of the posteromedial capsule called the posterior oblique ligament,[146,150,151] but there is disagreement in the literature on the exact anatomy, probably representing normal anatomic variations. The deep component of the MCL forms the medial joint capsule, blending with the peripheral aspect of the medial meniscus and inferiorly forming the meniscotibial ligament (also called the coronary ligament) and superiorly forming the meniscofemoral ligament.[146,149,152] The semimembranosus tendon also has a branch that forms the oblique popliteal ligament (of Winslow) of the posterior capsule, which is also reinforced by the medial limb of the arcuate ligament.[150,151] The posteromedial capsule is a restraint to internal rotation of the tibia.[153]

Injury

The MCL is injured as a result of valgus stress on the knee, often in combination with a rotational force, and therefore may be associated with injury of the menisci and cruciate ligaments. Isolated MCL injury due to pure valgus stress is less common. Injury is best appreciated on coronal fat-suppressed T2-weighted images. A grade I sprain, representing mild partial interstitial tearing, appears as edema surrounding an otherwise normal-appearing ligament. A grade II sprain, representing more extensive interstitial partial tearing, is manifest as surrounding edema with either thickening of the ligament with internal signal abnormality or thinning of the ligament due to more extensive partial tearing (Fig. 10.20). Complete rupture of the ligament, a grade III sprain, can occur from either the proximal or distal attachments and appears as focal discontinuity.[76,149,154] Bone bruises often are present, usually in the medial and lateral femoral condyles.[149]

The injured ligament sometimes heals with heterotopic ossification, which is radiographically visible and is referred to as Pellegrini-Stieda disease. It may be seen on MR images as a signal void in the ligament, best appreciated on T2-weighted gradient echo sequences, but may also occasionally demonstrate high signal intensity of fatty marrow on T1-weighted images if the ossification is mature.[155]

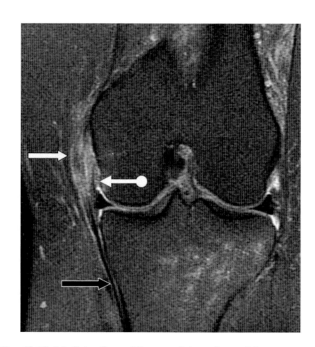

FIG. 10.20. Medial collateral ligament injury. Coronal fat-suppressed T2-weighted image shows extensive partial tearing of the proximal aspect of the medial collateral ligament (straight white arrow) manifested by thickening, poor definition and edema-like signal intensity. The distal aspect of the medial collateral ligament is intact (black arrow). There is also mild sprain of the meniscofemoral ligament of the medial joint capsule manifest by surrounding edema and poor definition (round tail white arrow).

Edema may also be present around the MCL in knees with degenerative arthritis, mimicking a traumatic sprain, but the edema is caused by chronic friction of medial osteophytes against the ligament, rather than by acute injury.[156]

Injury to the posteromedial capsule, potentially leading to anteromedial rotatory instability of the knee, always involves the posterior oblique ligament (POL).[151] Sims and Jacobson,[151] in a series of 93 patients, described three patterns of injury: (1) injury of the POL and the contributing component of the semimembranosus, occurring in 70% of cases; (2) injury of the POL and peripheral meniscal detachment, occurring in 30% of cases; and (3) injury of the POL and semimembranosus and peripheral meniscal detachment.[151] Other injuries in their series included the tibial collateral ligament in 33% of cases and meniscotibial and meniscofemoral ligaments in 83%, and the most common causes of posteromedial injury were football, basketball, and skiing. Injury is manifested as edema in the posteromedial aspect of the knee or disruption of these structures.[150] The semimembranosus tendon may also be avulsed from the tibia by the same mechanism of flexion and internal rotation of the tibia that produces a rupture of the ACL (see above). Isolated rupture of the semimembranosus tendon has been reported, but is uncommon.[150,157]

The sartorius, gracilis, and semitendinosus tendons are located in the superficial aspect of the posteromedial region, and comprise the pes anserinus. These tendons insert as a conjoined tendon on the medial aspect of the tibia, superficial and anterior to the attachment of the medial collateral ligament and are separated from the MCL by the pes anserinus bursa. They are flexors of the knee and assist in medial rotation of the tibia. They also have aponeurotic extensions that blend with the adjacent superficial fascial layer of the knee (layer 1) to provide medial stability.[158] Injury of these tendons is rare,[159] but the bursa may become inflamed by overuse or a single traumatic event (see below).

Posterolateral Stabilizers

Anatomy

The knee is restrained from posterolateral rotatory instability (varus angulation and external rotation of the tibia) by a complex group of posterolateral ligaments and tendons. Static stabilization is provided by the fibular collateral ligament (also called the lateral collateral ligament), which originates on the superolateral aspect of the lateral femoral condyle and inserts on the lateral aspect of the fibular head; the arcuate ligament, which arises from the fibular head and has a lateral limb that blends superiorly with the joint capsule and a medial limb that runs superomedially and blends with the oblique popliteal ligament of Winslow; the popliteus tendon; the popliteofibular ligament, which connects the popliteus tendon to the fibular head; and the fabellofibular ligament, which reinforces the posterior joint capsule even if the fabella is congenitally absent. Dynamic stabilization is provided by the popliteus muscle,

biceps femoris muscle, and lateral gastrocnemius muscle. The distal tendon of the biceps femoris and the fibular collateral ligament blend together at their insertion on the fibular head to form the conjoined tendon[134,160,161] (Figs. 10.3B and 10.21). Of all these stabilizers, the fibular collateral ligament, popliteofibular ligament, and popliteus muscle and tendon are the most important.[162] The normal fibular collateral ligament and popliteus muscle and tendon are consistently visualized with MRI, but the normal popliteofibular ligament was seen in only 57% of cases in one series.[163]

Injury

Isolated injury of the posterolateral structures is due to pure hyperextension, but this is unusual. More often the mechanism of injury is a combination of hyperextension with either varus force or external rotation, leading to injury of the posterolateral stabilizers and a variable combination of other structures, such as the PCL, ACL, MCL, menisci, and bone bruises.[134,160,162,164] The peroneal nerve may also be injured by the offending mechanism of injury.[134,162]

Injury to these stabilizers can be missed at physical examination, especially in the presence of injury to other ligaments such as the ACL and PCL. In Miller et al.'s[160] series of 30 patients with posterolateral corner injury, most of whom had accompanying variable injuries of the ACL, MCL, menisci, and PCL, only three instances of posterolateral injury were clinically suspected. Clinically unrecognized instability of the posterolateral corner of the knee can lead to failure of subsequent ACL and PCL reconstruction.[160]

Injury is best assessed on fat-suppressed T2-weighted MR images, looking for soft tissue edema surrounding these

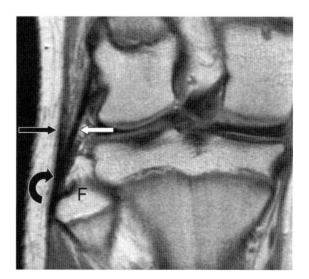

FIG. 10.21. Normal posterolateral aspect of the knee. Coronal proton-density image shows the normal fibular collateral ligament (white arrow) and biceps femoris tendon (straight black arrow). These two structures combine to form a conjoined tendon (curved black arrow), which inserts on the lateral aspect of the fibular head (F).

structures, which suggests mild sprain; thickening or thinning of these structures with internal edema, suggesting moderate sprain; or frank discontinuity of these structures, indicating rupture[160] (Fig. 10.22). In a prospective study of 20 patients with posterolateral injury and subsequent surgical confirmation, LaPrade et al.[165] found the MRI had 94% sensitivity and 100% specificity for identifying the injured fibular collateral ligament, and 69% sensitivity and 68% specificity for the injured popliteofibular ligament. Coronal images may be optimized by obliquing the plane along the course of the fibular collateral ligament.[165,166] Injury of the popliteus muscle usually occurs at the musculotendinous junction or muscle belly,[160,167] and appears as feathery high signal intensity in the muscle, disruption of muscle fibers, and swelling of the muscle.

Injury to the posterolateral stabilizers is also suggested on radiographs by the "arcuate sign," an avulsion fracture of the fibular head,[168] representing the avulsed attachment of the biceps femoris tendon and fibular collateral ligament. Associated injuries that have been noted in patients with this sign at subsequent MRI or surgery involve the cruciate ligaments, popliteofibular ligament, arcuate ligament, and menisci, as well as bone bruises in the anterior aspects of the medial femoral condyle and medial tibial plateau.[169–171] Thus, similar to the Segond fracture, this small avulsion fracture of the fibular head indicates major soft tissue injury and internal derangement.

Surgical techniques for reconstruction of the posterolateral corner are quite variable, and include anterior and distal advancement of the fibular attachment, tenodesis of the distal biceps femoris tendon to the lateral femoral condyle, thus converting the tendon from a dynamic to a static stabilizer,

primary repair of the injured structures, or reconstruction of either the fibular collateral ligament alone or including the popliteal tendon and popliteofibular ligament.[134,162,164] Typically, reconstruction requires a long graft, for which the Achilles tendon, anterior or posterior tibial tendon, or semitendinosus tendon may be used.

Iliotibial Band

Anatomy

The iliotibial band (ITB) is a long fibrous tract that originates at the level of the hip from fusion of the aponeuroses of the gluteus maximus, gluteus medius, and tensor fascia lata muscles, and courses distally to insert at the knee; it has a deep layer that attaches to the lateral femoral condyle, and a superficial layer that inserts on Gerdy's tubercle of the tibia.[159,165]

Injury

The ITB may become injured by the same varus and external rotation mechanisms that damage the posterolateral stabilizers, and the MR appearance of acute injury is the same as that of the structures of the posterolateral aspect and of the MCL. Accuracy of MRI for diagnosing injury to the ITB in these patients is 86% to 95%.[165,172]

More commonly, though, injury of the ITB is an overuse phenomenon, typically in long-distance runners, bicyclists, and rowers.[173,174] The mechanism of injury in these patients has traditionally been thought to be rubbing of the ITB, particularly the posterior aspect, against the lateral femoral condyle during repetitive flexion and extension of the knee,

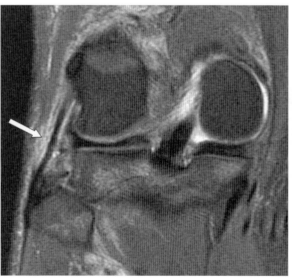
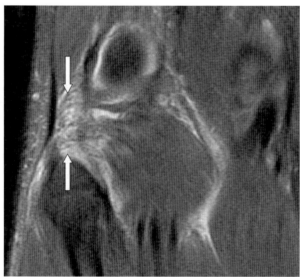

A   B

Fig. 10.22. Posterolateral corner injury. (A) Coronal fat-suppressed T2-weighted image shows a mild sprain of the fibular collateral ligament manifest by surrounding soft tissue edema (arrow). (B) Coronal fat-suppressed T2-weighted image in the same patient posterior to A shows feathery edema involving the arcuate ligament (arrows).

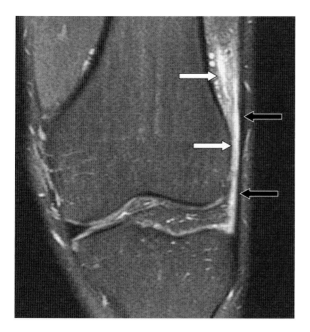

FIG. 10.23. Iliotibial band friction syndrome. Coronal fat-suppressed T2-weighted image shows high signal intensity edema (white arrows) deep to the iliotibial band (black arrows).

leading to painful inflammation, called the "iliotibial band friction syndrome."[175,176] Pain is maximal at 30 degrees of knee flexion, and patients with this syndrome have high signal intensity edema between the ITB and lateral femoral condyle and occasionally superficial to the ITB on coronal fat-suppressed T2-weighted MR images[177,178] (Fig. 10.23). However, a recent anatomic and clinical study has suggested that the syndrome is actually due to repetitive compression of fat between the ITB and lateral femoral condyle[174] rather than frictional rubbing, since the deep layer of the ITB anchors the band to the lateral femoral condyle and prevents it from rubbing back and forth against the condyle. Instead, as the knee flexes to 30 degrees the tibia internally rotates and brings the ITB against the lateral femoral condyle, thus compressing the intervening fat, which is well innervated and vascularized, and as the knee extends the tibia rotates externally thus moving the ITB away from the condyle and releasing the compression of the fat.

The Extensor Apparatus

Anatomy

The extensor apparatus consists of the quadriceps tendon, the patella, the patellar tendon, and the medial and lateral patellar retinacula.[179,180] The quadriceps tendon is the conglomeration of the distal tendons of the quadriceps muscle, and usually has a striated appearance on sagittal MR images, with the anterior striation representing the contribution from the rectus femoris, the middle striations representing the vastus lateralis and medialis, and the deep striation representing the vastus inter-

medius muscles. The quadriceps tendon inserts on the anterior aspect of the superior pole of the patella, but the anterior fibers of the tendon, usually mostly composed of the rectus femoris contribution, continue over the anterior aspect of the patella to become the patellar tendon. The patellar tendon is normally less than 75% of the thickness of the quadriceps tendon, has parallel surfaces, and exhibits uniformly low signal intensity, except at it proximal attachment, where there may be a V-shaped focus of high signal intensity on T1-weighted images[181,182] (Fig. 10.24).

The patella is the largest sesamoid bone in the body, and its purpose is to protect the extensor tendon apparatus from friction against the femur during knee flexion and to give mechanical advantage to the apparatus by lifting it away from the joint itself. The patellar articular cartilage is the thickest articular cartilage in the body, and engages the articular cartilage of the femoral trochlear groove as the knee flexes. The patella is normally composed of three facets: the lateral, which is long and shallowly oriented and is the predominant articular surface in extension; the medial facet, which is shorter and more steeply oriented and is the predominant articular surface in flexion;

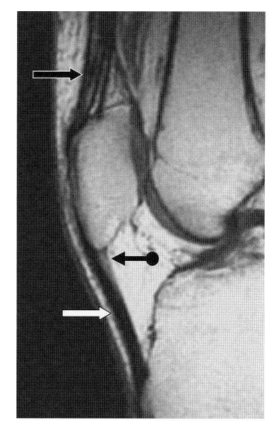

FIG. 10.24. Normal extensor mechanism. Sagittal T1-weighted image shows the normal striated appearance of the quadriceps tendon (straight black arrow). The patellar tendon (white arrow) is straight, thinner than the quadriceps tendon, and uniformly low signal intensity except for the normal V-shaped signal along the deep aspect of the proximal portion (round tail black arrow).

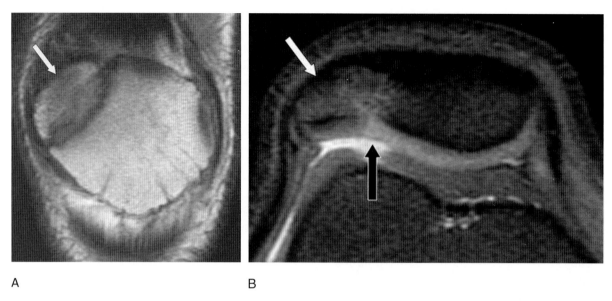

FIG. 10.25. Bipartite patella. (A) Coronal proton-density image shows the bipartite appearance, with the accessory center located in the upper lateral quadrant of the patella (arrow). Note that the ossification center does not fit perfectly like a puzzle piece with the remainder of the patella, as would a fracture. (B) Axial fat-suppressed T2-weighted image in the same patient shows the accessory ossification center (white arrow). Note that the articular cartilage (black arrow) covers the entire surface of the bipartite patella.

and the odd facet, which is the smallest and the most medially located, and is the predominant articular surface in extreme degrees of flexion (greater the 135 degrees).[179]

A bipartite patella is a normal variant in which there is a separate ossification center of the upper, outer quadrant of the patella, but the overlying articular cartilage surface remains uniform and unbroken (Fig. 10.25). The bipartite patella is present in approximately 2% of the population and is usually asymptomatic, but can become painful due to stress across the synchondrosis between the ossicle and patella resulting from repetitive pull by the vastus lateralis muscle.[183] Clinically, the patient's pain can be elicited by tapping over the symptomatic ossicle.

Medial and lateral stability of the patella is provided by the bony confines of the femoral trochlear groove and by the medial and lateral patellar retinacula. The retinacula are broad bands of fascial tissue that sweep forward from the medial and lateral sides of the knee to insert on the patella. They have both superficial and deep components, giving a bilaminar appearance on axial MRI[184] (Fig. 10.26). The superficial layer of the lateral retinaculum is formed by fascial tissue from the iliotibial band and vastus lateralis muscle and inserts on the patella and patellar tendon. The deep component is composed of a transverse band, which arises from the deep surface of the iliotibial band and inserts on the lateral side of the patella proximal to the inferior pole; the patellotibial band, which connects the tibia and lateral meniscus to the lateral margin of the patella inferior to the transverse band; and the epicondylopatellar band, which connects the lateral epicondyle to the patella, proximal to the transverse band. The superficial

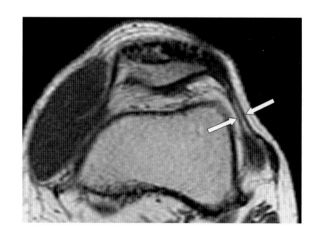

FIG. 10.26. Normal lateral retinaculum. Axial T1-weighted image shows the bilaminar appearance of the lateral retinaculum (arrows) with contributions from the iliotibial band (superficial) and vastus lateralis muscle (deep).

layer of the medial retinaculum is formed by a confluence of the anterior aspects of the first and second layers of the medial side of the knee (see Medial and Posteromedial Stabilizers, above). The deep portion is also composed of three ligaments, the largest, most superior, and clinically most important of which is the medial patellofemoral ligament, which originates from the adductor tubercle of the medial condyle and blends with the superficial layer as it inserts on the patella. The two other components of the deep layer are the patellomeniscal ligament, which is also clinically important to patellar stabilization and courses obliquely from the medial meniscus and meniscotibial (coronary) ligament to the tibia; and the patel-lotibial ligament, which is the most inferiorly located and least important functionally, extending from the anteromedial tibia to the patella.[184]

Injury

The quadriceps and patellar tendons are subject to both rupture and chronic degeneration due to overuse. The quadriceps tendon is more prone to tear, while the patellar tendon is more prone to overuse injury.

Rupture is usually seen in the unconditioned "weekend" athlete; in people with systemic disease such as diabetes, chronic renal failure, or rheumatoid arthritis; and in people on chronic steroid therapy. The mechanism of injury can be trivial, such as walking up or down stairs, but is usually due to stumbling, in which there is an eccentric contraction of the extensor mechanism as the flexing knee tries to extend against the weight of the stumbling person. While the diagnosis is usually made clinically, it is not always easy to determine a partial tear, which can be treated conservatively, from a complete rupture, which may be treated surgically. Both sagittal T2-weighted MR images and longitudinal sonographic images can be used to assess the degree of tendon rupture and retraction. Rupture typically appears as a balled-up and mildly retracted tendon edge with surrounding soft tissue edema and edema/hemorrhage in the tendon gap (Fig. 10.27). Some cases of nonretracted quadriceps tendon rupture can be difficult to distinguish from a partial tear using routine MRI of the extended knee; sonography can be helpful in such cases by

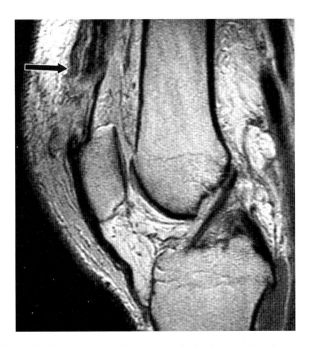

Fig. 10.27. Quadriceps tendon rupture. Sagittal proton-density image shows rupture of the distal quadriceps tendon and the retracted torn tendon edge (arrow). Some of the deep fibers remain apposed to the retracted edge.

imaging the patient in both the extended and flexed positions, looking for separation or retraction of the torn tendon edge in the flexed position.[185,186]

"Jumper's knee," or patellar tendinosis, is an overuse injury of the proximal aspect of the patellar tendon[187] and is characterized by degeneration of the collagen fibers of the tendon and subsequent partial tearing which can be painful,[188,189] but may also be asymptomatic.[190] Jumper's knee gets its name because it is commonly seen in basketball and volleyball players, but other athletes are also susceptible.[189] The term *tendinitis* is a misnomer since there is mucoid degeneration and angiofibroblastic proliferation rather than acute inflammation histologically.[188] On sagittal and axial T2-weighted MR images there is swelling of the proximal aspect of the patellar tendon with focal internal high signal intensity, with occasional edema in the adjacent fat pad and inferior pole of the patella[191] (Fig. 10.28). Sinding-Larsen-Johansson syndrome represents an abnormality of the proximal patellar tendon with radiographically visible areas of heterotopic ossification near the patellar attachment and is thought to be due to partial avulsion of the tendon,[192] but which may also be due to chronic degeneration.

Osgood-Schlatter disease is degeneration and partial tearing of the distal aspect of the patellar tendon near its insertion on the tibial tubercle,[193] and consists of the triad of pain, soft tissue swelling, and radiographically visible ossification in the distal aspect of the patellar tendon. On sagittal MRI the distal aspect of the patellar tendon may be enlarged, with low signal intensity foci of heterotopic ossification. There may also be distention of the deep infrapatellar bursa, manifest as fluid located between the anterior cortex of the tibia and the deep surface of the patellar tendon (Fig. 10.29).

The patellar tendon can exhibit other manifestations of chronic degeneration on sagittal MRI, most commonly focal areas of intermediate signal intensity on T1 and T2-weighted images without focal tendon thickening. The degenerated tendon may also appear "wrinkled," or may be diffusely thickened.[181,182] A patellar tendon that is as thick as the quadriceps tendon is abnormal.

Lateral dislocation of the patella occurs from a rotational force. Usually the patella spontaneously reduces and patients do not know that it dislocated, but they know that they "twisted the knee" and that it now hurts. Fat-suppressed T2-weighted MRI in the axial plane typically shows offset bone bruises in the medial aspect of the patella and the lateral aspect of the lateral femoral condyle, which occur as the patella spontaneously reduces. There may be associated partial tearing of the medial retinaculum manifest as thickening and internal high signal intensity, and associated tear of the distal aspect of the vastus medialis oblique muscle, manifest by feathery high signal intensity within this muscle on T2-weighted sequences[194,195] (Fig. 10.30). In addition, the lateral retinaculum can get stripped from its femoral and tibial attachments, and the medial patellofemoral ligament may be avulsed from the adductor tubercle. In patients with such forceful dislocation that the medial retinaculum ruptures completely,

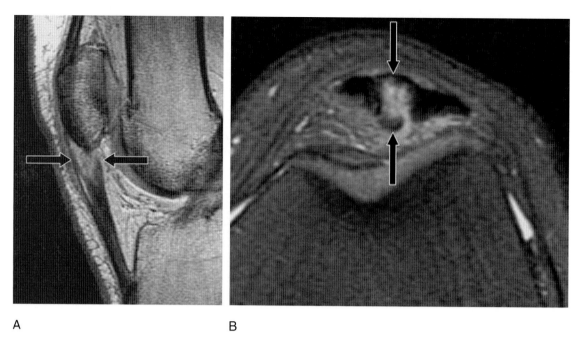

A   B

FIG. 10.28. Jumper's knee. (A) Sagittal proton-density image shows marked swelling of the proximal aspect of the patellar tendon (arrows) and abnormal high signal intensity. (B) Axial fat-suppressed T2-weighted image in this same patient shows the focal area of degeneration and partial tearing involving the central third of the patellar tendon (arrows).

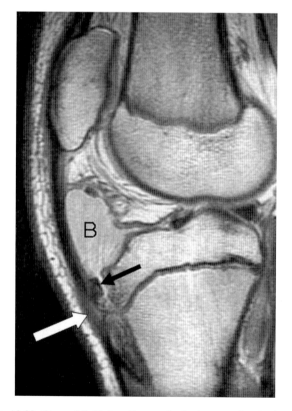

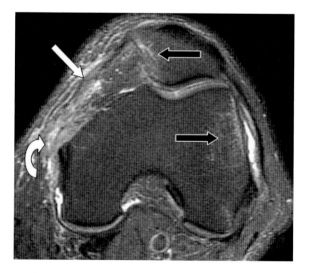

FIG. 10.30. Lateral dislocation of the patella. Axial fat-suppressed T2-weighted image shows faint offset bone bruises in the medial aspect of the patella and lateral aspect of the lateral femoral condyle (black arrows). The medial retinaculum is ill-defined (straight white arrow) with surrounding soft tissue edema. The medial patellofemoral ligament (curved white arrow) is not well seen and is replaced by high signal intensity edema.

FIG. 10.29. Osgood-Schlatter disease. Sagittal proton-density image shows thickening of the distal aspect of the patellar tendon (white arrow), with focal low signal intensity heterotopic ossification (black arrow). Note also the distended deep infrapatellar bursa (B).

the offset bone bruises are absent since there is no restraining medial tissue to bring the patella back into place.

Patellar maltracking and abnormal contact stress can occur if the patella is too high (patella alta) or too low (patella infera) within the femoral trochlear groove or if the patella is too medially or laterally located within the groove. Miller et al.[196] have shown that the Insall and Salvati[197] method of measuring patellar height can be applied to sagittal MRI, using an image with the longest patellar length and an image through the middle of the patellar tendon; patella alta is suggested when the ratio of tendon length to patellar length is 1.3 or greater (Fig. 10.31). In addition to altered contact stress between the patella and femur, patella alta may also be associated with the patellar tendon–lateral femoral condyle friction syndrome, which is an overuse injury in which the patellar tendon chronically rubs against the lateral femoral condyle or compresses the lateral aspect of Hoffa's fat pad between itself and the lateral condyle[198]; MRI demonstrates focal edema in the lateral aspect of Hoffa's fat pad.

It is not uncommon to see the patella mildly laterally subluxed relative to the femoral trochlear sulcus or slightly laterally tilted on routine axial MRI, and this positioning is usually of no clinical importance because the patella will align correctly as the knee flexes and the patella engages the trochlear groove. However, in some patients the patellar tilt or subluxation occurs during flexion and is painful or leads to recurrent dislocation. Causes of patellar maltracking include muscle imbalance, "tight" retinacula, or a congenitally shallow femoral trochlear groove or a flat patellar articular surface. Patellar

tracking is assessed in the axial plane using either CT or MRI, and can be evaluated statically or dynamically. Static assessment is performed by scanning the patient's patellofemoral joint at 0 degrees of flexion (i.e., full extension), 15 degrees of flexion both at rest and active extension, and 30 degrees both at rest and active extension.[199–202] (Fig. 10.32). Flexion is achieved with either a bolster or rolled-up blanket, and active extension is achieved by placing a strap across the ankle joints and having patients try to straighten their legs against the strap while being scanned. Inclusion of the contralateral knee in the field of view is helpful for comparison if it is normal. The dynamic assessment is performed by having the knees flexed over a bolster to 30 degrees, choosing a single slice location through the patellofemoral articulation, and scanning continuously in that same location while patients slowly and smoothly raise and lower their legs. Such kinematic imaging can be performed with MRI using gradient echo sequences, and with helical CT scanning by having the tube continually spin. The images are then placed in a cine loop for continuous viewing of patellar motion. Thirty degrees is chosen as the maximum amount of flexion for assessment of patellar tracking studies because soft tissue restraints like muscles and retinacula provide stability between 0 degrees and approximately 20 degrees of flexion, and the patella engages the femoral trochlear groove at 20 to 30 degrees.

The excessive lateral pressure syndrome refers to lateral tilt of the patella, which causes anterolateral knee pain. The patella is typically only tilted, not subluxed, and the tilt does

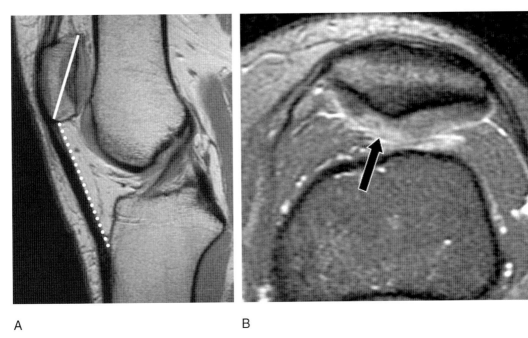

A   B

FIG. 10.31. Patella alta. (A) Sagittal proton-density image shows the maximal length of the patella (solid white arrow) compared to the length of the inner aspect of the patellar tendon (dotted arrow). In this case the patellar tendon length is more than 1.3 times the length of the patella. (B) Axial fat-suppressed T2-weighted image through the patella in this same patient shows focal chondromalacia (arrow) manifested by signal abnormality within the cartilage of the patellar apex and medial patellar facet as a result of the abnormal contact stress caused by the high-riding patella.

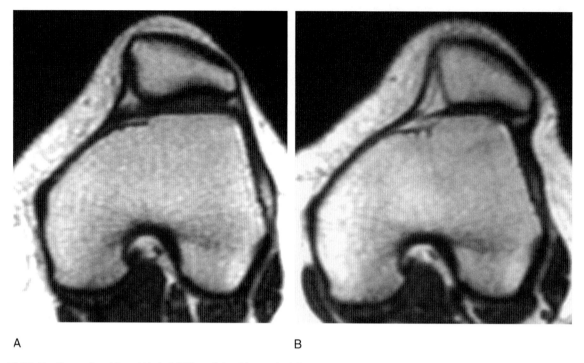

A   B

Fig. 10.32. Patellar maltracking. (A) Axial T1-weighted image in full extension at rest shows mild lateral tilt of the patella but no evidence of lateral subluxation. (B) Axial T1-weighted image through the same level of the same patient with the knee flexed 15 degrees and with active contraction of the quadriceps muscles shows lateral subluxation of the patella in addition to lateral tilt.

not change with knee flexion.[203] The cartilage over the lateral patellar facet may be eventually worn away by the excessive pressure. Patella infera is suggested when the patellar tendon length is less than 0.8 of the patellar length.[203]

Bursitis

Bursae are synovial-lined sacs typically located between a tendon and bone or between two tendons in order to reduce friction. Numerous bursae occur around the knee joint and any one of them can become distended or inflamed and thereby symptomatic. Some bursae, such as the suprapatellar bursa and deep infrapatellar bursa, are actually extensions of the knee joint itself, and therefore the term *bursa,* though commonly used, is actually a misnomer.

Other than a joint effusion in the suprapatellar recess, the most commonly seen fluid collection around the knee is the semimembranosus–medial gastrocnemius bursa, also called a Baker cyst. This cavity is a potential space located between the semimembranosus tendon and the medial head of the gastrocnemius muscle.[204] It has a communication with the posterior aspect of the joint capsule of the knee in adults, which allows fluid to be squeezed from the joint into the bursa. While there is a higher prevalence of these cysts in people who have rheumatoid arthritis, degenerative arthritis, joint effusion, or internal derangement of the knee,[205] there is a baseline level of prevalence in the general population.[206] This distended bursa is best appreciated on axial MRI, appearing

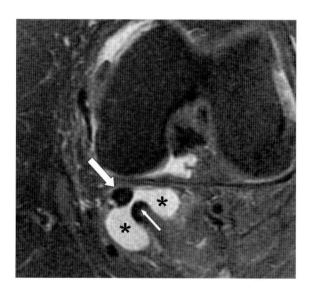

Fig. 10.33. Baker's cyst. Axial fat-suppressed T2-weighted image shows the comma-shaped Baker's cyst (asterisks). The neck of the cyst is located between the tendon of the medial gastrocnemius muscle (small white arrow) and the semimembranosus tendon (large white arrow).

comma shaped, with its neck extending between the tendon of the medial gastrocnemius and the semimembranosus tendon (Fig. 10.33). When the cysts are large, the patient may complain of pain or tightness in the back of the knee, and the cysts may track superiorly into the posterior aspect of the thigh or inferiorly into the calf, especially in patients with rheumatoid

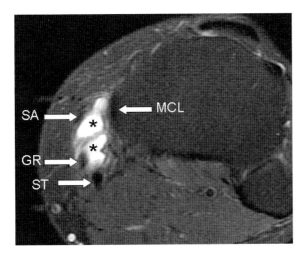

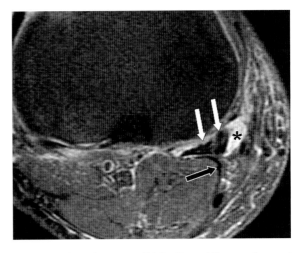

Fig. 10.34. Pes anserinus bursa. Axial fat-suppressed T2-weighted image through the proximal aspect of the tibia shows a septated pes anserinus bursa (asterisks) located between the medial collateral ligament (MCL), and the sartorius tendon (SA), gracilis tendon (GR), and semitendinosus tendon (ST).

Fig. 10.35. Semimembranosus–tibial collateral ligament bursa. Axial fat-suppressed T2-weighted image at the level the tibial plateau shows a mildly distended bursa (asterisk) adjacent to the semimembranosus tendon (white arrows). Note that this bursa is not interposed between the semimembranosus tendon and medial gastrocnemius tendon (black arrow), as would be a Baker cyst.

arthritis. The cysts may leak or rupture, best appreciated on axial fat-suppressed T2-weighted images as ill-defined soft tissue edema adjacent to the distal aspect of the cyst, thus exposing the surrounding tissue to irritative synovial fluid, which can cause severe pain and swelling, mimicking a deep venous thrombosis. These cysts can also actually cause deep venous thrombosis due to frank compression of the popliteal vein or rupture or leakage, since the irritative synovial fluid can cause a reactive thrombophlebitis. In children, cysts in the semimembranosus–medial gastrocnemius bursa do not communicate with the knee joint, are not associated with internal derangements, and are more appropriately called popliteal cysts rather than Baker cysts.[206,207]

Bursae that occur posteromedially are the pes anserinus and the semimembranosus–tibial collateral ligament bursae. The pes anserinus bursa is located between the tendons of the pes anserinus and the distal aspect of the medial collateral ligament[208] (Fig. 10.34). The semimembranosus–tibial collateral ligament bursa is located along the medial side of the distal aspect of the semimembranosus tendon (Fig. 10.35), and can be distinguished from the Baker cyst by the fact that it is medial to the semimembranosus tendon whereas the Baker cyst is lateral to the semimembranosus tendon, and it should be distinguished from the pes anserinus bursa by the fact that the semimembranosus–tibial collateral ligament bursa is adjacent to the semimembranosus tendon and follows the tendon's course[208,209] (Fig. 10.35). The Baker cyst, pes anserinus bursa, and semimembranosus–tibial collateral ligament bursa do not communicate with each other. The tibial collateral ligament bursa, located within the MCL, is rarely seen but may mimic a meniscocapsular separation on coronal T2-weighted images if it is distended (Fig. 10.36).

Two bursae of clinical concern in the anterior aspect of the knee are the prepatellar bursa and the superficial infrapatellar

bursa.[56] The prepatellar bursa is located anterior to the patella, and the superficial infrapatellar bursa is located anterior to the tibial tubercle and the distal aspect of the patellar tendon. Magnetic resonance imaging demonstrates these two structures as low signal intensity on T1-weighted sequences and high signal intensity on T2-weighted sequences (Fig. 10.26). Prepatellar bursitis is also called "housemaid's knee," because in the days when housemaids used to scrub floors on their hands and knees, the irritation of the patella rubbing against the hard surface of the floor would cause inflammation and

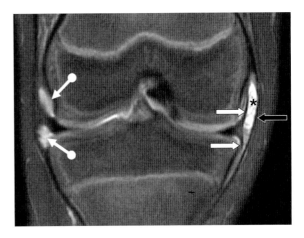

Fig. 10.36. Tibial collateral ligament bursa. Coronal fat-suppressed T2-weighted image through the knee of a child shows the distended tibial collateral ligament bursa (asterisk) located between the superficial aspect of the medial collateral ligament (black arrow) and the deep surface of the medial collateral ligament, which is the joint capsule (straight white arrows). Note the normal amount of fluid in the redundant meniscosynovial recesses of the lateral side of the knee (round tail arrows).

distention of this bursa. The symptomatic superficial infrapatellar bursa is called "preacher's knee" since this bursa is compressed between the tibial tubercle and the wooden bench on which the preacher kneels.

Cartilage and Osteochondral Injury

Because of the prevalence of degenerative arthritis and its concomitant health care costs, extensive research has been focused on imaging of articular cartilage. Numerous types of MRI sequences and techniques have been described both for the detection of gross defects as well as for detection of earliest chemical changes.[210–217] Most of these efforts have been performed with 1.5-T magnets, but as 3-T and higher field strength units become more widespread, efforts to evaluate ultrastructure will broaden. A trilaminar appearance of hyaline articular cartilage has been described on MRI, but does not perfectly correspond histologically to the true anatomic layers of articular cartilage.[218] There is no single standard cartilage imaging sequence, and many musculoskeletal radiologists have their own particular sequences that they routinely use, but the Articular Cartilage Imaging Committee of the International Cartilage Repair Society advocates proton density or T2-weighted fast spin echo sequences (with or without fat suppression) and T1-weighted three-dimensional (3D) spoiled gradient echo sequences (with fat suppression or water excitation).[219] On the fast spin echo techniques cartilage is low to intermediate signal intensity, and water, either in the joint or in the degenerating cartilage, is high signal intensity, while on the spoiled gradient echo sequence the cartilage is high signal intensity and water is low intensity. If metal instrumentation or metal debris is present from prior knee surgery, the fast spin echo technique is preferable since it is not as susceptible to dephasing as the gradient echo technique.

T2 mapping is a technique that uses the water content of articular cartilage as the biochemical marker for the earliest degenerative changes of cartilage, based on water bound to proteoglycans, which are in turn held in place by the extracellular collagen framework. These early changes are microscopic, consisting of breakdown of the collagen framework and loss of collagen orientation with resultant increase in water content of cartilage. The T2 map displays the transverse relaxation time of the cartilage based on the water content, with increased T2 in sites of increased water; color is then applied to the data to make a qualitative color map of regions of high water content.[214]

Chondromalacia patellae is a Latin term meaning "softening of the cartilage of the patella," and it is a syndrome of retropatellar pain in a teenager or young adult[203] but it represents a spectrum of cartilage degeneration, ranging from collagen breakdown and release of free water, to frank full-thickness loss of the cartilage.[220,221] In teenagers and young adults, this patellar cartilage degeneration may be an isolated finding as a result of the altered contact stress at the patellofemoral articulation due to patellar alta, patella infera, or

patellar maltracking (see Fig. 10.31), but in the older adult it is part of the larger picture of degenerative arthritis that usually also affects the cartilage of the femorotibial compartments. The early stages of this condition are seen on proton density or T2-weighted MRI as signal heterogeneity within the cartilage (stage I) and surface blistering (stage II), but have poor correlation with arthroscopic observation due to the fact that the arthroscopist cannot see the inside of the cartilage and may fail to appreciate focal early softening of the surface, seen arthroscopically as dulling of the otherwise shiny cartilage surface. The higher grades of this process, with frank cartilage defects (stage III, not full thickness; stage IV, full thickness), have better correlation between the MR appearance and arthroscopy[222,223] (Fig. 10.37).

Osteochondral injury runs the gamut from focal cartilage contusion (manifest as focal high signal intensity on T2-weighted images) to a loose osteochondral fragment, and the most common location in the knee is the lateral side of the weight-bearing portion of the medial femoral condyle. The imaging challenge of an osteochondral fragment is to determine its stability. Appearances suggestive of instability on conventional MRI are T2-weighted fluid signal intensity extending from the articular surface into and around the interface between the fragment and donor pit, and cystic change adjacent to the donor pit[224–226] (Fig. 10.38). Occasionally, MRA or CTA may be needed to clarify the integrity of the cartilage surface and the nature of the fragment–donor interface, with instability suggested if contrast insinuates into the fragment–pit interface.[227]

Caution should be exercised when interpreting subchondral bony irregularity of the femoral condyles of children because normal variations of ossification may mimic low-grade osteochondral injuries. These variations of subchondral ossification may be a single "puzzle piece" or a spiculated surface with or without accessory ossifications, and the clues to the fact that

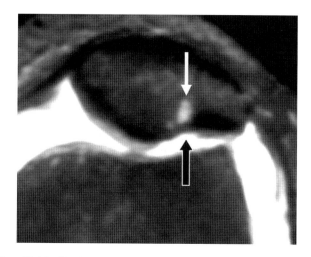

FIG. 10.37. Grade IV chondromalacia. Axial fat-suppressed T2–weighted image shows a full-thickness cartilage defect (black arrow) outlined by high signal intensity fluid in the joint. Degenerative fibrocystic change is present deep to the cartilage defect (white arrow).

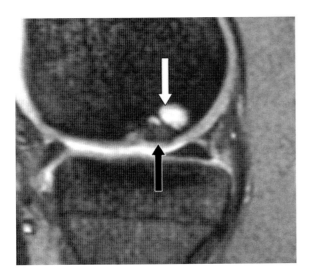

FIG. 10.38. Unstable osteochondral injury. Sagittal gradient echo T2-weighted image through the medial femoral condyle shows an osteochondral fragment in situ (black arrow) with adjacent cystic change (white arrow) indicating instability.

they are normal variations in growth and not osteochondral injuries are their posterior location in the femoral condyles, lack of associated marrow edema, and normal overlying cartilage.[228]

The need for surgical repair of osteochondral injuries depends on the size of the lesion, its depth, and its stability. Common surgical techniques for repair include marrow stimulation by drilling or microfracture, autologous osteochondral transplantation (AOT, mosaicplasty) or allograft osteochondral transplantation, and autologous chondrocyte implantation (ACI). It should be stressed that these procedures are performed for focal defects, not as therapies for generalized osteoarthritis, and that the affected knee must be stable (i.e., without ligamentous injury or meniscal tear) in order for the graft to heal. After surgery, MRI is often used to monitor noninvasively the healing and incorporation of the graft material.

Regardless of the type of cartilage repair procedure performed, Marlovits et al.[229] recommend that the following features of the repair tissue be assessed on MRI: (1) the degree of filling of the defect (e.g., complete, in which the articular surface of the graft cartilage is level with the adjacent cartilage; incomplete, in which the level of graft is lower; or hypertrophic, in which the graft surface is proud); (2) integration of the graft to the border of the adjacent cartilage (e.g., complete, in which there is no visible split between at the interface); (3) surface of the repair tissue (e.g., intact or fibrillated/ulcerated); (4) structure of the graft (e.g., normal layers of cartilage or inhomogeneity and cleft formation); (5) signal intensity of the repair tissue compared to adjacent normal cartilage; (6) subchondral bone plate (e.g., intact or broken); (7) subchondral bone (e.g., normal, or demonstrating edema, cysts, or sclerosis); (8) adhesions (i.e., fibrous bands attached to the repair site); and (9) synovitis of the joint.

In situ fragments may be pinned or drilled in order to stimulate healing of the underlying donor pit. Alternatively, the fragment may be debrided and microfracture may be performed of the underlying bone. This technique is usually used on lesions that are smaller than those for which AOTs or ACI are performed. The goal of microfracture is to stimulate bleeding in the defect site, with pluripotential stem cells in the blood eventually differentiating into cartilage. However, the cartilage that is formed is fibrocartilage, not articular hyaline cartilage, and the pluripotential cells may differentiate into bone instead of cartilage. The new bone that is formed may partially fill the defect, leading to a thinner layer of overlying reparative cartilage.[230] The reparative cartilage itself usually shows higher signal intensity than adjacent cartilage.[230,231] Patients with incomplete filling tended to have decreasing clinical functional scores over time in one series,[231] and another series found that only about 50% of athletes with this procedure were able to return to their preinjury level of activity compared to over 90% of athletes after the AOTs procedure.[232]

In the autologous osteochondral transplant procedure, cylindrical plugs of hyaline articular cartilage and underlying bone are harvested from non–weight-bearing areas, such as the posterior aspects of the femoral condyles, and embedded in the osteochondral defect. Within the first 4 weeks of implantation, the bony plugs have fatty signal intensity; at 4 to 6 weeks after implantation the plugs will demonstrate an edema-like signal intensity and will enhance with intravenous gadolinium, all of which suggests revascularization of the plugs; by 1 year the signal intensity of the plugs should return to normal, although small foci of edema-like signal intensity may remain.[219,233,234] Lack of enhancement with contrast suggests osteonecrosis, although this does not necessarily correlate with graft failure or symptoms.[234] The signal intensity of the articular cartilage of the plugs should remain normal,[234] although high signal intensity may occasionally occur.[23] The signal intensity of the fibrocartilage that develops to fill in the gaps between the hyaline cartilage surfaces of the plugs may give the entire graft a mildly heterogenous signal intensity.[219] Ideally, the surface of the plug should be level with the adjacent articular surface. The development of cystic change adjacent to the implant can be a sign of plug instability or loosening.[219] Joint effusions are common and may be present at least up to 10 months, but are usually small. Synovial enhancement may also be present, but the prevalence of effusion and synovitis decreases 2 to 3 years after the procedure.[234,235]

In the chondrocyte implantation technique, the patient's chondrocytes are harvested, cultured in vitro, and then injected into the defect. Several variations of the basic technique exist, such as using or not using an overlying covering membrane and the type of membrane used (e.g., autologous periosteum, porcine collagen membrane), using or not using a cell carrier matrix, and variation in the type of cell carrier used (e.g., fibrin, collagen, hyaluronic acid, and man-made polymers).[236–238] Ideally, the mature graft should fill the entire defect by 2 years after implantation and be flush with the adjacent articular

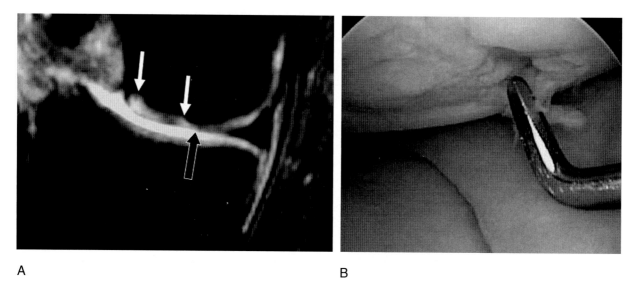

A   B

FIG. 10.39. Autologous chondrocyte implantation. (A) Coronal fat-suppressed T2-weighted image through the medial aspect of the knee 6 years after an autologous chondrocyte implantation (ACI) procedure shows focal thinning of cartilage (black arrow) and areas of abnormal high signal intensity within the transplanted cartilage (white arrows). (B) Arthroscopic image of the transplanted cartilage of the same patient shows the fibrillation, irregular surface, and defect of the cartilage. (Courtesy of Dr. Robert Pedowitz).

surface, and MRI can demonstrate if the site is underfilled or hypertrophied.[238] Techniques without a periosteal covering are sometimes used in order to avoid periosteal hypertrophy and periosteal-induced arthrofibrosis. Trattnig et al.[238] stress the importance of serial MR examinations, since several of their patients had either incomplete filling or hypertrophy within the first few months after implantation, which subsequently resolved. The signal intensity of the graft is variable, with both Tins et al.[239] and Recht et al.[219] reporting that the repair tissue generally has signal intensity lower than fluid or adjacent normal cartilage, but Henderson et al.[240] reported normal or near-normal signal intensity in 93% of their patients at 1 year, as did Wada et al.[241] While Roberts et al.[242] found a correlation between the MR appearance of the ACI graft and histology, Tins et al.[239] found no relationship between the signal intensity, thickness, surface smoothness, or bony integration of the graft and its histologic appearance 1 year after implantation. Similarly, the presence of underlying marrow edema is variable at 1 year, with 56% of 41 patients in Tins et al.'s series having edema, but only 9% of Henderson et al.'s[240] 57 patients demonstrating it. Linear fluid-like signal intensity occurring at the junction of a mature graft and underlying bone suggests poor integration or delamination[219] (Fig. 10.39), and Plank et al.[243] recommend indirect MRA for better evaluation of the integrity of the cartilage surface.

Arthritis and Arthropathy

Magnetic resonance imaging, because of its tomographic nature, is able to demonstrate osteophytes more readily than radiographs, and because of its capability of demonstrating soft tissue, it can demonstrate degenerative cartilage thinning or inflammatory synovitis that radiographs cannot.

The MRI features of degenerative arthritis are thinning or loss of articular cartilage, osteophytes, and subchondral signal intensity changes such as sclerosis, edema, or fibrocysts (Fig. 10.40). These findings exist in varying combinations and degrees of severity, and careful examination of articular cartilage throughout the knee joint should be performed, looking for signal abnormality or surface irregularity as

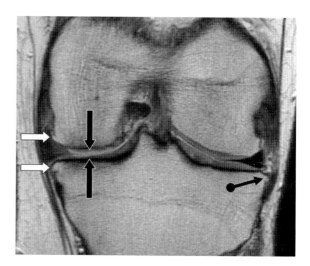

FIG. 10.40. Degenerative arthritis. Sagittal proton-density image shows marked thinning of cartilage of the medial femoral condyle and medial tibial plateau (black arrows) compared to the cartilage of the lateral compartment. Note also small osteophytes in the medial compartment (white arrows) and in the lateral compartment (black round tail arrow).

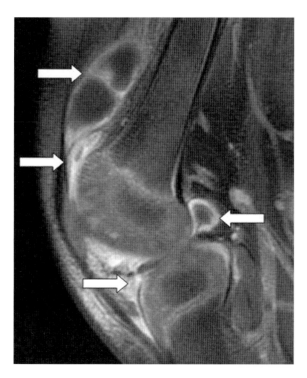

FIG. 10.41. Inflammatory arthritis. Sagittal fat-suppressed T1-weighted image after intravenous contrast in a child with juvenile chronic arthritis shows marked synovial thickening and enhancement (white arrows). The effusion in the posterior aspect of the knee and in the suprapatellar recess does not enhance.

early indicators of osteoarthritis. The MRI appearances of an inflammatory arthritis are synovial thickening and enhancement, effusion, and occasionally erosions (depending on the chronicity of the process), but MRI cannot distinguish septic inflammation from noninfectious inflammation such as rheumatoid arthritis (Fig. 10.41).

The infrapatellar fad pad (called Hoffa's fat pad) is intracapsular but extrasynovial, and there are numerous diseases and abnormalities that affect it and that can be causes of pain or locking. As outlined by Jacobson et al.[244] and Saddik et al.,[245] the abnormalities can be grouped according to intrinsic processes, such as impingement (Hoffa's disease), focal nodular synovitis, and postarthroscopy/postsurgical fibrosis, and extrinsic causes, which encompass any abnormality that involves the knee joint such as meniscal cysts and synovitides. Hoffa's disease is inflammation and enlargement of the fat pad due to single traumatic episode or repetitive overuse, such as during extension or rotation; the enlarged fat pad then gets impinged between the tibia and femur, further exacerbating the inflammation and enlargement.[245]

Plicae, remnants of fetal mesenchymal tissue as the knee forms by cavitation, are common but usually asymptomatic incidental findings on MRI. They may be infrapatellar (the so-called ligamentum mucosum)[246,247] (Fig. 10.42), suprapatellar,[248,249] and medial parapatellar[250] in decreasing order of prevalence.[250] All three types can become symptomatic,

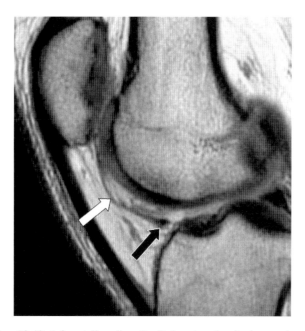

FIG. 10.42. Infrapatellar plica. Sagittal proton-density image shows the ligamentum mucosum, also called the infrapatellar plica (white arrow) in Hoffa's fat pad. The transverse meniscal ligament is also seen in cross section (black arrow).

causing anterior knee pain with or without snapping, but it is the medial type that is most often symptomatic. The medial plica can be symptomatic if it is complete, forming a shelf from the medial side of the joint capsule to the infrapatellar fat pad; it can then rub against the anterior aspect of the medial femoral condyle, becoming thickened, inflamed, and painful (Fig. 10.43). This is typically an overuse injury, associated with such sports as running and bicycling. It is best appreciated on axial T2-weighted MR images, particularly

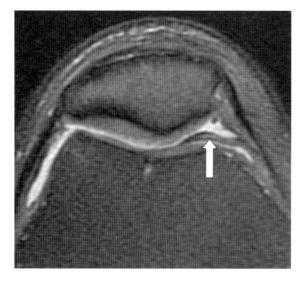

FIG. 10.43. Medial parapatellar plica. Axial fat-suppressed T2-weighted image shows a thick complete medial plica (arrow) with mild high signal intensity internally.

if there is a joint effusion or contrast to outline the low signal intensity plica extending across the medial aspect of the knee joint.[251] While a symptomatic complete plica tends to be thickened due to the chronic irritation against the medial condyle, Boles et al.[250] found no features of medial plicae on MRI that could predict which ones would get resected at arthroscopy. The symptomatic infrapatellar plica will display linear edema-like signal intensity in Hoffa's fat pad,[247] and very rarely, the suprapatellar plica is imperforate, causing fluid in the suprapatellar recess to become trapped and mimicking a mass clinically.

Two common arthropathies of the knee are pigmented villonodular synovitis and synovial chondromatosis. Pigmented villonodular synovitis is an idiopathic hemorrhagic proliferative synovitis, and has both diffuse and focal forms.[252–254] Focal villonodular synovitis, whether pigmented or not, tends to occur in Hoffa's fat pad. The MRI hallmark of the diffuse pigmented form is thick linear or globular foci of marked low signal intensity within the joint due to hemosiderin deposition, but in the early phase of the disease only synovial thickening may be present.[254] Moreover, hemosiderin deposition and synovial thickening are also features of hemophiliac arthropathy. Synovial chondromatosis is an idiopathic chondroid metaplasia of the synovium, yielding masses of globular or punctate synovium with high signal intensity on T2-weighted images.[255] If the metaplastic synovium mineralizes (synovial osteochondromatosis), the masses will have a punctate low signal intensity appearance.

Abnormalities of Bone

Abnormalities of the bones themselves can also cause pain, and entities that are often encountered on MRI of the knee are bone bruises, avascular necrosis, and subchondral insufficiency fractures.

Bone bruises are a spectrum of medullary injury, ranging from marrow edema to frank trabecular microfracture and hemorrhage.[256] They are due to an impaction injury, usually accompanying other injuries in and around the knee joint, and their pattern of location is often a clue to the mechanism of injury.[257] They may also occur as isolated injuries and be the sole cause of pain. They exhibit low signal intensity on T1-weighted images and high signal intensity on fat-suppressed T2-weighted sequences, and two typical patterns exist: (1) geographic—a crescentic focus located subarticularly; and (2) stellate—a reticular pattern not related to subchondral bone.[101] If the adjacent cortex is broken, the abnormality should be interpreted as an incomplete fracture rather than a bone bruise. The signal abnormality of bone bruises usually resolves by about 4 months, although it may last longer in the multiply-injured or unstable knee.[256,258] Bone bruises are not necessarily innocuous; subsequent thinning of the articular cartilage overlying the foci of bruised bone and subchondral depression have been documented on follow-up MRI.[100,101,256]

Bone ischemia has a spectrum of pathology and MR appearances. Initially, ischemia produces a large area of ill-defined marrow edema, usually involving a single condyle and mild adjacent soft tissue edema. If the ischemic event is transient and without frank osteonecrosis, the edema will resolve over a period of approximately 2 months, leaving a normal-appearing condyle.[259] Occasionally, the ischemic region of marrow edema will migrate to different locations with the knee, usually over a period of 2 to 4 months, indicating intraarticular regional migratory osteoporosis.[260] If osteonecrosis occurs during the ischemic event, then the demarcated zone of necrosis will become evident as the marrow edema subsides. Zones of necrosis occurring in the subchondral portions of bone are referred to as "avascular necrosis," while those occurring elsewhere in the bone are referred to as "infarcts." The zone of necrosis may have a single or double rim of demarcation from the adjacent normal bone, and the involved segment may have the appearance of fat, edema, blood, or sclerosis.[261] Avascular necrosis is a rare complication of arthroscopic surgery,[262–266] perhaps due to altered weight-bearing forces, although some of the reported cases may actually represent insufficiency fractures.

The entity previously known as spontaneous osteonecrosis of the knee (SONK) is actually now considered a subchondral insufficiency fracture of the knee (SIFK).[267–269] That the abnormality is an insufficiency fracture makes sense given that it occurs in elderly and thus presumably osteoporotic patients, and that the location of the lesion is the weight-bearing portion of the medial femoral condyle. Moreover, radiographic and histologic examinations of the affected areas show a subchondral fracture as the primary event, with osteonecrosis only occurring secondarily as part of the fracture process.[268] Magnetic resonance imaging demonstrates the collapsed cortex, the low signal intensity subchondral linear component, representing the fracture itself, and surrounding marrow edema[267] (Fig. 10.44).

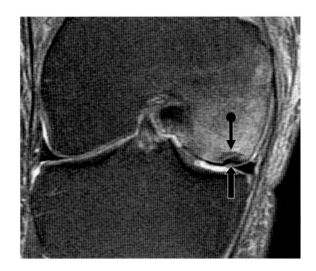

FIG. 10.44. Subchondral insufficiency fracture. Coronal fat-suppressed T2-weighted image shows collapse and condensation of the cortex of the medial femoral condyle (straight black arrow). The crescentic insufficiency fracture line itself is visualized (round tail arrow). Marked high signal intensity marrow edema is present.

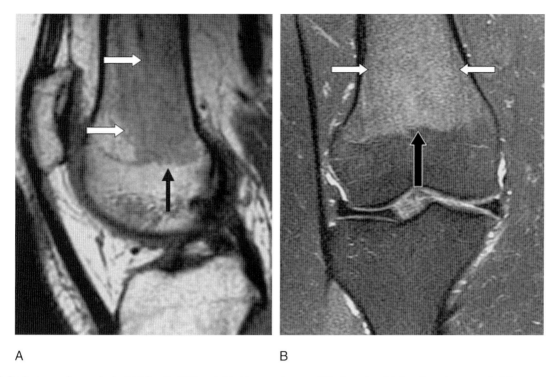

A   B

FIG. 10.45. Red marrow hyperplasia. (A) Sagittal T1-weighted image shows mildly low signal intensity red marrow (white arrows). Note that it does not extend distal to the physeal scar (black arrow). (B) Coronal fat-suppressed T2-weighted image of the same patient shows the mildly high signal intensity of the red marrow (white arrows). The marrow does not extend distal to the physeal scar (black arrow).

Physiologic red marrow persistence or hyperplasia is seen often on MRI of the knee and may occur due to anemia, chronic disease, smoking, aerobic conditioning, and obesity.[270–273] It has signal intensity similar to muscle on T1-weighted images and becomes mildly high signal intensity on fat-suppressed T2-weighted images (Fig. 10.45). It is usually of no clinical significance, and can be distinguished from an infiltrative neo-plastic process like myeloma or lymphoma by the fact that it does not extend across the physeal scar into the end of the bone and does not have a uniform, consolidated appearance. However, in patients with sickle cell disease or thalassemia, or in patients taking marrow stimulation medication, the red marrow reconversion will extend past the physeal scar to the end of the bone.

B. Orthopedic Perspective: Knee Disorders

Robert A. Pedowitz, Ali Dalal, Catherine Robertson, and Ryan Serrano

Ligaments

Knee ligament injuries occur frequently, and suspected ligamentous injury is a common indication for MRI. Ligamentous injuries occur after both contact and noncontact events. The mechanism of injury may suggest a specific diagnosis, for example, PCL tear after a dashboard injury. The clinical history and physical examination are often sufficient to establish an accurate ligament-related diagnosis, though MRI is often used to confirm the diagnosis and to identify related pathology. After a ligament injury is diagnosed, conservative treatment or surgery is chosen based on the known natural history of the specific injury, patient characteristics, and the degree of instability. The physical exam, treatment, and imaging of knee ligament injuries were reviewed recently by Cummings and Pedowitz.[274]

Anterior Cruciate Ligament

Anterior cruciate ligament injury is one of the most common traumatic internal derangements of the knee. There are roughly 100,000 new ACL injuries every year in the United States alone, and it is estimated that 1 in every 3000 Americans will experience an ACL injury in their lifetime. The ACL's primary role is to stabilize the knee by preventing anterior translation of the tibia relative to the femur. The ACL originates in the posterior lateral wall of the intercondylar notch of the femur and inserts onto the anterior tibial plateau. The ligament is made up of two bundles, the anteromedial and the posterolateral (Fig. 10.46). This organization of the ACL allows for stabilization of the knee through its entire range of motion as the anteromedial bundle tightens during flexion and the posterolateral bundle tightens during extension.

Anterior cruciate ligament injuries can occur as a result of contact or, more commonly, noncontact activity. The stereotypical noncontact ACL injury is associated with an abrupt change of direction, pivoting, or sudden deceleration, while the classic contact pattern of ACL injury occurs when the patient is struck on the lateral aspect of the knee with the foot planted. Anterior cruciate ligament injuries are more common in sports in which there is a high amount of friction between the playing surface and the athlete's shoe. "Cutting" in football provides a classic noncontact pattern of injury, with a similar mechanism accounting for the frequent ACL injuries observed in basketball and soccer. Anatomic

and biologic factors also increase the risk of ACL injury. A narrow femoral intercondylar notch and increased joint laxity are correlated with higher occurrences of ACL injury. Females experience ACL injury four to 10 times more frequently than males. The scientific basis for the gender difference in ACL injury risk has not been clearly established, although theories abound, including hormonal differences, anatomic differences, and differences in strength and conditioning. At this time, it appears that neuromuscular factors, such as quadriceps/hamstring balance and muscle firing patterns, are the most likely etiologic factors.

For 60% of patients, a "pop" is heard at the moment of ACL injury. Pain generally precludes return to play. Acute ACL injury is typically followed by rapid and profound swelling of the knee joint due to hemarthrosis. In the subsequent phases after injury, patients should be queried about experiences of instability with activities, particularly once the acute pain and swelling have resolved, especially with activities that involve planting and cutting maneuvers.

The specific tests that comprise the physical examination for ACL injury are the Lachman, the anterior drawer, and the pivot shift tests. The Lachman test is relatively easy to perform and is the most sensitive examination maneuver; however, the patient must be able to relax in order for the exam to be accurate (Fig. 10.47 and Table 10.2). The rationale behind each test is to determine whether there is abnormal anterior translation of the tibia with respect to the femur due to ACL insufficiency. Patients should also be examined to assess range of motion and evidence of concordant ligamentous or meniscal injury, including a careful examination of the posterolateral corner. Objective measurements of the sagittal plane movement of the tibia with respect to the femur can be obtained with an arthrometer (Fig. 10.48).

Imaging

A thorough physical exam performed by an experienced practitioner is usually sufficient to diagnose an ACL tear. Plain radiographs are useful in identifying secondary signs of ACL injury such as avulsion fractures of the tibial eminence or Segond fractures of the lateral tibial plateau. It is also important to rule out concomitant tibial plateau injury. Since physical examination can be very accurate for diagnosis of an ACL tear, MRI may not be required for clinical decision making in many cases. However, when imaging is required, MRI is

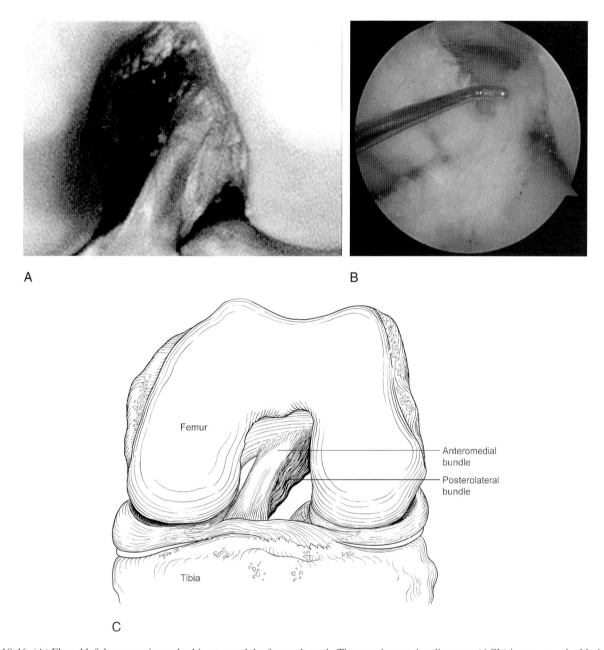

Fig. 10.46. (A) Flexed left knee specimen, looking toward the femoral notch. The anterior cruciate ligament (ACL) is seen as a double-bundle structure. The posterolateral bundle is relatively oblique, with a femoral origin that is more posterior on the femoral condyle (lower on this image) than the anteromedial bundle. With the knee flexed the posterolateral bundle appears relatively lax; this structure becomes taut with knee extension. (B) Arthroscopic image of a left knee with a tear of the anteromedial bundle of the ACL (which has been removed). The tip of the probe points to the preserved posterolateral bundle, and the posterior cruciate ligament (PCL) sits behind the shaft of the probe. (C) The posterolateral bundle is lax with the knee in a flexed position.

the current imaging modality of choice for evaluation of ACL injury. The 100% sensitivity and 90% specificity of MRI in detecting complete tears of the ACL is comparable to the 100% sensitivity and 99% specificity of the combination of all the tests that comprise the clinical exam in diagnosing ACL damage.[275,276] A study by Duc et al.[277] showed that MRI is not as reliable in diagnosing partial ACL tears compared to complete ACL tears. Bone bruises are commonly associated with ACL tears, and are caused by compression of the posterior

aspect of the lateral tibial plateau against the anterior aspect of the lateral femoral condyle. These common secondary signs of ACL rupture will be discussed separately.

There are several clinical indications for the use of MRI in diagnosing ACL tears. Magnetic resonance imaging is an ideal diagnostic tool for a treating physician who might be inexperienced with the clinical exam, particularly if that provider has easier access to an MRI than to an orthopedic specialist. Magnetic resonance imaging can be used when a

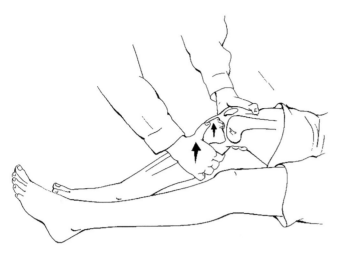

FIG. 10.47. The Lachman exam is performed with the patient supine and the knee in 20 to 30 degrees of flexion. The examiner stabilizes the femur and applies an anteriorly directed force at the posterior proximal tibia to note anterior translation of the tibia. (From Pedowitz R, O'Connor J, Akeson W, eds. Daniel's Knee Injuries. Ligament and Cartilage Structure, Function, Injury, and Repair. Philadelphia: Lippincott Williams & Wilkins, 2003:350, with permission).

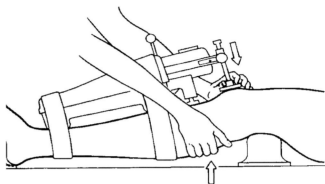

FIG. 10.48. Arthrometry of the knee using the KT-1000. An anteriorly directed force is applied to the tibia (right hand) while the arthrometer is stabilized relative to the femur with a posterior load applied via the patella (left hand). Tibial translation is measured by the arthrometer, with the most useful information being the comparison with the normal contralateral knee. (From Pedowitz R, O'Connor J, Akeson W, eds. Daniel's Knee Injuries. Ligament and Cartilage Structure, Function, Injury, and Repair. Philadelphia: Lippincott Williams & Wilkins, 2003:387, with permission).

compensation cases), and for satisfaction of patient expectations for advanced imaging.

Treatment

The decision to perform ACL reconstruction depends on a number of factors, including the presence of symptomatic instability, the magnitude of knee laxity, the patient's age and desired level of activity, associated limb alignment, and the presence and magnitude of knee arthrosis. Conservative management of an ACL tear consists of a guided, progressive program in order to regain range of motion, muscle power, neuromuscular performance, and sports-specific skills. Functional bracing may be considered; however, these devices cannot completely prevent subluxation events under high load conditions. Athletes should be encouraged to watch for episodes of recurrent instability after ACL injury, and if they occur, a decision should be made at that point about surgical reconstruction versus activity modification. Recurrent giving way should not be ignored due to the potential for cumulative and often irreversible damage to cartilage and meniscus.

Anterior cruciate ligament reconstruction is often indicated in active patients at an early stage after injury, due to the known poor natural history of untreated knee instability. This is particularly relevant to athletes participating in sports that involve a high degree of cutting and pivoting, such as soccer, basketball, and football. Patient age is a covariable since younger patients tend to participate in these kinds of sports more regularly than older patients. However, with modern reconstruction and rehabilitation methods, the morbidity of ACL surgery has decreased to the point that early surgical treatment can be considered at any age, given the presence of the most important indications for reconstructive surgery

TABLE 10.2. Physical examination for ACL injury.

Test	Patient position	Task performed by examiner	Sensitivity and specificity
Lachman	Supine with knee at 20 to 30 degrees of flexion		Torg et al.[311]: sensitivity 95% Jackson et al.[294]: specificity 90%
Anterior drawer test	Supine, hip flexed 45 degrees, knee flexed 90 degrees	Foot is stabilized; anteriorly directed force applied to proximal tibia	Jackson et al.[294]: sensitivity 56%, specificity 92%
Pivot shift test	Supine, knee extended	Knee flexed from an extended position with valgus force; pivot shift noted as tibia reduces	Jackson et al.[294]: sensitivity 31%, specificity 97%

patient is too guarded due to pain to undergo an accurate physical examination (this scenario may occur in the hands of very experienced examiners). It may also be useful when assessment of anterior tibial translation is difficult or impossible due to a displaced bucket-handle meniscus tear. It is also helpful when multiligament injury is suspected or when full range of motion is not recovered within 4 weeks of injury. This may be a sign of mechanical blockage of the intercondylar notch caused by an unreduced meniscus tear or ACL fragment.[278] In addition to these clinical indications, MRI is also sometimes necessary for documentation purposes (medical-legal; workers' (magnitude of knee laxity and desired level of sports/activities that might precipitate giving way episodes).

In contrast to this very early postinjury prognostic challenge, decision making is relatively straightforward in patients who have recurrent giving way episodes with routine simple sports or activities of daily living (regardless of age). In these cases, ACL reconstruction should be a strong consideration since long-term functional bracing is an impractical and relatively ineffective solution. In cases of chronic ACL insufficiency, it is important to look for evidence of moderate to severe arthrosis, because the presence of cartilage disease significantly affects expectations in regard to subsequent pain and function (despite a perfectly done ACL reconstruction). Plain radiographs and MRI can be useful for preoperative assessment of osteoarthrosis.

In addition to the benefit of functional improvement, knee stabilization should also be considered in the context of the potential adverse effects of recurrent instability upon intraarticular structures. However, even though successful ACL reconstruction can decrease the risk of subsequent meniscus tears, there are no convincing data available proving a substantial decrease in the long-term risk of arthrosis (compared to nonsurgical management). Patients should be counseled about the potential for osteoarthritis after ACL injury, despite what we would consider successful ACL surgery.[279,280]

Detailed presentations of the technical details of ACL reconstruction are outside the scope of this book. However, several issues are relevant to the use of MRI in the postoperative setting. Anterior cruciate ligament reconstruction involves placement of a ligament substitute (a graft), with the goals of anatomic and functional restoration (Fig. 10.49). There are multiple graft alternatives, including autografts (patellar

tendon with bone plugs from distal patella and tibial tubercle, semitendinosis with or without gracilis tendons, quadriceps tendon with a patellar bone plug) and allografts (patellar tendon, quadriceps tendon, Achilles tendon, tibialis anterior or posterior, hamstring tendons). More graft alternatives, including collagen-based synthetic scaffolds or processed xenografts, are likely to be available in the future; however, the basic biologic processes remain the same after surgery. These grafts should be considered collagen scaffolds that facilitate revascularization and cellular migration, ultimately leading to remodeling of a new ligamentous structure, coined "ligamentization." The time course involves early healing at the graft–bone interface, which occurs in the first few months after surgery (a bit slower with soft tissue grafts compared to bone plug grafts), and subsequent tissue remodeling (which can take 1 to 2 years for autografts and may be incomplete after allograft reconstruction). To this point noncollagenous synthetic grafts have been long-term clinical failures because they do not allow for biologic remodeling.

Most anatomic reconstructive methods involve placement of the graft via bone tunnels that are drilled within the femur and tibia, with a wide variety of fixation devices at the surgeon's disposal. These devices may be metallic, bioabsorbable, plastic, and even machined cortical bone, and surely more materials and designs will be available in the future. Some techniques involve intraosseous fixation (such as interference screws) while others exploit cortical or surface fixation. The point is that optimal interpretation of a postoperative MRI is facilitated by an understanding of the surgical technique, graft, and implants, and this knowledge should be shared between surgeon and radiologist if at all possible. Knowledge of prior surgical details is also critical in preparation for revision ACL surgery, and in such cases MRI can be particularly useful for surgical strategy in regard to bone tunnel position, osteolysis, and prior implant management.

The most important technical determinants of successful ACL reconstruction are the location of the graft within the knee (i.e., tunnel position) and the adequacy of fixation. The goal is rigid fixation that resists failure with early cyclic load (i.e., a stiff fixation construct), but there are many fixation devices that can be used to achieve these goals. Recent studies suggest little outcome variation for a given ACL graft comparing different high-quality fixation alternatives.[281–283] The specific graft choice is not the major determinant of success, assuming the other goals are achieved.[284–286]

Although single-bundle ACL reconstruction is the most common procedure at the moment, double-bundle ACL reconstruction has been popularized in the last decade with the goal of more anatomic restoration and, it is hoped, better functional outcome. It should be noted that although these procedures may improve the opportunity for peak surgical outcome (yet to be proven in long-term clinical studies), they may also increase the variability of clinical outcome or the rate of surgical complications across the population at large (due to increased complexity or inconsistent surgical method-

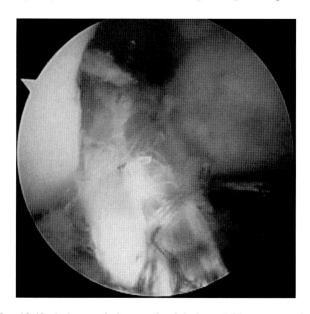

FIG. 10.49. Arthroscopic image of a right knee ACL reconstruction using hamstring autograft. The blue ink indicates the entry point of the graft into the tibial tunnel. The metal probe (on the right) sits between the ACL graft and the native PCL.

ology). Such procedures may also make failures more difficult to manage, since multiple bone tunnels and fixation devices will need to be handled at the time of revision surgery. It seems certain that new surgical methods, grafts, and implants will be developed in the future, since our current techniques are good but certainly not perfect.[287] Surgeons and radiologists need to communicate about these advances in order to maximize the accuracy and utility of imaging data.

Medial Collateral Ligament

The MCL originates at the medial epicondyle of the femur and inserts distally onto the tibia underneath the gracilis and semitendinosus tendons. The MCL is composed of a deep layer of capsular fibers that are in close opposition with the medial meniscus and a superficial layer that extends surprisingly distal, with a broad insertional area on the tibia (Fig. 10.50). The MCL acts as the primary stabilizer against valgus force applied to the knee, with posteromedial capsular thickening (the posterior oblique ligament) playing an important role in valgus stability at full knee extension.

The mechanism of MCL injury is a valgus force to the knee. Contact MCL injuries outnumber noncontact injuries, and are commonly seen in sports such as football. Cruciate ligament injuries can also be associated with tears of the MCL, given a sufficient magnitude of deforming force. Patellar dislocation and subluxation can also be caused by the same valgus/flexion mechanism as MCL injury.

Patients presenting with MCL injuries typically report pain or swelling localized to the medial side of the knee and valgus laxity on exam. Physical examination of MCL injury is generally reliable and sufficient for clinical management, although in the very early stage patients may have a difficult time relaxing for the exam due to pain and apprehension. Table 10.3 presents a common strategy for grading MCL injuries. This grading system is not particularly important in terms of surgical decision making, since most MCL tears are treated nonsurgically with good clinical results. This grading scheme is useful in terms of anticipated speed of recovery and return to play, and can also be helpful for decisions about early functional bracing.

Imaging

Plain radiograph should be obtained in the setting of acute MCL tears, specifically to rule out bony injuries such as lateral plateau fractures. These injuries can significantly affect clinical management and prognosis, and should be documented early in order to avoid later controversy about the time course of a displaced tibial plateau injury (for example any suggestion that a depressed fracture could have been due to premature weight bearing after injury). Plain radiographs may show acute epicondylar avulsion fracture, which should be fixed surgically when displaced, or in chronic cases calcification at or proximal to the epicondyle (the Pellegrini-Stieda lesion).

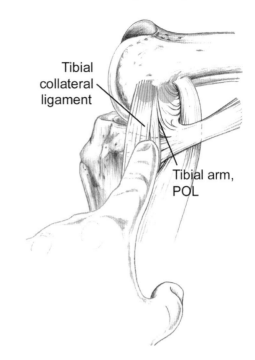

FIG. 10.50. Anatomy of the medial side of the knee, with the tibial collateral ligament (also known as the medial collateral ligament) and the posterior oblique ligament. (From Fanelli GC, ed. Posterior Cruciate Ligament Injuries: A Practical Guide to Management. New York: Springer, 2001:51, with permission).

TABLE 10.3. Medial collateral ligament (MCL) injury grading system.

Grade	Medial joint opening	End point
I	5 mm or less	Solid
II	6–10 mm	Good end point
III	10 mm or more	Soft

Isolated injuries of the MCL usually do not require MRI for diagnosis. However, MRI may be helpful to rule out other injuries, such as meniscal tears, cruciate tears, occult tibial plateau fractures, severe bone contusions, and (rarely) entrapment of the MCL within the joint. Extensive bone edema can make MRI interpretation difficult, in terms of distinguishing between a major bone contusion versus a nondisplaced or minimally displaced plateau fracture. In such cases, plain radiographs should be scrutinized, and occasionally a follow-up film can demonstrate a healing fracture. If plain radiographs are insufficient for early surgical decision making, CT scanning should be used to definitively assess bony anatomy.

Treatment

Treatment of MCL injury is generally nonsurgical, since this extraarticular structure has a good healing potential due to its richly vascularized tissue envelope (in contrast to the healing potential of the intraarticular ACL). Grade I injuries require little specific management, other than limitation of sports activity until full range of motion and comfortable weight bearing are achieved (typically within a few weeks after injury). Grade II injuries are managed similarly, with the expectation that return to sports will probably take a month or so, and early lightweight functional bracing may be helpful for comfort. Grade III injuries (complete tears) are often treated with a hinged range of motion brace, which can facilitate pain relief and early weight bearing. A short period of splinting may be helpful for comfort (on the order of days); however, long periods of immobilization should be avoided in order to decrease the chance of subsequent knee stiffness. Early knee range of motion does not interfere with MCL healing. Straight leg exercises and quadriceps exercises are encouraged from the beginning. Return to activity is gradual, with the expectation that a grade III injury will require 3 to 4 months for recovery. Impact loading should be avoided until the region is nonpainful with palpation and valgus stress testing, and the athlete is comfortable during strength training and light functional exercise (in order to minimize the chance of early reinjury).

Magnetic resonance imaging can be useful in some cases of grade III MCL tear in order to rule out concomitant ACL injury,[288] particularly when the physical examination is difficult. In this setting, some surgeons prefer early brace management of the MCL, with later ACL reconstruction with or without MCL surgery in the case of residual medial laxity. Others prefer early surgical repair of the MCL and early ACL reconstruction for combined injuries, even though recovery of knee range of motion can be quite challenging with this approach. Early surgery is indicated in patients with an incarcerated MCL, a large displaced epicondylar avulsion fragment, a displaced meniscus tear, and often in the setting of MCL tear and bicruciate ligament tear (i.e., acute knee dislocation).

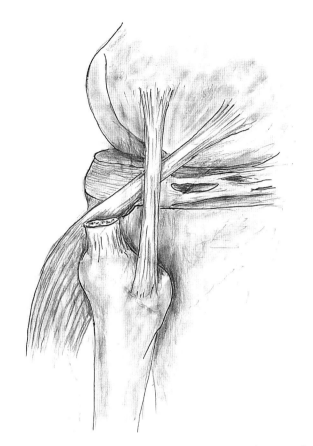

FIG. 10.51. Anatomy of the lateral side of the knee, demonstrating the oblique course of the popliteus tendon, which runs under and then just anterior to the fibular collateral ligament to insert on the lateral femur. Note the relatively small insertional area of the fibular collateral on the anterior portion of the fibula, with the posterior insertion of the biceps tendon (cut in this image). (From Fanelli GC, ed. Posterior Cruciate Ligament Injuries: A Practical Guide to Management. New York: Springer, 2001:36, with permission).

Lateral Collateral Ligament

The lateral collateral ligament (LCL) originates at the lateral epicondyle of the femur and inserts onto the superior aspect of the proximal fibula (Fig. 10.51). The LCL is the primary stabilizer against varus stress of the knee. Other posterolateral corner structures, such as the popliteus tendon, popliteofibular ligament, and arcuate complex provide additional varus stability, as these structures are the key stabilizers against posterolateral rotational forces. Excessive varus stress is accordingly the etiology of isolated LCL tears, although various injury mechanisms can cause LCL tear in combination with cruciate ligament injuries. Isolated LCL tears are much less common than isolated MCL tears, since a varus blow to the medial knee is relatively difficult to achieve due to the protective effect of the contralateral lower limb.

Patients with isolated LCL injuries generally present with lateral-sided pain and instability or pain with weight bearing or side-to-side movements. The patient may also have lateral tenderness, swelling, or ecchymosis. Isolated LCL tears are generally treated in a similar fashion to isolated MCL tears, with bracing and gradual return to activity. However, it should be emphasized that isolated LCL tears are relatively rare, and it is up to the clinician to rule out other types of significant pathology that may require surgical attention.

As with other ligamentous injury, plain radiographs should be obtained, in this case, to rule out proximal fibular avulsion fractures (treated surgically when displaced) and medial tibial plateau fractures. Since isolated LCL injuries are relatively rare, MRI should be considered in order to evaluate other ligamentous and periarticular structures. Magnetic resonance imaging can be particularly helpful with an acutely injured LCL when physical examination is hampered by pain.

Particular attention should be directed at the posterolateral corner on physical examination (the dial test), and, if need be, by advanced imaging. Early surgical repair of posterolateral corner injuries is generally thought to have better results than late reconstruction, and should be performed if possible within a few weeks of injury (prior to extensive scar formation). Magnetic resonance imaging can show extensive lateral fluid changes that are indicative of an acute lateral or posterolateral injury, and this information is useful for alerting the treating physician. This can be especially helpful for triage decisions from the primary care to the specialist setting, and the aware radiologist should directly communicate the potential for posterolateral injury in order to facilitate early referral and treatment. However, current MRI protocols make precise pathoanatomic diagnosis of the posterolateral corner quite challenging, and therefore specific surgical strategy requires very careful physical examination, including examination under anesthesia prior to surgery, and direct exploration in order to delineate and specifically repair damaged structures.

Posterior Cruciate Ligament

The PCL originates at the lateral wall of the medial femoral condyle and inserts onto the proximal posterior tibia (Fig. 10.52). The two-bundle organization of the PCL allows it to perform its primary function of preventing posterior translation of the tibia throughout its entire range of motion. The PCL is a

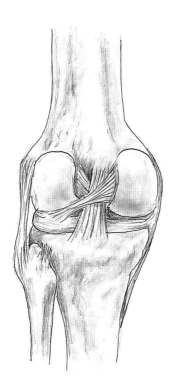

FIG. 10.52. Anatomy of the posterior aspect of the knee, demonstrating the ligament of Wrisberg coursing behind the posterior cruciate ligament (PCL). Note the insertional area of the PCL, which extends down the proximal tibia to the level of the inflection of the tibia (where the tibial metaphysis curves back in an anterior direction). (From Fanelli GC, ed. Posterior Cruciate Ligament Injuries: A Practical Guide to Management. New York: Springer, 2001:36, with permission).

secondary stabilizing structure against external rotation of the tibia relative to the femur.

Posterior cruciate ligament tears may result from low-energy impact as seen in sports or high-energy impact as seen in motor vehicle accidents. The most common mechanism of PCL injury is a posteriorly directed force on the tibia with the knee flexed. This scenario is seen on the playing field when an athlete falls on a flexed knee with the foot in plantar flexion and in motor vehicle accidents when the flexed knee strikes a dashboard. A hyperextension event may also result in a PCL tear.

Patients with PCL injury usually present with the typical findings of a swollen and painful knee, although sometimes hemarthrosis is not apparent because the injury causes posterior capsular venting into the popliteal region and proximal calf. In some cases, symptoms after PCL tear can be remarkably minimal. In contrast to ACL tears, PCL tears are often relatively well tolerated/compensated by the athlete. In chronic cases, patients may complain of symptomatic giving way and feelings of hyperextension instability. However, in many cases of chronic PCL tear, patients present with complaints of pain, which is often related to advancing chondrosis, and they have little or no awareness of a preexisting ligament injury. This is in contradistinction to the patient who has pain related to chronic ACL injury, because most of these patients report discrete episodes of symptomatic giving way.

Diagnosis of PCL tear is relatively easy on physical examination, assuming the physician spends a few moments to look for the injury. The posterior drawer test, the posterior sag test, and the quadriceps active test are used to evaluate the PCL (Table 10.4). The rationale behind the physical exam is diagnosis of abnormal posterior tibial translation with respect to the femur, a sign of PCL insufficiency (Fig. 10.53). The grading scheme is similar in concept to the grading

TABLE 10.4. Physical examination for posterior cruciate ligament (PCL) injury.

Test	Patient position	Task performed by examiner	Sensitivity and specificity
Posterior drawer test	Supine with test hip flexed at 45 degrees and knee flexed at 90 degrees	A posteriorly directed force is applied to anterior proximal tibia	Sensitivity: 90% Specificity: 99%
Posterior sag test	Supine with hip flexed to 45 degrees and knee flexed at 90 degrees	Notes the loss of step off due to posteriorly directed force of gravity	Sensitivity: 79% Specificity: 100%
Quadriceps active test	Supine with knee flexed at about 70 degrees (the "quad neutral angle")	Resisted slide of foot on table; quad contraction causes increased anterior tibial translation	Sensitivity: 54% Specificity: 97%

Source: Malanga et al.,[297] with permission of the *Archives of Physical Medicine and Rehabilitation*.

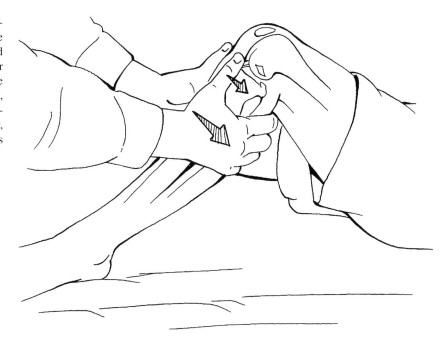

FIG. 10.53. The posterior drawer test is performed by stabilizing the foot against the examination table with the knee in a flexed position. Tibial translation relative to the femur is assessed during posterior load applied to the proximal tibia. (From Pedowitz R, O'Connor J, Akeson W, eds. Daniel's Knee Injuries. Ligament and Cartilage Structure, Function, Injury, and Repair. Philadelphia: Lippincott Williams & Wilkins, 2003:349, with permission).

TABLE 10.5. PCL Injury Grading System.

Grade	Posterior translation of the tibia	Tibia position at posterior drawer test endpoint	Type of tear
I	<5 mm	Maintained anterior step off	Partial ligament tear
II	5–10 mm	Tibial plateau flush with femoral condyle or slightly posterior with a solid endpoint	Partial ligament tear
III	>10 mm	Tibial plateau posterior to femoral condyle with a soft endpoint	Complete ligament tear

of MCL tears (Table 10.5). However, PCL tears are underdiagnosed because of a low index of clinical suspicion compared to other knee disorders. A major diagnostic pitfall is incorrect attribution of anterior tibial translation to a presumed ACL tear, when such translation is actually due to a posterior tibial starting point on the Lachman exam due to a PCL tear. Obviously such misunderstanding can lead to an error in surgical management (i.e., ACL reconstruction when in fact there is a PCL tear).

Imaging

Plain radiographs are helpful in acute PCL injuries to identify avulsion of the tibial PCL insertion, a condition that may require open intervention. Computed tomography may also assist in surgical planning required for treatment of PCL avulsion injuries. Magnetic resonance imaging is the imaging modality of choice in evaluation of in-substance PCL injuries. In a study by Gross et al.,[289] PCL tears were detected with a sensitivity and specificity of 100% by MRI. Although differentiation between complete and partial-thickness PCL tears by MRI criteria alone is more problematic, complete tears are more likely to show focal areas of discontinuity and partial tears are more likely to show at least some intact fibers.[278] As the PCL is the largest and strongest of the cruciate ligaments, associated injuries are common with acute PCL tears and may be evaluated by MRI.[290]

Grade I and II PCL injuries generally respond to conservative management with initial protected weight bearing and quadriceps strengthening. Grade III injuries undergo a similar acute treatment but require a longer absence from play and more commonly result in later surgical intervention. In contradistinction to ACL tears, many athletes perform very well despite complete PCL tears, and initial nonsurgical management of complete PCL tears is therefore generally recommended. Early surgery for young or high-caliber athletes may be considered, but there is little consensus about the specific indications for early PCL reconstruction. Posterior cruciate ligament functional bracing is generally not as effective as ACL bracing, because the restraining force of the brace must be applied to the thick muscle mass behind the proximal tibia (as opposed to the subcutaneous anterior proximal tibia with ACL braces).

Most would agree that PCL reconstruction is reasonable for persistent instability despite conservative management. The biologic processes of graft healing and remodeling after PCL reconstruction are the same as for ACL reconstruction; however, surgical results are somewhat less predictable. This is probably due to the greater technical challenges of PCL surgery (i.e., the posterior neurovascular structures), relatively small worldwide clinical experience relative to the predominance of ACL surgery, and perhaps due to insufficient reproduction of the true anatomy of the PCL with most single bundle reconstructive methods.[290]

Multiligament Injuries of the Knee: Knee Dislocation

Multiligament injuries of the knee are significant injuries that may be associated with limb-threatening vascular injury and long-term morbidity. Essentially all possible combinations of injury of the four major ligament complexes have been described. Three ligament and four ligament injuries are generally considered forms of knee dislocation, even if the knee is not dislocated on presentation.

Although knee dislocation most often occurs after a high-energy trauma such as a motor vehicle accident, a seemingly simple twisting injury or fall may also result in this severe injury. Moreover, knee dislocations often reduce spontaneously, such that the severity of the injury may not be obvious on initial evaluation or radiographs. Untreated neurovascular damage caused by knee dislocation can cause significant tissue ischemia that may ultimately lead to limb amputation.

Diagnosis of multiligament knee injury requires vigilance and a high index of suspicion. In most cases, patients present with a swollen and painful knee, and guarding can interfere with accurate clinical assessment of the pattern of ligament injury. Sometimes the capsular rupture is so large that the knee joint essentially vents, such that hemarthrosis will not be apparent at the time of presentation. A thorough neurovascular exam should be performed including clinical comparison of distal pulses with the contralateral limb. Better objective information can be obtained by determination of the ankle–brachial index (ABI), which is a ratio of the systolic pressures at these locations. Normal distal perfusion and an ABI >0.8 is sufficient evidence to preclude angiography; however, diligence must be maintained due to the potential for late vascular occlusion caused by an intimal flap tear. Otherwise, digital angiography or MRA should be performed for anatomic evaluation, with immediate vascular intervention initiated in order to restore or maintain distal perfusion. However, in the case of complete distal ischemia, critical time must not be lost in the process of imaging at the expense of emergent definitive intervention.

Plain radiographs can be used to establish subluxation, dislocation, and fractures that are associated with the dislocation. In these complex cases, MRI provides a relatively complete picture of multiligament damage,[291] and may also demonstrate co-injuries that can affect surgical decision making. Although multiple injuries decrease the diagnostic sensitivity and specificity of MRI, Rubin and coworkers[291] found that MRI was still able to diagnose multiple ligament injuries with a sensitivity and specificity of 88% and 84%, respectively. However, definitive imaging of the complex anatomy of the posterolateral corner is still challenging, particularly when the region is awash with acute hematoma/edema. Mechanisms of injury that cause damage to the popliteus tendon and peroneal nerve,

both easily identified by MRI, are highly correlated with vascular damage and should prompt heightened observation for ischemic changes in the limb.[292]

Treatment

An ischemic limb should be reduced promptly, using traction-countertraction methods, and the vascular status should be reassessed. If pulses return, radiographs and arteriography can be performed. Temporary stability may be provided by a splint, but sometimes the limb is so unstable that external fixators may be required. Persistent limb ischemia must be treated emergently. Successful surgical revascularization is confirmed by angiography. Irreducible dislocations are also treated surgically, but definitive ligamentous reconstruction is generally delayed in order to stabilize the patient's medical status and to provide time for an optimal surgical plan to be developed.

Nonsurgical management of knee dislocation consists of closed reduction and 6 weeks of immobilization in a hard cast. Nonsurgical management has largely been abandoned because many of these patients eventually require surgery anyway, to address either persistent instability or chronic loss of knee motion related to extended periods of immobilization. Earlier definitive surgical management of knee dislocation has become a better treatment alternative. The keys to success are accurate delineation of the injury pattern, recognition of co-injuries, appropriate timing of surgery, and anatomic restoration. Surgery is generally delayed for 10 to 14 days after injury in order to decrease swelling and to allow for some capsular healing, which can help to minimize fluid extravasation during arthroscopic treatment. This is also an appropriate time for careful and strategic clinical decision making (including consideration of tertiary referral), and is often the ideal time to obtain MRI. Detailed presentation of the surgical management of these difficult injuries is beyond the scope of this book. However the recent trend is toward reconstruction or repair of all injured structures,[293] as opposed to staged or partial reconstruction.

Meniscus

The menisci are fibrocartilaginous structures that absorb shock and add conformity to the knee. The peripheral 10% to 30% of the menisci are vascularized "red zones," fed by the peripheral capillary plexus (Fig. 10.54). These regions have the best intrinsic capacity to heal after injury or surgery. The inner portions of both menisci are avascular "white zones" and are much less amenable to repair.

Meniscal pathology can be related to traumatic, degenerative, or congenital factors. Traumatic meniscal tears usually occur after the knee is twisted with the foot planted or with a squatting maneuver. A sudden load and torque causes a tear to propagate within the fibrocartilage.[294] Large displaced tears (bucket-handle tears) can displace centrally, thereby blocking

FIG. 10.54. Vascular supply of the meniscus. Coronal drawing demonstrates perfusion of the peripheral third of the meniscus via a capillary network. (Modified from Arnoczky SP, Warren RF. Microvasculature of the human meniscus. Am J Sports Med 1982;10(2):90–95, with permission).

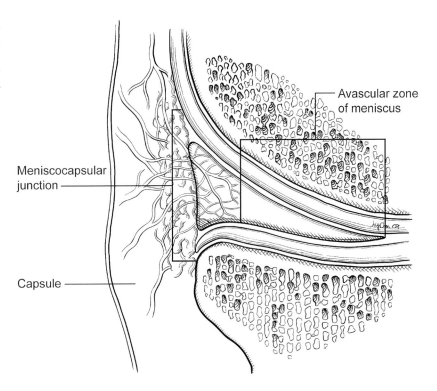

Avascular zone of meniscus

Meniscocapsular junction

Capsule

knee extension when they jam in the region of the intercondylar notch. Degenerative meniscus tears often occur without a specific notable mechanism of injury. The discoid meniscus is a morphologic variant that sometimes tears; however, incidental observation of an asymptomatic and intact discoid meniscus (on MRI or at the time of arthroscopy) should not prompt surgical resection. Various types of meniscus tears are noted at the time of arthroscopy, such as flap tears, oblique tears, and horizontal tears, but the most important distinction is between acute, longitudinal tears and degenerative patterns, since this is what affects decisions about repair versus resection (Fig. 10.55).

Meniscus cysts are usually associated with an adjacent meniscus tear (but not always), with extravasation of fluid into parameniscal soft tissues that eventually create a cyst cavity.[295] Meniscus cysts may be symptomatic, but they can be difficult to pick up on physical examination, particularly in the deep regions of the posteromedial corner of the knee. Magnetic resonance imaging is very sensitive for diagnosis and anatomic description of meniscus cysts, and it can be extremely helpful for surgical planning. In rare cases meniscal cysts may cause local erosion of the tibial plateau.

Patients presenting with meniscal tears may feel or hear a "pop" at the time of injury, much like an ACL tear, or may have pain after a twist or fall. Knee swelling after meniscal injury usually develops gradually, unlike the rapid swelling seen with an ACL tear. After the injury, mechanical symptoms such as clicking, catching, and locking may be present, and pain associated with squatting, twisting, and stair climbing is not uncommon.[296]

The physical examination of meniscus tears involves palpation of the joint line and maneuvers that are intended to elicit pain or a mechanical click as the torn meniscus fragment catches between the femoral condyle and the tibial plateau. Four physical exam tests are commonly used: the joint line tenderness test, the McMurray test, the Apley grind test, and the bounce home test (Table 10.6). An excellent review of all the physical examination tests of the knee is provided by Malanga et al.[297]

The most important diagnostic information for decision making is gleaned from a good history and physical examination. However, imaging studies provide important adjunctive information of meniscus pathology.[298] Plain radiographs may demonstrate osseous abnormalities and are particularly important for diagnosis of osteoarthrosis, because articular cartilage disease markedly affects treatment expectations for the meniscus. The diagnostic accuracy of MRI is very good[298] and is presented in detail in the imaging subsection that precedes this. It is important not to overread the MR images of adolescents because in this developmental stage, peripheral meniscus hypervascularity can mimic a vertical meniscus tear.

Although MRI is not required for clinical management (assuming the treatment plan is obvious from clinical factors alone), imaging can change the course of injury management. Preoperative MRI can assist surgical planning in some cases. In a study of 121 diagnosed meniscal tears, synovitis was diagnosed in 16 patients (13%), articular cartilage damage in 10 patients (8%), bone bruise injuries in 10 patients (8%), osteochondritis dissecans in three patients (2%), disruption of the inner layer of the medial collateral ligament

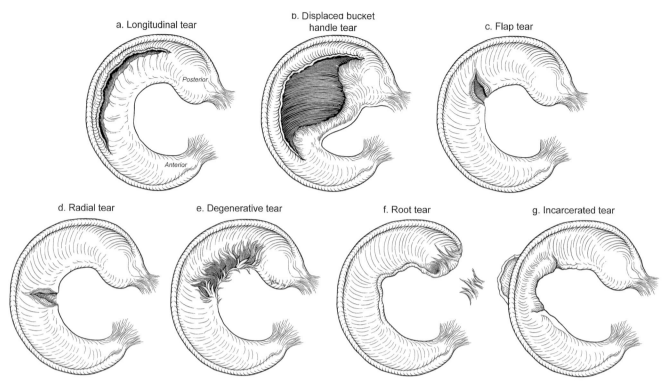

FIG. 10.55. Variants of meniscus tears encountered at arthroscopy (from upper left, moving clockwise): longitudinal, oblique, degenerative, horizontal, radial. (Adapted from Ciccotti MG, Shields CL, El Attrache NS. Meniscectomy. In: Fu FH, Harner CD, Vince KG, eds. Knee Surgery, vol 1. Baltimore: Williams & Wilkins, 1994:591–613, with permission).

TABLE 10.6. Tests of the meniscal physical examination.

Test	Patient position	Exam maneuver	Sensitivity/ specificity
Joint line tenderness	Supine, knee flexed	Palpation of the tibiofemoral joint space	Malanga et al.[297]: sensitivity 55% specificity 67%
McMurray test	Supine	Knee flexed with varus/valgus and simultaneous rotatory load; classic finding is pain with associated pop, but pain alone can be suggestive	Malanga et al.[297]: sensitivity 29% specificity 95%
Apley grind test	Prone	Tibiofemoral rotation with the knee at 90 degrees flexion with simultaneous distraction; increased pain with tibiofemoral compression suggests meniscus tear	Malanga et al.[297]: sensitivity 16% specificity 80%
Bounce home test	Supine	Knee extension from a semi-flexed position (by gravity) allows the knee to "bounce home," causing pain or a rubbery endpoint	NA

in three patients (2%), and osteonecrosis in one patient. The detection of associated pathologies allows the surgeon to construct a plan that addresses multiple abnormalities, and may also offer the patient better prognostic counseling. The use of MRI in this study also deemed arthroscopy unnecessary for 34 patients (28%).[299]

Magnetic resonance imaging is also useful in diagnosing bucket-handle tears of the meniscus and detecting meniscal cysts. Large displaced bucket-handle tears usually present with nonspecific clinical findings such as extension block, but are detected by MRI with high sensitivity.[300] Parameniscal cysts are usually associated with meniscal tears,[295] yet MRI should be used when meniscal cysts are suspected because only 15% of patients present with clinically palpable lesions. Magnetic resonance imaging allows cysts to be detected with 90% accuracy,[295] and preoperative MRI can help with surgical planning (with regard to all-arthroscopic versus open extirpation of the cyst).[301]

The utility of MRI should be discussed in reference to the clinical experience and diagnostic acumen of the specific treating physician. For example, an experienced orthopedic/arthroscopic surgeon may have little difficulty with clinical decision making based on clinical history, chronicity, and physical examination, when the plan is to perform arthroscopic surgery regardless of MR findings. In this situation, arthroscopic assessment is entirely sufficient for diagnosis and management of the range of possible meniscus pathologies. On the other hand, a less experienced, generalist physician may wish to use MRI of the meniscus for triage decisions, whereby the presence of a meniscus tear on MRI prompts referral (or not) to an orthopedic surgeon. This is a reasonable approach for meniscus tears, since the sensitivity of MRI of the meniscus is relatively good (i.e., a negative MRI has good predictive value). The algorithm for meniscus tears should be contrasted with other entities, such as subtle articular cartilage injuries, in which current MR techniques are much less sensitive, and therefore less reliable as a screening measure.

Treatment

Treatment options for meniscal tears include nonoperative management, partial meniscectomy, and meniscal repair. The choice of treatment is dependent on patient characteristics, symptomatology, and the morphology of the tear. Patient characteristics to consider include activity level, age, and other injuries. For example, a young, active athlete may benefit from earlier surgical intervention, while an older, sedentary individual may be more willing to wait several months to see if symptoms resolve. Many persons are asymptomatic with meniscus tears, particularly when the meniscus weakens as a part of the typical degenerative processes, so a positive MRI is not an indication for arthroscopic surgery (in and of itself). Pain or some kind of mechanical symptoms, even if intermittent in nature, should generally be present in order to justify surgery. Surely meniscus tears that block knee motion should be addressed to avoid permanent motion loss or focal pressure-related cartilage damage. There is no compelling evidence that the presence of a degenerative meniscus tear will affect long-term results (in terms of the meniscus fragment accelerating cartilage damage) or that partial meniscectomy somehow protects the cartilage from subsequent degeneration. In the setting of an unstable knee, meniscus tears are more likely to progress over time, and in these cases, surgical stabilization with concurrent meniscus treatment is usually the treatment of choice.

Conservative treatment includes initial activity modification, local care such as ice and antiinflammatories, and physical therapy to restore motion and strength if needed. Arthroscopy is indicated in patients with persistent symptoms consistent with the injury, for a displaced bucket-handle tear, or in patients with associated ligamentous injury. The majority of meniscal tears are treated with partial meniscectomy. This is a debridement of the torn portion of the meniscus to a stable rim. In the absence of chondrosis or other risk factors, the vast majority of patients benefit significantly from this procedure, with reduction of pain and mechanical symptoms.

Although most meniscal tears are not amenable to repair, long-term outcomes are improved when meniscus healing can be achieved. This is particularly true in large tears because total and subtotal meniscectomy are clearly associated with the development of osteoarthritis. The commonly accepted criteria for meniscal repair include (1) a complete vertical longitudinal tear >10 mm long; (2) a tear within the peripheral 10% to 30% of the meniscus or within 3 or 4 mm of the meniscocapsular junction; (3) a tear that can be displaced by probing, thus demonstrating instability; (4) a tear without secondary degeneration or deformity; and (5) a stable knee or a knee that is undergoing concurrent stabilization.[302] Meniscal healing can be facilitated by arthroscopic application of a fibrin clot, which is created as a precipitate from venous blood. A fibrin clot is not needed when meniscus repair is performed in conjunction with ACL reconstruction, due to the inherent hemarthrosis caused by the ligament surgery. Creation of a fibrin clot is relatively inexpensive (venous blood is gently stirred with a frosted glass rod in a plastic specimen bowl), but it can be a bit tricky to deliver from a technical perspective. The fibrin clot contains platelets and growth factors that affect local biologic processes, but the duration of action is not well known. More recent (and expensive) strategies include application of platelet-rich plasma or specific growth factors. It is likely that technically practical and cost-effective biologic manipulations will be developed in order to make meniscus repair more reliable (and therefore increase our ability to preserve this important structure).

Cartilage

Anatomy, Biology, and Function

Articular cartilage is a 2- to 5-mm-thick layer of tissue that covers the condylar surface of the femur, the posterior face of the patella, and the tibial plateau. It is composed of actively metabolizing chondrocytes that are embedded in their own intricately organized extracellular matrix of collagen and proteoglycans.[303] The main function of articular cartilage is to minimize friction at the interface between bones. More detailed descriptions of articular cartilage and imaging aspects are provided elsewhere in this book.

Mechanisms of Pathology

Articular cartilage damage occurs in a number of patterns, including microdamage, chondral damage, osteochondral fracture, and degenerative damage. Microdamage of cartilage can be due to a single excessive load on chondral tissue or may be related to repetitive submaximal loads. Chondrocyte death and loss of matrix can occur without an appreciable change in the appearance of the articular surface itself, which is relevant to both arthroscopic and MRI evaluation. Interestingly, increased muscle mass in the quadriceps and a favorable strength to body weight ratio has been correlated with better cartilage health in the knee, possibly due to the shock attenuation provided by muscle.[304] Chondral injuries are completely contained in the articular surface while osteochondral lesions also affect the subchondral bone (Fig. 10.56). Although the mechanisms of chondral and osteochondral injuries are similar, treatment options differ. Unfortunately, the most common mechanism of cartilage pathology is age-related degeneration.

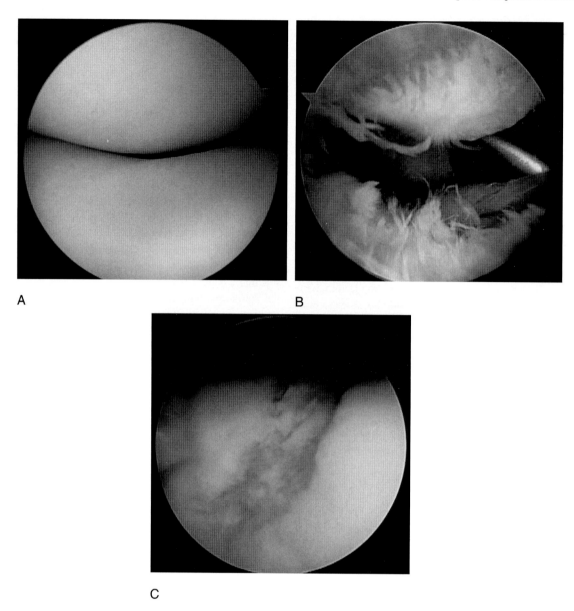

FIG. 10.56. Articular cartilage seen at arthroscopy. (A) Normal cartilage of patellofemoral articulation with a smooth, pearly white appearance. (B) Degenerative articular cartilage, with a rough, fibrillated appearance, with the patella seen above and the trochlea below. (C) Severe cartilage lesion of the femoral trochlea with exposure of subchondral bone.

With age, the metabolic activity of terminally differentiated chondrocytes decreases, causing decreased turnover of matrix materials and an overall decrease in articular cartilage quality. This slow deceleration in chondrocyte activity is the leading cause of osteoarthritis, a disease that ultimately affects 60% of men and 70% of women over 65.[303]

Presentation and Physical Examination

Physical examination is often vague with cartilage injury. Pain, swelling, crepitus, and deformity are late findings. Effusion is a very important early sign of cartilage injury, and may be the only finding on physical examination or MRI that suggests early chondrosis. Chronic chondral pathology is often associated with significant thigh muscle atrophy. Significant cartilage damage is characterized by coarse crepitus and by diminishing range of motion. Nonsurgical strategies, therefore, should include efforts to improve range of motion and strength, and, in fact, such efforts are often rewarded by a significant reduction of pain (even though this approach clearly does not cure the osteoarthritic process).

Imaging

Although radiologic imaging can provide some insight into the nature of knee chondral defects, currently nothing beats the diagnostic accuracy of arthroscopy (at least for surface assessment). Plain radiographs can show large osteochondral defects but will not pick up superficial defects restricted to articular cartilage. In late stages, radiographs will show joint space narrowing and other characteristic changes associated with osteoarthritis. Computed tomography can be used to identify loose bodies caught in synovial folds, and its excellent contrast between bone and soft tissue can be helpful in isolating strictly bony defects.[305] Magnetic resonance imaging provides the best noninvasive evaluation of articular cartilage. It has been shown to have a sensitivity of 33% and specificity of 98% in detecting isolated articular cartilage lesion; however, MRI cannot reliably define the size and depth of chondral lesions.[305] The use of MRA can provide heightened specificity and sensitivity in comparison to nonenhanced, standard MRI. There are a number of very exciting MR strategies that are being developed for articular cartilage assessment (see Chapter 2). When fully developed and validated, these approaches will be very important not only from the diagnostic perspective, but also as powerful research tools that should allow us to longitudinally follow and assess various therapeutic efforts.

Treatment

Currently, there are no definitive curative treatments available for knee chondrosis once the process begins. We essentially treat the symptoms, but cannot cure this disease. Nonsurgical treatment of cartilage injury consists of activity modification, maintenance of range of motion, bracing in some cases, and nonsteroidal antiinflammatory drug (NSAID) usage to provide symptomatic relief. A number of surgical treatments have been proposed to treat cartilage lesions, with variable success.

Arthroscopic debridement and lavage is a relatively benign and low-risk treatment for cartilage disorders, but its long-term effectiveness is subject to debate. Microfracture can be used for full-thickness chondral lesions and involves penetrating subchondral bone to induce clot formation and mesenchymal cell activation to create a fibrocartilage scar. One study showed that 75% of patients who underwent microfracture had an improvement in pain after a 7-year follow-up.[306] Mosaicplasty aims to repair the cartilage surface with donor osteochondral dowel plugs. Osteochondral allografting uses cadaveric plugs in a similar fashion to restore cartilage defects. Allografts have the advantage of avoiding donor site morbidity and can fill larger defects but are more logistically complicated than autografts, and allografts carry a small risk of disease transmission that may be unacceptable for some patients. Autologous chondrocyte implantation, either under a periosteal patch or as part of an implanted bioscaffold, is an example of one of the earliest clinical applications of tissue bioengineering. More detailed discussions are available in the cartilage sections of this book. It should be emphasized that evidence-based development of resilient cartilage treatments are significantly hampered by the lack of good, noninvasive monitoring techniques. At this time, it appears that MRI will become an increasingly important and powerful tool for critical evaluation of future treatment strategies.

Special Topics

Pigmented Villonodular Synovitis

Pigmented villonodular synovitis (PVNS) is a disease of the synovium of largely unknown etiology that affects roughly 1 in 500,000 people.[307] Histologic examination of PVNS reveals lipid-filled macrophages, multinucleated giant cells, and the presence of iron-rich hemosiderin in the synovium. The knee is the joint most commonly affected. There are two forms of PVNS, the localized (LPVNS) and diffuse (DPVNS) presentations. At arthroscopy, LPVNS lesions are discrete and pedunculated (Fig. 10.57), whereas DPVNS has a diffuse villous

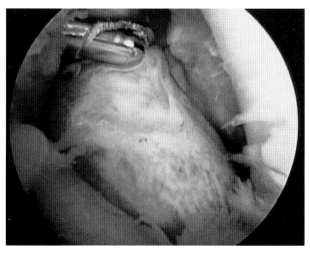 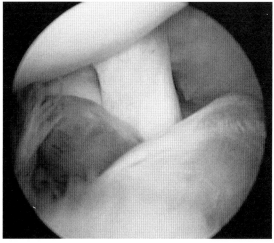

A B

Fig. 10.57. Arthroscopic images in two patients of localized pigmented villonodular synovitis in the anterior compartment of the knee. Both patients complained of pain with terminal knee extension. (A) Left knee, the articular cartilage of the lateral femoral notch appears in the upper right. (B) Right knee, the ACL is the vertical structure in the center of the image, with the lateral femoral articular cartilage to the upper left.

appearance across the synovium. They vary in their clinical presentation, prognosis, and response to treatment.

Localized PVNS occurs most commonly in the anterior knee compartment and mimics meniscal pathology. Patients present with joint pain and swelling along with locking catching and instability. Localized PVNS has a favorable prognosis, especially when the lesions are surgically excised early. It has an 8% recurrence rate.[307] Untreated LPVNS causes continued pain and discomfort and in rare cases has been noted to convert into the more debilitating diffuse form.

The onset of DPVNS is insidious, with gradual development of pain, swelling, and stiffness. It is often misdiagnosed as osteoarthritis or rheumatoid arthritis. It has a fairly poor prognosis. Thorough surgical excision of DPVNS (whether arthroscopic or open) is technically more challenging and historically less successful than treatment of LPVNS, with reported recurrence rates of 46%.[307] Synovial ablation, either chemically or by radiation therapy, may improve the natural history in severe cases of DPVNS. However, in some instances, total joint arthroplasty is the only reasonable recourse for severe pain and joint destruction.

Imaging

Since clinical diagnosis of PVNS can be quite difficult, imaging is key to preoperative assessment. Plain radiographs may show periarticular erosions and joint space narrowing, but the findings are nonspecific and insensitive. Magnetic resonance imaging is the imaging modality of choice because of its characteristic appearance and ability to localize the disease. Distinguishing between the two disease processes is essential because patients with DPVNS, especially those with extensive posterior compartment involvement, should be managed by a thoughtful and sometimes complex surgical algorithm. This includes multiportal arthroscopic treatment or open, multi-incision synovectomy.[307] Tertiary referral may be particularly appropriate for patients with DPVNS.

Patellar Tendinosis

Patellar tendinosis, or "jumper's knee," is a condition of anterior knee pain that is common in elite and recreational athletes alike. It is a repetitive strain injury seen in sports in which running, kicking, and jumping are common. Basketball is the sport most frequently associated with patellar tendinosis in the United States.[308] Histologic examination of the tendon reveals necrosis, degeneration, and microtears of the tissue. Patients report pain in the patellar tendon near its attachment to the patella. In the early stages, pain usually occurs after heavy training. As the disease progresses, patients feel pain while performing the offending sports activity and sometimes with activities of daily living. Complete rupture of the patellar tendon can occur due to chronic overuse, but this is rare.

Patellar tendinosis can be diagnosed relatively easily with a careful history and physical examination. The tendon is typically focally tender to palpation near the inferior pole of the patella. Although ultrasound can detect tendon abnormality, MRI is preferred for demonstration and localization of cystic or mucoid degeneration of the tendon. Better understanding of the pathoanatomy can be helpful for the occasional recalcitrant case that requires open surgical intervention.[308]

Other Diagnoses to Keep in Mind

In any clinical scenario it is important to consider all possible disease processes and to use the history and physical exam to form an efficient and thorough differential diagnosis. Table 10.7 presents a compilation of knee problems listed in order of

TABLE 10.7. Differential diagnosis of knee pain.

Type of injury	Conditions	Efficacy of clinical examination	Utility of MRI
Degenerative conditions	Osteoarthritis	Physical exam shows wide range, from subtle swelling to marked joint tenderness	Improving as cartilage-imaging techniques evolve
Mechanical derangement	Meniscal lesions, loose bodies, osteochondritis dissecans (OCD)	Meniscal injuries usually detected by physical exam; loose bodies sometimes palpable	MRI sensitive for meniscus lesions and helpful for prognosis with OCD lesions[311]
Instability	Single ligament or multiligament injuries	Clinical diagnosis highly accurate for experienced observer if patient can relax for exam	MRI very accurate for ligament injuries; helpful for detection of associated abnormalities
Extensor mechanism problems	Patellofemoral pain syndrome, patellar instability	Physical exam is mainstay, but findings can be vague	MRI detects bone bruises with patellar dislocation and MPFL tear; can be used to delineate patellar subluxation versus tilt
Extraarticular problems	Bursitis	Superficial bursitis relatively easy to diagnose on clinical examination	MRI helpful for detecting deeper bursal pathology
Inflammation or infectious problems	Rheumatoid arthritis (RA)	Physical exam detects inflammation, but biochemical tests better for definitive diagnosis	High-resolution MRI better than radiographs to detect bone erosion associated with RA[313]
Congenital problems		Clinical evaluation key for diagnosis and physical assessment of muscle imbalance and malalignment	
Tumors	Osteosarcoma, chondrosarcoma	Exam nonspecific; sometimes complaints of pain and swelling[314]	MRI effective for early detection and critical for definitive planning[315]

MPFL, medial patellofemoral ligament

the relative frequency with which they are seen in orthopedic practice.[309] In addition to these diagnoses, the physician must be alert for knee pain that might be related to hip disease, vascular dysfunction, or spine pathology.[310–315]

References

1. Fischer SP, Fox JM, Del Pizzo W. Accuracy of diagnosis from magnetic resonance imaging of the knee. A multi-center analysis of one thousand and fourteen patients. J Bone Joint Surg [Am] 1991;73:2–10.

2. Glynn N, Morrison WB, Parker L, et al. Trends in utilization: has extremity MR imaging replaced diagnostic arthroscopy? Skeletal Radiol 2004;33:272–276.

3. Bryan S, Bungay HP, Weatherburn G, et al. Magnetic resonance imaging for investigation of the knee joint: a clinical and economic evaluation. Int J Technol Assess Health Care 2004;20:222–229.

4. Gelb JH, Glasgow SG, Sapega AA. Magnetic resonance imaging of knee disorders. Clinical value and cost-effectiveness in a sports medicine practice. Am J Sports Med 1996;24:99–103.

5. Rose NE, Gold SM. A comparison of accuracy between clinical examination and magnetic resonance imaging in the diagnosis of meniscal and anterior cruciate ligament tears. Arthroscopy 1996;12:398–405.

6. Kocabey Y, Tetik O, Isbell WM. The value of clinical examination versus magnetic resonance imaging in the diagnosis of meniscal tears and anterior cruciate ligament rupture. Arthroscopy 2004;20:696–700.

7. Campbell JD. The evolution and current treatment trends with anterior cruciate, posterior cruciate, and medial collateral ligament injuries. Am J Knee Surg 1998;11:128–135.

8. Alioto RJ, Browne JE, Barnthouse CD. The influence of MRI on treatment decisions regarding knee injuries. Am J Knee Surg 1999;12:91–97.

9. Munshi M, Davidson M, MacDonald PB. The efficacy of magnetic resonance imaging in acute knee injuries. Clin J Sports Med 2000;10:34–39.

10. Treishmann HW Jr, Mosure JC. The impact of magnetic resonance imaging of the knee on surgical decision making. Arthroscopy 1996;12:550–555.

11. Twaddle BC, Hunter JC, Chapman JR. MRI in acute knee dislocation. J Bone Joint Surg [Br] 1996;78:573–579.

12. Sherman PM, Penrod BJ, Lane MJ. Comparison of knee magnetic resonance imaging findings in patients referred by orthopaedic surgeons versus nonorthopaedic practitioners. Arthroscopy 2002;18:201–205.

13. Bernstein J, Cain EL, Kneeland JB, et al. The incidence of pathology detected by magnetic resonance imaging of the knee: differences based on the specialty of the requesting physician. Orthopedics 2003;26:483–485.

14. Miller TT, Stein BE, Staron RB, et al. Relationship of the meniscofemoral ligaments of the knee to lateral meniscus tears: magnetic resonance imaging evaluation. Am J Orthop 1998;27:729–732.

15. Rankin M, Noyes FR, Barber-Westin SD, et al. Human meniscus allografts' in vivo size and motion characteristics: magnetic resonance imaging assessment under weightbearing conditions. Am J Sports Med 2006;34:98–107.

16. Vedi V, Williams A, Tennant SJ, et al. Meniscal movement. An in-vivo study using dynamic MRI. J Bone Joint Surg [Br] 1999;81:37–41.

17. Fukuta S, Masaki K, Korai F. Prevalence of abnormal findings in magnetic resonance images of asymptomatic knees. J Orthop Sci 2002;7:287–291.

18. Rohren EM, Kosarek FJ, Helms CA. Discoid lateral meniscus and the frequency of meniscal tears. Skeletal Radiol 2001;30:316–320.

19. Silverman JM, Mink JH, Deutsch AL. Discoid menisci of the knee: MR imaging appearance. Radiology 1989;173:351–354.

20. Singh K, Helms CA, Jacobs MT, et al. MRI appearance of Wrisberg variant of discoid lateral meniscus. AJR Am J Roentgenol 2006;187:384–387.

21. Araki Y, Tanaka H, Yamamoto H. MR imaging of pigmented villonodular synovitis of the knee. Radiat Med 1994;12:11–15.

22. Klingele KE, Kocher MS, Hresko MT. Discoid lateral meniscus: prevalence of peripheral rim instability. Pediatr Orthop 2004;24:79–82.

23. Bin SI, Kim JC, Kim JM. Correlation between type of discoid lateral menisci and tear pattern. Knee Surg Sports Traumatol Arthrosc 2002;10:218–222.

24. Stark JE, Siegel MJ, Weinberger E. Discoid menisci in children: MR features. J Comput Assist Tomogr 1995;19:608–611.

25. Araki Y, Ashikaga R, Fujii K. MR imaging of meniscal tears with discoid lateral meniscus. Eur J Radiol 1998;27:153–160.

26. Ryu KN, Kim IS, Kim EJ. MR imaging of tears of discoid lateral menisci. AJR 1998;171:963–967.

27. Park JS, Ryu KN, Yoon KH. Meniscal flounce on knee MRI: correlation with meniscal locations after positional changes. AJR Am J Roentgenol 2006;187:364–370.

28. De Smet AA, Norris MA, Yandow DR. MR diagnosis of meniscal tears of the knee: importance of high signal in the meniscus that extends to the surface. AJR 1993;161:101–107.

29. Crues JV 3rd, Mink J, Levy TL. Meniscal tears of the knee: accuracy of MR imaging. Radiology 1987;164:445–448.

30. Stoller DW, Martin C, Crues JV. Meniscal tears: pathologic correlation with MR imaging. Radiology 1987;163:731–735.

31. Anderson MW, Raghavan N, Seidenwurm DJ. Evaluation of meniscal tears: fast spin-echo versus conventional spin-echo magnetic resonance imaging. Acad Radiol 1995;2:209–214.

32. Magee T, Shapiro M, Williams D. Usefulness of simultaneous acquisition of spatial harmonics technique for MRI of the knee. AJR 2004;182:1411–1415.

33. Reeder JD, Matz SO, Becker L. MR imaging of the knee in the sagittal projection: comparison of three-dimensional gradient-echo and spin-echo sequences. AJR 1989;153:537–540.

34. Cotten A, Delfaut E, Demondion X, et al. MR imaging of the knee at 0.2 and 1.5 T: correlation with surgery. AJR Am J Roentgenol 2000;174:1093–1097.

35. James P, Buirski G. MR imaging of the knee: a prospective trial using a low field strength magnet. Australas Radiol 1990;34:59–63.

36. Magee T, Williams D. 3.0-T MRI of meniscal tears. AJR Am J Roentgenol 2006;187:371–375.

37. De Smet AA, Graf BK. Meniscal tears missed on MR imaging: relationship to meniscal tear patterns and anterior cruciate ligament tears. AJR 1994;162:905–911.

38. Jee WH, McCauley TR, Kim JM. Magnetic resonance diagnosis of meniscal tears in patients with acute anterior cruciate ligament tears. J Comput Assist Tomogr 2004;28:402–406.

39. Magee T, Shapiro M, Williams D. Prevalence of meniscal radial tears of the knee revealed by MRI after surgery. AJR 2004;182:931–936.

40. Weiss KL, Morehouse HT, Levy IM. Sagittal MR images of the knee: a low-signal band parallel to the posterior cruciate ligament caused by a displaced bucket-handle tear. AJR 1991;156:117–119.

41. Dorsay TA, Helms CA. Bucket-handle meniscal tears of the knee: sensitivity and specificity of MRI signs. Skeletal Radiol 2003;32:266–272.

42. Singson RD, Feldman F, Staron R. MR imaging of displaced bucket-handle tear of the medial meniscus. AJR 1991;156:121–124.

43. Lerer DB, Umans HR, Hu MX, et al. The role of meniscal root pathology and radial meniscal tear in medial meniscal extrusion. Skeletal Radiol 2004;33:569–574.

44. Costa CR, Morrison WB, Carrino JA. Medial meniscus extrusion on knee MRI: is extent associated with severity of degeneration or type of tear? AJR Am J Roentgenol 2004;183:17–23.

45. Brody JM, Lin HM, Hulstyn MJ, et al. Lateral meniscus root tear and meniscus extrusion with anterior cruciate ligament tear. Radiology 2006;239:805–810.

46. De Maeseneer M, Shahabpour M, Vanderdood K. Medial meniscocapsular separation: MR imaging criteria and diagnostic pitfalls. Eur J Radiol 2002;41:242–252.

47. Zanetti M, Pfirrmann CW, Schmid MR, et al. Patients with suspected meniscal tears: prevalence of abnormalities seen on MRI of 100 symptomatic and 100 contralateral asymptomatic knees. AJR Am J Roentgenol 2003;181:635–641.

48. Simonian PT, Sussmann PS, Wickiewicz TL, et al. Popliteomeniscal fasciculi and the unstable lateral meniscus: clinical correlation and magnetic resonance diagnosis. Arthroscopy 1997;13:590–596.

49. LaPrade RF, Konowalchuk BK. Popliteomeniscal fascicle tears causing symptomatic lateral compartment knee pain: diagnosis by the figure-4 test and treatment by open repair. Am J Sports Med 2005;33:1231–1236.

50. Johnson RL, De Smet AA. MR visualization of the popliteomeniscal fascicles. Skeletal Radiol 1999;28:561–566.

51. De Smet AA, Asinger DA, Johnson RL. Abnormal superior popliteomeniscal fascicle and posterior pericapsular edema: indirect MR imaging signs of a lateral meniscal tear. AJR Am J Roentgenol 2001;176:63–66.

52. Boxheimer L, Lutz AM, Zanetti M, et al. Characteristics of displaceable and nondisplaceable meniscal tears at kinematic MR imaging of the knee. Radiology 2006;238:221–231.

53. Vande Berg BC, Poilvache P, Duchateau F, et al. Lesions of the menisci of the knee: value of MR imaging criteria for recognition of unstable lesions. AJR Am J Roentgenol 2001;176:771–776.

54. Campbell SE, Sanders TG, Morrison WB. MR imaging of meniscal cysts: incidence, location, and clinical significance. AJR 2001;177:409–413.

55. McCarthy CL, McNally EG. The MRI appearance of cystic lesions around the knee. Skeletal Radiol 2004;33:187–209.

56. Tyson LL, Daughters TC Jr, Ryu RK. MRI appearance of meniscal cysts. Skeletal Radiol 1995;24:421–424.

57. Blair TR, Schweitzer M, Resnick D. Meniscal cysts causing bone erosion: retrospective analysis of seven cases. Clin Imaging 1999;23:134–138.

58. Lee W, Kim HS, Kim SJ. CT arthrography and virtual arthroscopy in the diagnosis of the anterior cruciate ligament and meniscal abnormalities of the knee joint. Korean J Radiol 2004;5:47–54.

59. Vande Berg BC, Lecouvet FE, Poilvache P. Anterior cruciate ligament tears and associated meniscal lesions: assessment at dual-detector spiral CT arthrography. Radiology 2002;223:403–409.

60. Vande Berg BC, Lecouvet FE, Poilvache P. Dual-detector spiral CT arthrography of the knee: accuracy for detection of meniscal abnormalities and unstable meniscal tears. Radiology 2000;216:851–857.

61. Deutsch AL, Mink JH, Fox JM. Peripheral meniscal tears: MR findings after conservative treatment or arthroscopic repair. Radiology 1990;176:485–488.

62. Lim PS, Schweitzer ME, Bhatia M. Repeat tear of postoperative meniscus: potential MR imaging signs. Radiology 1999;210:183–188.

63. Farley TE, Howell SM, Love KF. Meniscal tears: MR and arthrographic findings after arthroscopic repair. Radiology 1991;180:517–522.

64. Kent RH, Pope CF, Lynch JK. Magnetic resonance imaging of the surgically repaired meniscus: six-month follow-up. Magn Reson Imaging 1991;9:335–341.

65. Applegate GR, Flannigan BD, Tolin BS. MR diagnosis of recurrent tears in the knee: value of intraarticular contrast material. AJR 1993;161:821–825.

66. Sciulli RL, Boutin RD, Brown RR. Evaluation of the postoperative meniscus of the knee: a study comparing conventional arthrography, conventional MR imaging, MR arthrography with iodinated contrast material, and MR arthrography with gadolinium-based contrast material. Skeletal Radiol 1999;28:508–514.

67. Magee T, Shapiro M, Rodriguez J. MR arthrography of postoperative knee: for which patients is it useful? Radiology 2003;229:159–163.

68. Mutschler C, Vande Berg BC, Lecouvet FE. Postoperative meniscus: assessment at dual-detector row spiral CT arthrography of the knee. Radiology 2003;228:635–641.

69. Vives MJ, Homesley D, Ciccotti MG. Evaluation of recurring meniscal tears with gadolinium-enhanced magnetic resonance imaging: a randomized, prospective study. Am J Sports Med 2003;31:868–873.

70. White LM, Schweitzer ME, Weishaupt D. Diagnosis of recurrent meniscal tears: prospective evaluation of conventional MR imaging, indirect MR arthrography, and direct MR arthrography. Radiology 2002;222:421–429.

71. Hantes ME, Zachos VC, Zibis AH. Evaluation of meniscal repair with serial magnetic resonance imaging: a comparative study between conventional MRI and indirect MR arthrography. Eur J Radiol 2004;50:231–237.

72. Potter HG, Rodeo SA, Wickiewicz TL. MR imaging of meniscal allografts: correlation with clinical and arthroscopic outcomes. Radiology 1996;198:509–514.

73. Noyes FR, Westin-Barber SD, Rankin M. Meniscal transplantation in symptomatic patients less than fifty years old. J Bone Joint Surg 2004;86:1392–1404.

74. Verdonk PC, Verstraete KL, Almqvist KF,et al. Meniscal allograft transplantation: long-term clinical results with radiological and magnetic resonance imaging correlations. Knee Surg Sports Traumatol Arthrosc 2006;7:1–13.

75. Wirth CJ, Peters G, Milachowski KA. Long-term results of meniscal allograft transplantation. Am J Sports Med 2002;30:174–181.

76. Barry KP, Mesgarzadeh M, Triolo R. Accuracy of MRI patterns in evaluating anterior cruciate ligament tears. Skeletal Radiol 1996;25:365–370.

77. Lerman JE, Gray DS, Schweitzer ME, et al. MR evaluation of the anterior cruciate ligament: value of axial images. J Comput Assist Tomogr 1995;19:604–607.

78. Mellado JM, Calmet J, Olona M. Magnetic resonance imaging of anterior cruciate ligament tears: reevaluation of quantitative parameters and imaging findings including simplified method for measuring the anterior cruciate ligament angle. Knee Surg Sports Traumatol Arthrosc 2004;12:217–224.

79. Murao H, Morishita S, Nakajima M. Magnetic resonance imaging if the anterior cruciate ligament (ACL) tears: diagnostic value of ACL-tibial plateau angle. J Orthop Sci 3:1998;10–17.

80. Katahira K, Yamashita Y, Takahashi M. MR imaging of the anterior cruciate ligament: value of thin slice direct oblique coronal technique. Radiat Med 2001;19:1–7.

81. Hong SH, Choi JY, Lee GK. Grading of anterior cruciate ligament injury. diagnostic efficacy of oblique coronal magnetic resonance imaging of the knee. J Comput Assist Tomogr 2003;27:814–819.

82. Huang GS, Chain-Her K, Chan WP. Acute anterior cruciate ligament stump entrapment in anterior cruciate ligament tears: MR imaging appearance. Radiology 2002;225:537–540.

83. Chen WT, Shih TT, Tu HY. Partial and complete tear of the anterior cruciate ligament. Acta Radiol 20021;43:511–516.

84. Umans H, Wimpfheimer O, Haramati N. Diagnosis of partial tears of the anterior cruciate ligament of the knee: value of MR imaging. AJR 1995;165:893–897.

85. Yao L, Gentili A, Petrus L, et al. Partial ACL rupture: an MR diagnosis? Skeletal Radiol 1995;24:247–51.

86. Garcia-Alvarez F, Garcia-Pequerul JM, Avila JL. Ganglion cysts associated with cruciate ligaments of the knee: a possible cause of recurrent knee pain. Acta Orthop Belg 2000;66:490–494.

87. Krudwig WK, Schulte KK, Heinemann C. Intra-articular ganglion cysts of the knee joint: a report of 85 cases and review of the literature. Knee Surg Sports Traumatol Arthrosc 2004;12:123–129.

88. Recht MP, Applegate G, Kaplan P. The MR appearance of cruciate ganglion cysts: a report of 16 cases. Skeletal Radiol 1994;23:597–600.

89. McIntyre J, Moelleken S, Tirman S. Mucoid degeneration of the anterior cruciate ligament mistaken for ligamentous tears. Skeletal Radiol 2001;30:312–315.

90. Narvekar A, Gajjar S. Mucoid degeneration of the anterior cruciate ligament. Arthroscopy 2004;20:141–146.

91. Friedl W, Glaser F. Dynamic sonography in the diagnosis of ligament and meniscal injuries of the knee. Arch Orthop Trauma Surg 1991;110:132–138.

92. Gebhard F, Authenrieth M, Strecker W. Ultrasound evaluation of gravity induced anterior drawer following anterior cruciate ligament lesion. Knee Surg Sports Traumatol Arthrosc 1999;7:166–172.

93. Goldman AB, Pavlov H, Rubenstein D. The second fracture of the proximal tibia: a small avulsion that reflects major ligamentous damage. AJR 1988;151:1163–1170.

94. Davis DS, Post WR. Segond fractures: lateral capsular ligament avulsion. J Orthop Sports Phys Ther 1997;25:103–106.

95. Weber WN, Neumann CH, Barakos JA. Lateral tibial rim (Segond) fractures: MR imaging characteristics. Radiology 1991;180:731–734.

96. Remer EM, Fitzgerald SW, Friedman H. Anterior cruciate ligament injury: MR imaging diagnosis and patterns of injury. RadioGraphics 1992;12:901–915.

97. Snearly WN, Kaplan PA, Dussault RG. Lateral-compartment bone contusions in adolescents with intact anterior cruciate ligaments. Radiology 1996;198:205–208.

98. Lee K, Siegel MJ, Lau DM. Anterior cruciate ligament tears: MR imaging-based diagnosis in a pediatric population. Radiology 1999;213:697–704.

99. Johnson DL, Urban WP Jr, Caborn DN. Articular cartilage changes seen with magnetic resonance imaging-detected bone bruises associated with acute anterior cruciate ligaments rupture. Am J Sports Med 1998;26:409–414.

100. Costa-Paz M, Muscolo DL, Ayerza MA. Magnetic resonance imaging follow-up study of bone bruises associated with anterior cruciate ligament ruptures. Arthroscopy 2001;17:445–449.

101. Vellet AD, Marks PH, Fowler PJ. Occult posttraumatic osteochondral lesions of the knee: prevalence, classification, and short-term sequelae evaluated with MR imaging. Radiology 1991;178:271–276.

102. Chan KK, Resnick D, Goodwin D. Posteromedial tibial plateau injury including avulsion fracture of the semimembranosus tendon insertion site: ancillary sign of anterior cruciate ligament tear at MR imaging. Radiology 1999;211:754–758.

103. Kaplan PA, Gehl RH, Dussault RG. Bone contusions of the posterior lip of the medial tibial plateau (countercoup injury) and associated internal derangements of the knee at MR imaging. Radiology 1999;211:747–753.

104. Gentili A, Seeger LL, Yao L. Anterior cruciate ligament tear: indirect signs at MR imaging. Radiology 1994;193:835–840.

105. Robertson PL, Schweitzer ME, Bartolozzi AR. Anterior cruciate ligament tears: evaluation of multiple signs with MR imaging. Radiology 1994;193:829–834.

106. Tung GA, Davis LM, Wiggins ME. Tears of the anterior cruciate ligament: primary and secondary signs at MR imaging. Radiology 1993;188:661–667.

107. Vahey TN, Broome DR, Kayes KJ. Acute and chronic tears of the anterior cruciate ligament: differential features at MR imaging. Radiology 1991;181:251–253.

108. Dimond PM, Fadale PD, Hulstyn MJ. A comparison of MRI findings in patients with acute and chronic ACL tears. Am J Knee Surg 1998;11:153–159.

109. Nakauchi M, Kurosawa H, Kawakami A. Abnormal lateral notch in knees with anterior cruciate ligament injury. J Orthop Sci 2000;5:92–95.

110. Cobby MJ, Schweitzer ME, Resnick D. The deep lateral femoral notch: an indirect sign of a torn anterior cruciate ligament. Radiology 1992;184:855–858.

111. McCauley TR. MR imaging evaluation of the postoperative knee. Radiology 2005;234:53–61.

112. Tomczak RJ, Hehl G, Mergo PJ. Tunnel placement in anterior cruciate ligament reconstruction: MRI analysis as an important risk factor in the radiological report. Skeletal Radiol 1997;26:409–413.

113. Warden WH, Friedman R, Teresi LM. Magnetic resonance imaging of bioabsorbable polylactic acid interference screws during the first 2 years after anterior cruciate ligament reconstruction. Arthroscopy 1999;15:474–480.

114. Lajtai G, Noszian I, Humer K. Serial magnetic resonance imaging evaluation of operative site after fixation of patellar tendon graft with bioabsorbable interference screws

in anterior cruciate ligament reconstruction. Arthroscopy 1999;15:709–718.

115. Horton KL, Jacobson JA, Lin J. MR imaging of anterior cruciate ligament reconstruction graft. AJR 2000;175:1091–1097.

116. Hong SJ, Ahn JM, Ahn JH, et al. Postoperative MR findings of the healthy ACL grafts: correlation with second look arthroscopy. Clin Imaging 2005;29:55–59.

117. Ayerza MA, Muscolo L, Costa-Paz M. Comparison of sagittal obliquity of the reconstructed anterior cruciate ligament with native anterior cruciate ligament using magnetic resonance imaging. Arthroscopy 2003;19:257–261.

118. Fujimoto E, Sumen Y, Deie M. Anterior cruciate ligament graft impingement against the posterior cruciate ligament: diagnosis using MRI plus three-dimensional reconstruction software. Magnetic Resonance Imaging 2004;22:1125–1129.

119. Stockle U, Hoffmann R, Schwedke J. Anterior cruciate ligament reconstruction: the diagnostic value of MRI. Int Orthop 1998;22:288–292.

120. Vogl TJ, Schmitt J, Lubrich J. Reconstructed anterior cruciate ligaments using patellar tendon ligament grafts: diagnostic value of contrast-enhanced MRI in a 2–year follow-up regimen. Eur Radiol 2001;11:1450–1456.

121. Amiel D, Kleiner JB, Roux RD, et al. The phenomenon of "ligamentization": anterior cruciate ligament reconstruction with autogenous patellar tendon. J Orthop Res 1986;4:162–172.

122. Howell SM, Berns GS, Farley TE. Unimpinged and impinged anterior cruciate ligament grafts: MR signal intensity measurements. Radiology 1991;179:639–643.

123. Kanamiya T, Hara M, Naito M. Magnetic resonance evaluation of remodeling process in patellar tendon graft. Clin Orthop Relat Res 2004;419:202–206.

124. Jansson KA, Harilainen A, Sandelin J, et al. Bone tunnel enlargement after anterior cruciate ligament reconstruction with the hamstring autograft and endobutton fixation technique. A clinical, radiographic and magnetic resonance imaging study with 2 years follow-up. Knee Surg Sports Traumatol Arthrosc 1999;7:290–295.

125. McCauley TR, Elfar A, Moore A. MR arthrography of anterior cruciate ligament reconstruction grafts. AJR 2003;181:1217–1223.

126. May DA, Snearly WN, Bents R. MR imaging findings in anterior cruciate ligament reconstruction: evaluation of notchplasty. AJR 1997;169:217–222.

127. Bradley DM, Bergman AG, Dillingham MF. MR imaging of Cyclops lesions. AJR 2000;174:719–726.

128. Recht MP, Piraino DW, Cohen MA. Localized anterior arthrofibrosis (cyclops lesion) after reconstruction of the anterior cruciate ligament: MR imaging findings. AJR 1995;165:383–385.

129. Rispoli DM, Sanders TG, Miller MD. Magnetic resonance imaging at different time periods following hamstring harvest for anterior cruciate ligament reconstruction. Arthroscopy 2001;17:2–8.

130. Leis HT, Sander TG, Larsen KM. Hamstring regrowth following harvesting for ACL reconstruction: the lizard tail phenomenon. J Knee Surg 2003;16:159–164.

131. Svensson M, Kartus J, Ejerhed L. Does the patellar tendon normalize after harvesting its central third? Am J Sports Med 2004;32:34–38.

132. Patten RM, Richardson ML, Zink-Brody G, et al. Complete vs partial-thickness tears of the posterior cruciate ligament: MR findings. J Comput Assist Tomogr 1994 ;18:793–799.

133. Sonin AH, Fitzgerald SW, Hoff FL, et al. MR imaging of the posterior cruciate ligament: normal, abnormal, and associated injury patterns. Radiographics 1995;15:551–561.

134. Malone AA, Dowd GS, Saifuddin A. Injuries of the posterior cruciate ligament and posterolateral corner of the knee. Injury 2006;37:485–501.

135. Mair SD, Schlegel TF, Gill TJ, et al. Incidence and location of bone bruises after acute posterior cruciate ligament injury. Am J Sports Med 2004;32:1681–1687.

136. Escobedo EM, Mills WJ, Hunter JC. The "reverse Segond" fracture: association with a tear of the posterior cruciate ligament. AJR 2002;178:979–983.

137. Shelbourne KD, Jennings RW, Vahey TN. Magnetic resonance imaging of posterior cruciate ligament injuries: assessment of healing. Am J Knee Surg 1999;12:209–213.

138. Tewes DP, Fritts HM, Fields RD, et al. Chronically injured posterior cruciate ligament: magnetic resonance imaging. Clin Orthop Relat Res 1997;335:224–232.

139. Griffin LY, Burnett M, Milsap JH. Appearance of previously injured posterior cruciate ligaments on magnetic resonance imaging. South Med J 2002;95:1153–1157.

140. Servant CT, Ramos JP, Thomas NP. The accuracy of magnetic resonance imaging in diagnosing chronic posterior cruciate ligament injury. Knee 2004;11:265–270.

141. Mariani PP, Margheritini F, Christel P, et al. Evaluation of posterior cruciate ligament healing: a study using magnetic resonance imaging and stress radiography. Arthroscopy 2005;21:1354–1361.

142. Mariani PP, Adriano E, Bellelli A. Magnetic resonance imaging of tunnel placement in posterior cruciate ligament reconstruction. Arthroscopy 1999;15:733–740.

143. Bosch U, Kasperczyk WJ. Healing of the patellar tendon autograft after posterior cruciate ligament reconstruction–a process of ligamentization? An experimental study in a sheep model. Am J Sports Med 1992;20:558–66.

144. Mariani PP, Margheritini F, Camillieri G. Serial magnetic resonance imaging evaluation of the patellar tendon after posterior cruciate ligament reconstruction. Arthroscopy 2002;18:38–45.

145. de Abreu MR, Kim HJ, Chung CB, et al. Posterior cruciate ligament recess and normal posterior capsular insertional anatomy: MR imaging of cadaveric knees. Radiology 2005;236:968–73.

146. Robinson JR, Bull AM, Thomas RR, et al. The Role of the Medial Collateral Ligament and Posteromedial Capsule in Controlling Knee Laxity. Am J Sports Med 2006;34:1815–1823.

147. Warren LF, Marshall JL. The supporting structures and layers on the medial side of the knee: an anatomical analysis. J Bone Joint Surg [Am] 1979;61:56–62.

148. De Maeseneer M, Shahabpour M, Van Roy F, et al. MR imaging of the medial collateral ligament bursa: findings in patients and anatomic data derived from cadavers. AJR Am J Roentgenol 2001;177:911–917.

149. Schweitzer ME, Tran D, Deely DM. Medial collateral ligament injuries: evaluation of multiple signs, prevalence and location of associated bone bruises, and assessment with MR imaging. Radiology 1995;194:825–829.

150. Beltran J, Matityahu A, Hwang K, et al. The distal semimembranosus complex: normal MR anatomy, variants, biomechanics and pathology. Skeletal Radiol 2003;32:435–445.

151. Sims WF, Jacobson KE. The posteromedial corner of the knee: medial-sided injury patterns revisited. Am J Sports Med 2004;32:337–345.

152. De Maeseneer M, Van Roy F, Lenchik L, et al. Three layers of the medial capsular and supporting structures of the knee: MR imaging-anatomic correlation. Radiographics 2000;20:S83–89.

153. Amis AA, Bull AM, Gupte CM, et al. Biomechanics of the PCL and related structures: posterolateral, posteromedial and meniscofemoral ligaments. Knee Surg Sports Traumatol Arthrosc 2003;11:271–281.

154. Yao L, Dungan D, Seeger LL. MR imaging of tibial collateral ligament injury: comparison with clinical examination. Skeletal Radiol 1994;23:521–524.

155. Niitsu M, Ikeda K, Iijima T, et al. MR imaging of Pellegrini-Stieda disease. Radiat Med 1999;17:405–409.

156. Bergin D, Keogh C, O'Connell M, et al. Atraumatic medial collateral ligament oedema in medial compartment knee osteoarthritis. Skeletal Radiol 2002;31:14–18.

157. Alioto RJ, Browne JE, Barnthouse CD, Scott AR. Complete rupture of the distal semimembranosus complex in a professional athlete. Clin Orthop Relat Res 1997;336:162–165.

158. Mochizuki T, Akita K, Muneta T, et al. Pes anserinus: layered supportive structure on the medial side of the knee. Clin Anat 2004;17:50–54.

159. Bencardino JT, Rosenberg ZS, Brown RR, et al. Traumatic musculotendinous injuries of the knee: diagnosis with MR imaging. Radiographics 2000;20:S103–120.

160. Miller TT, Gladden P, Staron RB. Posterolateral stabilizers of the knee: anatomy and injuries with MR imaging. AJR 1997;169:1641–1647.

161. Harish S, O'Donnell P, Connell D, et al. Imaging of the posterolateral corner of the knee. Clin Radiol 2006;61:457–466.

162. Stannard JP, Brown SL, Robinson JT, et al. Reconstruction of the posterolateral corner of the knee. Arthroscopy 2005;21:1051–1059.

163. Munshi M, Pretterklieber ML, Kwak S, et al. MR imaging, MR arthrography, and specimen correlation of the posterolateral corner of the knee: an anatomic study. AJR Am J Roentgenol 2003,180.1095–1101.

164. Yoon KH, Bae DK, Ha JH, et al. Anatomic reconstructive surgery for posterolateral instability of the knee. Arthroscopy 2006;22:159–165.

165. LaPrade RF, Gilbert TJ, Bollom TS, et al. The magnetic resonance imaging appearance of individual structures of the posterolateral knee. A prospective study of normal knees and knees with surgically verified grade III injuries. Am J Sports Med 2000;28:191–199.

166. Yu JS, Salonen DC, Hodler J. Posterolateral aspect of the knee: improved MR imaging with a coronal oblique technique. Radiology 1996;198:199–204.

167. Brown TR, Quinn SF, Wensel JP, et al. Diagnosis of popliteus injuries with MR imaging. Skeletal Radiol 1995;24:511–514.

168. Shindell R, Walsh WM, Connolly JF. Avulsion fracture of the fibula: the "arcuate sign" of posterolateral knee instability. Nebr Med J 1984;69:369–371.

169. Juhng SK, Lee JK, Choi SS, et al. MR evaluation of the "arcuate" sign of posterolateral knee instability. AJR Am J Roentgenol 2002;178:583–588.

170. Lee J, Papakonstantinou O, Brookenthal KR, et al. Arcuate sign of posterolateral knee injuries: anatomic, radiographic, and MR imaging data related to patterns of injury. Skeletal Radiol 2003;32:619–627.

171. Huang GS, Yu JS, Munshi M, et al. Avulsion fracture of the head of the fibula (the "arcuate" sign): MR imaging findings predictive of injuries to the posterolateral ligaments and posterior cruciate ligament. AJR Am J Roentgenol 2003;180: 381–387.

172. Theodorou DJ, Theodorou SJ, Fithian DC, et al. Posterolateral complex knee injuries: magnetic resonance imaging with surgical correlation. Acta Radiol 2005;46:297–305.

173. Rumball JS, Lebrun CM, Di Ciacca SR, et al. Rowing injuries. Sports Med 2005;3:537–555.

174. Fairclough J, Hayashi K, Toumi H, et al. The functional anatomy of the iliotibial band during flexion and extension of the knee: implications for understanding iliotibial band syndrome. J Anat 2006;2 08:309–316.

175. Farrell KC, Reisinger KD, Tillman MD. Force and repetition in cycling: possible implications for iliotibial band friction syndrome. Knee 2003;10:103–109.

176. Orchard JW, Fricker PA, Abud AT, et al. Biomechanics of iliotibial band friction syndrome in runners. Am J Sports Med 1996;24:375–379.

177. Murphy BJ, Hechtman KS, Uribe JW. Iliotibial band friction syndrome: MR imaging findings. Radiology 1992;185:569–571.

178. Muhle C, Ahn JM, Yeh L. Iliotibial band friction syndrome: MR imaging findings in 16 patients and MR arthrographic study of six cadaveric knees. Radiology 1999;212:103–110.

179. Sonin AH, Fitzgerald SW, Bresler ME, et al. MR imaging appearance of the extensor mechanism of the knee: functional anatomy and injury patterns. Radiographics 1995;15:367–382.

180. Andrikoula S, Tokis A, Vasiliadis HS, et al. The extensor mechanism of the knee joint: an anatomical study. Knee Surg Sports Traumatol Arthrosc 2006;14:214–220.

181. Schweitzer ME, Mitchell DG, Ehrlich SM. The patellar tendon: thickening, internal signal buckling, and other MR variants. Skeletal Radiol 1993;22:411–416.

182. El-Khoury GY, Wira RL, Berbaum KS. MR imaging of patellar tendinitis. Radiology 199;184:849–854.

183. Vanhoenacker FM, Bernaerts A, Van de Perre S, et al. MRI of painful bipartite patella. JBR-BTR 2002;85:219.

184. Starok M, Lenchik L, Trudell D, et al. Normal patellar retinaculum: MR and sonographic imaging with cadaveric correlation. AJR Am J Roentgenol 1997;168:1493–1499.

185. Bianchi S, Zwass A, Abdelwahab IF. Diagnosis of tears of the quadriceps tendon of the knee: value of sonography. AJR 1994;162:1137–1140.

186. La S, Fessell DP, Femino JE. Sonography of partial-thickness quadriceps tendon tears with surgical correlation. J Ultrasound Med 2003;22:1323–1329.

187. Schmid MR, Hodler J, Cathrein P. Is impingement the cause of jumper's knee? Dynamic and static magnetic resonance imaging of patellar tendinitis in an open-configuration system. Am J Sports Med 2002;30:388–395.

188. Khan KM, Bonar F, Desmond PM. Patellar tendinosis (jumper's knee): findings at histopathologic examination, US, and MR imaging. Victorian Institute of Sports Tendon Study Group. Radiology 1996;200:821–827.

189. Lian OB, Engebretsen L, Bahr R. Prevalence of jumper's knee among elite athletes from different sports: a cross-sectional study. Am J Sports Med 2005;33:561–567.

190. Major NM, Helms CA. MR imaging of the knee: findings in asymptomatic collegiate basketball players. AJR 2002;179:641–644.

191. Peace KA, Lee JC, Healy J. Imaging the infrapatellar tendon in the elite athlete. Clin Radiol 2006;61:570–578.

192. Medlar RC, Lyne ED. Sinding-Larsen-Johansson disease. Its etiology and natural history. J Bone Joint Surg [Am] 1978;60:1113–1116.

193. Rosenberg ZS, Kawelblum M, Cheung YY. Osgood-Schlatter lesion: fracture or tendinitis? Scintigraphic, CT, and MR imaging features. Radiology 1992;185:853–858.

194. Elias DA, White LM, Fithian DC. Acute lateral patellar dislocation at MR imaging: injury patterns of medial patellar soft-tissue restraints and osteochondral injuries of the inferomedial patella. Radiology 2002;225:736–743.

195. Pope TL. MR imaging of patellar dislocation and relocation. Semin Ultrasound CT MR 2001;22:371–382.

196. Miller TT, Staron RB, Feldman F. Patellar height on sagittal MR imaging of the knee. AJR 1996;167:339–341.

197. Insall J, Salvati E. Patella position in the normal knee joint. Radiology 1971;101:101.

198. Chung CB, Skaf A, Roger B, et al. Patellar tendon-lateral femoral condyle friction syndrome: MR imaging in 42 patients. Skeletal Radiol 2001;30:694–697.

199. Shellock FG, Mink JH, Deutsch AL, et al. Kinematic MR imaging of the patellofemoral joint: comparison of passive positioning and active movement techniques. Radiology 1992;184:574–577.

200. Muhle C, Brinkmann G, Skaf A, et al. Effect of a patellar realignment brace on patients with patellar subluxation and dislocation. Evaluation with kinematic magnetic resonance imaging. Am J Sports Med 1999;27:350–353.

201. Dupuy DE, Hangen DH, Zachazewski JE, et al. Kinematic CT of the patellofemoral joint. AJR Am J Roentgenol 1997;169:211–215.

202. Niitsu M. Kinematic MR imaging of the knee. Semin Musculoskelet Radiol 2001;5:153–157.

203. Elias DA, White LM. Imaging of patellofemoral disorders. Clin Radiol 2004;59:543–557.

204. Ward EE, Jacobson JA, Fassell DP. Sonographic detection of Baker's cysts: comparison with MR imaging. AJR 2001;176:373–380.

205. Marti-Bonmati L, Molla E, Dosda E. MR imaging of Baker cysts- prevalence and relation to internal derangements of the knee. MAGMA 2000;10:205–210.

206. Miller TT, Staron RB, Koenigsberg T. MR imaging of Baker cysts: association with internal derangement, effusion, and degenerative arthropathy. Radiology 1996;201:247–250.

207. De Maeseneer M, Debaere C, Desprechins B. Popliteal cysts in children: prevalence, appearance, and associated findings at MR imaging. Pediatr Radiol 1999;29:605–609.

208. Forbes JR, Helms CA, Janzen DL. Acute pes anserine bursitis: MR imaging. Radiology 1995;194:525–527.

209. Rothstein CP, Laorr A, Helms CA. Semimembranosus-tibial collateral ligament bursitis: MR imaging findings. AJR 1996;166:875–877.

210. Bredella MA, Tirman PF, Peterfy CG. Accuracy of T2–weighted fast spin-echo MR imaging with fat saturation in detecting cartilage defects in the knee: comparison with arthroscopy in 130 patients. AJR 1999;172:1073–1080.

211. Gold GE, Fuller SE, Hargreaves BA. Driven equilibrium magnetic resonance imaging of articular cartilage: initial clinical experience. J Magn Reson Imaging 2005;21:476–481.

212. Kornaat PR, Doornbos J, van der Molen AJ. Magnetic resonance imaging of knee cartilage using a water selective balanced steady-state free precession sequence. J Magn Reson Imaging 2004;20:850–856.

213. Graichen H, Al-Shamari D, Hinterwimmer S. Accuracy of quantitative MRI in the detection of ex vivo focal cartilage defects. Ann Rheum Dis 2005;64:1120–1125.

214. Mosher TJ, Dardzinski BJ. Cartilage MRI T2 relaxation time mapping: overview and applications. Semin Musculoskelet Radiol 2004;8:355–368.

215. Potter HG, Linklater JM, Allen AA. Magnetic resonance imaging of articular cartilage in the knee. An evaluation with use of fast spin-echo imaging. J Bone Joint Surg [Am] 1998;80:1276–1284.

216. Tiderius CJ, Tjornstrand J, Akeson P. Delayed gadolinium-enhanced MRI of cartilage (dGEMRIC): intra-and interobserver variability in standardized drawing of regions of interest. Acta Radiol 2004;45:628–634.

217. Yoshioka H, Stevens K, Hargreaves BA. Magnetic resonance imaging of articular cartilage of the knee: comparison between fat-suppressed three-dimensional SPGR imaging, fat-suppressed FSE imaging, and fat-suppressed three-dimensional DEFT imaging, and correlation with arthroscopy. J Magn Reson Imaging 2004;20:857–864.

218. Modl JM, Sether LA, Haughton VM. Articular cartilage: correlation of histologic zones with signal intensity at MR imaging. Radiology 1991;181:853–855.

219. Recht M, White LM, Winalski CS. MR imaging of cartilage repair procedures. Skeletal Radiol 2003;32:185–2000.

220. Brown T, Quinn SF. Evaluation of chondromalacia of the patellofemoral compartment with axial magnetic resonance imaging. Skeletal Radiol 1993;22:325–328.

221. McCauley TR, Kier R, Lynch KJ. Chondromalacia patellae: diagnosis with MR imaging. AJR 1992;158:101–105.

222. van Leersum M, Schweitzer ME, Gannon F, et al. Chondromalacia patellae: an in vitro study. Comparison of MR criteria with histologic and macroscopic findings. Skeletal Radiol 1996;25:727–732.

223. Gagliardi JA, Chung EM, Chandnani VP, et al. Detection and staging of chondromalacia patellae: relative efficacies of conventional MR imaging, MR arthrography, and CT arthrography. AJR Am J Roentgenol 1994;163:629–636.

224. De Smet AA, Fisher DR, Graf BK. Osteochondritis dissecans of the knee: value of MR imaging in determining lesion stability and the presence of articular cartilage defects. AJR 1990;155:549–553.

225. De Smet AA, Ilahi OA, Graf BK. Reassessment of the MR criteria for stability of osteochondritis dissecans in the knee and ankle. Skeletal Radiol 1996;25:159–163.

226. Hinshaw MH, Tuite MJ, De Smet AA. "Dem bones": osteochondral injuries of the knee. Magn Reson Imaging Clin North Am 2000;8:335–348.

227. Brossmann J, Preidler KW, Daenen B. Imaging of osseous and cartilaginous intraarticular bodies in the knee: comparison of MR imaging and MR arthrography with CT and CT arthrography in cadavers. Radiology 1996;20:509–517.

228. Gebarski K, Hernandez RJ. Stage-I osteochondritis dissecans versus normal variants of ossification in the knee in children. Pediatr Radiol 2005;35:880–886.

229. Marlovits S, Striessnig G, Resinger CT, et al. Definition of pertinent parameters for the evaluation of articular cartilage repair

tissue with high-resolution magnetic resonance imaging. Eur J Radiol 2004;52:310–319.

230. Brown WE, Potter HG, Marx RG, et al. Magnetic resonance imaging appearance of cartilage repair in the knee. Clin Orthop Relat Res 2004;422:214–223.

231. Mithoefer K, Williams RJ 3rd, Warren RF, et al. The microfracture technique for the treatment of articular cartilage lesions in the knee. A prospective cohort study. J Bone Joint Surg [Am] 2005;87:1911–1920.

232. Gudas R, Stankevicius E, Monastyreckiene E, et al. Osteochondral autologous transplantation versus microfracture for the treatment of articular cartilage defects in the knee joint in athletes. Knee Surg Sports Traumatol Arthrosc 2006;14(9):834–842.

233. Sanders TG, Mentzer KD, Miller MD. Autogenous osteochondral "plug" transfer for the treatment of focal chondral defects: postoperative MR appearance with clinical correlation. Skeletal Radiol 2001;30:570–578.

234. Link TM, Mischung J, Wortler K, et al. Normal and pathological MR findings in osteochondral autografts with longitudinal follow-up. Eur Radiol 2006;16:88–96.

235. Koulalis D, Schultz W, Heyden M. Autologous osteochondral grafts in the treatment of cartilage defects of the knee joint. Knee Surg Sports Knee Surg Sports Traumatol Arthrosc 2004;12:329–334.

236. James SL, Connell DA, Saifuddin A, et al. MR imaging of autologous chondrocyte implantation of the knee. Eur Radiol 2006;16:1022–1030.

237. Krishnan SP, Skinner JA, Bartlett W, et al. Who is the ideal candidate for autologous chondrocyte implantation? J Bone Joint Surg [Br] 2006;88:61–64.

238. Trattnig S, Pinker K, Krestan C, et al. Matrix-based autologous chondrocyte implantation for cartilage repair with Hyalograft C: two-year follow-up by magnetic resonance imaging. Eur J Radiol 2006;57:9–15.

239. Tins BJ, McCall IW, Takahashi T. Autologous chondrocyte implantation in knee joint: MR imaging and histologic features at 1-year follow-up. Radiology 2005;234:501–508.

240. Henderson IJ, Tuy B, Connell D. Prospective clinical study of autologous chondrocyte implantation and correlation with MRI at three and 12 months. J Bone Joint Surg [Br] 2003;85:1060–1066.

241. Wada Y, Watanabe A, Yamashita T. Evaluation of articular cartilage with 3D-SPGR MRI after autologous chondrocyte implantation. J Orthop Sci 2003;8:514–517.

242. Roberts S, McCall IW, Darby AJ. Autologous chondrocyte implantation for cartilage repair: monitoring its success by magnetic resonance imaging and histology. Arthritis Res Ther 2003;5:R60–73.

243. Plank CM, Kubin K, Weber M, et al. Contrast-enhanced high-resolution magnetic resonance imaging of autologous cartilage implants of the knee joint. Magn Reson Imaging 2005;23:739–744.

244. Jacobson JA, Lenchik L, Ruhoy MK. MR imaging of the infrapatellar fat pad of Hoffa. RadioGraphics 1997;17:675–691.

245. Saddik D, McNally EG, Richardson M. MRI of Hoffa's fat pad. Skeletal Radiol 2004;33:433–444.

246. Boyd CR, Eakin C, Matheson GO. Infrapatella plica as a cause of anterior knee pain. Clin J Sport Med 2005;15:98–103.

247. Cothran RL, McGuire PM, Helms CA. MR imaging of infrapatellar plica injury. AJR 180:2003:1443–1447.

248. Base DK, Nam GU, Sun SD. The clinical significance of the complete type of suprapatellar membrane. Arthroscopy 1998;14:830–835.

249. Kim SJ, Shin SJ, Koo TY. Arch type pathologic suprapatellar plica. Arthroscopy 2001;17:536–538.

250. Boles CA, Butler J, Lee JA. Magnetic resonance characteristics of medial plica of the knee correlation with arthroscopic resection. J Comput Assist Tomogr 2004;28:397–401.

251. Kobayashi Y, Murakami R, Tajima H, et al. Direct MR arthrography of plica synovialis mediopatellaris. Acta Radiol 2001;42:286–290.

252. Asik M, Erlap L, Altinel L. Localized pigmented villonodular synovitis of the knee. Arthroscopy 2001;17:e23.

253. Kim RS, Lee JY, Lee KY. Localized pigmented villonodular synovitis attached to the posterior cruciate ligament of the knee. Arthroscopy 2003;19:e32–e35.

254. Cheng XG, You YH, Liu W. MRI features of pigmented villonodular synovitis (PVNS). Clin Rheumatol 2004;23:31–34.

255. Roberts D, Miller TT, Erlanger SM. Sonographic appearance of primary synovial chondromatosis of the knee. J Ultrasound Med 2004;23:707–709.

256. Mandalia V, Fogg AJ, Chari R, et al. Bone bruising of the knee. Clin Radiol 2005;60:627–636.

257. Sanders TG, Medynski MA, Feller JF, et al. Bone contusion patterns of the knee at MR imaging: footprint of the mechanism of injury. Radiographics 2000;20:S135–151.

258. Miller MD, Osborne JR, Gordon WT, et al. The natural history of bone bruises. A prospective study of magnetic resonance imaging-detected trabecular microfractures in patients with isolated medial collateral ligament injuries. Am J Sports Med 1998;26:15–19.

259. Lecouvet FE, Van de Berg BC, Maldague BE. Early irreversible osteonecrosis versus transient lesions of the femoral condyles: prognostic value of subchondral bone and marrow changes on MR imaging. AJR 1998;170:71–77.

260. Moosikasuwan JR, Miller TT, Math K. Shifting bone marrow edema of the knee. Skeletal Radiol 2004;33:380–385.

261. Mitchell DG, Steinberg ME, Dalinka MK. Magnetic resonance imaging of the ischemic hip. Alterations within osteonecrotic, viable, and reactive zones. Clin Orthop Relat Res 1989;244:60–77.

262. De Falco RA, Ricci AR, Balduini FC. Osteonecrosis of the knee after arthroscopic meniscectomy and chondroplasty: a case report and literature review. Am J Sports Med 2003;31:1013–1016.

263. Encalada I, Richmond JC. Osteonecrosis after arthroscopic meniscectomy using radiofrequency. Arthroscopy 2004;20:632–636.

264. Johnson TC, Evans JA, Gilley JA. Osteonecrosis of the knee after arthroscopic surgery for meniscal tears and chondral lesions. Arthroscopy 2000;16:254–261.

265. Prues-Latour V, Bonvin JC, Fritschy D. Nine cases of osteonecrosis in elderly patients following arthroscopic meniscectomy. Knee Surg Sports Traumatol Arthrosc 1998;6:142–147.

266. Athanasian EA, Wickiewicz TL, Warren RF. Osteonecrosis of the femoral condyle after arthroscopic reconstruction of a cruciate ligament. Report of two cases. J Bone Joint Surg [Am] 1995;77:1418–1422.

267. Ramnath RR, Kattapuram SV. MR appearance of SONK-like subchondral abnormalities in the adult knee: SONK redefined. Skeletal Radiol 2004;33:575–581.

268. Yamamoto T, Bullough PG. Spontaneous osteonecrosis of the knee: the result of subchondral insufficiency fracture. J Bone Joint Surg [Am] 2000;82:858–866.

269. Kidwai AS, Hemphill SD, Griffiths HJ. Radiologic case study: spontaneous osteonecrosis of the knee reclassified as insufficiency fracture. Orthopedics 2005;28:333–336.

270. Deutsch AL, Mink JH, Rosenfelt FP. Incidental detection of hematopoietic hyperplasia on routine knee MR imaging. AJR 1989;152:333–336.

271. Poulton TB, Murphy WD, Duerk JL. Bone marrow reconversion in adults who are smokers: MR imaging findings. AJR 1993;161:1217–1221.

272. Shellock FG, Morris E, Deutsch AL. Hematopoietic bone marrow hyperplasia: high prevalence on MR images of the knee in asymptomatic marathon runners. AJR 1992;158:335–338.

273. Wilson AJ, Hodge JC, Pilgram TK. Prevalence of red marrow around the knee joint in adults demonstrated on magnetic resonance imaging. Acad Radiol 1996;3:550–555.

274. Cummings JR, Pedowitz RA. Knee instability: the orthopedic approach. Semin Musculoskeletal Radiol 2005;9(1):1–16.

275. Bui-Mansfield LT, Youngberg RA, Warme W, Pitcher JD, Nguyen PL. Potential cost savings of MR imaging obtained before arthroscopy of the knee: evaluation of 50 consecutive patients. AJR 1997;168:913–918.

276. Rose NE, Gold SM. A comparison of accuracy between clinical examination and magnetic resonance imaging in the diagnosis of meniscal and anterior cruciate ligament tears. Arthroscopy 1996;12(4):398–405.

277. Duc SR, Zanetti M, Kramer J, Kach KP, Zollikofer, Wentz KU. Magnetic resonance imaging of anterior cruciate ligament tears: evaluation of standard orthogonal and tailored paracoronal images. Acta Radiol 46;7:729–733.

278. Patten RM, Richardson ML, Zink-Brody G, Rolfe BA. Complete versus partial thickness tears of the posterior cruciate ligament: MR findings. J Comput Assist Tomogr 1994;18(5):793–799.

279. Porat E, Roos M, Roos H. High prevalence of osteoarthritis 14 years after an anterior cruciate ligament tear in male soccer players: a study of radiographic and patient relevant outcomes. Ann Rheum Dis 2004;63:269–273.

280. Lohmander LS, Ostenberg A, Englund M, Roos H. High prevalence of knee osteoarthritis, pain, and functional limitations in female soccer players twelve years after anterior cruciate ligament injury. Arthritis Rheum 2004;50(10):3145–3152.

281. Harilainen A, Sandelin J, Jansson KA. Cross-pin femoral fixation versus metal interference screw fixation in anterior cruciate ligament reconstruction with hamstring tendons: results of a controlled prospective randomized study with 2-year follow-up. Arthroscopy 2005;21(1):25–33.

282. Fauno P, Kaalund S. Tunnel widening after hamstring anterior cruciate ligament reconstruction is influenced by the type of graft fixation used: a prospective randomized study. Arthroscopy. 2005;21(11):1337–1341.

283. Rose T, Hepp P, Venus J, Stockmar C, Josten C, Helmut. Prospective randomized clinical comparison of femoral transfixation versus bioscrew fixation in hamstring tendon ACL reconstruction—a preliminary report. Knee Surg Sport Trauma 2006;14(8):730–738.

284. Laxdal G, Kartus J, Hansson L, Heidvall M, Ejerhed L, Karlsson J. A prospective randomized comparison of bone-patellar

285. Svensson M, Sernert N, Ejerhed L, Karlsson J, Kartus J. A prospective comparison of bone-patellar tendon-bone and hamstring grafts for anterior cruciate ligament reconstruction in female patients. Knee Surg Sport Trauma 2006;14(3):278–286.

286. Harilainen A, Linko E, Sandelin J. Randomized prospective study of ACL reconstruction with interference screw fixation in patellar tendon autografts versus femoral metal plate suspension and tibial post fixation in hamstring tendon autografts: 5-year clinical and radiological follow-up results. Knee Surg Sports Traumatol Arthrosc 2006;14(6):517–528.

287. Getelman MH, Friedman MJ. Revision anterior cruciate ligament reconstruction surgery. J Am Acad Orthop Surg 1999;7:189–198.

288. Fetto JF, Marshall JL. MCL injuries of the knee: rationale for treatment. Clin Orthop Rel Res 1978;132:206–218.

289. Gross ML, Grover JS, Bassett LW, Seeger LL, Finerman GA. Magnetic resonance imaging of the posterior cruciate ligament. Clinical use to improve diagnostic accuracy. Am J Sports Med 1992;20(6):732–737.

290. Johnson DH, Fanelli GC, Miller MD. PCL 2002: indications, double bundle versus inlay technique and revision surgery. Arthroscopy 2002;18:40–52.

291. Rubin DA, Kettering JM, Towers JD, Britton CA. MR imaging of knees having isolated and combined ligament injuries. AJR 1998;170:1207–1213.

292. Yu JS, Goodwin D, Salonen D, et al. Complete dislocation of the knee, spectrum of associated soft tissue injuries depicted by MR imaging. AJR 1995;164(1):135–139.

293. Rihn JA, Cha PS, Groff YJ, Harner CD. The acutely dislocated knee: evaluation and management. J Am Acad Orthop Surg 2004;12:334–346.

294. Jackson JL, O'Malley PG, Kroenke K. Evaluation of acute knee pain in primary care. Ann Intern Med 2003;139(7) 575–588.

295. Campbell SE, Sanders TG, Morrison WB. MR imaging of meniscal cysts: incidence, location and clinical significance. AJR 2001;177:409–413.

296. Eren OT. The accuracy of joint line tenderness by physical examination in the diagnosis of meniscal tears. Arthroscopy 2003;19(8):850–854.

297. Malanga GA, Andrus S, Nadler SF, McLean J. Physical examination tests of the knee. Arch Phys Med Rehabil 2003;84(4):592–603.

298. Greis PE, Bardana DD, Holmstrom MC, Burks RT. Meniscal injury: I. Basic science and evaluation. J Am Acad Orthop Surg 2002;10(3):168–176.

299. Rangger C, Klestil T, Kathrein A, Inderster A, Laith H. Influence of magnetic resonance imaging on indications for arthroscopy of the knee. Clin Orthop Rel Res 1996;330:133–142.

300. Wright DH, De Smet AA, Norris M. Bucket-handle tears of the medial and lateral menisci of the knee: value of MR imaging in detecting displaced fragments. AJR 1995;165(3):621–625.

301. Pedowitz RA, Feagin JA, Rajagopalan S. A surgical algorithm for treatment of cystic degeneration of the meniscus. Arthroscopy 1996;12(2):209–216.

302. Greis PE, Holmstrom MC, Bardana DD, Burks RT. Meniscal injury: II. Management. J Am Acad Orthop Surg 2002;10(3):177–187.

303. Ulrich-Vinther, Maloney M, Schwarz EM, Rosier R, O'Keefe RJ. Articular cartilage biology. J Am Acad Orthop Surg 2003;11:421–430.

304. Wearing SC, Hennig EM, Byrne NM, Steele JR, Hills AP. Musculoskeletal disorders associated with obesity: a biomechanical perspective. Obes Rev 2006;7:239.

305. Bruce EJ, Hamby T, Jones DG. Sports related osteochondral injuries: clinical presentation, diagnosis and treatment. Prim Care Clin Office Pract 2005;32:253–276.

306. Browne JE, Branch TP. Surgical alternatives for treatment of articular cartilage lesions. J Am Acad Orthop Surg 2000;8(3):180–190.

307. Tyler WK, Vidal AF, Williams RJ, Healey JH. Pigmented villonodular synovitis. J Am Acad Orthop Surg 2006;12:376–385.

308. el-Khoury GY, Wira RL, Berbaum KS, Pope TL Jr, Monu JU. MR imaging of patellar tendinitis. Radiology 1992;184(3):849–854.

309. Khan KM, Bonar F, Desmond PM, et al. Patellar tendinosis (jumper's knee): findings at histopathologic examination, US, and MR imaging. Victorian Institute of Sport Tendon Study Group. Radiology 1996;200(3):821–827.

310. Larson RL, Grana WA. The Knee: Form, Function, Pathology and Treatment. Philadelphia: WB Saunders, 1993.

311. Torg JS, Conrad W, Kalen V. Clinical diagnosis of anterior cruciate ligament instability in the athlete. Am J Sports Med 1976;4:84–93.

312. Kocher MS, Tucker R, Ganley TJ, Flynn JM. Management of osteochondritis dissecans of the knee: current concepts overview. Am J Sports Med 2006;34(7):1181–1191.

313. Chen TS, Crues JV 3rd, Ali M, Troum OM. Magnetic resonance imaging is more sensitive than radiography in detecting change and size of erosions in rheumatoid arthritis. J Rheumatol 2006;33(10):1957–1967.

314. McGrath B, Schlatterer D, Mindell E. Case reports: osteogenic sarcoma of the patella spread to lateral meniscus after arthroscopy. Clin Orthop Rel Res 2006;444:250–255.

315. Huang H, Chen YP, Cao GH, Lin ZC. MRI and radiography for diagnosis of lower limb osteosarcoma: a comparison. Di Yi Jun YI Da Xue Xue Bao 2005;25(12):1552–1554.

11
Ankle

A. Radiologic Perspective: Magnetic Resonance Imaging of the Ankle

Jenny T. Bencardino and Zehava S. Rosenberg

Over the past two decades, magnetic resonance imaging (MRI) has become the imaging modality of choice for evaluating most soft tissue and osseous abnormalities in the ankle. The technique offers a noninvasive and expeditious diagnostic assessment of ankle injuries, which are often occult on conventional radiographs and computed tomography (CT). This chapter provides a brief review of the normal magnetic resonance (MR) anatomy and a detailed discussion of abnormalities around the ankle including tendons, ligaments, nerves, fascia, and bone.

Routine MR images are obtained in the axial, coronal, and sagittal planes (Fig. 11.1). We obtain the axial sequence immediately after a three-plane positioning scout. The coronal and sagittal planes are prescribed obliquely using the information acquired on the axial images. Thus, the coronal images are obtained parallel to the anterior margin of the talar dome, and the sagittal images parallel to the lateral wall of the calcaneus. Imaging the ankle is often performed with the patient supine and the ankle in neutral position.[1] The ankle in neutral position has an inherent 10 to 20 degrees of plantar flexion[2] and 10 to 30 degrees of external rotation. This mild degree of plantar flexion is useful for eliminating magic angle effect when examining the flexor and extensor tendons in the hindfoot and midfoot.[1] Increasing the fat planes between the peroneus brevis and peroneus longus tendons, and displacing the flexor and peroneal tendons away from the bones are other advantages of imaging the ankle in plantar flexion.[3] Mechanical stabilization of the ankle is paramount for good image quality.[4] Immobilization can be achieved using foam sponges between the ankle and the coil and Velcro straps on the leg outside the coil.

Dedicated phased-array extremity coils are currently utilized to perform most studies of the ankle.[5] This type of coil provides image homogeneity and an improved signal-to-noise ratio at depth. The main disadvantages are a lower signal-to-noise ratio in the periphery of the study part, and inability to cover the entire area of interest if the anatomy does not fit within the rigid structure of the coil.[5] Utilization of the knee coil provided with most available commercial systems is a common practice for examining the ankle.[1]

We utilize an imaging protocol that combines T1-weighted and fast spin echo T2-weighted images as well as fluid-sensitive T2-weighted sequences with fat saturation.

Tendons

Normal Magnetic Resonance Anatomy

Tendon morphology (Fig. 11.2), longitudinal splits, tendon sheath fluid, and adjacent soft tissue abnormalities are best depicted on axial MR images. The sagittal plane is most useful for depicting disease of the Achilles tendon, pre-Achilles fat pad, and sinus tarsi. The coronal plane is the least useful for assessing the tendons. The compact parallel arrangement of fibers and low water content account for the low signal homogeneity of tendons on all MR pulse sequences.[6] There are, however, exceptions to this general rule. The magic angle effect may produce spurious intrasubstance hyperintensity in normal tendons.[1] This phenomenon, only seen on low echo time (TE) sequences, occurs in tendons that have a 55-degree orientation to the magnetic field. The magic angle effect is quite common in the ankle tendons as they curve around the ankle joint. The distal portion of the posterior tibial tendon is particularly susceptible to the magic angle effect at its attachment to the navicular tuberosity. Absence of additional pathologic findings and the presence of hyperintensity only on short TE images without correlation on other sequences are highly suggestive of this phenomenon. Imaging the patient in the prone position has been recommended in order to avoid the magic angle effect.[7]

A small amount of tenosynovial fluid, frequently seen within the flexor sheaths, may cause T2 prolongation around tendons. A normal anatomic communication between the flexor hallucis longus tendon sheath and the ankle joint is

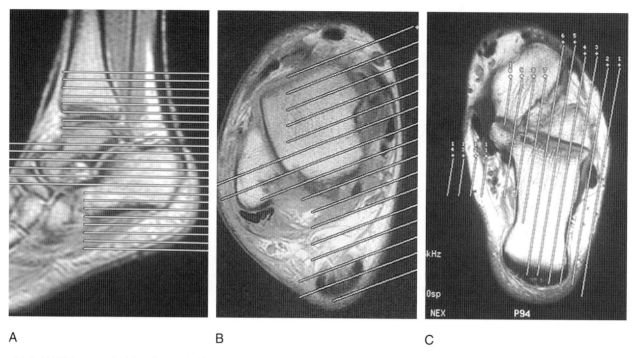

FIG. 11.1. (A) Using a sagittal localizer, axial images are prescribed covering the Achilles tendon and entire calcaneus. The ankle is in neutral position with 20 degrees of plantar flexion. (B) Based on a transverse image, the coronal plane is prescribed parallel to the anterior margin of the talar dome. (C) Based on a transverse image, the sagittal plane should be aligned with the long axis of the calcaneus.

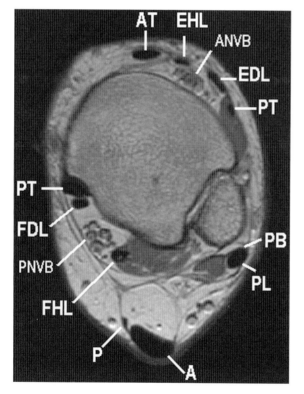

FIG. 11.2. Normal tendons. Axial proton density MR image depicting the normal low-signal intensity tendons. A, Achilles tendon; ANVB, anterior neurovascular bundle; AT, anterior tibial tendon; EDL, extensor digitorum longus tendon; EHL, extensor hallucis longus tendons; FHL, flexor hallucis longus tendon; FDL, flexor digitorum longus tendon; P, plantaris tendon; PB, peroneus brevis tendon; PL, peroneus longus tendon; PNVB, posterior neurovascular bundle; PT, peroneus tertius tendon; PTT, posterior tibial tendon.

responsible for the higher frequency of tenosynovial fluid in this location.[8] Fluid within the sheaths of the extensor tendons is quite uncommon and is almost always pathologic. Signal heterogeneity and striations are often seen at the insertion sites of some ankle tendons, particularly the posterior tibial and Achilles tendons.[9]

The tendons that are most commonly affected in the ankle and foot include the Achilles tendon, the posterior tibial tendon, peroneal tendons, and flexor hallucis longus tendon. The flexor digitorum longus tendon is rarely diseased. Similarly the extensor tendons, excluding the anterior tibial tendon are rarely injured.

Achilles Tendon

The Achilles tendon is formed by the confluence of the tendon fibers of the medial and lateral gastrocnemius and soleus muscles.[10] As the Achilles tendon descends, the anteriorly placed soleus fibers twist 90 degrees relative to the gastrocnemius fibers, resulting in medial insertion for the former and a lateral attachment for the latter into the posterior calcaneus. This spiral twist results in an area of increased internal stress and decreased vascularity upon contraction of the tendon.[11,12]

The length of the Achilles tendon is best assessed on sagittal MR images. It ranges from 20 to 120 mm[13] (Fig. 11.3A,B). The anteroposterior dimension, measured at the greatest thickness of the tendon, fluctuates between 3.5 and 6.8 mm.[13] On axial MR images, most normal Achilles tendons have a flat or concave anterior margin (Fig. 11.2). Only 10% of the tendons may have a mild anterior convexity.[13] The spiraling of the soleus and gastrocnemius tendon fibers may

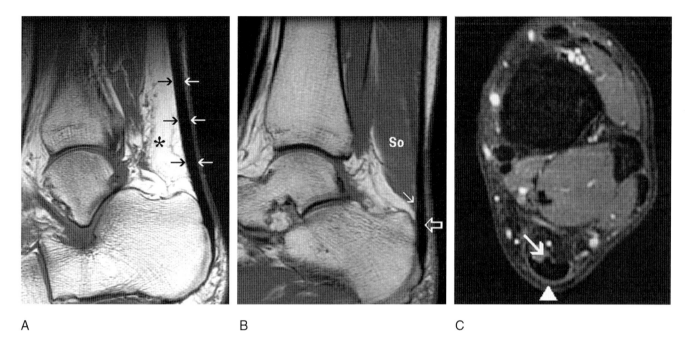

A B C

FIG. 11.3. Normal Achilles tendon. (A) Sagittal T1-weighted image demonstrates the normal parallel anterior (black arrows) and posterior (white arrows) margins of a normal hypointense Achilles tendon. The asterisk indicates pre-Achilles Kager's fat pad. (B) Sagittal T1-weighted image shows low incorporation of the soleus tendon (arrow) resulting in a short Achilles tendon (open arrow). Soleus. (C) Axial fat-suppressed T2-weighted image shows the wavelike anterior bulge of the Achilles tendon from incorporation of the soleus and gastrocnemius fibers. Arrowhead indicates the posterior paratenon.

create a wavelike bulge, which shifts from the lateral to the medial anterior margins of the Achilles tendon (Fig. 11.3C). The anterior and posterior margins of the Achilles tendon are typically parallel on sagittal MR images below the level of the soleus incorporation (Fig. 11.3A). Although the classical MR appearance of the Achilles tendon is that of homogeneous low signal on all pulse sequences, intrasubstance punctate and linear foci can also be seen on T1-weighted and proton-density images, and more pronounced toward the Achilles tendon insertion.[14] This MR signal heterogeneity is perhaps related to infoldings of the paratenon, resulting in connective tissue and vessels between the tendon fascicles.[15] However, hyperintensity on fluid-sensitive sequences should be regarded as highly suspicious for pathology.

The Achilles tendon lacks a tendon sheath and is covered by a gliding paratenon along its posterior, medial, and lateral sides.[16] A network of paratenon vessels extends within and outside the Achilles tendon. The paratenon can be easily identified on axial high-resolution MR images[17] (Fig. 11.3C). Adipose tissue interposed between the Achilles tendon and the deep ankle muscles has been termed Kager's fat pad[18] (Fig. 11.3A). Septa and vessels within this fat pad may account for signal heterogeneity on T1-weighted images. However, increased signal on fluid-sensitive images should be regarded as highly suspicious for pathology.[17]

The retrocalcaneal bursa is found between the distal Achilles tendon and the posterosuperior calcaneal tuberosity. The bursa, whose main function is to protect the distal Achilles ten-

don from frictional wear at its insertion, is a small, horseshoe-shaped structure limited anteriorly by Kager's fat pad. A small amount of retrocalcaneal fluid may be a normal MR finding. Excessive fluid in the retrocalcaneal bursa has been defined as greater than 2 mm in anteroposterior (AP) dimension.[19]

Posterior Tibial Tendon

The posterior tibial muscle has two heads of origin in the proximal third of the leg: the medial head arising from the posterior surface of the interosseous membrane and tibia, and the lateral head from the posterior surface of the fibula.[10] The posterior tibial tendon functions as an invertor and plantar flexor of the ankle and subtalar joints. It also provides support to the medial longitudinal arch of the foot.

The posterior tibial tendon crosses the flexor digitorum longus tendon a few centimeters above the ankle joint. At the level of the ankle, the tendon resides within the medial retromalleolar groove, posterior to the distal tibia. In this location, the tendon is subject to friction stress and ischemia.[20]

The posterior tibial tendon enters the foot through the tarsal tunnel, lying beneath the flexor retinaculum and superficial to the deltoid ligament. The distal insertion of the posterior tibial tendon is rather complex. The main attachment site is to the medial navicular tubercle. In 4% of the population, the bulk of the posterior tibial tendon inserts onto a true accessory navicular (Fig. 11.4A)[21] or a fused navicular ossicle (cornuate navicular) (Fig. 11.4B). Other multiple insertional

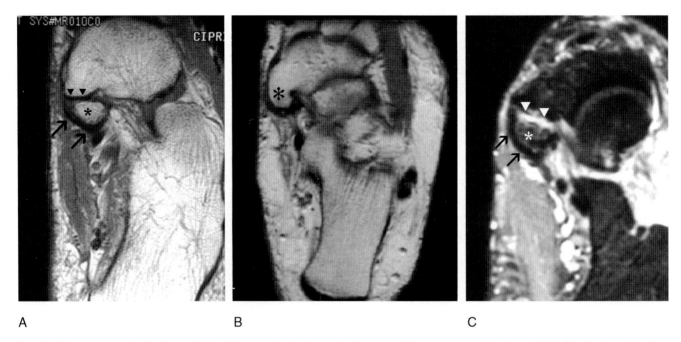

FIG. 11.4. Accessory navicular bone. (A) Axial proton-density image depicts a type II accessory navicular (asterisk) bridged via synchondrosis (arrowheads) to the medial navicular tuberosity. The posterior tibial tendon (arrows) is noted attaching to the accessory ossicle. (B) Axial proton-density image shows a cornuate navicular bone (type III) characterized by prominence of the navicular tuberosity secondary to a fully incorporated accessory navicular (asterisk). (C) A symptomatic accessory navicular. Axial fat suppressed T2-weighted image demonstrates cortical irregularity and increased signal at the synchondrosis between the navicular tuberosity and accessory navicular (arrowheads). Also noted are edematous changes of the accessory navicular (asterisk). The distal posterior tibial tendon (arrows) appears intact.

slips can be found extending to the sustentaculum tali, cuneiforms, and bases of the second, third, and fourth metatarsals. These distal insertion sites underscore the contribution of the posterior tibial tendon to the maintenance of the longitudinal arch of the foot.[10]

On axial MR images, the posterior tibial tendon is depicted as the most medial hypointense structure located behind the medial malleolus within a shallow medial retromalleolar groove shared with the flexor digitorum longus tendon. Signal heterogeneity in the distal tendon close to its insertion to the navicular is frequently noted on axial and sagittal MR images related to either the magic angle phenomenon (Fig. 11.5) or fat interposed between the tendon slips.[22] Signal heterogeneity in this location has also been attributed to the presence of intratendinous fibrocartilage or ossified type I accessory navicular ossicle, noted in 87.5% and 12.5%, respectively, of cadaveric feet.[23] A practical internal parameter for the normal caliber of the posterior tibial tendon, on axial MR images, is the adjacent flexor digitorum longus (FDL) tendon. In a healthy person, the posterior tibial tendon is roughly twice the size of the FDL[23] (Fig. 11.2). A small amount of tenosynovial fluid is commonly seen within the posterior tibial tendon sheath at the ankle level (Fig. 11.6). Since the very distal posterior tibial tendon lacks a synovial sheath, fluid noted in this location is considered abnormal and is likely related to metaplastic synovium and partial tearing.[24,25]

Flexor Hallucis Longus Tendon

The flexor hallucis longus muscle originates from the lower two thirds of the posterior surface of the fibula.[10] The main function of the flexor hallucis longus tendon is plantar flexion of the distal phalanx of the hallux. Secondarily, it provides weak plantar flexion and supination of the ankle. It also aids in supporting the longitudinal arch during walking.

At the level of the medial ankle, the flexor hallucis longus tendon is located underneath the flexor retinaculum, posterolateral to the flexor digitorum longus tendon. In this location, a small amount of tenosynovial fluid is often identified on axial and sagittal MR images due to a normal communication of the ankle joint with the sheaths of the flexor hallucis longus and flexor digitorum longus tendons. This communication is present in up to 20% of individuals.[8]

The flexor hallucis longus tendon descends toward the foot via a fibro-osseous tunnel formed by the medial and lateral talar tubercles; it then passes beneath the sustentaculum tali. In 7% to 14% of individuals, the lateral talar tubercle does not fuse to the talus forming the so-called os trigonum[26] (Fig. 11.7). The magic angle phenomenon can also affect the flexor hallucis longus tendon particularly as it curves underneath the sustentaculum tali and also in between the sesamoids.[21]

The flexor hallucis longus tendon converges medially as it advances in the midfoot. It sends an anastomotic tendinous slip to the flexor digitorum longus tendon in the region of

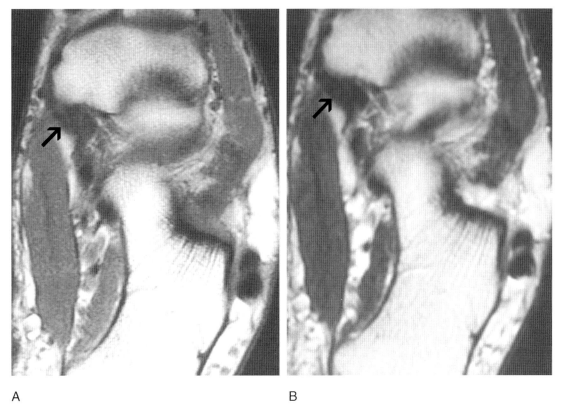

A   B

FIG. 11.5. Magic angle phenomenon. (A) Axial proton-density MR image demonstrates spurious increased signal involving the insertional slips of the posterior tibial tendon (arrow) adjacent to the navicular bone without associated pathologic findings. (B) Axial T2-weighted image at the same level (arrow) demonstrates normal homogeneous hypointensity confirming magic angle phenomenon.

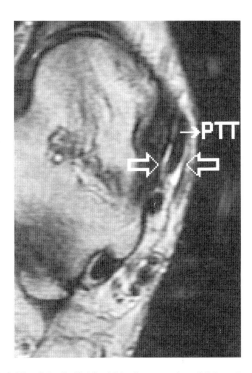

FIG. 11.6. Physiologic fluid within the posterior tibial tendon sheath. Axial fast spin echo T2-weighted image demonstrates the posterior tibial tendon (PTT) surrounded by minimal amount of fluid (open arrows).

the knot of Henry underneath the navicular bone.[27] Normal tenosynovial fluid often collects in this location.[22] The tendon then pierces the medial septum, entering the medial plantar compartment. Just proximal to the sesamoid tunnel the tendon lies superficial and in between the heads of the flexor hallucis brevis tendon. The flexor hallucis longus tendon inserts to the base distal phalanx of the great toe.

Peroneal Tendons

The peroneus longus and peroneus brevis muscles plantar flex the ankle joint and evert the foot at the subtalar and transverse tarsal joints. Another important function of the peroneal tendons is to stabilize the lateral ankle joint and aid in maintaining the lateral longitudinal and transverse arches of the foot.

The origin of the peroneus longus muscle is from the proximal two thirds of the fibula, intermuscular septum, and crural fascia. The peroneus brevis muscle arises from the lower two thirds of the fibula and intermuscular septum.[10]

The peroneus longus and peroneus brevis tendons descend into the foot through the peroneal tunnel behind the fibula, within the lateral retromalleolar groove. The floor of the peroneal tunnel is formed by a concave lateral retromalleolar or retrofibular groove, which is present in 82% of individuals.[28] Flat and convex retromalleolar grooves are found in 11% and 7% of individuals, respectively.[28] The superior peroneal retinaculum, responsible for

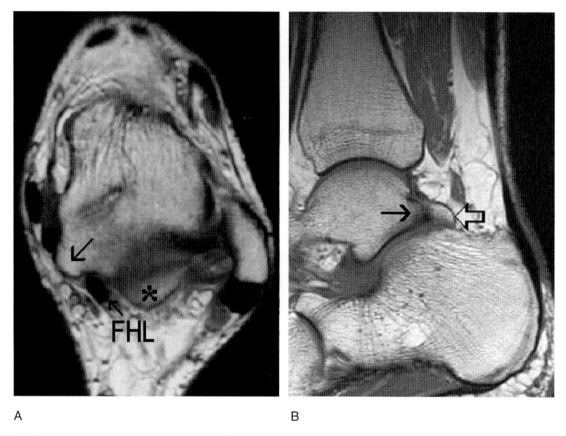

A   B

FIG. 11.7. Os trigonum. (A) Axial proton-density image demonstrates a separate secondary ossification center of the lateral tibial tubercle consistent with os trigonum (asterisk). The flexor hallucis longus (FHL) tendon is seen within the talar tunnel just lateral to the medial talar tubercle (arrow). (B) Sagittal T1-weighted image shows the os trigonum (open arrow) articulating to a somewhat sclerotic lateral talar tubercle (arrow).

the stability of the peroneal tendons,[29] constitutes the posterolateral border of the peroneal tunnel. It originates at the lateral malleolus and, in most cases, inserts into the lateral calcaneal wall in close proximity to the calcaneofibular ligament. Therefore, coexistent injuries of the calcaneofibular ligament and superior peroneal retinaculum may be seen following a lateral ankle sprain.

At the level of the peroneal tunnel, the peroneus brevis tendon can be seen on axial MR images just anterior to and slightly medial to the peroneus longus tendon (Fig. 11.8A). The peroneus brevis tendon has a flat to crescentic configuration as it conforms to the retromalleolar groove anteriorly and the peroneus longus tendon posteriorly.[30,31] In some patients the peroneus brevis tendon descends medial to the peroneus longus tendon, resulting in a more globular configuration to the former.[22] Distal to the peroneal tunnel, the peroneus brevis tendon descends adjacent to the lateral calcaneal wall, anterior to the peroneus longus tendon and peroneal tubercle (trochlea) (Fig. 11.7B). At this level, the peroneal tubercle and the inferior peroneal retinaculum create an osteoaponeurotic wall, which separates the peroneal tendons[29] (Fig. 11.8B). The peroneal tubercle is present in 32% to 97% of asymptomatic individuals and can be of a variable size.[32]

The distal insertion of the peroneus brevis tendon is at the base of the fifth metatarsal. The peroneus longus tendon con-tinues underneath the cuboid bone within a fibrous groove created by the long plantar ligament. In 20% of individuals, an ossified sesamoid embedded within the peroneus longus tendon, the so-called os peroneum, can be encountered at the point of contact with the edge of the cuboid bone.[28,30] The peroneus longus tendon inserts into the base of the first metatarsal and the medial cuneiform bone.

A common peroneal tendon sheath contains both peroneal tendons at the level of the lateral malleolus. As the tendons approach the inferior peroneal retinaculum, the sheath splits into two individual extensions. The common peroneal tendon sheath and the calcaneofibular ligament are in close proximity,[31] which explains fluid within the sheath on MRI in patients with tears of the calcaneofibular ligament.

Extensor Tendons

The extensor tendon group from medial to lateral includes the anterior tibial, extensor hallucis longus, extensor digitorum longus, and peroneus tertius tendons. The anterior tibial tendon is the strongest invertor and dorsiflexor of the foot.[10] The main origins of the anterior tibial muscle are from the lateral tibial condyle and proximal two thirds of the lateral surface of the tibia and the interosseous membrane. The anterior tibial tendon

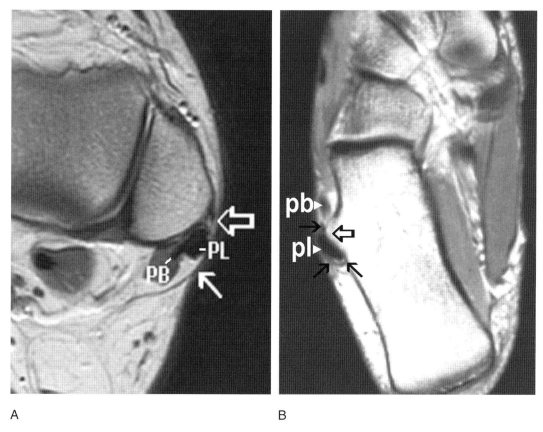

A   B

FIG. 11.8. Peroneal tendon anatomy. (A) Axial proton-density image at the level of the distal fibula demonstrates flat to crescentic configuration of the peroneus brevis tendon (PB) and the globular peroneus longus tendon (PL) posteriorly. The superior peroneal retinaculum (arrow) and fibular fibrocartilaginous ridge (open arrow) are also seen. (B) Axial proton-density image at the level of the lateral calcaneal wall shows a prominent peroneal tubercle (open arrow) and inferior peroneal retinaculum (black arrows) separating the peroneus brevis (pb) and the peroneus longus (pl) tendons.

courses along the anterior lower leg, passing beneath the extensor retinacula to insert into the dorsal and medial aspects of the first cuneiform and the first metatarsal base. The extensor digitorum longus and extensor hallucis longus muscles both arise from the fibula and interosseous membrane, with the former arising also from the lateral tibial condyle. The peroneus tertius, considered a part of the extensor digitorum longus, originates from the distal third of the anterior fibular cortex and the adjacent interosseous membrane. On axial MR images, the anterior tibial tendon is the thickest and most medial tendon[33] (see Fig. 11.2). The extensor hallucis longus and the extensor digitorum longus tendons are found lateral to it. The peroneus tertius is often seen as a distinct small low signal dot abutting the lateral margin of the flexor digitorum longus tendon.

Pathology

Repetitive microtrauma and overuse have been implicated as important etiologic factors for tendon injuries at the ankle. Excessive tensile strain and overstretching may result in failure of tendon fibers. The spectrum of tendon injuries can be categorized as tendinosis, peritendinitis/tenosynovitis, entrap-

ment, rupture, and dislocation.[34,35] There can be substantial overlap between these conditions, which may complicate the MR diagnosis.

There are several histologic types of tendinosis including fibromatous (hypoxic), lipoid, osseous/calcific, and myxoid.[36] The terms *tendinosis* and *tendinopathy* are preferred over *tendinitis* as minimal or absent inflammatory reaction is noted microscopically.[37] Tendinosis is often manifested on MR images by fusiform thickening of the involved tendon associated with intrasubstance signal heterogeneity on T1-weighted and proton-density–weighted images.

Peritendinitis, paratenonitis, and tenosynovitis are caused by inflammatory or mechanical irritation of the peritenon, paratenon, and tendon sheath, respectively.[38] Acute tenosynovitis typically results in tenosynovial effusion manifested on MRI as fluid accumulation within the tendon sheath often associated with synovial proliferation. Edematous changes of the adjacent fat may be noted. In chronic cases, stenosing tenosynovitis may develop. This is due to synovial proliferation and fibrosis leading to peritendinous scarring with subsequent tendon entrapment and even rupture.[38] Intermediate to low signal intensity scar engulfing the tendon can be seen

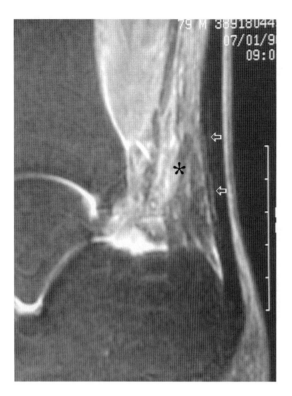

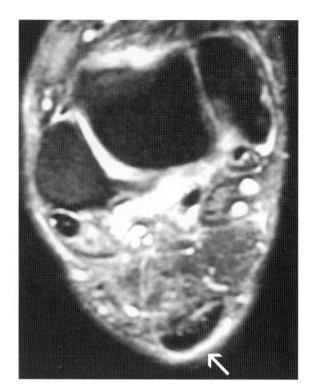

FIG. 11.9. Anterior Achilles peritendinitis. Sagittal fast spin echo short-tau inversion recovery (STIR) image demonstrates a reticular pattern of increased signal in the pre-Achilles fat pad reflecting edema (asterisk). Note intratendinous linear signal heterogeneity within the Achilles tendon and slight fusiform appearance of the tendon consistent with tendonopathy.

FIG. 11.10. Posterior Achilles paratenonitis. A discrete crescentic area of signal hyperintensity is demonstrated partially surrounding the Achilles tendon consistent with paratenonitis (arrow) in this axial fat suppressed T2-weighted image.

on all MR sequences. Pockets of tenosynovial fluid outlining areas of proliferative synovitis may also be noted.

Tendon ruptures typically occur in previously diseased tendons.[35,37] Tendon rupture may be acute or chronic, partial or complete. Acute tendon ruptures often demonstrate hyperintensity on fluid sensitive sequences within the tendon defect due to the presence of edema and hemorrhage. Conversely, chronic tendon ruptures may depict low signal intensity within the tendon gap related to scar tissue. Partial tendon tears are manifested by focal discontinuity of fibers outlined by fluid-like signal. Complete rupture is depicted as full-thickness disruption of the tendon fibers. The tendon gap may be filled with fluid, hemorrhage, or scar depending on the age of the tear.[23]

The three main tendons, which dislocate at the ankle, are the peroneals and, less commonly, the posterior tibial tendon. Flexor hallucis longus tendon dislocation, while rare, has also been described. Instability of the tendons whether subluxation or dislocation may be detected on conventional MRI. However, if there is clinical suspicion of tendon dislocation dynamic MRI or ultrasound is indicated, as the instability may not be depicted on nonstress images. The presence of associated osseous abnormalities such as shallow or convex grooves, injuries to the overlying retinacula, tendon entrap-

ment, and concomitant tendon rupture can also be assessed on MRI.[31,39,40]

Achilles Tendon

Overuse or traumatic injuries of the Achilles tendon are quite frequent in runners, tennis players, and ballet dancers.[34] Systemic diseases such as rheumatoid arthritis, collagen vascular diseases, gout, diabetes, and hyperparathyroidism may also cause Achilles tendon dysfunction.[41,42]

Achilles tendon injuries can be divided into noninsertional and insertional.[34,35,43] Noninsertional tendon dysfunction includes acute and chronic peritendinitis, paratenonitis, tendinosis, and rupture involving the Achilles tendon at 2 to 6 cm above the calcaneal insertion site. The clinical presentation of lesions involving the Achilles tendon itself versus isolated injury to the peritendinous structures can be quite similar. Therefore, accurate MRI diagnosis may have great impact in the management of these injuries.

Achilles peritendinitis, often associated with systemic inflammatory disease, is characterized by peritendinous edema and inflammation.[16] On MRI, linear or irregular areas of hyperintensity are typically seen within the pre-Achilles fat pad on fluid-sensitive sequences (Fig. 11.9).[17] In Achilles paratenonitis,

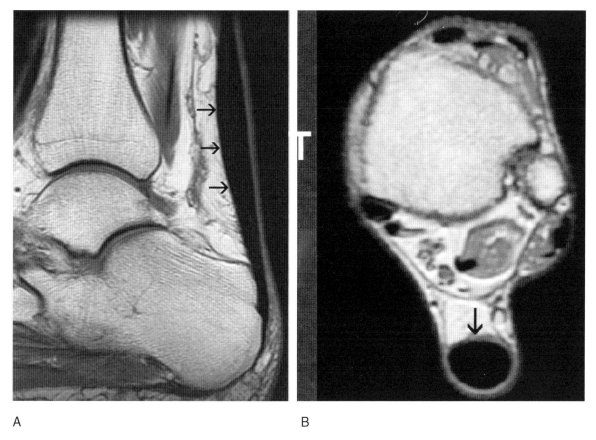

A   B

FIG. 11.11. Achilles tendinosis. Axial proton-density (A) and sagittal T1-weighted (B) images show fusiform thickening and loss of the anterior concavity of the Achilles tendon (arrows) without evidence of intrasubstance increased signal.

a discrete crescentic area of increased signal best appreciated medial, lateral, and posterior to the tendon can be seen.[17] Chronic peritendinitis/paratenonitis presents with irregular thickening of the paratenon and scarring of the pre-Achilles fat pad (Fig. 11.10).[44] Isolated peritendinous abnormalities of the Achilles tendon have a better prognosis than combined peritendinous and intratendinous injury.[17]

Chronic degenerative intrasubstance microtearing leads to Achilles tendinosis, which results in thickening of the tendon on cross-sectional and sagittal MRI. Magnetic resonance imaging manifestations of tendinosis include loss of the anterior concave or flat surface of the Achilles tendon and fusiform thickening (Fig. 11.11). In tendinosis, the intrasubstance signal is typically low. Intrasubstance fluid-like signal areas are consistent with associated partial tearing. In Astrom et al's[45] study, a sagittal tendon diameter greater than 10 mm was associated with severe intratendinous signal abnormalities and found to be a useful discriminating factor between partial rupture and tendinopathy.

Distinction of partial versus complete ruptures can be easily performed using MRI. A history of preceding trauma is often found in patients with partial tear of the Achilles tendon. The orientation of partial tears is longitudinal in most cases. Better long-term results have been noted in surgically treated patients with chronic partial tears.[16] Magnetic resonance imaging manifestations of partial tear include thickening with focal areas of signal increased on fluid-sensitive images and heterogeneity without complete interruption (Fig. 11.12). Acute partial tears are usually found in the posterior aspect of the tendon. Differentiation between partial tear and severe chronic Achilles tendinosis may be difficult without the aid of clinical history. The presence of subcutaneous edema, hemorrhage within the pre-Achilles fat, and peritendinitis contiguous with the area of tendon involvement has been reported in as much as two thirds of cases with partial tears.[17]

Complete rupture of the Achilles tendon by indirect trauma is more often seen in middle-aged men than in women.[46] The clinical diagnosis can be misleading since one of four patients with full-thickness Achilles tendon rupture present clinically with obscuration of the tendon gap due to swelling and retained weak plantar flexion (false-negative Thompson test).[47] Magnetic resonance imaging can provide invaluable information as to the location of the tear, size of the tendon gap, and chronicity of the injury. Complete Achilles tendon rupture is depicted on MRI as discontinuity with fraying and retraction of the torn edges of the tendon (Fig. 11.13).[48] The tendon gap may be filled with fluid, blood, scar, or fat. Care should be taken to include a sagittal sequence with large field of view including the Achilles tendon in its entirety and the distal soleus muscle belly.[14] In acute tears, imaging in plantarflexion has been proposed as a way

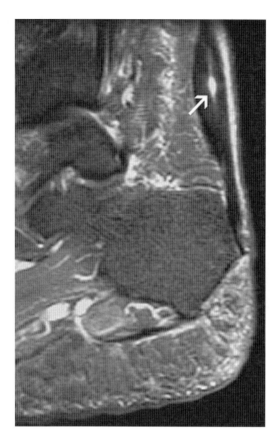

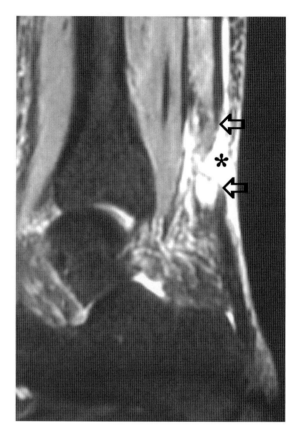

FIG. 11.12. Partial tear of the Achilles tendon. Sagittal fast spin echo (FSE) STIR image demonstrates longitudinal intrasubstance partial-thickness tear of the Achilles tendon (arrow) associated with focal widening of the sagittal diameter of the tendon.

FIG. 11.13. Complete tear of the Achilles tendon. Sagittal FSE STIR image depicts complete disruption and retraction of the torn ends of the Achilles tendon (open arrows) with a fluid-filled gap (asterisk).

of approximating the torn ends and providing the surgeon with information regarding the length of the remaining tendon gap.

On postoperative MR images, evaluation of the extent of tendon union and healing can be obtained (Fig. 11.14). It is important to keep in mind that postoperative intratendinous signal will decrease as the tendon heals gradually over a period of months or even a year.[49] However, permanent residual thickening of the tendon can be seen even after normal signal intensity has been regained.[50] In a recent study, the degree of tendon thickening noted on MRI correlated with increased tendon elongation (increased dorsiflexion) as compared to the contralateral uninjured leg.[51] The rate of Achilles tendon retear is ten times higher in patients treated conservatively (30%) as compared to those treated surgically (2–5%).[52] Surgical repair can be achieved via either open or percutaneous techniques. Direct repair or tendon transfers are among the surgical options. The development of intratendinous and peritendinous calcifications after open Achilles tendon repair was found in 36% of patients in a recent study.[52] Calcifications larger than 10 mm were associated with chronic swelling, decreased range of motion, and increased pain.

Insertional Achilles tendon dysfunction includes insertional Achilles tendinosis with or without calcification, calcification or ossification without tendinosis, and Haglund's syndrome.

Insertional Achilles tendinosis and partial tears in athletes are typically related to overuse. The MR findings include thickening and heterogeneity of the distal tendon often associated with areas of intratendinous calcifications, fibrosis, and insertional enthesophytes (Fig. 11.15). This type of Achilles tendon injury appears to have a worse prognosis than any other subgroup of overuse pathology.[17]

Haglund's syndrome is characterized by the presence of a prominent posterosuperior calcaneal tuberosity (Haglund's deformity) associated with distension of the retrocalcaneal bursa and insertional Achilles tendinosis or tear (Fig. 11.16). Marrow edema within the calcaneal tuberosity may also be encountered. Haglund's deformity can be assessed on T1-weighted images using the parallel pitch lines method (Fig. 11.16A).[53] Success rates of 71% and 100% following surgery of insertional tendinosis with and without Haglund deformity have been reported, respectively.[43]

Isolated retrocalcaneal bursitis is considered a distinct clinical entity from insertional Achilles tendinosis.[19] However, both entities can coexist. On MR images, excessive retrocalcaneal bursal fluid has been defined as greater than 2 mm in the AP dimension.[19] Magnetic resonance imaging allows differential diagnosis between isolated retrocalcaneal bursitis,

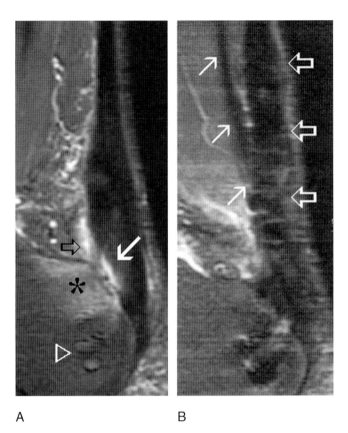

A   B

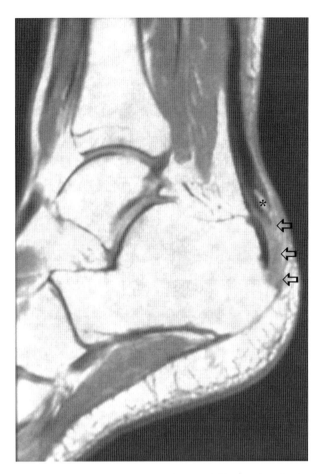

FIG. 11.14. Achilles tendon postinsertional repair. (A) Sagittal FSE STIR images shows postoperative changes at the insertion of the Achilles into the calcaneus (open arrowhead). Note re-tear of the insertional portion (white arrow) associated with retrocalcaneal bursitis (open arrow) and reactive calcaneal edema (asterisk). (B) Sagittal FSE STIR image in the same patient obtained following surgical revision with flexor hallucis longus tendon transfer (arrows). Note near-signal homogeneity of the postoperative thickened Achilles (open arrows).

FIG. 11.15. Insertional partial tear of the Achilles tendon. Sagittal T1-weighted image shows a high-grade partial tear at the insertion of the Achilles tendon (open arrows) with a retracted osseous fragment (asterisk).

insertional tendinosis/retrocalcaneal bursitis, and calcaneal marrow pathology.

Xanthomas of the Achilles tendon may be found in patients with familial hyperlipidemia. Intrasubstance reticulation and stippling are typically seen and are related to infiltration of the tendon by lipid-filled xanthoma cells, extracellular cholesterol, and inflammatory response. The cholesterol and cholesterester are typically devoid of signal, while the bright signal is often related to triglycerides and inflammation. Therefore, the lack of increased signal in the Achilles tendon does not necessarily preclude the presence of a xanthoma. Diffuse thickening and abnormal configuration of the Achilles tendon may be noted but are not mandatory. The MR appearance of xanthomas can occasionally be indistinguishable from tendinosis and partial tearing of the Achilles tendon.[54]

Posterior Tibial Tendon Dysfunction

Acute or chronic dysfunction of the posterior tibial tendon encompasses a spectrum of abnormalities ranging from teno-synovitis, to tendinosis, to partial and complete rupture. Acute, symptomatic tenosynovitis of the posterior tibial tendon without any structural change of the hindfoot is frequently seen in the athletic population as a result of overuse.[43,55] On MRI, the tendon is surrounded by fluid without significant associated morphologic changes (Fig. 11.17A). Chronic stenosing teno-synovitis is characterized by nodular or diffuse thickening as well as scarring of the tendon sheath (Fig. 11.17B).

Mild to severe signal heterogeneity and thickening of the posterior tibial tendon are typical features of tendino-sis. Microscopically, intratendinous degeneration, localized necrosis, and hypocellularity without inflammation may be found. Progressive and continuous microtearing eventually leads to macroscopic disruption of the tendon.

The most common clinical presentation of posterior tibial tendon tearing is a progressive and painful flatfoot deformity in middle-aged and elderly women with no significant history of previous trauma. Underlying systemic conditions that increase the risk of posterior tibial tendon dysfunction include many entities such as rheumatoid arthritis, obesity, systemic

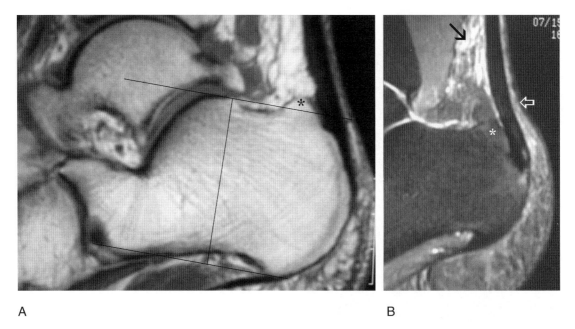

A

B

FIG. 11.16. Haglund syndrome with Haglund deformity, Achilles insertional tendinosis, peritendinitis, and retro-Achilles bursitis. Sagittal T1-weighted image demonstrates a prominent posterior superior calcaneal tuberosity (asterisk) extending above the upper parallel pitch line. (B) Sagittal FSE STIR image demonstrates mild thickening and irregularity of the distal tendon consistent with insertional Achilles tendinosis associated with anterior Achilles peritendinitis (arrow) and retro-Achilles bursitis (open arrow). Note prominent and edematous posterior-superior calcaneal tuberosity (asterisk).

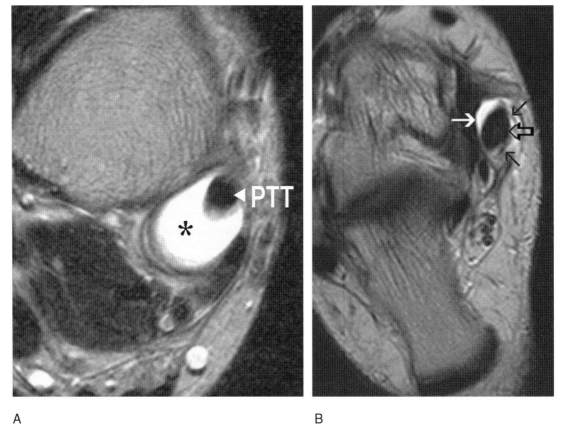

A

B

FIG. 11.17. Posterior tibial tenosynovitis. (A) Axial fast spin echo T2-weighted image demonstrates the posterior tibial tendon (PTT) surrounded by a large amount of fluid within the tendon sheath consistent with tenosynovitis. (B) Axial fast spin echo T2-weighted image shows asymmetric fluid collection (white arrow) associated with fibrous septa (black arrows) surrounding a thickened and heterogeneous posterior tibial tendon (open arrow) indicative of stenosing tenosynovitis and posterior tibial tendonopathy.

FIG. 11.18. Partial tear of the posterior tibial tendon. Axial fast spin echo T2-weighted image (A) and sagittal fast spin echo STIR image (B) demonstrate a focal intratendinous fusiform fluid-filled gap (open arrows) consistent with partial tearing. Associated peritendinous fluid is noted (closed arrow).

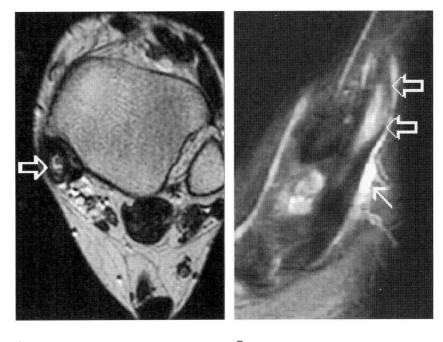

A   B

lupus erythematosus, gout, hypertension, and seronegative spondyloarthropaties.[41,56] The presence of a type II accessory navicular, cornuate navicular, or developmental pes planovalgus deformity is important predisposing factors. In the presence of a type II accessory navicular deformity, the posterior tibial tendon more commonly inserts directly into the ossicle without extending to the sole of the foot.[57] This results in loss of function of the posterior tibial tendon as a supporter of the longitudinal arch.

Distinction of advanced tendinosis and partial tear by MRI may be difficult due to the histopathologic overlap in the two conditions. Increased biomechanical stress as the posterior tibial tendon descends behind the medial malleolus into the foot is likely the main reason for the high frequency of tears in this location. There are three patterns of posterior tibial tears at the medial malleolus, which correlate well with the surgical classification of ruptured tendons.[58] Type I tears, which overlap histologically with tendinosis, are characterized by fusiform enlargement of the tendon associated with intrasubstance longitudinal splitting (Fig. 11.18). On MRI, the tendon is hypertrophic and can be 5 to 10 times as large as the adjacent flexor digitorum longus tendon.[58] Punctate intrasubstance heterogeneity may be noted on T1- and T2-weighted images. Type II is a more severe incomplete tear with focal attenuation of the caliber of the tendon. On MRI, the posterior tibial tendon may be equal to or smaller than the adjacent flexor digitorum longus tendon. Heterogeneity of the attenuated tendon is usually absent. Full-thickness rupture of the tendon fibers is found in type III posterior tibial tendon tears (Fig. 11.19). On MRI, the proximal and distal tendon ends can be identified with fluid, hemorrhage, or granulation tissue filling the gap, depending on the chronicity of the injury. Grading of the

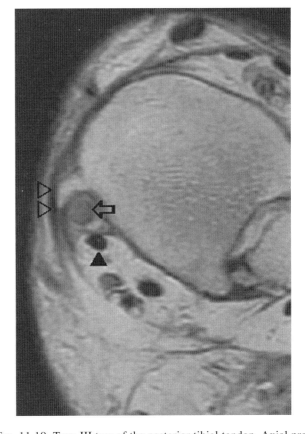

FIG. 11.19. Type III tear of the posterior tibial tendon. Axial proton-density image shows absence of the posterior tibial tendon (open arrow) with minimal residual mucinoid degeneration within the sheath. Note the adjacent normal flexor digitorum longus tendon (black arrowhead). A large tibial spur (open arrowheads) is identified.

rupture by the interpreting radiologist is important for surgical planning. Type I injuries are initially treated conservatively. However, tenosynovectomy, release of the flexor retinaculum, and tendon augmentation may be required if the disease progresses. Depending on the extent and rigidity of the flat foot deformity, tendon reconstruction and calcaneal osteotomy may be indicated in more advanced types of rupture. With type III ruptures, bony arthrodesis may be required.

An MRI evaluation for associated soft tissue and osseous anomalies should be undertaken when treating a patient with posterior tibial dysfunction.[21,58] Sinus tarsi syndrome can occur concomitantly due to either increased biomechanical stress from acquired flat foot deformity or underlying inflammatory arthritis. Therefore, abnormal MRI signal within the sinus tarsi should raise the possibility of a diseased posterior tibial tendon.[59] Other associated soft tissue abnormalities include sprain/rupture of the spring (calcaneo-navicular) ligament, stretching of the deltoid ligament, plantar fasciitis, medial and lateral malleolar bursitis (Fig. 11.20), reactive tenosynovial effusion, and peritendinitis. With increasing hindfoot valgus the fibula becomes weight-bearing, and entrapment and tearing of the peroneal tendons may also develop. Hindfoot valgus, subtalar and talonavicular malalignment, and periostitis at the insertion of the flexor retinaculum to the tibia can be seen with posterior tibial tendon dysfunction. Tibial mar-

row edema in the region of the medial malleolus can also be encountered. A type II os naviculare and cornuate navicular tubercle have been implicated as predisposing factors for tendonopathy and tears.[60]

Twenty-five percent of posterior tibial tendon tears are found at the navicular insertion of the tendon (Fig. 11.21). This type of injury is often related to acute trauma in young, athletic patients.[61] Complete posterior tibial tendon avulsion can be seen in association with pronation-external rotation-type closed ankle fractures.[62] Distal tears may also be seen in patients with seronegative disorders. Degeneration and

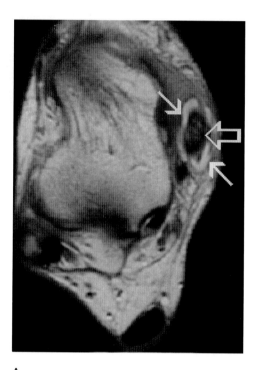

A

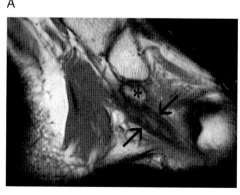

B

FIG. 11.21. Distal posterior tibial tendon partial tear. (A) Axial proton-density image at the level of the talar neck demonstrates marked thickening and heterogeneity of the posterior tibial tendon (open arrow) associated with tenosynovitis (closed arrows). (B) Sagittal T1-weighted image in the same patient shows a thickened a heterogeneous distal posterior tibial tendon (arrows) associated with a type II accessory navicular (asterisk).

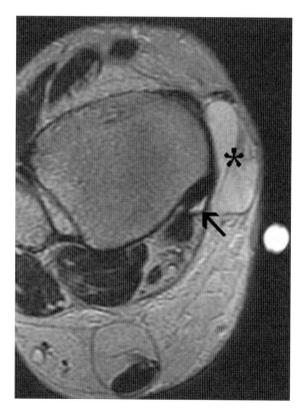

FIG. 11.20. Medial malleolar bursitis in a skater. Axial fast spin echo T2-weighted image shows marked distention of the medial malleolar bursa (asterisk) associated with a small posterior tibial tenosynovial effusion (arrow).

separation of the accessory navicular synchondrosis is in the differential diagnosis of posterior tibial tendon tear affecting its distal insertional portion.[63] Also, distinction of this type of tear with the normal signal heterogeneity and flaring of the posterior tibial tendon at its navicular insertion may be challenging.[22] Useful distinguishing features include the presence of edema or hemorrhage in and around the tendon fibers as well as the history of precedent trauma.

Posterior tibial tendon dislocation is quite rare. The injury occurs more often among young patients who have sustained significant trauma to the ankle.[64] It may also be seen in diabetic patients. The tendon slides out of its retromalleolar groove as a result of stripping or tear of the overlying flexor retinaculum.[39] An MR diagnosis of posterior tendon dislocation is straightforward with the tendon lying medial or anterior to the medial malleolus. In addition, avulsed or stripped flexor retinaculum, pressure erosion of the medial malleolus, shallow retromalleolar groove, and partial posterior tibial tendon tear may be seen.[39]

Flexor Hallucis Longus Tendon Injuries

The flexor hallucis longus tendon is susceptible to increased chronic wear and friction with secondary longitudinal splits and tenosynovitis as it travels within its three fibro-osseous tunnels: (1) between the medial and lateral talar tuberosities, (2) underneath the sustentaculum tali, and (3) between the hallucal sesamoids.

Athletes such as soccer players and ballet dancers who perform extreme plantar flexion and push-off maneuvers from the forefoot are susceptible to injuries at the talar fibro-osseous tunnel.[65] Acute tenosynovitis in this location may be followed by chronic and extensive inflammation of the tendon sheath leading to stenosing tenosynovitis, tendon nodularity and longitudinal splits with secondary entrapment of the tendon sheath, and functional hallux rigidus or checkrein deformity.[66] Posterior tibial and calcaneal fracture fragments may also lead to post-traumatic adhesions of the flexor hallucis longus tendon.[67]

The magic angle phenomenon may affect the flexor hallucis longus tendon when it curves underneath the sustentaculum tali and also in between the hallucal sesamoids.[22] Absence of clinical symptoms and lack of morphologic tendon abnormalities help to distinguish the magic angle effect from true disease. Flexor hallucis longus tendon injuries are best visualized on axial and sagittal MR images. Tenosynovitis and partial longitudinal tear of the flexor hallucis longus tendon have a different prevalence depending on the patient population. Partial tears are twice as common in dancers as compared to nondancers.[65] Complete rupture of the flexor hallucis longus tendon at the level of the ankle is quite rare.

Tenosynovial effusion surrounding an otherwise intact flexor hallucis longus tendon is characteristic of tenosynovitis, particularly if little ankle joint fluid is noted (Fig. 11.22). Tendon sheath fluid in the presence of a large ankle joint effusion most likely reflects a normal communication between the two structures and is usually of no clinical significance.

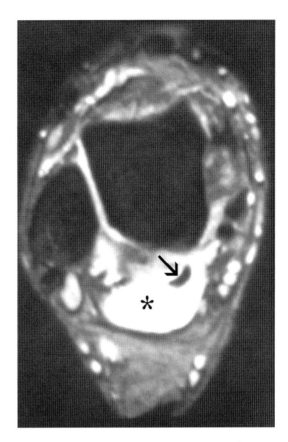

Fig. 11.22. Flexor hallucis longus tenosynovitis. Axial fat-suppressed T2-weighted image demonstrates a large amount of fluid (asterisk) within the tendon sheath of the flexor hallucis longus tendon (arrow). The amount of fluid is disproportionate to the fluid within the ankle joint indicative of true pathology and pseudocyst formation.

Nonfusion of the lateral talar tubercle, constituting the so-called os trigonum, can be seen in 7% to 14% of individuals.[26] In patients with os trigonum syndrome, the ossicle can wedge the flexor hallucis longus tendon between the tibia and the calcaneus, producing tenosynovitis. Entrapment of the ossicle may result in disruption of the cartilaginous synchondrosis and pseudarthrosis between the os trigonum and the lateral talar tubercle (Fig. 11.23). Contusion and compression fractures of the ossicle and opposing bony surfaces of the talus may also develop.[68] The MR findings include fragmentation, sclerosis, and bone marrow edema in the os trigonum or lateral talar tubercle, flexor hallucis longus tenosynovial effusion, posterior ankle and subtalar joint effusions, and posterior soft tissue edema (Fig. 11.24).[69] The clinical presentation of a pseudocyst of the flexor hallucis longus tendon may manifest on MRI as quite a large amount of tendon sheath fluid, which may extend proximal to the ankle joint and plantar to the tarsal bones (Fig. 11.22). This may produce a "dumbbell" appearance to the fluid column with narrowing at the level of the talar fibro-osseous tunnel.

Posterior ankle impingement and flexor hallucis longus tenosynovitis can also be related to the presence of a large

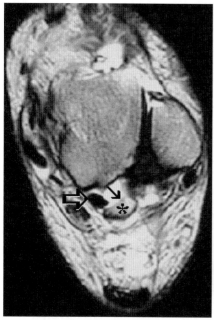 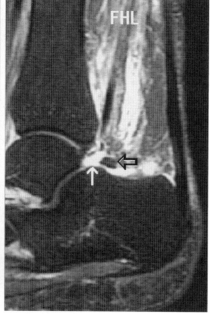

FIG. 11.23. Avulsed os trigonum. (A) Axial fast spin echo T2-weighted image shows a posteriorly displaced os trigonum (closed arrow) partly entrapping the flexor hallucis longus tendon (open arrow). (B) Sagittal fast spin echo STIR image shows the separated os trigonum (open arrow) outlined by fluid interposed between the lateral talar tubercle and the ossicle (arrow). Note associated edema within the flexor hallucis longus muscle (FHL).

A   B

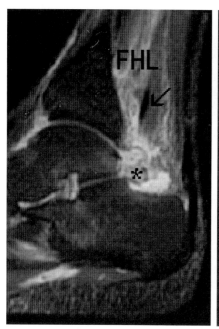 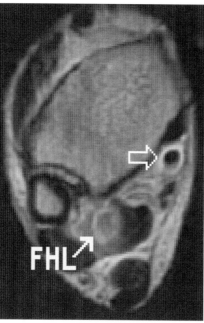

FIG. 11.24. Os trigonum fracture. Sagittal fast spin echo STIR (A) and axial fast spin echo T2-weighted (B) images demonstrate a fractured, edematous os trigonum (asterisk) associated with intramuscular edema and hematoma (closed arrow) of the flexor hallucis longus (FHL) muscle. Reactive tenosynovitis of the adjacent flexor digitorum longus tendon (open arrow) is seen.

A   B

Stieda process, ankle intraarticular bodies, tibial or calcaneal fracture fragments, prominent posterior intermalleolar ligament, hypertrophy or tearing of the transverse tibiofibular ligament (inferior portion of the posterior tibiofibular ligament) (Fig. 11.25), accessory flexor digitorum longus,[70] or a combination of these injuries.[71] Flexor hallucis longus tendon thickening, intrasubstance signal heterogeneity, and longitudinal splitting are indicative of tendinosis and partial tear, which can be found in the following sites in decreasing order of frequency: (1) behind or just below the tibiotalar joint,

(2) between the hallucal sesamoids, and (3) under the base of the first metatarsal in the region of Henry's knot.[65,72,73]

Complete rupture of the flexor hallucis longus tendon is a rare condition that occurs as a result of acute dorsiflexion or laceration injuries.[65] A connecting fibrous slip between the flexor hallucis longus and flexor digitorum longus tendons at Henry's knot provides an anatomic landmark for assessing the site of rupture. Recoiling of the tendon indicates rupture of the flexor hallucis longus proximal to the fibrous slip, while rupture distal to the slip limits the recoil to the forefoot.

FIG. 11.25. Posterolateral impingement syndrome in a ballet dancer. Axial proton-density (A) and coronal fast spin echo fat suppressed T2-weighted (B) images depict a globular scarring originating from the inferior transverse ligament (open arrow).

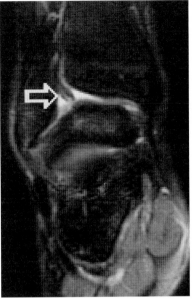

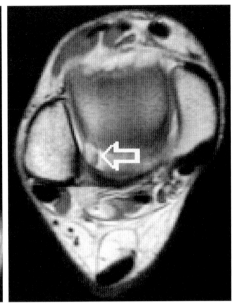

A   B

Intermittent dislocation of the flexor hallucis longus is a very unusual condition at the level of the intertubercular talar tunnel, but it has been reported in a synchronized swimmer.[74]

Hypertrophied or low-lying flexor hallucis longus muscle fibers may extend into the tunnel in between the talar tubercles. This prevents normal sliding of the tendon during ankle dorsiflexion, resulting in the corking-bottle effect. This condition is manifested on MRI as distal extension of muscle fibers into and beyond the talar tubercles.

Peroneal Tendons

Peroneal peritendinitis and tenosynovitis present clinically with swelling and tenderness along the common tendon sheath from the lateral malleolus distally, and may be visible due to the superficial course of the tendons. Increased biomechanical stress around fixed pulleys including the retrofibular groove, the peroneal tubercle, and the undersurface of the cuboid bone is the most likely etiology of peroneal tenosynovitis.[22,75,76] The MR characteristics of peritendinitis and tenosynovitis include scarring around the tendon and fluid within the common tendon sheath best seen on axial and sagittal MR images.[77] Large tenosynovial effusion with preserved morphology of the tendons is diagnostic of isolated tenosynovitis.[78] The differential diagnosis includes reactive tenosynovial effusion from tearing of the adjacent calcaneofibular ligament.

Overuse is the most common etiology for peroneal tendinosis and ensuing longitudinal splits. Other causes of peroneal tendinosis include underlying rheumatoid arthritis, other seronegative arthritides, and diabetes.[79] On MRI, thickening and increased intrasubstance signal are characteristic. Associated tenosynovitis is frequently seen. In patients presenting with nonspecific lateral ankle pain, MRI can differentiate peroneal tendinosis/tears from lateral collateral ligament injuries.

Longitudinal splits of the peroneus brevis tendon may occur in both the young and the elderly as well as in recreational and professional athletes.[80–82] In younger athletes, these tears are commonly symptomatic. Associated recurrent inversion injury and ligamentous sprains are frequently found.[81,83] In the elderly, peroneus brevis tendon tears are presumably due to chronic attrition and compressive wedging of the peroneus brevis tendon between the peroneus longus tendon and the fibular malleolus. Associated conditions include ligamentous sprain, superior peroneal retinacular injury,[81] prominent calcaneofibular ligament, mechanical crowding within the peroneal tunnel due to a low-lying peroneus brevis muscle belly or a peroneus quartus muscle,[84–86] convex or flat retromalleolar groove,[28] and peroneal tendon dislocations.[83,87]

The clinical diagnosis of peroneus brevis tendon longitudinal splits is not always straightforward. Therefore, MRI can be of great benefit to the clinician to help distinguish tears of the tendon from other entities that affect the lateral ankle as well as revealing the type and extent of the tear.

Longitudinal tears of the peroneus brevis tendon are best visualized on axial MR images. The central portion of the tendon becomes progressively thin as two or more globular limbs migrate medial and lateral to the peroneus longus tendon (Fig. 11.26). This classical arrangement gives the torn peroneus brevis tendon a characteristic C-shaped configuration. Complete disruption and retraction of the tendon fibers is rare although not unseen.[88] As the tendon descends along the lateral calcaneal wall, reconstitution into one single, nonsplit tendon is typical. Care should be taken to distinguish a true peroneus brevis tear from the normally splayed or crescentic appearance of the peroneus brevis tendon within the retromalleolar groove. A peroneus quartus tendon should also be distinguished from a peroneus brevis tendon tear. Other MRI findings of peroneus brevis tear include contour irregularity, signal heterogeneity,

FIG. 11.26. Peroneus brevis tendon tear. Axial proton-density images at the level of the distal fibula (A) and lateral calcaneal wall (B) demonstrate the C-shaped appearance and longitudinal tearing of the peroneus brevis tendon (arrows). Note a convex retromalleolar groove (arrowhead).

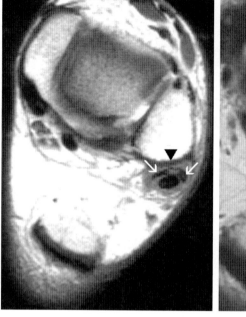
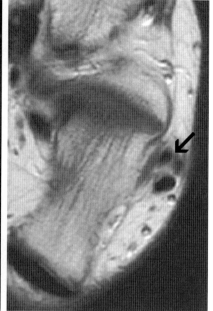

A

B

and clefts within the tendon. Associated peroneus longus tendinosis and splitting may also be encountered.

Conservative treatment of peroneus brevis tendon tears includes antiinflammatory medication, rest, orthotics, and cast immobilization.[80,82] Refractory cases may require surgical intervention such as end-to-end anastomosis or tenodesis to the adjacent peroneus longus tendon.[79,89] Surgical repair of a torn superior peroneal retinaculum, reconstruction and deepening of a shallow or convex retromalleolar groove, and resection of fibular spurs and muscle variants that may cause overcrowding of the peroneal tunnel are vital for successful surgical repair of peroneus brevis tendon tears.

Peroneus longus tendon tears can be either isolated or associated with peroneus brevis tendon tears. In the latter, the tears usually occur at the level of the retrofibular groove and tend to be longitudinal splits rather than complete discontinuity of the tendon. The peroneus longus tendon migrates anteriorly in between the torn limbs of the torn peroneus brevis tendon and thus becomes susceptible to increased friction against the fibula.

Isolated ruptures of the peroneus longus tendon are most frequently seen at the midfoot level due to chronic attrition and increased biomechanical stress as the peroneus longus tendon curves around a hypertrophic peroneal tubercle and around the cuboid bone (Fig. 11.27).[90] The etiology of an enlarged

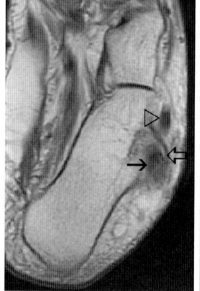
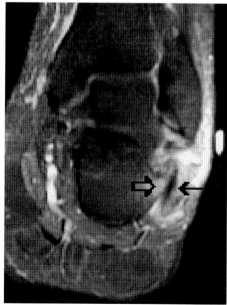

FIG. 11.27. Partial tear of the peroneus longus tendon associated with hypertrophic peroneal tubercle. Axial proton-density (A) and coronal fat-suppressed T2-weighted (B) images demonstrate longitudinal tearing of the peroneus longus tendon (black arrow) at the level of a prominent peroneal tubercle (open arrow). Note associated reactive edematous marrow changes in the peroneal tubercle and overlying soft tissues.

A

B

FIG. 11.28. Partial tear of the peroneus longus tendon at the level of the cuboid tunnel. Sagittal fat-suppressed (A) and axial proton-density (B) images depict heterogeneity of the peroneus longus tendon (arrow) and reactive marrow edema in the cuboid (C).

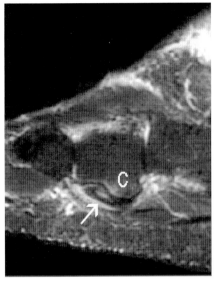
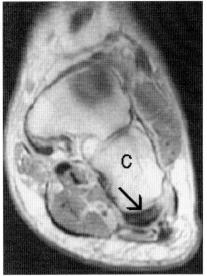

A   B

peroneal tubercle is unknown and may be developmental.[75] Trauma, altered biomechanics, and inflammatory pathology of the overlying peroneal tendons are among possible related factors.[30,32] Tears of the peroneus longus tendon are also associated with fractures of the calcaneus or acute direct crushing injury to the calcaneocuboid joint.[91] Acute tear due to avulsion fracture through the os peroneum following inversion or forced eversion of a supinated foot has been reported.[92]

Midfoot peroneus longus tendon tears often present with nonspecific symptoms. Magnetic resonance imaging should be performed whenever persistent lateral ankle and plantar foot pain are present. Coronal MR images of the midfoot should be extended distally to the metatarsal area when a tear of the peroneus longus tendon is suspected.[86] Magnetic resonance imaging findings include intrasubstance signal heterogeneity, thickening/thinning, longitudinal splitting, and discontinuity of the tendon, as well as associated lateral calcaneal/cuboid marrow edema (Fig. 11.28),[93] erosions, and a hypertrophic peroneal tubercle. Complete discontinuity of the peroneus longus tendon is more common at the level of the peroneal tubercle and under the cuboid compared to at the level of the lateral malleolus (Fig. 11.29).

FIG. 11.29. Proximal peroneus longus tendon tear. Axial proton-density (A) and coronal fat-suppressed T2-weighted (B) images demonstrate almost full-thickness disruption of the peroneus longus tendon (arrows). Minimal residual lateral fibers are noted. Asterisk points to edema within the muscle.

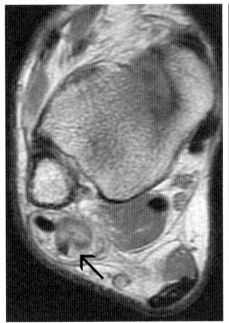
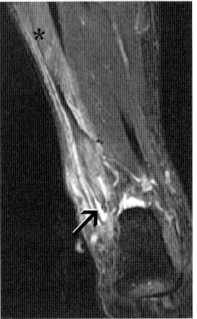

A   B

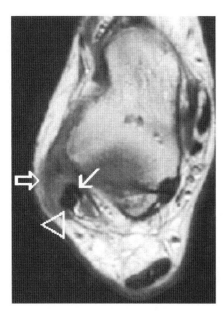

FIG. 11.30. Chronic superior peroneal retinacular (SPR) injury. Axial proton-density image shows marked scarring of the SPR partly encasing the peroneus brevis (arrow) and peroneus longus (arrowhead) tendons.

Symptomatic partial tears of the peroneus longus tendon often respond to conservative treatment with antiinflammatory medication and immobilization, followed by physical or orthotic therapy. If symptoms persist, surgical debridement with direct repair of the tendon and tenosynovectomy may be indicated. A complete tear of the peroneus longus tendon often requires a surgical repair, especially in young symptomatic patients. Removal of an os peroneum or hypertrophic peroneal tubercle, if present, is important for a successful outcome.[94]

Peroneal tendon dislocations are the most common dislocations at the ankle joint. Acute dislocation is often misdiagnosed as an ankle sprain, and thus the diagnosis is frequently delayed. Recurrent snapping and popping about the ankle and positive provocative maneuvers may provide clues to the diagnosis. Once chronic peroneal tendon dislocation ensues, the clinical diagnosis is more easily established but again can be mistaken for chronic lateral ankle instability.

Insufficiency of the superior peroneal retinaculum, whether congenital laxity or posttraumatic tearing, leads to peroneal tendon instability. Traumatic injury to the superior peroneal retinaculum is produced by a sudden dorsiflexion injury with either inversion or eversion of the foot. Increased strain and attenuation of the retinaculum can also be related to inversion injuries and ankle instability. Chronic ankle instability associated with superior peroneal retinacular laxity is considered a predisposing condition for peroneal tendon dislocation (Fig. 11.30).[95]

Magnetic resonance imaging allows direct assessment of the position of the peroneal tendons relative to the fibular retromalleolar groove. Axial images easily demonstrate subluxation or dislocation of the peroneal tendons anterior and lateral to the distal fibula (Fig. 11.31). Stripping of the superior peroneal retinaculum is more frequent as compared to complete avulsion.[40] The dislocated peroneal tendons are often located within a pouch formed by the stripped-off superior peroneal retinaculum fibular periosteum (Fig. 11.32). Predisposing factors for peroneal tendon instability such as a flattened or convex posterior fibular contour, stripped, torn, or absent superior peroneal retinaculum, and crowding by either a peroneus quartus (Fig. 11.33)[85,95] or low-lying peroneus brevis muscles can also be evaluated on MRI.[31,86]

A stable peroneal tendon dislocation may not require any treatment. Conversely, repair of the superior peroneal retinac-

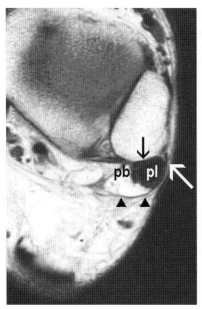

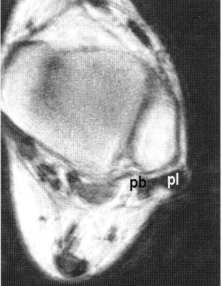

FIG. 11.31. Peroneal tendon instability demonstrated on dynamic MRI. (A) Axial proton-density image through the distal fibula in neutral position depicts a convex retrofibular groove associated with minimal medial shift of the peroneus brevis (pb) and peroneus longus (pl) tendons. The superior peroneal retinaculum (arrowheads) and fibular fibrocartilaginous ridge (white arrow) originate quite far laterally. (B) Axial proton-density image in forced dorsiflexion elicited lateral subluxation of the peroneus longus tendon.

A   B

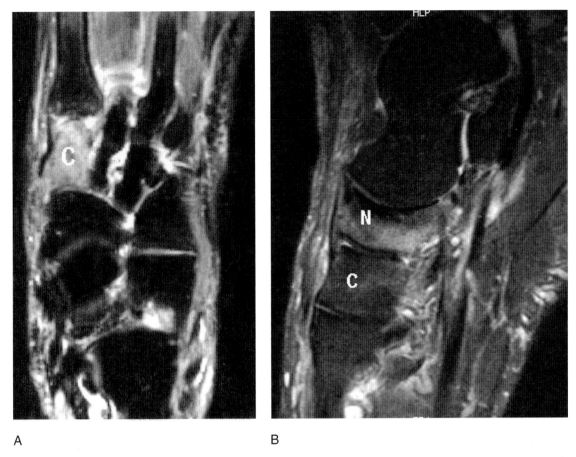

A

B

FIG. 11.56. Transient bone marrow edema. (A) Axial fat-suppressed T2-weighted image of the midfoot demonstrates diffuse marrow edema involving the medial cuneiform bone (C). (B) Follow-up sagittal FSE STIR image obtained 5 months later reveals interval near complete resolution of edematous changes in the medial cuneiform (C). Migratory edema pattern now involving the navicular bone (N), lateral cuneiform (not shown) and cuboid (not shown) is seen.

Miscellaneous

Plantar Fasciitis

The plantar fascia is a fibrous aponeurosis formed by the blending of three cords—medial, central and lateral. The central cord is the most important component emanating from the medial calcaneal tuberosity and inserting distally to the soft tissues and periosteum at the bases of the proximal phalanges of the five toes. Plantar fasciitis typically involves the proximal portion of the central cord adjacent to its origin on the calcaneal tuberosity.

Repetitive trauma and mechanical stress resulting in microtears and inflammation of the fascia and perifascial soft tissues are likely etiologic factors for plantar fasciitis. Runners and obese patients are frequently affected.[200,201] Patients with plantar fasciitis present with pain at the origin of the plantar fascia, typically more severe in the morning. Exacerbation of the pain can be elicited by dorsiflexion of the toes.

Calcaneal spurs are often found on lateral radiographs of patients with plantar fasciitis. However, this finding is not specific since it can be seen in about 25% of the asymptomatic population. Also, the spurs are more commonly found at the origin of the flexor digitorum brevis muscle than at the origin of the plantar fascia. Bone scintigraphy may demonstrate increased uptake in the region of the calcaneus, probably reflecting periosteal inflammation of the calcaneus.[200]

Magnetic resonance imaging is useful in distinguishing plantar fasciitis from other causes of heel pain such as calcaneal stress fracture, plantar fibromatosis, plantar fascia rupture, and tendinosis (Figs. 11.57 and 11.58).[200,201] The normal plantar fascia can be identified on sagittal and coronal MR images as a linear hypointense structure extending anteriorly from the calcaneal tuberosity. The plantar fascia flares slightly at the calcaneal insertion, and its thickness ranges between 2 and 4 mm. In plantar fasciitis, thickening of up to 7 to 8 mm, more pronounced at or near the fascia's insertion to the calcaneus, can be seen. The plantar fascia exhibits intermediate signal on T1-weighted and proton-density–weighted images and hyperintensity on fluid-sensitive sequences. Magnetic resonance imaging can easily provide information regarding the presence and extent of plantar fasciitis and also evaluate for associated findings such as soft tissue edema, perifascial edema, calcaneal bone marrow edema, and plantar heel spur.[202–204]

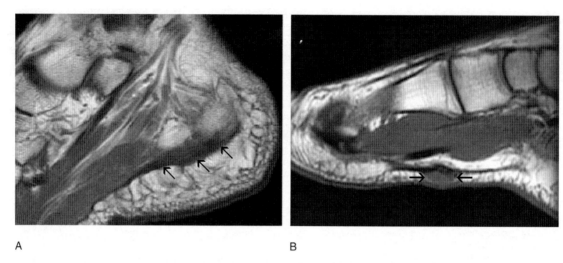

FIG. 11.57. Plantar fasciitis (A) and plantar fibroma (B). (A) Sagittal T1-weighted image shows diffuse fusiform thickening (arrows) of the medial cord of plantar fascia consistent with fasciitis (arrows). (B) Sagittal T1-weighted image demonstrates focal nodular thickening along the non–weight-bearing portion of the medial plantar fascial slip to the great toe consistent with fibroma (arrows).

The thickening in plantar fasciitis is often fusiform as opposed to focal/nodular thickening typical of plantar fibromatosis (Fig. 11.57). A tear of the fascia is manifested by discontinuity of the fibers associated with focal edema and hemorrhage. Treatment of plantar fasciitis is initially conservative and includes physical therapy orthotics and nonsteroidal antiinflammatory agents. In more severe cases local injection of steroids or resection of the fascia may be required. Extracorporeal shock wave therapy (ESWT) has been utilized in plantar fasciitis in order to elicit an acute inflammatory response, which may lead to healing of this chronic disorder. In a recent study, MR features related to ESWT included increased severity and extent of soft tissue and perifascial edema.[205] Preexisting bone marrow edema, plantar heel spur, the thickness of the plantar fascia, and the signal intensity of the plantar fascia were not significantly affected by ESWT.[205]

The inflammatory reaction associated with plantar fasciitis and heel spurs may produce entrapment of the inferior calca-

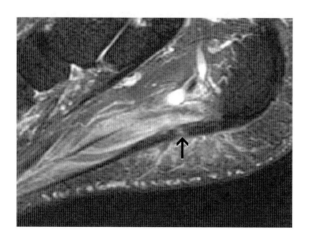

FIG. 11.58. Partial tear of the plantar fascia. A focal tear of the central cord of the plantar fascia (arrow) is noted on this sagittal FSE STIR image.

neal nerve, or first branch of the lateral plantar nerve (Baxter's neuropathy).[206] This can manifest on MRI as muscle denervation alterations within the abductor digiti minimi muscle, best seen on coronal images of the ankle.

Tarsal Tunnel Syndrome

The tarsal tunnel is a medial, fat-filled space bounded laterally (from superior to inferior) by the medial malleolus, talus, calcaneus, and quadratus plantae muscle, and medially first by the deep aponeurosis of the leg and then, more distally, by the flexor retinaculum. The tarsal tunnel is traversed by the posterior tibial tendon, flexor digitorum longus tendon, and flexor hallucis longus tendon; by the posterior tibial nerve and its branches; and by the accompanying posterior tibial vessels. The posterior tibial nerve trifurcates above or at the level of the flexor retinaculum into the medial calcaneal nerve and the medial and lateral plantar nerves. The medial calcaneal nerve innervates the medial plantar heel. The medial plantar nerve carries most of the sensation from the medial two thirds of the plantar aspect of the midfoot and forefoot but innervates only four muscles: the first lumbrical, the abductor hallucis, the flexor digitorum brevis, and the flexor hallucis brevis muscles. The lateral plantar nerve carries sensation from the lateral third of the plantar midfoot and forefoot and supplies motor innervation to most of the plantar muscles of the foot, including the quadratus plantae, flexor digiti minimi brevis, all the interossei, and the second to fourth lumbricals.

Compression or entrapment of the posterior tibial nerve and its branches results in a constellation of clinical findings consistent with the tarsal tunnel syndrome. There are a few major causes for compression, including trauma, space-occupying lesions, and foot deformities. The cause of the tarsal tunnel remains obscure in up to 40% of cases. Additionally, the clinical symptoms vary depending on the site of compression.[207]

Intrinsic and extrinsic lesions to the tarsal tunnel may cause direct compression of the posterior tibial nerve. Some intrinsic causes include accessory muscles,[208] ganglion cysts, neurogenic tumors, varicose veins, tumors, synovial hypertrophy, tenosynovial osteochondromatosis,[209] tendon tear,[210] and scar tissue. Talocalcaneal coalition,[211] flatfoot deformity,[212] accessory soleus,[208] accessory ossicle (os trigonum), and bony fragments as well as excessive pronation during the practice of some sports (sprinting, jumping, judo) are just a few of the extrinsic causes of this syndrome.[212] Failure of the medial longitudinal arch support related to posterior tibial tendon and plantar fascia dysfunction may also result in traction injury to the posterior tibial nerve.[213] The combination of posttraumatic lower back injury and tarsal tunnel syndrome underscores the possibility of double crush syndrome in the lower extremities.[214] The cause of tarsal tunnel syndrome remains obscure in about 50% of cases.

Clinically, patients present with insidious onset of pain, paresthesia, a tingling and burning sensation, as well as positive Tinnel's sign along the plantar and medial aspects of the foot and great toe. The heel is often spared. Pain is exacerbated with exercise possibly due to venous engorgement. Electromyographic studies are positive in most cases, but in early situations they may be falsely negative. Magnetic resonance imaging has been shown to be useful in the preoperative assessment of space-occupying lesions within the tarsal tunnel (Fig. 11.59). It may also play a role in clinically and electrodiagnostically inconclusive cases by displaying denervation injury manifested by diffuse hyperintensity or atrophy of the affected muscle(s) on fluid-sensitive sequences (Fig. 11.59). Contrast-enhanced images may be of additional value, highlighting the denervated muscles.

Relief of symptoms in idiopathic tarsal tunnel syndrome following retinacular release is frequently seen. In a recent study, decreased volume associated with increased tarsal tunnel pressure was noted when the foot and ankle were positioned in eversion or inversion, two positions that may aggravate symptoms of posterior tibial nerve entrapment.[215] Therefore, neutral immobilization of the foot and ankle is recommended in order to minimize pressure on the nerve and maximize tarsal tunnel volume available for the nerve.[215]

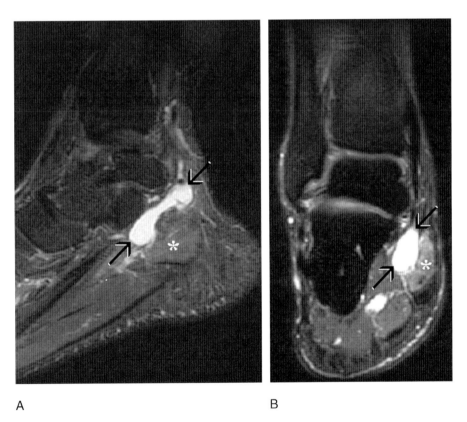

A   B

FIG. 11.59. Tarsal tunnel syndrome. Sagittal (A) and coronal (B) STIR images demonstrate a bilobed ganglion cyst occupying the tarsal tunnel (arrows). Note the denervation-related increased signal within the abductor hallucis muscle (asterisk).

B. Orthopedic Perspective: Foot and Ankle Clinical Applications

Alastair S.E. Younger and Margie Pohl

Magnetic resonance imaging is able to differentiate signal changes primarily in soft tissue. It is therefore an imaging technique that outlines soft tissue injuries and disease. Magnetic resonance imaging is a non–weight-bearing investigation, and should be preceded by weight-bearing views of the foot or ankle. The images should be interpreted in light of both investigations and the history and physical. In the clinical scenario, patients may present with an MRI diagnosis. In some cases no other investigations have been performed. For the clinician to use the information from the MRI in context, the patient, all other images, and the MRI films should be reviewed at the same time. Inconsistencies in the clinical picture can then be easily recognized and resolved.

In some cases the diagnosis is easy; a patient may present with a history of an ankle sprain a year prior. The patient points to the ankle as the main source of pain related to exercise, and clinical exam confirms tenderness at the ankle joint margins with swelling. The plain radiographs show an osteochondral defect consistent with an MRI with a lesion in the same area. In such a patient the diagnosis is clear.

However in many cases the diagnosis is not clear. An MRI may show a lesion remote to the area of clinical pain (a false-positive investigation), or the MRI may not show a cartilage defect in the ankle that is clinically suspected and proven by an ankle arthroscopy (false-negative investigation).[216]

While the MRI is an indispensable treatment tool, it must always be taken in context with the physical findings and the complaint. To this end, the physician should understand some basic research with regard to diagnostic techniques.

Test-retest reliability is the ability of an investigation repeated on separate occasions to diagnose the same disease. This may test the ability of the same scanner to provide the same result, or different scanners and interpreters to provide the same result. An MRI scan may be sensitive and specific in diagnosing a lesion, for example an osteochondral defect, cited in a study performed at a single institution with one scanner and a set protocol using one set of films read by different observers on two occasions. However, a clinician may find that his local MRI clinic has missed a few lesions he has picked up arthroscopically. This may be because of a difference in diagnostic accuracy of the machine and different radiologists used in the study and in the local clinic. Factors such as sequences, resolution, size of the magnet, surface coil use, and experience of the radiologist all come into play. The Hawthorne effect, the improvement of performance simply as a result of being involved in a study, may also have an effect. So clinicians must accept that the diagnostic accuracy of the local clinic may not be the same as that cited in published studies. This means that the locally performed MRI scan is still a good test, but it must be interpreted with caution and in conjunction with the history and physical examination. In the case when there is a discrepancy between the clinical examination and the MRI scan, the clinical examination may be more accurate, as shown in one study on Morton's neuroma.[217]

Some lesions may be more reliably diagnosed than others. For example, osteochondral defects of the ankle may be more reliably diagnosed than chondral injuries alone.[218] Staging of the osteochondral injury, and hence selecting the appropriate treatment may not be accurate.[219] Tendon tears may be more reliably diagnosed than ligament tears. In some cases the films may show the lesion and the radiologist may miss the lesion or misinterpret the anatomy. In our clinical practices we have seen osteochondral defects on review of the films that were not reported. We have found intraoperative ruptured posterior tibial tendons that have been reported as intact, complete ruptures of the Achilles tendons that have been reported as partial ruptures, and complete tears of the deltoid ligament that are not visible on the MRI on retrospective review of the films with the radiologist. We have also seen second metatarsophalangeal joint synovitis that has been reported as a Morton's neuroma. For these reasons patients are reviewed with their actual images to ensure consistency of diagnosis and treatment. When relevant, these inconsistencies must be reported to insurance carriers, disability providers, and team physicians. Abnormalities can be found on MR scanning of asymptomatic athletes, including fluid on the flexor hallucis longus tendon, bone marrow edema, and signal changes in the Achilles tendon.[220] The physics of MRI have been discussed extensively and will not be repeated in this chapter.

The Role of Magnetic Resonance Imaging in the Management of the Athlete with Foot or Ankle Pain

Diagnostic algorithms can be useful for the management of the athlete with foot pain. These tend to be specific for individual surgeons. However, in principle, the patient should be worked up with standing radiographs, a history, and a physical exam. If the diagnosis is not clear at this point, further imaging is required. For a likely soft tissue injury, MRI is the next investigation of choice. The plain radiographs are often complementary to the MRI exam and should be performed in every case. For bone lesions CT scan may be a more appropriate investigation, as bone defects and anatomy are best seen.

Ankle Instability

Lateral ankle instability can be associated with a number of pathologies. These include peroneal tendon tears[221] (around 16%), osteochondral defects,[222-224] and anterolateral impingement.[224-227] Magnetic resonance imaging is a useful diagnostic test more for ruling out associated injuries rather than diagnosing lateral ankle instability, for which the physical exam and history remain the mainstays of diagnosis.[228] If the associated lesion such as osteochondral injuries is treated without stabilization of the ankle, the outcome will be worse.[224] In cases when the pain after ankle instability appears atypical, or when an osteochondral defect or peroneal tendon tear is suspected on clinical examination, then the MRI can help with this diagnosis. Sometimes this can assist with surgical planning. We routinely perform arthroscopy of the ankle in all patients with instability, but the surgeon may choose to arthroscope the ankle based on the result of the MRI. Some surgeons choose to arthroscope the ankle based on clinical symptoms. A decision to explore the peroneal tendons may also be made based on the results of the MRI.[221] Some surgeons perform the ankle arthroscopy at a separate surgery, while others perform the arthroscopy and ligament reconstruction at the same sitting.[229] Medial ankle pain may also occur after ankle instability associated with a medial chondral injury.[230]

Imaging of Specific Conditions

Osteochondral and Cartilage Injuries of the Ankle

The Berndt and Harty classification was used to describe the types of defect associated with osteochondral injuries. More recent classification systems use the Berndt and Harty classification as the template. An MRI classification system has been described.[226,231,232] However, it may be simpler to consider the injury as chondral, osseous, or both (Fig. 11.60). The degree of signal change on MRI is affected by the time since the original injury. It is our experience that MRI often poorly visualizes chronic isolated cartilage injuries. Magnetic resonance imaging is much better at defining the extent and size of a bone injury regardless of the overlying cartilage injury.[218] It enables good determination of the stability of an osteochondral defect.[233] An MR arthrogram may be better at determining cartilage integrity. In many cases, if the patient is symptomatic and has well localized pain within the ankle, an ankle arthroscopy may be a better alternative for determining the extent and integrity of the cartilage defect. An MRI, therefore, is not required prior to many ankle arthroscopies. A patient with ankle pain and a negative MRI can often benefit from an ankle arthroscopy.

On occasion a subchondral cyst can form from repetitive load (Fig. 11.61). A small cartilage defect can result in a large cyst deep to the joint surface. This can be best visualized by MRI as the T2 signal will outline the fluid-filled cyst penetrating to the joint line.

An acute injury can cause a bone bruise within the ankle similar to those seen in the knee with an anterior cruciate ligament (ACL) injury.

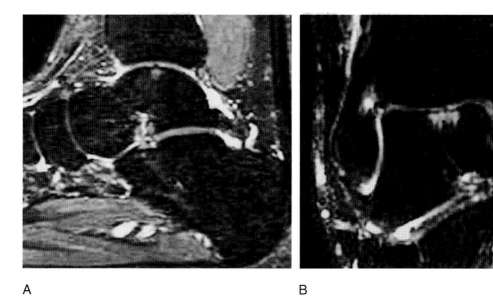

A   B

FIG. 11.60. Central osteochondritis dissecans (OCD) talus in a 51-year-old athletic man with ankle discomfort. Sagittal (A) and coronal (B) MR shows an osteochondral defect mid-talar dome and anterior lateral tibial plafond. Definitive comment on the status of the overlying cartilage is difficult as minimal or no joint fluid is present.

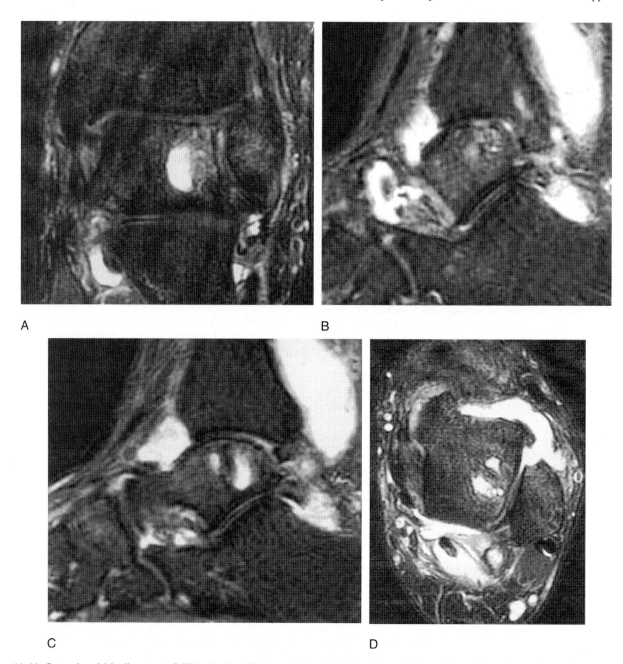

FIG. 11.61. Osteochondritis dissecans (OCD) talus in a 22-year-old skateboarder with multiple ankle sprains and ongoing pain and swelling. Cononal (A), parasagittal (B), mid sagittal (C), and transverse (D) MR images show a large osteochondral defect in the posterolateral aspect of the talar dome. There are large cystic components within this osteochondral defect. A large ankle effusion is present.

Osteochondral injuries occur often with lateral ligament instability, and are associated therefore indirectly with peroneal tendon injuries; both should be reviewed on the MRI to determine if an associated injury has occurred.

The MRI can assist in the treatment of osteochondral defects by determining the nature of the overlying cartilage and the age of the injury. Occasionally, a plain radiograph shows an osteochondral injury of unknown duration and significance. The MRI determines the status of the overlying cartilage and the degree of bone edema present. In cases with edema, the osteochondral defect is more acute. In cases with cartilage disruption, the treatment is more likely to be surgical.

Anterior Impingement Syndrome

Pain may be present on the anterior and lateral side of the ankle. This can occur after an ankle sprain, osteochondral injury, or fracture.[224,234] The anterior talofibular ligament can impinge on the anterior tibiofibular ligament, or the anterior talofibular ligament may be hypertrophied.[226] With ankle dorsiflexion the synovium on the anterior aspect of the ankle can impinge and cause pain. Debridement can allow athletes to return to their sport.[235,236]

The clinical examination and history show that patients have pain at the junction of the tibia, fibula, and talus. Dorsiflexion of the ankle may aggravate the pain on clinical examination. On occasion, impingement may be associated with anterior osteophytes that can be imaged by plain radiographs or CT scan. Standing radiographs of the ankle may show anterior osteophytes, and their relationship to the talar neck can be seen on the standing lateral view. However, in the absence of osteophytes, MRI is the only imaging modality available for assessing the anterior lateral impingement syndrome.[237–239] Studies show reasonable correlation with arthroscopic findings. Magnetic resonance imaging may be able to distinguish the difference between anterior impingement and damage to the talofibular ligament, although both injuries may coexist.[240]

Anterior Osteophytes and Impingement

Some athletes are predisposed by their sport to form anterior osteophytes within the ankle. These osteophytes can be associated with synovitis and impingement (Fig. 11.62). The talar osteophytes tend to occur on the medial side of

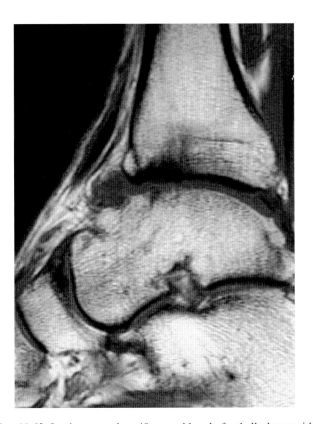

FIG. 11.62. Impingement in a 40-year-old male football player with gradual onset of ankle pain and stiffness. MR shows significant impingement from the anterior osteophytes along with synovitis and an osteochondral lesion.

the ankle while the tibial osteophytes occur on the lateral side.[241] While the osteophytes themselves are poorly imaged by MRI and are best defined by CT or weight-bearing or oblique radiographs,[241] the inflammation associated with the soft tissue impingement can be assessed by MRI.[242] The soft tissue inflammation may also be a major source of pain. These osteophytes can also be visualized by an oblique radiograph.[243] Removal of the osteophytes enables athletes to return to their sport so long as there is no joint space narrowing or osteoarthritic change.[236,244]

Impingement can occur on both the lateral side of the ankle and the medial side in the corner between the medial maleolus and tibia. Impingement can also affect the gutters, particularly if osteophytes form on the talar neck or on the anterior aspects of the medial and lateral maleoli.

Ligament Injuries

Our understanding of ligament injuries around the ankle is gradually expanding. Injuries to the lateral collateral ligaments are the most common injury associated with an ankle sprain. Injuries to the syndesmosis are associated with an external rotation injury of the foot on the ankle. A deep deltoid ligament injury in the fibers joining the talus to medial maleolus may occur at the same time, allowing the talus to translate laterally.[245]

Injuries to the deltoid ligament region are less well understood. Injuries to the deep deltoid ligament can be associated with syndesmosis injuries or may occur on their own. A deep deltoid ligament injury may allow the medial side of the ankle to anteriorly rotate, causing the ankle joint to become unstable on the medial side. A deep deltoid ligament injury may occur in isolation (Fig. 11.63).

Injuries to the superficial deltoid ligament are associated with a planovalgus foot deformity. Continuation of this tear may extend to the spring ligament. These injuries can occur acutely. The chronic tear is not visible on MRI using standard sequences, but may be visible in the acute phase or may be visible on MRA.

On the lateral side of the ankle injuries may occur to the anterior talofibular ligament (preventing anterior rotation of the talus on the tibia) or the calcaneofibular ligament (preventing inversion of both the calcaneus on the talus at the subtalar joint and the talus on the tibia at the ankle joint).

Visualization of the lateral ligament complex in the chronic setting may be unreliable to diagnose an insufficient ligament. After an acute injury there will be edema and bleeding in the lateral collateral ligament complex with excellent sensitivity and specificity.[246,247] After healing, the deficient ligaments can be in continuity, making the insufficiency hard to visualize once the acute swelling has settled. An MR arthrogram may show fluid in continuity through the lateral ligament complex, confirming the diagnosis (Fig. 11.64).

All ligament injuries may be associated with synovitis in the ankle if recurrent injuries are occurring. Anterior lateral

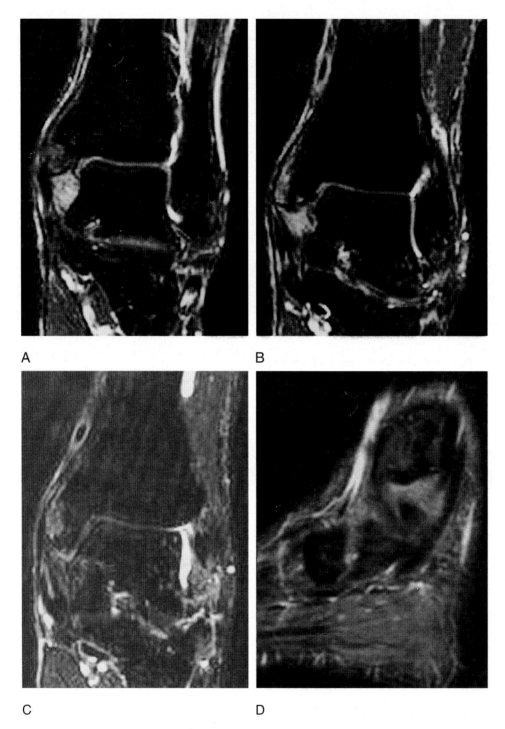

A   B

C   D

FIG. 11.63. Deltoid ligament injury in a 31-year-old football player with acute ankle sprain with medial tenderness. Sequential coronal (A-C) and sagittal (D), MR images show thickening and increased signal intensity in the region of the posterior tibiotalar ligament of the deltoid ligament compatible with injury. The remainder of the deltoid ligament appears intact.

impingement may also complicate ankle instability and can be viewed on MRI.[240]

Syndesmosis injuries can occur without an ankle fracture. These injuries present as an injury to the planted foot with an external rotation force, distinct to the inversion injury.[248]

Synovial Impingement

Synovial impingement is invariably associated with an inciting cause, such as ankle instability, loose bodies, repetitive injury to the anterior ankle, or entrapment between

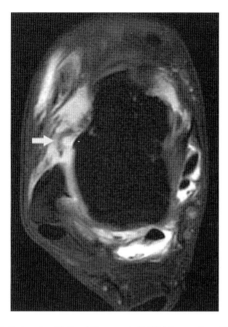

FIG. 11.64. Lateral collateral ligament (LCL) injury in a 28-year-old male snowboarder with lateral ankle pain and instability. MR arthrogram delineates the disrupted anterior talofibular ligament (arrow).

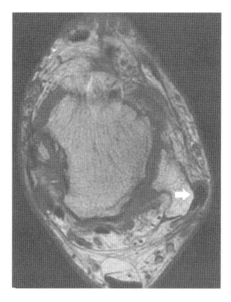

FIG. 11.65. Peroneal tendon dislocation in a 36-year-old male skater who developed lateral ankle discomfort following a twisting fall 6 months prior. MR shows that the peroneus brevis and longus tendons are dislocated laterally (arrow). Metal wear is present from a previous unrelated injury.

osteophytes or ligaments.[249] Patients present with localized tenderness on palpation worse on activity. Patients may localize the pain well to the anterior medial, anterior lateral, or posterior margins of the ankle depending on the location of the discomfort.

An MRI may assist in determining the location and degree of synovitis present.

Peroneal Tendon Disease

The peroneal tendons run behind the lateral maleolus. The brevis tendon inserts onto the base of the fifth metatarsal and runs anterior to a bone prominence on the lateral side of the calcaneus. The longus tendon runs posterior to the bone prominence and inferior to the cuboid. The tendon turns around the cuboid with a sesamoid in its substance at that level, before decussating and inserting into multiple bones on the medial border of the foot.

The peroneal tendons can be injured in sports. Forceful eversion of the ankle against resistance can disrupt the peroneal retinaculum, allowing the tendons to sublux or dislocate anterior to the fibula.[250] Injury of the peroneal retinaculum can be associated with a shallow fibular groove visible on MRI (Fig. 11.65). The tendons may also sublux one on another in the peroneal groove.

Tears can occur in the peroneal tendons (Fig. 11.66). These tears are associated with lateral ankle instability and may be associated with overload from a cavus foot position. Tears tend to occur in the region of the tendon undergoing maximum strain. The peroneus brevis can tear behind the fibula.[221] The longus tendon can tear as it crosses the cuboid. An acute rupture can occur through the os perineum when it fractures.[251]

In peroneal instability the brevis tear can span the tip of the fibula.

Magnetic resonance imaging can diagnose peroneal tendon dislocation by demonstrating the position of the tendons with respect to the fibula. Peroneal tendon tears can also be seen on MRI.[221] Tears are often longitudinal while the tendon is in continuity. Occasionally the tendon can rupture. Acute peroneal tendon ruptures are rare, and may be associated with avulsion off the fifth metatarsal base. Peroneus quartus muscles can also cause some confusion both in injury and surgery. This accessory muscle and tendon can be effectively visualized only with MRI.

Planovalgus Feet in Sports

Some athletes have planovalgus feet, which may cause pain during athletic activity. A planovalgus foot causes overload of the medial structures of the foot, and potential impingement laterally. On the medial side, the tibialis posterior tendon works to maintain the arch. It inserts onto the tuberosity of the navicular. An accessory navicular may be a reflection of chronic overpull of the tendon as accessory naviculars are seen in 2% of the population in general and in 33% of patients with planovalgus feet. Pain may occur due to the avulsion of the insertion with bone, or secondary to synovitis and tears of the overloaded tendon. If the foot becomes flatter after injury, then a tear of the deltoid or spring ligament may have occurred.[252] Tears can occur in the posterior tibial tendon.[253] Tears may occur in the plantar aspect of the navicular cuneiform joint, or there may be impingement on the dorsal side of the navicular cuneiform joint.

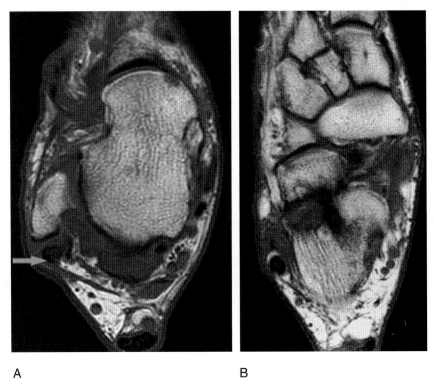

A   B

Fɪɢ. 11.66. Peroneus brevis tear in a 68-year-old man who is an active curler with posterolateral ankle pain and swelling. (A) Transverse MR demonstrates peroneus brevis abnormal morphology at the level of the lateral malleolus (arrow), where it is thin, and demonstrates a semilunar configuration. The tendon is split as it courses around the lateral malleolus. The peroneus longus tendon is unremarkable. (B) Coronal image of the foot shows that he also has moderate osteoarthritis of the middle and posterior subtalar joints.

Impingement may occur on the lateral side of the ankle.[254] With increased subtalar eversion the contents of the sinus tarsi may be crushed, causing pain. An MRI may confirm increased signal in the sinus tarsi region. Impingement occurs as the anterior process of the talus translates forward. Bony impingement between the talus and calcaneus may occur in severe planovalgus feet.

Patients with a flat foot and minimal or no subtalar motion may have a tarsal coalition. On occasion an acute injury may break down a previously asymptomatic solid tarsal coalition and cause it to become symptomatic. In these patients the MRI may demonstrate loss of the medial subtalar facet or a fibrous coalition with acute signal change during the recovery phase.

Achilles Tendon Disease

The Achilles tendon can restrict athletic activity because of recurrent injury or underlying disease in older athletes. The heel counter on shoes can cause inflammation of the Achilles paratenon. This may occur in isolation, or be associated with deep changes to the Achilles tendon, or its insertion.[255] The Achilles bursa can also be associated with inflammation and damage associated with sports. In ice hockey the retrocalcaneal bursa can be inflamed by irritation of the heel counter of the skate. The MRI may not visualize the associated Hagelund

deformity, but the inflammation of the bursa and fluid within the bursa will be seen.

Disease around the insertion of the Achilles tendon can include concomitant insertional Achilles tendonitis, Achilles bursitis, and a prominent posterior process of the calcaneus. Acute injuries to the Achilles tendon complex can result in muscle tears, or partial or complete ruptures of the tendon. The functional length of the Achilles is the determinant of outcome of the Achilles rupture. The tendon rupture can be transverse, resulting in easier imaging of the rupture. An oblique rupture plane may make a complete rupture appear incomplete on imaging. In this scenario clinical examination will differentiate the partial from complete tear. On the affected side, if excessive dorsiflexion is seen compared to the noninjured side, then the tendon is functionally long. In many patients the Thompson test may indicate an intact tendon in patients with a functionally long tendon. These patients include those with a partial rupture that is functionally healed, a healed missed rupture, or an acute rupture with an intact plantaris (Figs. 11.67 and 11.68). The MRI is useful in diagnosing a missed Achilles rupture, as the scar of the missed rupture will be visualized. The rupture may occur through a preexisting degenerative zone in the tendon.[256] Tears may occur in the proximal Achilles at the muscle tendon junction. Ultrasound is not as good as MRI in detecting these injuries.[257] Many patients may present with preexisting Achilles tendon disease. This may present as

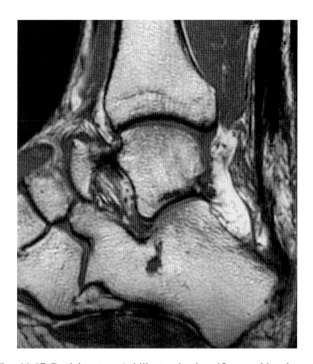

FIG. 11.67. Partial rupture Achilles tendon in a 45-year-old male runner 1 year following an unresolved Achilles tendon injury. There is fusiform thickening of the Achilles tendon beginning 2 cm superior to its insertion and extending more superiorly for approximately 7 cm. Within the tendon there is some intermediate T1 signal that is hyperintense on T2-weighted images, likely indicating edema. The tendon is grossly intact. The findings are consistent with a partial tear of the Achilles tendon.

an acute or subacute injury, where the MRI will show preexisting deformity (Fig. 11.69).

Flexor Hallucis Tendonitis

The flexor hallucis longus tendon passes posterior to the ankle joint in a fibro-osseous tunnel bordered anteriorly by the talus. This bony and fibrous constriction can constrict the tendon of the flexor hallucis longus, resulting in pain.[258,259] An accessory muscle can cause similar symptomatology.[259] Ultrasound and MRI remain the imaging techniques of choice. Surgical release of the fibro-osseous tunnel may resolve symptoms. The release can be done arthroscopically reducing the recovery time.

Heel Pain and Plantar Fasciitis

Heel pain can cause significant down time for athletes, usually associated with a chronic stress injury. Heel pain can be caused by injury to the heel pad, or secondary to plantar fasciitis. The diagnosis may be made by clinical examination, and can be assisted by MRI. The MRI visualizes the origin of the plantar fascia, with edema of the plantar fascia, its insertion, or the bone confirming plantar fasciitis.

Most heel pain settles with activity modification and nonsurgical treatment. Treatment initially includes physiotherapy (stretching), orthotics[260,261] (over the counter, prefabricated,

and custom all have a similar effectiveness), and nonsteroidal antiinflammatory medication. If this fails, night splints[262] and shock wave therapy may be considered as a noninvasive treatment that appears to be as effective as surgery.[263–265]

Plantar fascia release can be performed endoscopically or as an open procedure. Analysis of outcomes show both procedures to have the same outcome and treatment effect.[266–274] A less invasive procedure would therefore be preferable in patients failing nonoperative treatment.

Disorders of the First Metatarsophalangeal Joint

The first metatarsophalangeal (MTP) joint is prone to sports injury. It can suffer cartilage injuries from direct trauma. Injuries can be divided into hyperextension injuries, hyperflexion injuries, and dislocations.[274] The flexor tendons of the first MTP joint are quite complex. The flexor hallucis longus tendon runs in a tunnel between the sesamoids and inserts into the base of the distal phalanx. The flexor hallucis brevis muscle splits and each head inserts into the sesamoids. The adductor hallucis and abductor hallucis tendons insert on the lateral and medial sides of the sesamoids. A common flexor tendon then goes from each sesamoid and inserts onto the base of the proximal phalanx. The sesamoids and their tendons therefore stabilize the proximal phalanx on the metatarsal head, and allow transmission of force from the ground through the metatarsal head.

Injuries of the flexor tendons can include fractures of the sesamoids (Fig. 11.70) or avulsions of the tendons from the sesamoids (turf toe) (Fig. 11.71). Magnetic resonance imaging is often required to define the anatomic structures injured. Initial management is conservative. A cast with a great toe spica will allow appropriate immobilization. Late problems include ongoing first MTP joint pain, traumatic hallux valgus, and secondary degeneration.

Treatment options are limited, as the first MTP joint has a complex structure. If the disruption includes the sesamoid, an early or late open reduction can help to restore integrity to the plantar structures. However, the results of such reconstructions have not been evaluated and the ability to return an athlete to high-level sport remains questionable.

Tarsal Tunnel Syndrome

Tarsal tunnel syndrome causes compression of the tibial nerve as it passes from the deep posterior compartment of the leg into the foot. The clinical history may be difficult to define, as the signs may resolve during rest. Tarsal tunnel syndrome in an athlete may be associated with other pathology within the tarsal canal. A planovalgus foot can cause increased stretch on the tibial nerve.[275] Local tissue and tumors can also compress the nerve.[276] Ganglion cysts, fibro-osseous bands, and vascular anomalies can impinge on the nerve causing compression.

Investigation should include standing radiographs. Electromyography (EMG) changes are not always consistently present. Prior to surgery an MRI enables three-dimensional visualization of the nerve and facilitates diagnosis of any

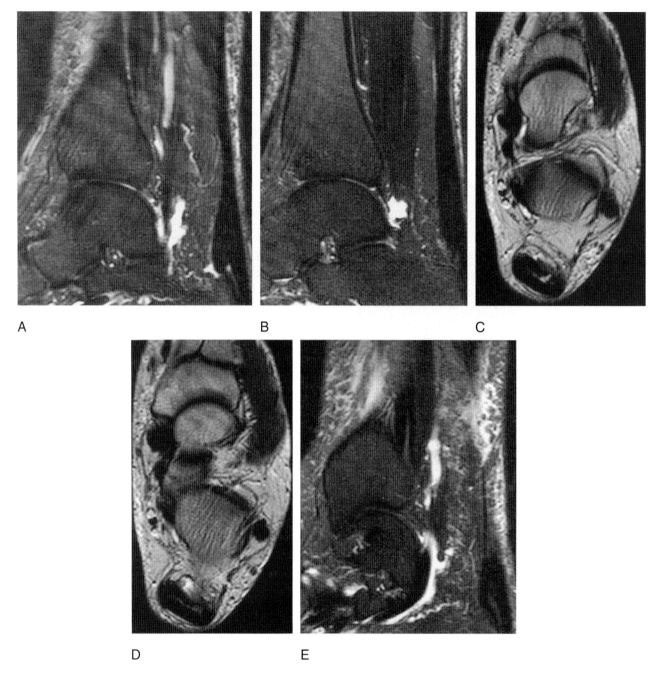

FIG. 11.68. Partial rupture Achilles tendon in a 65-year-old avid golfer and hill walker with complaints of Achilles tendon weakness and limited push-off strength. MR shows there is a mild irregularity of the osseous insertion of the Achilles tendon. The distal Achilles tendon is thickened. On the T2 images, there is a high signal within the distal Achilles tendon which surfaces anteriorly, just before its insertion. This represents a partial-thickness tear of the Achilles.

impingement. Changes within the nerve can be visualized on MRI.

Exercise-Induced Compartment Syndromes

Patients may present with muscle cramps or discomfort associated with exercise. The symptoms and signs resolve with rest so the diagnosis can be hard to make. Invasive pressure monitoring during exercise can be done. However, muscle edema can also occur after exercise and the development of

compartment syndrome assisting in the diagnosis. In some cases MRI can diagnose the muscle injury immediately after the injury period.[277]

Other Tendonopathies

Magnetic resonance imaging demonstrates tendon disease. Tendons that may be involved in athletes include the peroneal tendons, the tibialis posterior tendon, the tibialis anterior tendon in runners, and the flexor hallucis longus tendon in ballet

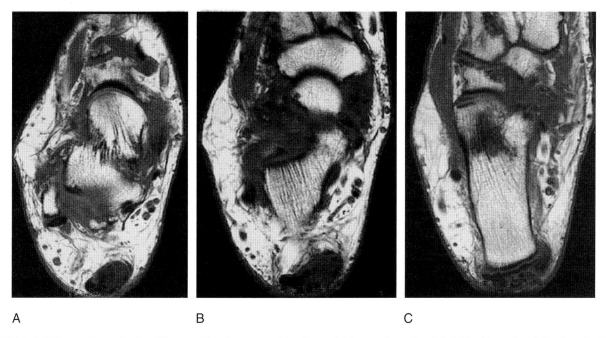

A   B   C

Fig. 11.69. Achilles tendinopathy in a 65-year-old male runner with a 6-month history of exertional Achilles discomfort following significant increase in mileage. Sequential coronal MR images (A-C) show there is marked enlargement and abnormal signal in the entire visualized portion of the Achilles tendon, consistent with chronic Achilles tendinopathy.

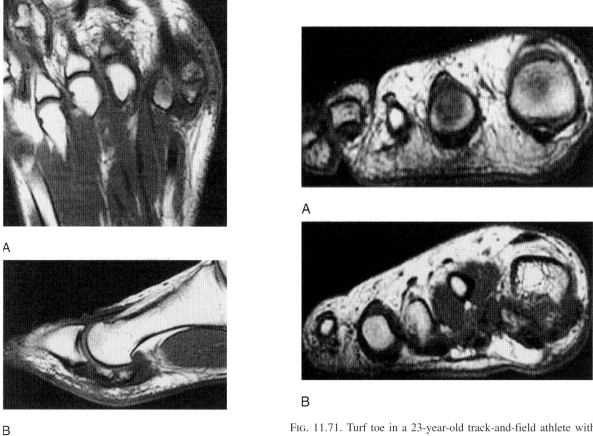

A

B

Fig. 11.70. Medial sesamoid nonunion in a 20-year-old female gymnast with an 18-month history of medial sesamoid pain on weight bearing. Coronal (A) and sagittal (B) MR images show transverse fracture centrally in the medial sesamoid.

Fig. 11.71. Turf toe in a 23-year-old track-and-field athlete with a 3-month history of persistent discomfort following toe sprain. On MR the normal low signal intensity band of the plantar plate inserting onto the proximal phalanx in the medial aspect of the first metatarsophalangeal (MTP) joint is not visualized. This is consistent with a plantar plate injury of the medial aspect of the first MTP joint.

dancers. Peroneal tendon disease is associated with an unstable ankle.[278] Patients with a high arch foot are more likely to injure the lateral tendons, as they will use the muscle to centralize the joint reaction force in the ankle. The posterior tibial tendon is more likely to be injured in a patient with a planovalgus foot.

Assessment therefore requires a standing examination of the foot and ankle. Observation of gait and single heel raise will assist in determining the function of the foot. Standing plain radiographs assist in determining the alignment of the foot. The angle between the talus and the first ray is the most sensitive radiographic measure of arch height.

Stress Fractures

The diagnosis of stress fracture should be considered if the patient has had increased localized pain, particularly if there has been a change in training routine. Changes in training routine may include change of surface or a change in intensity or duration of exercise.

Early in the history of the fracture, the patient may have localized pain and a normal radiograph. In some cases waiting and repeating radiographs may confirm the diagnosis. In other cases the diagnosis is harder to make. However, these fractures are well visualized early on with MRI as the edema in the bone can be picked up. If the fracture is not diagnosed then the fracture may go on to displace. Magnetic resonance imaging, therefore, is an important investigation in the workup of the radiographic-negative patient.

Stress fractures seen in the foot and ankle are multiple. At-risk activities include running, ballet dancing, and aerobics. Stress fractures can occur in the sesamoids (Fig. 11.72). Changes in training surface can precipitate the fracture. Localized pain is elicited over the medial or lateral sesamoid. The second through fourth metatarsal can fracture through the shaft (Fig. 11.73). Pain is localized over the metatarsal shaft. The shaft fracture occurs in the region of biomechanical load. Predisposing factors for second metatarsal fracture include tight heel cords, an elevated or mobile first ray, or an excessively long second ray. Lateral metatarsal fractures may be associated with a cavus foot.

The medial cuneiform may fracture at the base of the first ray. This fracture may occur in ballet dancers.

Navicular stress fractures occur in runners (Fig. 11.74). The fracture may occur at the navicular at the level of the middle

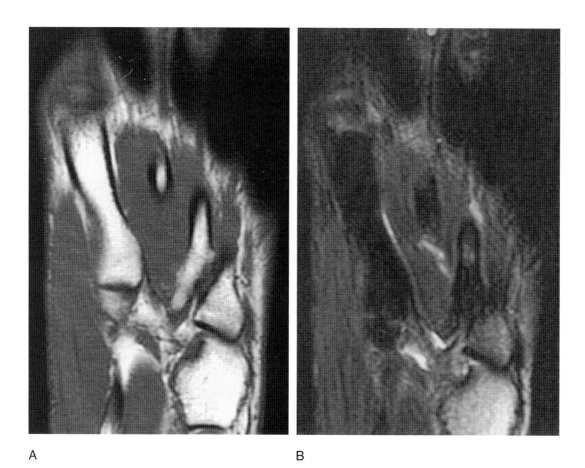

A   B

FIG. 11.72. (A) Stress injury in the third metatarsal in a 25-year-old elite 800-m runner with a 3-month history of well-localized metatarsalgia involving the third metatarsal. MR shows an abnormal T2 high signal (B) present within the proximal portion of the third metatarsal, which represents a stress injury.

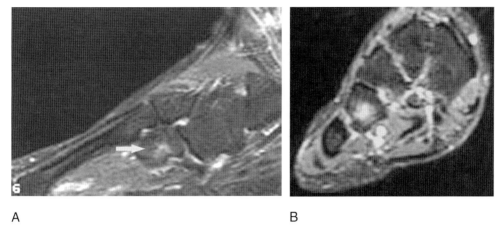

A   B

FIG. 11.73. Sagittal (A) and transverse (B) images show a stress injury in the fourth metatarsal in a 50-year-old athletic hill walker with a 1-year history of gradual onset of pain localized to the fourth metatarsal. High signal is present in the bone marrow at the base of the fourth metatarsal (arrow).

and lateral cuneiforms. These fractures may be more amenable to surgical treatment, as nonoperative treatment may be prolonged. Displacement may occur on occasion. The calcaneus can fracture at the junction of the tuberosity with the body. The ankle can fracture with a vertical shear fracture from the medial maleolus. The distal tibia can fracture at the metaphyseal to diaphyseal junction.

Forefoot Pain

Athletes may have forefoot pain from repetitive strain. Patients with overloaded second metatarsals may present with discomfort at the second metatarsal phalangeal joint. The end result of second metatarsal overload depends on the age and load characteristics for that patient. Some patients develop osteonecrosis of the second metatarsal head (Freiberg's infraction).

Others damage the plantar plate and may sublux or dislocate the second metatarsal phalangeal joint. Other patients have a stress fracture of the metatarsal shaft. Other patients damage the second MTP joint (Fig. 11.75). Often this pain is poorly localized within the foot, and in early stages there may be minimal findings on plain radiographs. However, an underlying biomechanical cause may be apparent on plain radiographs, such as long second metatarsal or elevated first ray. Magnetic resonance imaging enables correct identification of the zone of injury and enables the physician to choose the best line of treatment. Chronic strain of this joint can damage the plantar plate, and cause synovitis. These changes can be visualized with MRI.

A standing plain radiograph of the foot enables assessment of the functional relationships of the metatarsal heads. All the

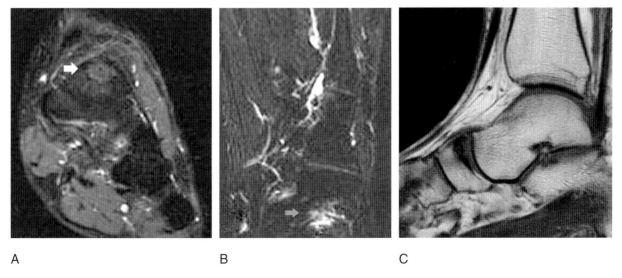

A   B   C

FIG. 11.74. Navicular stress in a 22-year-old female runner with discomfort localized to the navicular. X-rays showed no abnormality. Transverse (A), coronal (B), and sagittal (C) MR images reveals a stress fracture of the navicular (arrow).

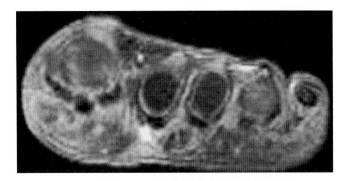

A

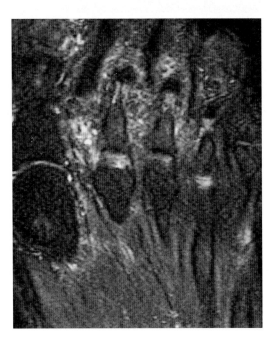

B

FIG. 11.75. Second metatarsal synovitis in a 38-year-old athletic female with a 6-month history of pain under the second metatarsal head. Clinical examination revealed a hypermobile first ray. Transverse (A) and Coronal (B) MR images demonstrate features of second metatarsal overload with synovitis and plantar plate disruption.

metatarsal heads should be the same length if force is to be transmitted equally through the metatarsal heads at toe off. All need to be the same height if force is to be transmitted equally during stance.

Orthotics facilitate redistribution of forefoot load and reduce symptoms. In resistant cases an osteotomy and shortening or plantar flexion of the metatarsal heads allows redistribution of load.

Forefoot pain is also associated with a tight gastrocnemius muscle. Stretching exercises assist in the treatment. Occasionally a gastrocnemius recession enables resolution of symptoms, potentially at the risk of some loss of Achilles strength.

Acute Injuries

Outside of standard trauma care and fractures, athletes may suffer injuries to the foot and ankle with minimal radiographic change. Injuries to the midfoot at the Lisfranc joint level, anterior lateral process fractures of the talus, anterior calcaneal process fractures, and avulsion fractures of the medial and lateral maleoli can all be overlooked on plain radiographs. Ruptures of the tibialis anterior and Achilles tendons may occur in older athletes and can be easily overlooked. Failure to immobilize these tendon injuries may cause separation of the tendon ends and require surgical apposition. Syndesmosis injuries can be subtle and involve the deltoid and syndesmosis ligaments.[248]

Subtalar dislocations can also occur and spontaneously reduce. In patients with significant injury and bruising with continued disability, an MRI early in the injury progression may facilitate early diagnosis and treatment of these conditions. While subtalar dislocations require early remobilization, midfoot subluxation or Lisfranc injuries require early reduction and treatment. Achilles tendon ruptures and syndesmosis injuries also require early diagnosis and treatment. The MRI can also be used to screen for fractures of the distal tibia and talar dome that may require immobilization to prevent displacement.

References

1. Erickson SJ, Cox IH, Hyde JS, et al. Effect of tendon orientation on MR imaging signal intensity: A manifestation of the "magic angle" phenomenon. Radiology 1991;181:389–92.
2. Farooki S, Sokoloff RM, Theodorou DJ, et al. Visualization of ankle tendons and ligaments with MR imaging: influence of passive positioning. Foot Ankle Int 2002;23:554–9.
3. Bencardino J, Rosenberg ZS. MRI of the ankle and hindfoot. In: Current Protocols in Magnetic Resonance Imaging. New York: John Wiley, 2002;A25.1:1–12.
4. Kneeland JB. Technical considerations for magnetic resonance imaging of the ankle and foot. Magn Reson Imaging Clin North Am 1994;2:23–28.
5. Zlatkin MB. Techniques for MR imaging of joints in sports medicine. Magn Reson Imaging Clin North Am 1999;7:1–21.
6. Beltran J, Noto AM, Herman LJ, et al. Tendons: high-field strength, surface coil MR imaging. Radiology 1987;162:735–40.
7. Mengiardi B, Pfirrmann CW, Schottle PB, et al. Magic angle effect in MR imaging of ankle tendons: influence of foot positioning on prevalence and site in asymptomatic subjects and cadaveric tendons. Eur Radiol 2006;16(10):2197–2206.
8. Schweitzer ME, Van Leersum M, Ehrlich SS, et al. Fluid in normal and abnormal ankle joints: Amount and distribution as seen on MR images. AJR 1994;162:111–4.
9. Klein MA. Reformatted three-dimensional Fourier transform gradient-recalled echo MR imaging of the ankle: Spectrum of normal and abnormal findings. AJR 1993;161:831.
10. Jenkins DB. The leg. In: Jenkins DB, ed. Hollingshead's Functional Anatomy of the Limbs and Back. Philadelphia: WB Saunders, 1991:283–305.
11. Pufe T, Petersen WJ, Mentlein R, Tillmann BN. The role of vasculature and angiogenesis for the pathogenesis of degenerative tendons disease. Scand J Med Sci Sports 2005;15:211–22.

12. Kvist M, Jozsa L, Jarvinen M. Vascular changes in the ruptured Achilles tendon and paratenon. Int Orthop 1992;16:377–82.

13. Soila K, Karjalainen PT, Aronen HJ, et al. High-resolution MR imaging of the asymptomatic Achilles tendon; new observations. AJR 1999;173:323–28.

14. Schweitzer ME, Karasick D. MR imaging of disorders of the Achilles tendon. AJR 2000;175:612–25.

15. Mantel D, Falutre B, Bastian D, et al. Structural MRI study of the Achilles tendon: correlation with microanatomy and histology [French]. J Radiol 1996;77;261–5.

16. Kvist M. Achilles tendon injuries in athletes. Sports Med 1994;18:173–201.

17. Karjalainen PT, Soila K, Aronen JH, et al. MR imaging of overuse injuries of the Achilles tendon. AJR 2000;175: 251–60.

18. Theobald P, Bydder G, Dent C, Nokes L, Pugh N, Benjamin M. The functional anatomy of Kager's fat pad in relation to retrocalcaneal problems and other hindfoot disorders. J Anat 2006;208:91–7.

19. Bottger BA, Schweitzer ME, El-Noueam KI, et al. MR imaging of the normal and abnormal retrocalcaneal bursae. AJR 1998;170:1239–1241.

20. Mann RA, Thompson FM. Rupture of the posterior tibial tendon causing flat foot. J Bone Joint Surg 1995;67A:556–61.

21. Lim PS, Schweitzer ME, Deely DM, et al. Posterior tibial tendon dysfunction: secondary MR signs. Foot Ankle Int 1997;18: 658–63.

22. Rosenberg ZS, Bencardino J, Mellado JM. Normal variants and pitfalls in magnetic resonance imaging of the foot and ankle. Top Magn Reson Imaging 1998;9:262–72.

23. Delfault EM, Demondion X, Bieganski A, et al. The fibrocartilaginous sesamoid: a cause of size and signal variation in the normal distal posterior tibial tendon. Eur Radiol 2003;13:2642–9.

24. Lovell AGH, Tanner HH. Synovial membranes, with special reference to those related to the tendons of the foot and ankle. J Anat 1988;42:414–423.

25. Nazarian LN, Rawool NM, Martin CE, et al. Synovial fluid in the hindfoot and ankle: detection of amount and distribution with US. Radiology 1995;197:275–8.

26. Grogan DP, Walling AK, Odgen JA. Anatomy of the os trigonum. J Pediatr Orthop 1990;10:618–22.

27. O'Sullivan E, Carare-Nnadi R, Greenslade J, et al. Clinical significance of variations in the interconnections between flexor digitorum longus and flexor hallucis longus in the region of the knot of Henry. Clin Anat 2005;18:121–5.

28. Edwards ME. The relations of the peroneal tendons to the fibula, calcaneus and cuboideum. Am J Anat 1928;42:213–53.

29. Sarrafian SK. Myology. In: Sarrafian SK, ed. Anatomy of the Foot and Ankle: Descriptive, Topographic, Functional, 2nd ed. Philadelphia: JB Lippincott, 1993:235–9.

30. Wang XT, Rosenberg ZS, Mechlin MB, Schweitzer ME. Normal variants and diseases of the peroneal tendons and superior peroneal retinaculum: MR imaging features. Radiographics 2005;25:587–602.

31. Rosenberg ZS, Beltran J, Cheung YY, et al. MR features of longitudinal splits of the peroneus brevis tendon. AJR 1997;168: 141–7.

32. Hyer CF, Dawson JM, Philbin TM Berlet GC, Lee TH. The peroneal tubercle: description, classification, and relevance to peroneus longus tendon pathology. Foot Ankle Int 2005;26: 947–50.

33. Rosenberg ZS, Beltran J, Bencardino JT. MR imaging of the ankle and foot. Radiographics 2000;20:S153–79.

34. Teitz CC, Garrett WE, Mioniaci A, et al. Tendon problems in athletic individual. J Bone Joint Surg 1997;79A:138–52.

35. Trevino S, Ford Baumhauer J. Tendon injuries of the foot and ankle. Clin Sports Med 1992;11:727–39.

36. Józsa L, Balint BJ, Reffy A, et al. Hypoxic alterations of tenocytes in degenerative tendinopathy. Arch Orthop Trauma Surg 1982;99(4):234–246.

37. Kannus P, Jozsa L. Histopathological changes preceding spontaneous rupture of tendon: a controlled study of 891 patients. J Bone Joint Surg 1991;73A:1507–25.

38. Duddy RK, Meredith R, Visser HJ, Brooks JS. Tendon sheath injuries of the foot and ankle. J Foot Surg 1991;30:179–86.

39. Bencardino J, Rosenberg ZS, Beltran J, et al. Dislocation of the posterior tibial tendon: MR imaging. AJR 1997;169:1109–1112.

40. Rosenberg ZS, Bencardino J, Astion D, Schweitzer ME, Rokito A, Sheskier S. MRI features of chronic injuries of the superior peroneal retinaculum. AJR Am J Roentgenol 2003;181:1551–7.

41. Stiskal M, Szolar DH, Stenzel I, et al. Magnetic resonance imaging of Achilles tendon in patients with rheumatoid arthritis. Invest Radiol 1997;32:602–8.

42. Erdem CZ, Sarikaya S, Erdem LO. MR imaging features of foot involvement in ankylosing spondylitis. Eur J Radiol 2005;53: 110–9.

43. McDermott EP. Basketball injuries of the foot and ankle. Clin Sports Med 1993;12:373–93.

44. Lehto MU, Jarvinen M, Suominen P. Chronic Achilles peritendinitis and retrocalcaneal bursitis. Long-term follow-up of surgically treated cases. Knee Surg Sports Traumatol Arthrosc 1994;2:182–5.

45. Astrom M, Gentz CF, Nilsson P, Rausing A, Sjoberg S, Westlin N. Imaging in chronic Achilles tendinopathy: a comparison of ultrasonography, magnetic resonance imaging and surgical findings in 27 histologically verified cases. Skeletal Radiol 1996;25:615–20.

46. Hattrup SJ, Johnson KA. A review of rupture of the Achilles tendon. Foot Ankle 1985;6:34–38.

47. Scioli MW. Achilles tendinitis. Orthop Clin North Am 1994;25:133–182.

48. Keene JS, Lash EG, Fisher DR, et al. Magnetic resonance imaging of Achilles tendon ruptures. Am J sports Med 1989;17: 333–7.

49. Panageas E, Greenberg S, Franklin PD, et al. Magnetic resonance imaging of pathologic conditions of the Achilles tendon. Orthop Rev 1990;19:975–80

50. Dillon EH, Pope CF, Barber V, et al. Achilles tendon healing: 12 month follow-up with MR imaging. Radiology 1990;177:306.

51. Wagnon R, Akayi M. The Webb-Bannister percutaneous technique for acute Achilles' tendon ruptures: a functional and MRI assessment. J Foot Ankle Surg 2005;44:437–44.

52. Kraus R, Stahl JP, Meyer C, Pavlidis T, Alt V, Horas U, Schnettler R. Frequency and effects of intratendinous and peritendinous calcifications after open Achilles tendon repair. Foot Ankle Int 2004;25:827–32.

53. Pavlov H, Heneghan MA, Hersh A, et al. The Haglund syndrome: initial and differential diagnosis. Radiology 1982;144:83–8.

54. Dussault RG, Kaplan PA, Roederer G. MR imaging of Achilles tendon in patients with familial hyperlipidemia: Comparison with plain films, physical examination, and patients with traumatic tendon lesions. AJR 1995;164:403–7.

55. Conti SF. Posterior tibial tendon problems in athletes. Orthop Clin North Am 1994;25:109–21.

56. Holmes GB Jr, Mann RA. Possible epidemiological factors associated with rupture of the posterior tibial tendon. Foot Ankle 19992;13:70–9.

57. Kiter E, Gunal I, Karatosun V, Korman E. The relationship between the tibialis posterior tendon and the accessory navicular. Ann Anat 2000;182:65–8.

58. Rosenberg ZS, Cheung YY, Jahss MH, et al. Rupture of posterior tibial tendon: CT and MR imaging with surgical correlation. Radiology 1988;169:229–35.

59. Anderson MW, Kaplan PA, Dussault RG. Association of posterior tibial tendon abnormalities with abnormal signal intensity in the sinus tarsi on MR imaging. Skeletal Radiol 2000;29:514–9.

60. Schweitzer Me Caccese R, Karasick D. Posterior tibial tendon tears: Utility of secondary signs for MR imaging diagnosis. Radiology 1993;188:655–9.

61. Marcus RE, Good fellow DB, Pfister ME. The difficult diagnosis of posterior tibialis tendon rupture in sports injuries. Orthopedics 1995;715–21.

62. Rocco Monto R, Moorman CT, Mallon WJ, et al. Rupture of the posterior tibial tendon associated with closed ankle fracture. Foot Ankle Int 1991;11;400–3.

63. Chen YJ, Hsu RW, Liang SC. Degeneration of the accessory navicular synchondrosis presenting as rupture of the posterior tibial tendon. J Bone Joint Surg 1997;79A:1791–8.

64. Loncarich DP, Clapper M. Dislocation of posterior tibial tendon. Foot Ankle Int 1998;19:821–4.

65. Sammarco GJ, Cooper PS. Flexor hallucis longus tendon injury in dancers and nondancers. Foot Ankle Int 1998;19:356–62.

66. Michelson J, Dunn L. Tenosynovitis of the flexor hallucis longus: a clinical study of the spectrum of presentation and treatment. Foot Ankle Int 2005;26:291–303.

67. Carr JB. Complications of calcaneus fractures entrapment of the flexor hallucis longus: report of two cases. J Orthop Trauma 1990;4:166–168.

68. Karasick D, Schweitzer Me. The os trigonum syndrome: imaging features. AJR 1996;166:125–9.

69. Lo LD, Schweitzer ME, Fan JK, et al. MR imaging findings of entrapment of the flexor hallucis longus tendon. AJR 2001;176:1145–8.

70. Eberle CF, Moran B, Gleason T. The accessory flexor digitorum longus as a cause of flexor hallucis syndrome. Foot Ankle Int 2002;23:51–5.

71. Bureau NJ, Cardinal E, Hobden R, et al. Posterior ankle impingement syndrome: MR imaging findings in seven patients. Radiology 2000;215:497–503.

72. Sanhudo JA. Stenosing tenosynovitis of the flexor hallucis longus tendon at the sesamoid area. Foot Ankle Int 2002;23:801–3.

73. Boruta PM, Beauperthuy GD. Partial tear of the flexor hallucis longus at the knot of Henry: presentation of three cases. Foot Ankle Int 1997;18:243–6.

74. Renard M, Simonet J, Bencteux P, et al. Intermittent dislocation of the flexor hallucis longus tendon. Skeletal Radiol 2003;32:78–81.

75. Boles MA, Lomasney LM, Demos TC, et al. Enlarged peroneal process with peroneus longus tendon entrapment. Skeletal Radiol 1997;26:313–315.

76. Pierson JL, Inglis AE. Stenosing tenosynovitis of the peroneus longus tendon associated with hypertrophy of the peroneal tubercle and an os peroneum. J Bone Joint Surg [Am] 1992;74:440–442.

77. Mota J, Rosenberg ZS. Magnetic resonance imaging of the peroneal tendons. Top Magn Reson Imaging 1998;9:273–285.

78. Bencardino J, Rosenberg ZS. MR imaging in sports injuries of the foot and ankle. MR Imag Clin North Am 1999;7:131–149.

79. Sammarco GJ. Peroneal tendon injuries. Orthop Clin North Am 1994;25:135–145.

80. LeMelle DP, Janis LR. Longitudinal rupture of the peroneus brevis tendon: a study of eight cases. J Foot Surg 1989;28:132–136.

81. Sammarco GJ, DiRaimondo CV. Chronic peroneus brevis tendon lesions. Foot Ankle 1989;9:163–170.

82. Sobel M, Geppert MJ, Olson EJ, et al. The dynamics of peroneus brevis tendon splits: a proposed mechanism, technique of diagnosis and classification of injury. Foot Ankle 1992;13:413–422.

83. Larsen E. Longitudinal rupture of the peroneus brevis tendon. J Bone Joint Surg Br 1987;69:340–341.

84. Buschmann WR, Cheung Y, Jahss MH. Magnetic resonance imaging of anomalous leg muscles: accessory soleus, peroneus quartus, and the flexor digitorum longus accessorius. Foot Ankle 1991;12:109–116.

85. Cheung YY, Rosenberg ZS, Ramsinghani R, et al. Peroneus quartus muscle: MR imaging features. Radiology 1997;1202:745–750.

86. Rademaker J, Rosenberg ZS, Beltran J, et al. Alterations in the distal extension of the musculus peroneus brevis with foot movement. AJR 1997;168:787–789.

87. Sobel M, Bohne WH, O'Brien SJ. Peroneal tendon subluxation in case of anomalous peroneus brevis muscle. Acta Orthop Scand 1992;63:682–684.

88. Springer KR. Isolated rupture of the peroneus brevis treated with a free split thickness tendon graft. J Foot Surg 1992;31:595–8.

89. Karlsson J, Brandsson S, Kalebo P, et al. Surgical treatment of concomitant chronic ankle instability and longitudinal rupture of the peroneus brevis tendon. Scand J Med Sci Sports 1998;8:42–49.

90. Rademaker J, Rosenberg ZS, Delfaut EM, et al. Tear of the peroneus longus tendon: MR imaging features in nine patients. Radiology 2000;214:700–704.

91. Goodwin MI, O'Brien PJ, Connell DG. Intra-articular fracture of the calcaneus associated with rupture of the peroneus longus tendon. Injury 1993;24:269–71.

92. Peacock KC, Resnick EJ, Thoder JJ. Fracture of the os perineum with rupture of the peroneus longus tendons: a case report and review of the literature. Clin Orthop Relat Res 1986;202:223–6.

93. O'Donnell P. Saifuddin A. Cuboid oedema due to peroneus longus tendinopathy: a report of four cases. Skeletal Radiol 2005;34:381–388.

94. Wander DS, Galli K, Ludden JW, et al. Surgical management of a ruptures peroneus longus tendon with a fractured multipartite os perineum. J Foot Ankle Surg 1994;33:124–8.

95. Sobel M, Geppert MJ, Warren RF. Chronic ankle instability as a cause of peroneal tendon injury. Clin Orthop 1993;296:187–91.

96. Mason RB, Henderson JP. Traumatic peroneal tendon instability. Am J Sports Med 1996;24:652–8.

97. Oden RR. Tendon injuries about the ankle resulting from skiing. Clin Orthop Rel Res 1997;216:63–9.

98. Mengiardi B, Pfirrmann CWA, Vienne P, et al. Anterior tibial tendon abnormalities, MR imaging findings. Radiology 2005;235:977–84.

99. Otte S, Klinger HM, Lorenz F, Haerer T. Operative treatment in case of a closed rupture of the anterior tibial tendon. Arch Orthop Trauma Surg 2002;122:188–90.

100. Erickson SJ, Smith JW, Ruiz ME, et al. MR imaging of the lateral collateral ligament of the ankle. AJR 1991;156:131–6.

101. Chandnani VP, Harper MT, Ficke JR, et al. Chronic ankle instability: evaluation with MR arthrography, MR imaging, and stress radiography. Radiology 1994;192:189–94.

102. Lee SH, Jacobson J, Trudell D, et al. Ligaments of the ankle: normal anatomy and MR arthrography. J Comput Assist Tomogr 1998;22:807–13.

103. Farroki S, Sokoloff RM, Theodorou DJ, et al, Visualization of ankle tendons and ligaments with MR imaging: influence of passive positioning. Foot Ankle Int 2002;23:554–559.

104. Mengiardi B, Zanetti M, Schottle PB, et al. Spring ligament complex: MR imaging anatomic correlation and findings in asymptomatic subjects. Radiology 2005;237:242–9.

105. Sarrafian S. Syndesmology. In: Sarrafian S, ed. Anatomy of the Foot and Ankle: Descriptive Topographic, Functional. Philadelphia: Lippincott Williams & Wilkins, 1993:159–217.

106. Brown KW, Morrison WB, Schweitzer ME, et al. MRI findings associated with distal tibiofibular syndesmosis injury. AJR 2004;182:131–6.

107. Milner CE, Soames RW. The medial collateral ligaments of the human ankle joint: anatomical variations. Foot Ankle Int 1998;19:289–92.

108. Pankovich AM, Shivaram MS. Anatomical basis of variability in injuries of the medial malleolus and the deltoid ligament. I. Anatomical studies. Acta Orthop Scand 1979;50:217–223.

109. Rasmussen O, Kromann-Andersen C, Boe S. Deltoid ligament. Functional analysis of the medial collateral ligamentous apparatus of the ankle joint. Acta Orthop Scand 1983;54:36–44.

110. Klein MA. MR imaging of the ankle: normal and abnormal findings in the medial collateral ligament. AJR 1994;162:377–83.

111. Koulouris G, Connell D, Schneider T, et al. Posterior tibiotalar ligament injury resulting in posteromedial impingement. Foot Ankle Int 2003;24:575–83.

112. Muhle C, Frank LR, Rand T, et al. Collateral ligaments of the ankle: high-resolution MR imaging with a local gradient coil and anatomic correlation in cadavers. Radiographics 1999;19:673–83.

113. Toye LR, Helms CA, Hoffman BD, et al. MRI of spring ligament tears. AJR 2005;184:1475–80.

114. Harper MC. The lateral ligamentous support of the subtalar joint. Foot Ankle 1991;11:354–8.

115. Garrick JG. The frequency of injury, mechanism of injury, and epidemiology of ankle sprains. Am J Sports Med 1977;5:241–2.

116. Cass J. Ankle instability current concepts, diagnosis and treatment. Mayo Clinic Proc 1984;59:165–70.

117. Holmer P, Sondergaard L, Konradsen L, et al. Epidemiology of sprains in the lateral ankle and foot. Foot Ankle Int 2994;15:72–4.

118. Jackson DW, Ashley RL, Powell JW. Ankle sprains in young athletes. Relation of severity and disability. Clin Orthop Rel Res 1974;101:201–15.

119. Gerber JP, Williams GN, Scoville CR, et al. Persistent disability associated with ankle sprains: a prospective examination of an athletic population. Foot Ankle Int 1998;19:653–60.

120. Labovitz JM, Schweitzer ME, Larka UB, et al. Magnetic resonance imaging of ankle ligament injuries correlated with time. J Am Podiatr Med Assoc 1998;88:387–93.

121. Kreitner KF, Ferber A, Grebe P, et al. Injuries of the lateral collateral ligaments of the ankle: assessment with MR imaging. Eur Radiol 1999;9:519–24.

122. Povacz P, Unger SF, Miller WK, et al. A randomized, prospective study of operative and non-operative treatment of injuries of the fibular collateral ligaments of the ankle. J Bone Joint Surg 1998;80A:345–51.

123. Frank C, Amiel D, Woo SL, et al. Normal ligament properties and ligament healing. Clin Orthop Rel Res 1985;196:15–25.

124. Labovitz JM, Schweitzer ME. Occult osseous injuries after ankle sprains: incidence, location, pattern, and age. Foot Ankle Int 1998;19:661–7.

125. Breitenseher MJ, Trattnig S, Kukla C, et al. MRI versus lateral stress radiography in acute lateral ankle ligament injuries. J Comput Assist Tomogr 1997;21:280–5.

126. Schaffler GJ, Tirman PF, Stoller DW, et al. Impingement syndrome of the ankle following supination external rotation trauma. Eur Radiol 2003;13:1357–62.

127. Hauger O, Moinard M, Lasalarie JC, et al. Anterolateral compartment of the ankle in the lateral impingement syndrome: appearance on CT arthrography. AJR 1999;173:685–90.

128. Liu SH, Raskin A, Osti L, et al. Arthroscopic treatment of anterolateral ankle impingement. Arthroscopy 1994;10:215–18.

129. Rubin DA, Tishkoff NW, Britton CA, Conti SF, Towers JD. Anterolateral soft-tissue impingement in the ankle: diagnosis using MR imaging. AJR 1997;169:829–835.

130. Farooki S, Yao L, Seeger LI. Anterolateral impingement of the ankle: Effectiveness of MR imaging. Radiology 1998;207:357–360.

131. Jordan LK, Helms CA, Cooperman AE, et al. Magnetic resonance imaging findings in anterolateral impingement of the ankle. Skeletal Radiol 2000;29:34–39.

132. Urguden M, Soyuncu Y, Ozdemir H, et al. Arthroscopic treatment of anterolateral soft tissue impingement of the ankle: evaluation of factors affecting outcome. Arthroscopy 2005;21:317–22.

133. Boytim MJ, Fischer DA, Neumann L. Syndesmotic ankle sprains. Am J sports Med 1991;19:294–8.

134. Ono A, Nishikawa S, Nagao A, et al. arthroscopically assisted treatment of ankle fractures; arthroscopic findings and surgical outcomes. Arthroscopy 2004;20:627–31.

135. Mosier-LaClair S, Pike H, et al. Syndesmosis injuries: acute, chronic, new techniques for failed treatment. Foot Ankle Clin 2002;7:551–65.

136. Leeds HC, Ehrlich MG. Instability of the distal tibiofibular syndesmosis after bimalleolar and trimalleolar ankle fractures. J Bone Joint Surg 1984;66A:490–503.

137. Oae K, Takao M, Naito K, et al. Injury of the tibiofibular syndesmosis; value of MR imaging for diagnosis. Radiology 2003;227:155–61.

138. Ogilvie-Harris DJ, Reed Sc. Disruption of the ankle syndesmosis: diagnosis and treatment by arthroscopic surgery. Arthroscopy 1994;10:561–8.

139. Harper MC. Deltoid ligament: an anatomical evaluation of function. Foot Ankle 1987;8:19–22.

140. Roberts CS, DeMaio M, Larkin JJ, et al. Eversion ankle sprains. Orthopedics 1995;18:299–304.

141. Michelson JD, Varner KE, Checcone M. Diagnosing deltoid injury in ankle fractures: the gravity stress view. Clin Orthop Rel Res 2001;387:178–182.

142. Mosier-La Clair SM, Monroe MT, Manoli A. Medial impingement syndrome of the anterior tibiotalar fascicle of the deltoid ligament on the talus. Foot Ankle Int 2000;21:385–391.

143. Egol Ka, Parisien JS. Impingement syndrome of the ankle caused by a medial meniscoid lesion. Arthroscopy 1997;13:522–25.

144. Conti S, Michelson J, Jahss M. Clinical significance of magnetic resonance imaging in preoperative planning for reconstruction of posterior tibial tendon ruptures. Foot Ankle 1992;13:208–214.

145. Gazdag AR, Cracchiolo A 3rd. Rupture of the posterior tibial tendon. Evaluation of injury of the spring ligament and clinical assessment of tendon transfer and ligament repair. J Bone Joint Surg 1997;79A:675–81.

146. Yao L, Gentili A, Cracchiolo A. MR imaging findings in spring ligament insufficiency. Skeletal Radiol 1999;28:245–50.

147. Balen PF, Helms CA. Association of posterior tibial tendon injury with spring ligament injury, sinus tarsi abnormality, and plantar fasciitis on MR imaging. AJR 2001;176:1137–43.

148. Tochigi Y, Yoshinaga K, Wada Y, et al. Acute inversion injury of the ankle: magnetic resonance imaging and clinical outcomes. Foot Ankle Int 1998;19:730–4.

149. Klein MA, Spreitzer AM. MR imaging of the tarsal sinus and canal: normal anatomy, pathologic findings, and features of the sinus tarsi syndrome. Radiology 1993;186:233–40.

150. Lektrakul N, Chung CB, Lai Y, et al. Tarsal sinus: arthrographic, MR imaging, MR arthrographic, and pathologic findings in cadavers and retrospective study data in patients with sinus tarsi syndrome. Radiology 2001;219:802–10.

151. Anderson MW, Kaplan PA, Dussault RG, et al. Association of posterior tibial tendon abnormalities with abnormal signal intensity in the sinus tarsi on MR imaging. Skeletal Radiol 2000;29:514–9.

152. Muthukumar T, Butt SH, Cassar-Pullicino VN. Stress fractures and related disorders in foot and ankle: plain films, scintigraphy, CT and MR imaging. Semin Musculoskelet Radiol 2005;9:210–26.

153. Umans H, Pavlov H. Insufficiency fracture of the talus: diagnosis with MR imaging. Radiology 1995;197:439–442.

154. Kathol MH, El-Khoury GY, Moore TE, Marsh JL. Calcaneal insufficiency avulsion fractures in patients with diabetes mellitus. Radiology 1991;180:725–729.

155. Franco M, Albno L, Kacso I, Gaid H, Jaeger P. An uncommon cause of foot pain: the cuboid insufficiency stress fracture. Joint Bone Spine 2005;72:76–8.

156. Chantelau E, Richter A, Schmidt-Grigoriadis P, Scherbaum VA. The diabetic Charcot foot: MRI discloses bone stress injury as trigger mechanism of neuroarthropathy. Exp Clin Endocrinol Diabetes 2006;114:118–23.

157. Maenpaa H, Lehto MU, Belt EA. Stress fractures of the ankle and forefoot in patients with inflammatory arthritides. Foot Ankle Int 2002;23:833–7.

158. Stafford SA, Rosenthal KI, Gebhardt MC, Brady TJ, Scott JA. MRI in stress fracture. AJR 1986;147:553–556.

159. Berger PE, Ofstein RA, Jackson DW, Morrison DS, Silvin N, et al. MRI demonstration of radiographically occult fractures: What have we been missing? RadioGraphics 1989;9:407–436.

160. Lee JK, Yao L. Occult intraosseous fractures: Detection with MR imaging. Radiology 1988;168:749–750.

161. Lynch TCP, Crues JV, Morgan FW, Sheeha WE, Harter LP, et al. Bone abnormalities of the knee: Prevalence and significance at MR imaging. Radiology 1989;171:761–766.

162. Flick AB, Gould N. Osteochondritis dissecans of the talus (transchondral fractures of the talus): review of the literature and new surgical approach for medial dome lesions. Foot Ankle 1985;5:165–185.

163. De Smet AA, Fisher DR, Burnstein MI, Graf BK, Lange RH. Value of MR imaging in staging osteochondral lesions of the talus (osteochondritis dissecans): results in 14 patients. AJR 1990;154:555–558.

164. Berndt AL, Harty M. Transchondral fractures (osteochondritis dissecans) of the talus. J Bone Joint Surg [Am] 1959;41:988–1020.

165. Hepple S, Winson IG, Glew D. Osteochondral lesions of the talus: a revised classification. Foot Ankle Int 1999;20:789–93.

166. Taranow WS, Bisignani GA, Towers JD, et al. Retrograde drilling of osteochondral lesions of the medial talar dome. Foot Ankle Int 1999;20:474–80.

167. Mintz DN, Tashjian GS, Connel DA, et al. Osteochondral lesions of the talus: a new magnetic resonance grading system with arthroscopic correlation. Arthroscopy 2003;19:353–9.

168. Shelton ML, Pedowitz WJ. Injuries to the talar dome, subtalar joint, and mid foot. In: MH Jahss, ed. Disorders of the Foot and Ankle. Philadelphia: WB Saunders, 1991:2274–2292.

169. Zengerink M, Szerb I, Hangody L, Dopirak RM, Ferkel RD, van Dijk CN. Current concepts: treatment of osteochondral ankle defects. Foot Ankle Int 2006;11:331–59.

170. Sasaki K, Ishibashi Y, Sato H, Toh S. Arthroscopically assisted osteochondral autogenous transplantation for osteochondral lesion of the talus using a transmalleolar approach. Arthroscopy 2003;19:922–7.

171. Koulalis D, Schultz W, Psychogios B, Papagelopoulos PJ. Articular reconstruction of osteochondral defects of the talus through autologous chondrocyte transplantation. Orthopedics 2004;27:559–61.

172. Giannini S, Buda R, Grigolo B, Vannini F, De Franceschi L, Facchini A. The detached osteochondral fragment as a source of cells for autologous chondrocyte transplantation (ACI) in the ankle joint. Osteoarthritis Cartilage 2005;13:601–7.

173. Schibany N, Ba-Ssalamah A, Marlovits S, et al. Impact of high field (3.0 T) magnetic resonance imaging on diagnosis of osteochondral defects in the ankle joint. Eur J Radiol 2005;55:283–8.

174. Verhagen RA, Maas M, Dijkgraaf MG, Tol JL, Krips R, van Dijk CN. Prospective study on diagnostic strategies in osteochondral lesions of the talus. Is MRI superior to helical CT? J Bone Joint Surg [Br] 2005;87:41–6.

175. Mesgarzadeh M, Sapega AA, Bonakdarpour A Revesz G, Moyer RA, et al. Osteochondritis dissecans: Analysis of mechanical stability with radiography, scintigraphy, and MR imaging. Radiology 1987;165:775–780.

176. Nelson DW, DiPaola J, Colville M, Schmidgall J. Osteochondritis dissecans of the talus and knee: prospective comparison of MR and arthroscopic classifications. J Comput Assist Tomogr 1990;14:804–808.

177. Yulish BS, Mulopulos GP, Goodfellow DB, Bryan PJ, Modic MT, et al. MR imaging of osteochondral lesions of the talus. J Comput Assist Tomogr 1987;11:296–301.

178. De Smet A, Ilahi O, Graf B. Reassessment of the MR criteria for stability of osteochondritis dissecans of the femoral condyles: prediction of patient outcome using radiographic and MR findings. Skeletal Radiol 1997;26:463.

179. Scranton PE Jr, Frey CC, Feder KS. Outcome of osteochondral autograft transplantation for type-V cystic osteochondral lesions of the talus. J Bone Joint Surg Br 2006; 88:614–9.

180. Elias I, Jung JW, Raikin SM, Schweitzer MW, Carrino JA, Morrison WB. Osteochondral lesions of the talus: change in MRI findings over time in talar lesions without operative intervention and implications for staging systems. Foot Ankle Int 2006;27:157–66.

181. Resnick D, Niwayama G. Osteonecrosis: Diagnostic techniques, specific situations, and complications. In: Resnick D, Niwayama G, eds. Diagnosis of Bone and Joint Disorders. Philadelphia: WB Saunders, 1988:3238–3288.

182. Pearce DH, Mongiardi CN, Fornasier VL, Daniels TR. Avascular necrosis of the talus: a pictorial essay. Radiographics 2005;25:399–410.

183. Haller J, Sartoris DJ, Resnick D, et al. Spontaneous osteonecrosis of the tarsal navicular in adults: imaging findings. AJR 1988;151:355–8.

184. Neary MT, Jones RO, Sushein K, et al. Avascular necrosis of the first metatarsal head following Austin osteotomy: a follow-up study. J Foot Ankle Surg 1993;32:530 5.

185. Abrahimzadeh R, Klein RM, Leslie D, et al. Characteristics of calcaneal bone infarction: An MR imaging investigation. Skeletal Radiol 1998;27:231–324.

186. Li KCP, Hiette P. Contrast-enhanced fat saturation magnetic resonance imaging for studying the Pathophysiology of osteonecrosis of the hips. Skeletal Radiol 1992;21:375–79.

187. Nadel Sn, Debatin JF, Richardson WJ, et al. Detection of acute avascular necrosis of the femoral head in dogs; Dynamic contrast-enhanced MR imaging vs. spin-echo and STIR sequences. AJR 1992;159:1255–61.

188. Raikin SM. Stage VI: massive osteochondral defects of the talus. Foot Ankle Clin 2004;9:737–44.

189. Toms AP, Marshall TJ, Becker E, Donell ST, Lobo-Mueller EM, Barker T. Regional migratory osteoporosis: a review illustrates by five cases. Clin Radiol 2005;60:425–38.

190. Miltner O, Niedhart C, Piroth W, Weber M, Siebert CH. Transient osteoporosis of the navicular bone in a runner. Arch Orthop Trauma Surg 2003;123:505–8.

191. Beaulieu JG, Razzano CD, Levine RB. Transient osteoporosis of the hip in pregnancy: review of the literature and a case report. Clin Orthop 1976;115:165–8.

192. Rozenbaum M, Zinman C, Nagel AM, Pollak S. Transient osteoporosis of the hip joint with liver cirrhosis. J Rheumatol 1984;11:241–243.

193. Coates PT, Tie M, Russ GR, et al. Transient bone marrow edema in renal transplantation: a distinct post-transplantation syndrome with a characteristic MRI appearance. Am J Transplant 2002;2:467–70.

194. Goffin E, Vande Berg B, Devogelaer JP, et al. Post-renal transplant syndrome of transient lower limb joint pain: description under a tacrolimus-based immunosuppression. Clin Nephrol 2003;59:98–105.

195. Pinals RS, Jabss JM. Type-IV hyperlipoproteinemia and transient osteoporosis. Lancet 1972;II:929.

196. Rodriguez S, Paniagua O, Nugent KM, Phy MP. Regional transient osteoporosis of the foot and vitamin C deficiency. Clin Rheumatol 2007;26(6):976–978.

197. Gigena LM, Chung CB, Nittaya Lektrakul, Pfirrmann CWA, Sung MS, Resnick D. Transient bone marrow edema of the talus: MR imaging findings in five patients. Skeletal Radiol 2002;31:202–7.

198. Ringe JK, Dorst A, Faber H. Effective and rapid treatment of painful localized transient osteoporosis (bone marrow edema) with intravenous ibandronate. Osteoporos Int 2005;16: 2063–8.

199. Meizer R, Radda C, Stolz G, et al. MRI-controlled analysis of 104 patients with painful bone marrow edema in different joint localizations treated with the prostacyclin analogue iloprost. Wien Klin Wochenschr 2005;117:278–86.

200. Berkowitz JF, Kier R, Rudicel S. Plantar fasciitis: MR imaging. Radiology 1991;179:665–667.

201. Grasel RP, Schweitzer ME, Kovalovich AM, et al. MR imaging of plantar fasciitis: edema, tears and occult abnormalities correlated with outcome. AJR 1999;173:699–701.

202. Narvaez JA, Narvaez J, Ortega R, Aguilera C, Sanchez A, Andia E. Painful heel: MR imaging findings. Radiographics 2000;20:333–52.

203. Theodorou DJ, Theodorou SJ, Daditsubata Y, et al. Plantar fasciitis and fascial rupture: MR findings in 26 patients supplemented by anatomic data in cadavers. Radiographics 2000;20: S181–97.

204. Yu JS. Pathologic and post-operative conditions of the plantar fascia: review of MR imaging appearances. Skeletal Radiol 2000;29:491–501.

205. Zhu F, Johnson JE, Hirose CB, Bae KT. Chronic plantar fasciitis: Acute changes in the heel after extracorporeal high-energy shock wave therapy—observations at MR imaging. Radiology 2005;234:206–10.

206. Baxter DE, Pfeffer GB. Treatment of chronic heel pain by surgical release of the first branch of the lateral plantar nerve. Clin Orthop Rel Res 1992;279:229–36.

207. Erickson SJ, Quinn SF, Kneeland JB, et al. MR imaging of the tarsal tunnel and related spaces: normal and abnormal findings with anatomic correlation. AJR 1990;155:323–328.

208. Kinoshita M, Okuda R, Morikawa J, Abe M. Tarsal tunnel syndrome associated with an accessory muscle. Foot Ankle Int 2003;24:132–6.

209. Sugimoto K, Iwai M, Kawate K, Yajima H, Takakura Y. Tenosynovial osteochondromatosis of the tarsal tunnel. Skeletal Radiol 2003;32:99–102.

210. Mezrow CK, Sanger JR, Matloub HS. Acute tarsal tunnel syndrome following partial avulsion of the flexor hallucis longus muscle: a case report. J Foot Ankle Surg 2002;41:243–6.

211. Lee MF, Chan PT, Chau LF, Yu KS. Tarsal tunnel syndrome caused by talocalcaneal coalition. Clin Imaging 2002;26: 140–3.

212. Kinoshita M, Okuda R, Yasuda T, Abe M. Tarsal tunnel syndrome in athletes. Am J Sports Med 2006;34:1307–12.

213. Labib SA, Gould JS, Rodriguez-del-Rio FA, Lyman S. Heel pain triad (HPT): the combination of plantar fasciitis, posterior tibial tendon dysfunction and tarsal tunnel syndrome. Foot Ankle Int 2002;23:212–20.

214. Golovchinsky V. Double crush syndrome in lower extremities. Electromyogr Clin Neurophysiol 1998;38:115–20.

215. Bracilovic A, Nihal A, Houston VL, Beattie AC, Rosenberg ZS, Trepman E. Effect of foot and ankle position on tarsal tunnel compartment volume. Foot Ankle Int 2006;27:431–7.

216. Kirkwood BR, Sterne JAC, Medical Statistics, 2nd ed. Malden, MA: Blackwell, 2003.

217. Sharp RJ, Wade CM, Hennessy MS, et al. The role of MRI and ultrasound imaging in Morton's neuroma and the effect of size of lesion on symptoms. J Bone Joint Surg [Br] 2003;85(7): 999–1005.

218. Verhagen RA, Maas M, Dijkgraaf MG, et al. Prospective study on diagnostic strategies in osteochondral lesions of the talus. Is MRI superior to helical CT? J Bone Joint Surg [Br] 2005;87(1):41–6.

219. Radke S, Vispo-Seara J, Walther M, et al. [Osteochondral lesions of the talus—indications for MRI with a contrast agent]. Z Orthop Ihre Grenzgeb 2004;142(5):618–24.

220. Lohman M, Kivisaari A, Vehmas T, et al. MRI abnormalities of foot and ankle in asymptomatic, physically active individuals. Skeletal Radiol 2001;30(2):61–6.

221. Karlsson J, Brandsson S, Kalebo P, et al. Surgical treatment of concomitant chronic ankle instability and longitudinal rupture of the peroneus brevis tendon. Scand J Med Sci Sports 1998;8(1):42–9.

222. Hintermann B, Boss A, Schafer D, Arthroscopic findings in patients with chronic ankle instability. Am J Sports Med 2002;30(3):402–9.

223. Schafer D, Hintermann B. Arthroscopic assessment of the chronic unstable ankle joint. Knee Surg Sports Traumatol Arthrosc 1996;4(1):48–52.

224. Ogilvie-Harris DJ, Gilbart MK, Chorney K. Chronic pain following ankle sprains in athletes: the role of arthroscopic surgery. Arthroscopy 1997;13(5):564–74.

225. Bonnin M, Bouysset M. Arthroscopy of the ankle: analysis of results and indications on a series of 75 cases. Foot Ankle Int 1999;20(11):744–51.

226. Ferkel RD, Chams RN. Chronic lateral instability: arthroscopic findings and long-term results. Foot Ankle Int 2007;28(1):24–31.

227. Ferkel RD, Fasulo GJ. Arthroscopic treatment of ankle injuries. Orthop Clin North Am 1994;25(1):17–32.

228. Helgason JW, Chandnani VP. MR arthrography of the ankle. Radiol Clin North Am 1998;36(4):729–38.

229. Boyer D, Younger AS. Anatomic lateral ligament reconstruction using the gracilis tendon. Foot Ankle Clin 2006;11(3):585–595.

230. van Dijk CN, Bossuyt PM, Marti RK. Medial ankle pain after lateral ligament rupture. J Bone Joint Surg [Br] 1996;78(4):562–7.

231. Hepple S, Winson IG, Glew D. Osteochondral lesions of the talus: a revised classification. Foot Ankle Int 1999;20(12): 789–93.

232. Mintz DN, Tashjian GS, Connell DA, et al. Osteochondral lesions of the talus: a new magnetic resonance grading system with arthroscopic correlation. Arthroscopy 2003;19(4):353–9.

233. De Smet AA, Ilahi OA, Graf BK. Reassessment of the MR criteria for stability of osteochondritis dissecans in the knee and ankle. Skeletal Radiol 1996;25(2):159–63.

234. Jordan LK 3rd, Helms CA, Cooperman AE, et al. Magnetic resonance imaging findings in anterolateral impingement of the ankle. Skeletal Radiol 2000;29(1):34–9.

235. Biedert R. Anterior ankle pain in sports medicine: aetiology and indications for arthroscopy. Arch Orthop Trauma Surg 1991;110(6):293–7.

236. Amendola A, Petrik J, Webster-Bogaert S. Ankle arthroscopy: outcome in 79 consecutive patients. Arthroscopy 1996;12(5):565–73.

237. Rubin DA, Tishkoff NW, Britton CA, et al. Anterolateral soft-tissue impingement in the ankle: diagnosis using MR imaging. AJR Am J Roentgenol 1997;169(3):829–35.

238. Masciocchi C, Catalucci A, Barile A. Ankle impingement syndromes. Eur J Radiol 1998;27(suppl 1):S70–3.

239. Farooki S, Yao L, Seeger LL. Anterolateral impingement of the ankle: effectiveness of MR imaging. Radiology 1998;207(2):357–60.

240. Schaffler GJ, Tirman PF, Stoller DW, et al. Impingement syndrome of the ankle following supination external rotation trauma: MR imaging findings with arthroscopic correlation. Eur Radiol 2003;13(6):1357–62.

241. Berberian WS, Hecht PJ, Wapner KL, et al. Morphology of tibiotalar osteophytes in anterior ankle impingement. Foot Ankle Int 2001;22(4):313–7.

242. Huh YM, Suh JS, Lee JW, et al. Synovitis and soft tissue impingement of the ankle: assessment with enhanced three-dimensional FSPGR MR imaging. J Magn Reson Imaging 2004;19(1):108–16.

243. Tol JL, Verhagen RA, Krips R, et al. The anterior ankle impingement syndrome: diagnostic value of oblique radiographs. Foot Ankle Int 2004;25(2):63–8.

244. Coull R, Raffiq T, James LE, et al. Open treatment of anterior impingement of the ankle. J Bone Joint Surg [Br] 2003;85(4):550–3.

245. Miller CD, Shelton WR, Barrett GR, et al. Deltoid and syndesmosis ligament injury of the ankle without fracture. Am J Sports Med 1995;23(6):746–50.

246. Breitenseher MJ, Trattnig S, Kukla C, et al. MRI versus lateral stress radiography in acute lateral ankle ligament injuries. J Comput Assist Tomogr 1997;21(2):280–5.

247. Verhaven EF, Shahabpour M, Handelberg FW, et al. The accuracy of three-dimensional magnetic resonance imaging in the diagnosis of ruptures of the lateral ligaments of the ankle. Am J Sports Med 1991;19(6):583–7.

248. Uys HD, Rijke AM. Clinical association of acute lateral ankle sprain with syndesmotic involvement: a stress radiography and magnetic resonance imaging study. Am J Sports Med 2002;30(6):816–22.

249. Ferkel RD, Karzel RP, Del Pizzo W, et al. Arthroscopic treatment of anterolateral impingement of the ankle. Am J Sports Med 1991;19(5):440–6.

250. Niemi WJ, Savidakis J Jr, DeJesus JM. Peroneal subluxation: a comprehensive review of the literature with case presentations. J Foot Ankle Surg 1997;36(2):141–5.

251. Peacock KC, Resnick EJ, Thoder JJ. Fracture of the os peroneum with rupture of the peroneus longus tendon. A case report and review of the literature. Clin Orthop 1986(202): 223–6.

252. Nelson DR, Younger A. Acute posttraumatic planovalgus foot deformity involving hindfoot ligamentous pathology. Foot Ankle Clin 2003;8(3):521–37.

253. Marks RM, Schon LC. Posttraumatic posterior tibialis tendon insertional elongation with functional incompetency: a case report. Foot Ankle Int 1998;19(3):180–3.

254. Malicky ES, Crary JL, Houghton MJ, et al. Talocalcaneal and subfibular impingement in symptomatic flatfoot in adults. J Bone Joint Surg [Am] 2002;84–A(11):2005–9.

255. Kamel M, Eid H, Mansour R. Ultrasound detection of heel enthesitis: a comparison with magnetic resonance imaging. J Rheumatol 2003;30(4):774–8.

256. Bleakney RR, White LM. Imaging of the Achilles tendon. Foot Ankle Clin 2005;10(2):239–54.

257. Kayser R, Mahlfeld K, Heyde CE. Partial rupture of the proximal Achilles tendon: a differential diagnostic problem in ultrasound imaging. Br J Sports Med 2005;39(11):838–42; discussion 842.

258. Tuite MJ. MR imaging of the tendons of the foot and ankle. Semin Musculoskelet Radiol 2002;6(2):119–31.

259. Eberle CF, Moran B, Gleason T. The accessory flexor digitorum longus as a cause of Flexor Hallucis Syndrome. Foot Ankle Int 2002;23(1):51–5.

260. Landorf KB, Keenan AM, Herbert RD. Effectiveness of foot orthoses to treat plantar fasciitis: a randomized trial. Arch Intern Med 2006;166(12):1305–10.

261. Pfeffer G, Bacchetti P, Deland J, et al. Comparison of custom and prefabricated orthoses in the initial treatment of proximal plantar fasciitis. Foot Ankle Int 1999;20(4):214–21.

262. Barry LD, Barry AN, Chen Y. A retrospective study of standing gastrocnemius-soleus stretching versus night splinting in the treatment of plantar fasciitis. J Foot Ankle Surg 2002;41(4):221–7.

263. Rompe JD, Schoellner C, Nafe B. Evaluation of low-energy extracorporeal shock-wave application for treatment of chronic plantar fasciitis. J Bone Joint Surg [Am] 2002;84–A(3):335–41.

264. Sems A, Dimeff R, Iannotti JP. Extracorporeal shock wave therapy in the treatment of chronic tendinopathies. J Am Acad Orthop Surg 2006;14(4):195–204.

265. Wang CJ, Wang FS, Yang KD, et al. Long-term results of extracorporeal shockwave treatment for plantar fasciitis. Am J Sports Med 2006;34(4):592–6.

266. Hogan KA, Webb D, Shereff M. Endoscopic plantar fascia release. Foot Ankle Int 2004;25(12):875–81.

267. Jerosch J. Endoscopic release of plantar fasciitis—a benign procedure? Foot Ankle Int 2000;21(6):511–3.

268. Saxena A. Uniportal endoscopic plantar fasciotomy: a prospective study on athletic patients. Foot Ankle Int 2004;25(12):882–9.

269. Conflitti JM, Tarquinio TA. Operative outcome of partial plantar fasciectomy and neurolysis to the nerve of the abductor digiti minimi muscle for recalcitrant plantar fasciitis. Foot Ankle Int 2004;25(7):482–7.

270. Baxter DE. Release of nerve to abductor digiti quinti. In: Johnson KA, ed. Master Techniques in Orthopaedic Surgery. Philadelphia: Lippincott-Raven, 1994:333–40.

271. Jarde O, Diebold P, Havet E, et al. Degenerative lesions of the plantar fascia: surgical treatment by fasciectomy and excision of the heel spur. A report on 38 cases. Acta Orthop Belg 2003;69(3):267–74.

272. Boyle RA, Slater GL. Endoscopic plantar fascia release: a case series. Foot Ankle Int 2003;24(2):176–9.

273. Ogilvie-Harris DJ, Lobo J. Endoscopic plantar fascia release. Arthroscopy 2000;16(3):290–8.

274. Watson TS, Anderson RB, Davis WH. Periarticular injuries to the hallux metatarsophalangeal joint in athletes. Foot Ankle Clin 2000;5(3):687–713.

275. Bracilovic A, Nihal A, Houston VL, et al. Effect of foot and ankle position on tarsal tunnel compartment volume. Foot Ankle Int 2006;27(6):431–7.

276. Tsai CC, Lin TM, Lai CS, et al. Tarsal tunnel syndrome secondary to neurilemoma—a case report. Kaohsiung J Med Sci 2001;17(4):216–20.

277. Verleisdonk EJ, van Gils Avan der Werken C. The diagnostic value of MRI scans for the diagnosis of chronic exertional compartment syndrome of the lower leg. Skeletal Radiol 2001;30(6):321–5.

278. Vertullo C. Unresolved lateral ankle pain. It's not always "just a sprain." Aust Fam Physician 2002;31(3):247–53.

Index

Index

Index

Printed in the United States of America